S0-BMG-554

Mechanism and Control
of Animal Fertilization

This is a volume in
CELL BIOLOGY
A series of monographs

Editors: D. E. Buetow, I. L. Cameron, G. M. Padilla, and A. M. Zimmerman

A complete list of the books in this series appears at the end of the volume.

Mechanism and Control of Animal Fertilization

Edited by

John F. Hartmann

Department of Reproductive Biology
Merck Institute for Therapeutic Research
Rahway, New Jersey

1983

ACADEMIC PRESS
A Subsidiary of Harcourt Brace Jovanovich, Publishers
New York   London
Paris   San Diego   San Francisco   São Paulo   Sydney   Tokyo   Toronto

QP
273
.M43
1983

COPYRIGHT © 1983, BY ACADEMIC PRESS, INC.
ALL RIGHTS RESERVED.
NO PART OF THIS PUBLICATION MAY BE REPRODUCED OR
TRANSMITTED IN ANY FORM OR BY ANY MEANS, ELECTRONIC
OR MECHANICAL, INCLUDING PHOTOCOPY, RECORDING, OR ANY
INFORMATION STORAGE AND RETRIEVAL SYSTEM, WITHOUT
PERMISSION IN WRITING FROM THE PUBLISHER.

ACADEMIC PRESS, INC.
111 Fifth Avenue, New York, New York 10003

United Kingdom Edition published by
ACADEMIC PRESS, INC. (LONDON) LTD.
24/28 Oval Road, London NW1 7DX

Library of Congress Cataloging in Publication Data
Main entry under title:

Mechanism and control of animal fertilization.

(Cell biology)
Includes index.
1. Fertilization (Biology) I. Hartmann, John F.
II. Series.
QP273.M43 1983   599'.016   82-18493
ISBN 0-12-328520-8

PRINTED IN THE UNITED STATES OF AMERICA

83 84 85 86   9 8 7 6 5 4 3 2 1

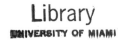
Library
UNIVERSITY OF MIAMI

9-30-93 PD

Contents

Contributors

Numbers in parentheses indicate the pages on which the authors' contributions begin.

J. MICHAEL BEDFORD (453), Department of Anatomy, Cornell University Medical College, New York, New York 10021

ANTHONY R. BELLVÉ (55), Department of Physiology and Biophysics and Laboratory of Human Reproduction and Reproductive Biology, Harvard Medical School, Boston, Massachusetts 02115

ERIC D. CLEGG (177), Division of Veterinary Biology, Virginia–Maryland Regional College of Veterinary Medicine, Blacksburg, Virginia 24061

BONNIE S. DUNBAR (139), Department of Cell Biology, Baylor College of Medicine, Houston, Texas 77030

BELA J. GULYAS (365), Pregnancy Research Branch, National Institute of Child Health and Human Development, National Institutes of Health, Bethesda, Maryland 20205

JOHN F. HARTMANN (325), Department of Reproductive Biology, Merck Institute for Therapeutic Research, Rahway, New Jersey 07065

JERRY L. HEDRICK (365), Department of Biochemistry and Biophysics, University of California, Davis, California 95616

ALINA C. LOPO (269), Department of Biological Chemistry, School of Medicine, University of California, Davis, California 95616

HARRY D. M. MOORE (453), The Zoological Society of London, Nuffield Laboratories of Comparative Medicine, Institute of Zoology, Regent's Park, London NW1 4RY, England

DEBORAH A. O'BRIEN (55), Department of Anatomy and Laboratory of Human Reproduction and Reproductive Biology, Harvard Medical School, Boston, Massachusetts 02115

JAMES W. OVERSTREET (499), Department of Human Anatomy, School of Medicine, University of California, Davis, California 95616

ELI D. SCHMELL (365), Biological Sciences Division, Office of Naval Research, Arlington, Virginia 22217

SHELDON S. SHEN (213), Department of Zoology, Iowa State University, Ames, Iowa 50011

PAUL M. WASSARMAN (1), Department of Biological Chemistry and Laboratory of Human Reproduction and Reproductive Biology, Harvard Medical School, Boston, Massachusetts 02115

DEBRA J. WOLGEMUTH (415), Department of Human Genetics and Development, College of Physicians and Surgeons, Columbia University, New York, New York 10032

Preface

The successful union of a sperm and egg, eventually resulting in the formation of a new individual, is an impressive example among biological phenomena of the operation of sensitive control mechanisms. Indeed, Professor Einstein's famous admonition to the quantum physicists of his day that "God does not throw dice" finds dramatic application in describing the harmonious interactions required of fertilization.

An understanding of the molecular mechanisms involved in animal fertilization has just begun. Studies of invertebrate gamete interactions, particularly those of the sea urchin, have laid much of the groundwork toward acquiring an understanding of these systems. The availability of large numbers of gametes capable of undergoing synchronous fertilization in an inexpensive medium has been a blessing for students of fertilization and early development for more than a century. Those working with mammalian gametes, on the other hand, have had to struggle with less than abundant quantities of cells and artificial *in vitro* systems, the use of which have, nevertheless, begun to yield answers. Of course mammalian fertilization does not occur in the test tube (normally), so a complete understanding of this phenomenon must take into account the influence of the *in vivo* environment, still a formidable consideration.

As is so common in science, methodological difficulties discourage many from entering a given field of study; mammalian fertilization is no exception. However, with the development of systems for increasing the yield of gametes, in particular of the egg, combined with highly sensitive analytical techniques, both of which are discussed in some of the chapters in this volume, it is hoped that more investigators will be induced to enter this area.

The purpose of this book is to review many of the contributions that the study of both invertebrate and vertebrate systems has made toward elucidating the mechanism of animal fertilization. The majority of the chapters deals with the mammal, which simply reflects the current prejudice of the editor. Informally, the chapters can be grouped into the following sections: (1) formation of gametes (oogenesis and spermiogenesis), (2) composition and response of gamete surfaces (zona pellucida, sperm capacitation, and membrane behavior as reflected by ionic movements in invertebrate egg), (3) prepenetration interactions between sperm and eggs of both invertebrates and mammals, (4) early postfertilization changes (block to polyspermy in the invertebrate, mammalian, and anuran egg; early synthetic and other changes in the fertilized mammalian egg), and, finally, (5) aspects of *in vivo* fertilization in the mammal (interaction of sperm and egg and gamete transport in the female reproductive tract).

John F. Hartmann

1

Oogenesis: Synthetic Events in the Developing Mammalian Egg

PAUL M. WASSARMAN

I. INTRODUCTION

The unfertilized mammalian egg represents the culmination of oogenesis, a complex developmental process that begins in the fetus and terminates with ovulation by sexually mature offspring. As a result of the process of oogenesis each ovulated egg has the potential to

Mechanism and Control of Animal Fertilization
Copyright © 1983 by Academic Press, Inc.
All rights of reproduction in any form reserved.
ISBN 0-12-328520-8

give rise to a new individual who will express and maintain the characteristics of the species.

Among the consequences of oogenesis are an increase in genotypic variation due to crossing over and recombination, a decrease in gamete ploidy to the haploid state, and the accumulation of macromolecules and organelles that will be used to regulate and sustain early embryogenesis. It is the latter aspect of mammalian oogenesis that will be emphasized here. In particular, this chapter reviews synthetic events that occur during oocyte growth and during conversion of oocytes into unfertilized eggs in the mouse. This chapter is not intended to be a comprehensive survey of the field or of all of the relevant literature. Rather, it is intended to be more of an introduction to this important aspect of mammalian developmental biology.

II. OOGENESIS IN THE MOUSE: A PRÉCIS

A brief description of oogenesis in the mouse is presented below and is summarized in Fig. 1. The information presented is drawn from a variety of sources to which the reader is referred for a more detailed account of the subject (Parkes, 1956; Zuckerman, 1962; Austin and Short, 1972; Biggers and Schuetz, 1972; Zuckerman and Weir, 1977; Jones, 1978; Van Blerkom and Motta, 1979). The text edited by Jones (1978) is, perhaps, the most up-to-date, comprehensive treatment of mammalian oogenesis available.

A. Appearance of Oocytes during Fetal Development

Oogenesis in the mouse begins with the formation of primordial germ cells in presomite embryos. In the 8-day-old embryo, containing four pairs of somites, about 100 primordial germ cells are recognizable due to their distinctive morphology. These large cells are found in that region of the allantois arising from the primitive streak. Consequently, the embryonic rudiment of the allantois and the caudal end of the primitive streak may be considered the regions of primordial germ cell formation. The primordial germ cells migrate by ameboid movement into the endoderm and then along the dorsal mesentery of the genital ridges found in the roof of the coelom. These primordial germ cells are the sole source of adult germ cells. In the 13-day-old embryo (52–60 pairs of somites), containing a differentiated ovary, migration of primordial germ cells is complete, with virtually all of the cells converted to actively multiplying oogonia ($\simeq$ 95% of the germ cells) or

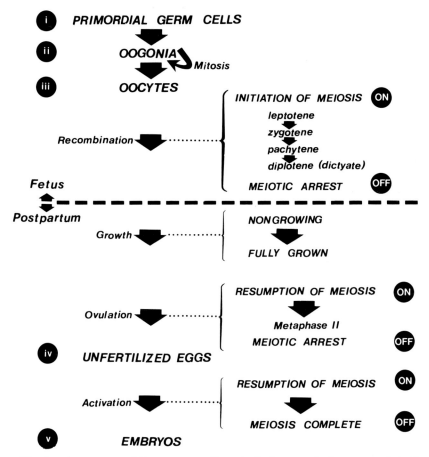

Fig. 1. A summary of the sequence of events that occurs during oogenesis in the mouse. For details see Section II,A–D.

to oocytes ($\simeq$ 5% of the germ cells) in leptotene of the first meiotic prophase. By day 14 of embryogenesis (61–62 pairs of somites) the germ cell population is about equally divided between oogonia and oocytes, and by day 17 (full quota of 65 pairs of somites) the ovary contains only oocytes at various stages of the first meiotic prophase.

As early as day 12 of embryogenesis, a few oogonia enter the preleptotene and then leptontene stage of the first meiotic prophase. It is during preleptotene (interphase following the last mitotic division of oogonia) that the final DNA synthesis takes place in preparation for meiosis. This synthetic activity signals the transformation of oogonia into oocytes. Oocytes progress rapidly through leptotene (3–6 hours) and then take 12–40 hours to complete zygotene. During zygotene homologous chromosomes pair and synapse to form what often appear to be single chromosomes but are actually bivalents composed of four chromatids. By day 16 of embryogenesis nearly all oocytes are in pachytene of the first meiotic prophase; a stage that lasts about 60 hours and involves genetic crossing over and recombination. Therefore, nuclear progression from leptotene through pachytene takes approximately 4 days to complete. The first oocytes in the diplotene stage of the first meiotic prophase are seen by day 18 of embryogenesis, with their chromosomes exhibiting the chiasmata that result from crossing over. By the time of parturition a majority of oocytes have entered the late diplotene, or so-called dictyate stage, and by day 5 postpartum nearly all ooctyes have reached the dictyate stage where they will remain until stimulated to resume meiosis at the time of ovulation.

B. Growth of Oocytes and Follicles

Shortly after birth, the mouse ovary is populated with thousands ($\simeq$ 11,000) of small ($\simeq$ 12 μm in diameter), primary oocytes arrested in late prophase of meiosis and enclosed within several squamous follicular cells. There is a loss of about 50% ($\simeq$ 6000) of these oocytes during the first 2 weeks after birth, attributable in large measure to oocytes leaving the ovary through the surface epithelium. However, in the first 2 weeks after birth more oocytes begin to grow ($\simeq$ 600 oocytes, or $\simeq$ 10% of the total population) than at any other period in the lifetime of the mouse. Commencement of oocyte growth is apparently regulated within the ovary, the number of oocytes entering the growth phase being a function of the size of the pool of nongrowing oocytes. The oocyte and its surrounding follicle grow coordinately, progressing through a series of definable morphological stages. The oocyte completes its growth in the adult mouse before the formation of the follicular antrum; consequently, the vast majority of follicle growth occurs after the oocyte has stopped growing. Growth is continuous, ending either in ovulation of a matured oocyte (unfertilized egg) or degeneration (atresia) of the oocyte and its follicle.

Completion of oocyte growth in the mouse takes approximately 2 weeks, a relatively short period of time in comparison to the months or years required for completion of oocyte growth in many nonmammalian animal species. The oocyte grows from a diameter of about 12 μm (volume of $\simeq$ 0.9 pl) to a terminal diameter of about 85 μm (volume of $\simeq$ 320 pl), not including the zona pellucida. Therefore, during its growth phase, while continually arrested in dictyate of the first meio-

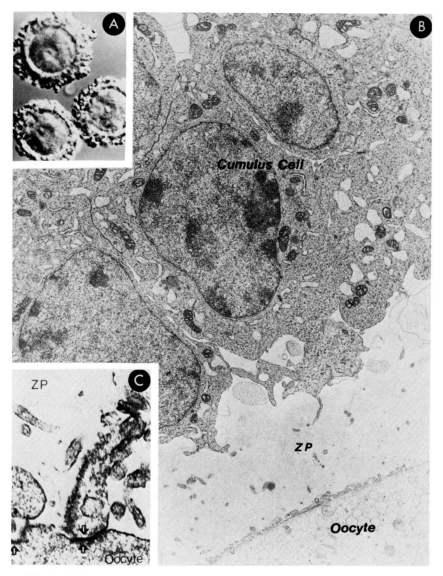

Fig. 2. Light (A) and transmission electron (B,C) micrographs of isolated, fully grown mouse oocytes with their adherent cumulus cells. The arrows in panel C indicate the positions of junctions between plasma membranes of an oocyte and an innermost cumulus cell. zp, Zona pellucida.

TABLE I

Ultrastructural Changes Accompanying Growth of Mouse Oocytes

Organelle or inclusion	Stage of oocyte growth (diameter)		
	Early ($\approx$ 20–40 μm)	Middle ($\approx$ 40–60 μm)	Late ($\approx$ 60–85 μm)
Nucleoli	Fibrillogranular	Larger, fibrillar	Very large, very dense
Mitochondria	Elongated, transverse cristae ("orthodox")	Smaller, round, columnar cristae	Round or oval, concentric cristae ("unorthodox")
Golgi complex	Flattened stacks of parallel lamellae	Parallel lamellae, vacuoles, granules	Swollen lamellae, highly vacuolated, granular
Zona pellucida	Thin, diffuse	Thicker, denser	Very thick, very dense
Endoplasmic reticulum	Smooth	Moderately vesicular	Highly vesicular
Lipid droplets	+	+ +	+ + + +
Multivesicular bodies	+	+ +	+ + + +
Cytoplasmic lattices	—	+ + +	+ + + + + +
Cortical granules	—	+	+ + +

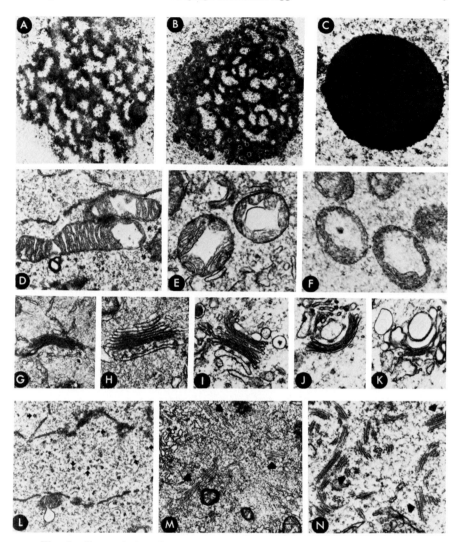

Fig. 3. Transmission electron micrographs of isolated mouse oocytes at various stages of growth. (A–C) The nucleolus at early (A), middle (B), and late (C) stages of oocyte growth. (D–F) Mitochondria at early (D), middle (E), and late (F) stages of oocyte growth. (G–K) The Golgi complex at early (G,H), middle (I,J), and late (K) stages of oocyte growth. (L) The presence of abundant polysomes (arrows) and absence of cytoplasmic lattices during the early stages of oocyte growth. (M,N) The appearance of cytoplasmic lattices (arrows) during the middle (M) and late (N) stages of oocyte growth. For details, see Wassarman and Josefowicz, 1978.

tic prophase, the mouse oocyte undergoes more than a 300-fold increase in volume. Each oocyte is contained within a cellular follicle (initially ≃ 17 μm in diameter) that grows concomitantly with the oocyte, from a single layer of a few flattened cells to three layers of cuboidal granulosa cells (≃ 900 cells; follicle ≃ 125 μm in diameter) by the time the oocyte has completed its growth. The theca is first distinguishable, outside of and separated by a basement membrane from the granulosa cells, when the granulosa region is two cell layers thick (≃ 400 cells; follicle ≃ 100 μm in diameter). During a period of several days, while the fully grown oocyte remains a constant size, the follicle cells undergo rapid division, increasing to more than 50,000 cells and resulting finally in a Graafian follicle greater than 600 μm in diameter. The follicle exhibits an incipient antrum when it is several layers thick (≃ 6000 cells; follicle ≃ 250 μm in diameter) and, as the antrum expands, the oocyte takes up an acentric position surrounded by two or more layers of granulosa cells. The innermost layer of granulosa cells becomes columnar in shape and constitutes the corona radiata (Fig. 2).

During its growth phase (≃ 2 weeks) the mouse oocyte undergoes an impressive ultrastructural reorganization of its organelles and inclusions (summarized in Table I and Fig. 3). Progressive changes in the oocyte's nucleus (germinal vesicle), nucleoli, ribosomes, mitochondria, endoplasmic reticulum, Golgi complex, and surface all support the idea that growth of the oocyte involves not just enlargement of the cell, but extensive alterations in its overall metabolism as well. Certain structures, such as cortical granules, cytoplasmic lattice arrays, and zona pellucida, first appear during oocyte growth, while changes in the appearance of other organelles, such as nucleoli and Golgi complex, are indicative of a period of active synthesis of intracellular and secretory products.

C. Meiotic Maturation of Oocytes

In sexually mature female mice, fully grown oocytes in Graafian follicles resume meiosis and complete the first meiotic reductive divi-

---

Fig. 4. (Part I). Meiotic maturation of fully grown mouse oocytes during culture *in vitro*. (A–C) Nomarski interference microscopy of (A) oocytes arrested at dictyate of the first meiotic prophase, (B) oocytes that have undergone germinal vesicle breakdown (GVBD) and chromosome condensation following the resumption of meiosis, and (C) unfertilized eggs arrested at metaphase II following the completion of meiotic maturation. (D,E) Geimsa-stained chromosome spreads from oocytes before (D) and after (E) chromosome condensation during meiotic maturation *in vitro;* the arrows (E) indicate twenty bivalents. n, Nucleolus; gv, germinal vesicle; zp, zona pellucida; pb, polar body.

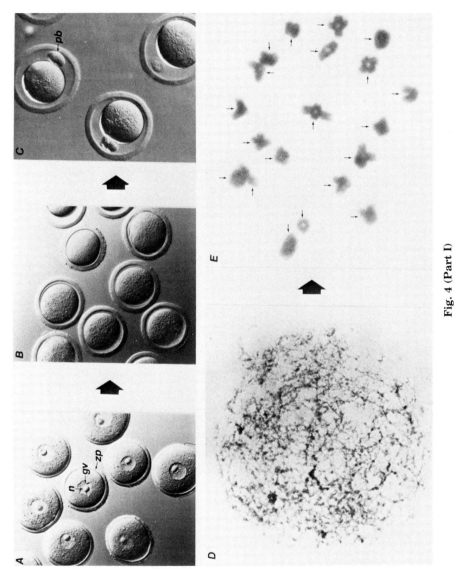

Fig. 4 (Part I)

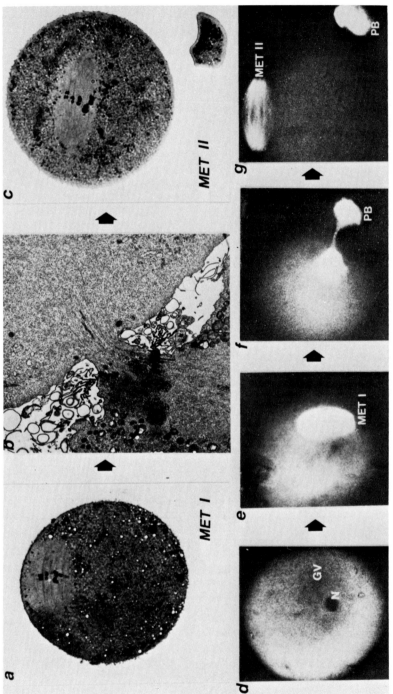

Fig. 4 (Part II)

sion just prior to ovulation. Therefore, oocytes may remain arrested in dictyate of the first meiotic prophase from only a few weeks to more than 18 months following birth; in humans, this period of meiotic arrest can persist for more than 40 years. The resumption of meiosis can be mediated by a hormonal stimulus *in vivo* or simply by the release of oocytes from their ovarian follicles into a suitable culture medium *in vitro*. The oocytes undergo nuclear progression from dictyate of the first meiotic prophase (with four times the haploid DNA complement) to metaphase II (with two times the haploid DNA complement) and remain at this stage of meiosis in the oviduct, or in culture, until triggered to complete meiosis when either fertilization or parthenogenetic activation takes place. Progression from the dictyate (oocyte) to the metaphase II (unfertilized egg) stage is termed meiotic maturation, a process characterized by dissolution of the nuclear, or germinal vesicle (GV) membrane, condensation of diffuse chromatin into distinct bivalents, separation of homologous chromosomes and emission of the first polar body, and arrest of meiosis at metaphase II (Fig. 4). Meiotic maturation is of fundamental importance in mammalian development since it is only after reaching metaphase II that the female gamete is competent to be fertilized. It should be noted that mouse oocytes matured and fertilized *in vitro* have developed into viable fetuses following transplantation to the uteri of foster mothers.

D. Epilogue

From the preceding, it should be apparent that mammalian oogenesis is an exquisitely programmed cellular process that begins very early in fetal development and may not end until quite late in adulthood. A fundamental aspect of this process is the tremendous growth of oocytes (> 300-fold increase in volume) over a relatively short time span ($\simeq 2$ weeks) just prior to meiotic maturation, ovulation, and fertilization for it is during its growth phase that mammalian oocytes, like oocytes of nonmammalian animal species (Davidson, 1977), are mobi-

---

Fig. 4. (Part II). Meiotic maturation of fully grown mouse oocytes during culture *in vitro*. (a–c) Light micrographs of toluidine blue-stained thick sections of (a) an oocyte arrested at metaphase I, and (c) an unfertilized egg arrested at metaphase II. (b) Transmission electron micrograph of cleavage furrow of an oocyte undergoing polar body emission. The condensed chromosomes and meiotic spindles are visible in (a) and (c). (d–g) Changing patterns of fluorescein-labeled antitubulin IgG staining during meiotic progression of oocytes from dictyate (d), through metaphase I (e), polar body emission (f), to metaphase II (g). n, Nucleolus; gv, germinal vesicle; pb, polar body. For details, see Wassarman and Fujiwara, 1978.

lized to synthesize and accumulate a large macromolecular store to be used during early embryogenesis.

III. MACROMOLECULAR STORES OF THE EGG

Unfertilized mouse eggs, while small in comparison with eggs from many nonmammalian animal species, are extraordinarily large relative to nearly all mammalian somatic cells. During a 2-week period, the growing oocyte increases in diameter at a rate of about 5 μm per day, reaching a terminal diameter, exclusive of the zona pellucida, of about 85 μm. Consequently, oocyte volume increases at a rapid rate, from about 2 pl per day at the beginning of the growth phase to more than 50 pl per day in the final stages of oocyte growth (all values calculated exclusive of microvilli). In the final 3 to 4 days of growth the oocyte actually doubles in volume, from about 160 to 320 pl.

TABLE II

Estimates of the DNA, RNA, and Protein Content of Mouse Eggs[a]

Macromolecule	Amount/egg
Nuclear DNA	6.0 ± 0.5 pg
Mitochondrial DNA	2.5 ± 0.5 pg
Total RNA	480 ± 130 pg
18 + 28 S RNA	285 ± 87 pg
4 + 5 S RNA	165 ± 34 pg
Informational RNA	30 ± 8 pg
Total protein	29 ± 1 ng
Zona pellucida protein	4 ± 0.5 ng
Mitochondrial protein	0.5 ± 0.2 ng

[a] These estimates were made with data taken from the following references: Lowenstein and Cohen, 1964; Brinster, 1967; Olds et al., 1973; Pikó and Chase, 1973; Bachvarova, 1974, 1981; Matsumoto et al., 1974; Jahn et al., 1974; Pikó and Matsumoto, 1976; Schultz and Wassarman, 1977a,b; Levey et al., 1978; Schultz et al., 1978; Bachvarova and DeLeon, 1980; Schultz and Wassarman, 1980; Brower et al., 1981; Sellens et al., 1981; Sternlicht and Schultz, 1981; Cascio and Wassarman, 1982; Pikó and Clegg, 1982.

The unusual size of fully grown mouse oocytes and unfertilized eggs is reflected in the macromolecular contents of these cells (Tables II and III). On a per cell basis, the fully grown mouse oocyte contains about 200 times more RNA, 60 times more protein, 1000 times more ribosomes, and 100 times more mitochondria than a typical mammalian somatic cell (e.g., liver). However, on a volume (per picoliter) basis, mouse oocytes are not unlike somatic cells with respect to RNA, protein, ribosome, and mitochondria concentration. In fact, a comparison of the macromolecular contents of mouse, sea urchin, and amphibian oocytes indicates that, although there is a large disparity in total contents, in each case, the concentrations of RNA, protein, ribosomes, and mitochondria are not very dissimilar from each other or from somatic cells. This conclusion is of considerable interest when one considers that during early cleavage the mass of egg cytoplasm is divided into a number of blastomeres without a significant increase in the total dry mass of the embryo. Therefore, for all intents and purposes, early cleavage simply results in a restoration of the egg's macromolecular stores to somatic cell levels by partitioning of cytoplasm among the blastomeres. In this manner the nutritional, synthetic, and energetic requirements of the early embryo can be met to varying degrees by the mature egg.

In the remainder of this chapter, the synthetic events that occur during oogenesis in the mouse, leading to the accumulation of a large macromolecular store in the unfertilized egg, will be reviewed.

TABLE III

Estimates of the Macromolecular Contents of Mouse, Sea Urchin, and Amphibian Eggs

Parameter	Mammalian liver cell	Mouse egg (*M. musculus*)	Sea urchin egg (*L. pictus*)	Amphibian egg (*X. laevis*)
Volume (pl)	5	320	700	1,250,000
RNA (pg/pl)	0.5	1.5	5.5	3.0
Protein (pg/pl)	95	80	20	20 (nonyolk)
Ribosomes				
Total number	10^5	10^8	10^9	10^{12}
Number/pl	6×10^4	3×10^5	1×10^6	8×10^5
Mitochondria				
Total number	10^3	10^5	10^5	10^6
Number/pl	260	300	320	2

IV. RIBONUCLEIC ACID SYNTHESIS DURING OOGENESIS

The fully grown mouse oocyte (85 μm) contains approximately 500 pg of RNA, or about 200 times the amount ($\simeq$ 2.5 pg) found in a somatic (liver) cell (Tables II and III). Nearly 15 years ago, autoradiography of sectioned ovaries from mice injected intraperitoneally with [³H]uridine demonstrated that oocytes synthesize RNA throughout their growth phase (Oakberg, 1967, 1968). Today it is clear that both growing and fully grown mouse oocytes synthesize and accumulate all classes of RNA (ribosomal, transfer, and informational RNA), and it is likely that this relatively large store of RNA plays an important role during early embryogenesis.

A. Overall Ribonucleic Acid Synthesis

The total amount of RNA in mouse oocytes increases dramatically during oocyte growth and exhibits biphasic kinetics of accumulation with respect to oocyte volume (Fig. 5); oocytes at about 65% of their final volume have accumulated about 95% of the total amount of RNA present in the fully grown oocyte (Sternlicht and Schultz, 1981). It can be estimated that, overall, there is approximately a 300-fold increase in the RNA content of mouse oocytes during their growth phase and there is a good correlation between oocyte nuclear (GV) and nucleolar sizes and extent of RNA synthesis during this period (Moore *et al.,* 1974; Moore and Lintern-Moore, 1974); it should be noted that the volume of the oocyte's nucleus (GV) and nucleolus increase about 10-fold and 100-fold, respectively, during the growth phase. The progressive changes in the size and ultrastructure of the growing oocyte's nucleolus or, in some cases, nucleoli (Table I and Fig. 3) are totally consistent with increasing levels of ribosomal RNA synthesis during oocyte growth (Chouinard, 1971; Palombi and Viron, 1977; Wassarman and Josefowicz, 1978). Similarly, measurements of the endogenous levels of RNA polymerase activities during oocyte growth are consistent with progressively increasing levels of RNA synthesis until the oocyte has reached about 70% of its final volume, at which time RNA polymerase levels and the rate of RNA accumulation decrease (Moore *et al.,* 1974; Moore and Lintern-Moore, 1978; Sternlicht and Schultz, 1981). RNA continues to be synthesized in fully grown oocytes, declining to barely detectable levels only after chromosome condensation and nuclear (GV) dissolution during meiotic maturation at the time of ovulation (Bloom and Mukherjee, 1971; Rodman and Bachvarova, 1976; Wassarman and Letourneau, 1976).

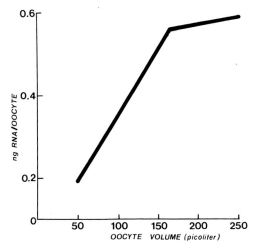

Fig. 5. The relationship between mouse oocyte growth and the accumulation of oocyte RNA. Adapted from Sternlicht and Schultz, 1981. It should be noted that overall there is nearly a 300-fold increase in RNA content during growth of mouse oocytes from about 12 to 85 μm in diameter. In these experiments the smallest oocytes examined were about 40 μm in diameter; the change in RNA content during growth of oocytes from 12 to 45 μm was not determined.

B. Synthesis of Specific Classes of Ribonucleic Acid

In recent years, a variety of experimental approaches have been used to assess the patterns of synthesis of specific classes of RNA during oocyte growth in the mouse. These approaches include the following. (1) A radiolabeled RNA precursor (e.g., [³H]uridine or [³H]adenosine) is injected into the ovarian bursa, followed by auto-radiographic and/or biochemical analyses of radiolabeled RNA in ovulated eggs collected at various times (from 1 to 24 days) after the injection. Since the major growth phase of the oocyte is known to occur between about 20 and 6 days prior to ovulation (see Section II,B), such analyses can provide information about the types of RNA synthesized and their stability during oocyte growth (e.g., Bachvarova, 1974; Jahn et al., 1976). (2) Denuded growing oocytes, cumulus–oocyte complexes, or follicle-enclosed oocytes are incubated in the presence of a radiolabeled RNA precursor in an appropriate culture medium in vitro, followed by autoradiographic and/or biochemical analysis of radiolabeled RNA (e.g., Brower et al., 1981; Bachvarova, 1981). (3) ³H-Labeled poly(U) is hybridized in situ to ovarian sections or fixed oocytes, followed by autoradiography, to permit estimation of the relative amounts and intracellular localization of poly(A)-containing RNA during oocyte growth (e.g., Sternlicht and Schultz, 1981; Pikó and Clegg, 1982). The results of experiments utilizing these different procedures have led to a clearer understanding of the pattern of synthesis and stability of various classes of RNA during oocyte growth in the mouse.

The time course of radiolabeling of RNA, following injection of [^{3}H]adenosine or [^{3}H]uridine into the ovarian bursa of the mouse, demonstrates that there is significant incorporation of radiolabeled precursor into oocyte RNA 7 to 19 days ($\simeq$ 2-week period) prior to ovulation (Bachvarova, 1974; Jahn et al., 1976). This time period corresponds very well to the major growth phase of the oocyte, from 6 to 20 days before ovulation (Pedersen, 1969, 1970; Section II,B). Furthermore, a minimum of 70% of newly synthesized RNA present at 19 hours and 82% of that present at 43 hours after bursal injection of radiolabeled precursor is retained until ovulation 10 to 20 days later. Therefore, the RNA synthesized in growing mouse oocytes is unusually stable. Biochemical analyses of the RNA on both sucrose gradients and polyacrylamide gels have revealed very similar distributions of radiolabel throughout oocyte growth, with 60 to 70% in ribosomal RNA (28 S and 18 S), 18 to 20% in 5 S plus transfer RNA (4 S), and 10 to 21% in heterogeneous RNA. Analyses of the distribution of radiolabel between poly(A)$^+$ and poly(A)$^-$ RNA by chromatography on poly(U)-Sepharose columns suggest that about 10% of the radiolabel is in the poly(A)$^+$ fraction for RNA synthesized at any time during oocyte growth, from 19 to 7 days before ovulation; this corresponds to about 8% ($\simeq$ 25 pg) of the mass of egg RNA (Bachvarova and DeLeon, 1980). Therefore, by these criteria, polyadenylated RNA is synthesized and accumulates throughout oocyte growth and is present in sufficient quantities to account for all polysomal informational RNA present in mouse eggs (Bachvarova and DeLeon, 1980).

The accumulation of poly(A)$^+$ RNA during oocyte growth has also been examined by in situ hybridization of ^{3}H-labeled poly(U) to ovarian sections, followed by autoradiography (Sternlicht and Schultz, 1981; Pikó and Clegg, 1982). By this method, the kinetics of accumulation of poly(A)$^+$ RNA during oocyte growth appear to be similar to the biphasic kinetics of accumulation of total RNA; i.e., about 95% of the poly(A)$^+$ RNA present in a fully grown oocyte is present in a growing oocyte when it is about 70% of its final volume (Sternlicht and Schultz, 1981). On the other hand, grain densities over the oocyte's cytoplasm indicate that there is a significant reduction ($\simeq$ twofold) in poly(A) content in the interval between completion of oocyte growth and ovulation (6–7 days) (Pikó and Clegg, 1982). Despite this reduction, which is consistent with reduced RNA polymerase II levels (Moore and Lintern-Moore, 1978), the relative concentration of poly(A) in the nucleus (GV) of the fully grown oocyte remains about two times that in the cytoplasm, suggesting that nuclear poly(A)$^+$ RNA synthesis continues following completion of oocyte growth. Hybridization with ^{3}H-labeled poly(U) in solution indicates that just before ovulation the fully grown oocyte contains about 1 pg of poly(A) [$\simeq$ 26 pg poly(A)$^+$ RNA], but that the poly(A) content falls to about 0.7 pg [$\simeq$ 19 pg poly(A)$^+$ RNA] in the unfertilized egg. These results, as well as others (Bachvarova and De-Leon, 1980), suggest that the amount of informational RNA in mouse oocytes and eggs (5–10% of total RNA) is unusually high relative to eggs of various nonmammalian animal species and to somatic cells.

Recently, RNA synthesis in growing mouse oocytes has been examined *in vitro* (1) in follicle-enclosed oocytes (Brower *et al.*, 1981) and (2) in denuded oocytes maintained in the presence of ovarian somatic cell monolayers (Bachvarova, 1981). In the former case, the percentage of poly(A)$^+$ RNA, determined by chromatography of [^{3}H]uridine-labeled RNA (5-hour culture period) on poly(U)-Sepharose, remains fairly constant at 40 to 50% of total newly synthesized RNA in growing oocytes ($\simeq$ 35–65 μm in diameter) and falls to about 20% in fully grown oocytes and unfertilized eggs. The ratios of the relative amounts of radiolabel associated with 28, 18, and 4 plus 5 S RNA, determined by agarose gel electrophoresis, remain essentially constant (2.4:1.0:1.6) for the follicle-enclosed oocytes at different stages of oocyte growth (consistent with Bachvarova, 1974; Bachvarova and DeLeon, 1980; see discussion above). Furthermore, these ratios change only slightly during a "chase" period of several days following a 5-hour "pulse" (28:18:4 plus 5 S, 2.7:1.0:1.3), suggesting that the relative stabilities of the various classes of RNA are quite similar. In fact, total RNA synthesized in follicle-enclosed growing oocytes is unusually stable, having a half-life of about 28 days (consistent with Bachvarova, 1974; Jahn *et al.*, 1976; see discussion above) so long as oocytes continue growing *in vitro*. (Note: Under conditions in which oocytes are viable, but do not grow, the half-life of total RNA is about 4.5 days.) Under these conditions, turnover of ribosomal, 4 and 5 S RNA is barely detectable, whereas poly(A)$^+$ RNA turns over slowly (half-life $\simeq$ 10 days), exhibiting kinetics suggestive of the existence of a relatively unstable species of high-molecular-weight, heterogeneous RNA (Brower *et al.*, 1981).

Examination of RNA synthesis in denuded oocytes at mid-growth ($\simeq$ 45 μm in diameter), cultured and radiolabeled with [^{3}H]uridine *in vitro* in the presence of ovarian somatic cell monolayers (conditions under which oocytes continue to grow; Bachvarova *et al.*, 1981), has permitted estimation of the rates of synthesis and half-lives of heterogeneous RNA (Bachvarova, 1981). Heterogeneous RNA in these oocytes includes material >36 S representative of heterogeneous nuclear RNA (HnRNA) and <36 S which undoubtedly includes cytoplasmic messenger RNA [poly(A)$^+$ RNA]. From the kinetics of [^{3}H]uridine incorporation into various RNA classes, the rates of synthesis, steady-state amounts, and stabilities of the two heterogeneous RNA classes can be estimated by assuming that ribosomal RNA is synthesized at about 0.2 ng per week and is completely stable throughout the radiolabeling period; the results of these calculations are summarized in Table IV. It would appear that heterogeneous RNA is synthesized at a relatively high rate ($\simeq$ 0.6 pg/min) and turns over rapidly (half-life $\simeq$ 20 minutes) during oocyte growth; however, because of a high rate of synthesis, the steady state amount of nuclear heterogeneous RNA (>36 S) is quite large ($\simeq$ 17 pg). Approximately 2% of the total heterogeneous RNA is conserved, reaches the oocyte's cytoplasm, and accumulates at about 50% of the rate of ribosomal RNA ($\simeq$ 0.01 pg/min) (Bachvarova, 1981).

C. Accumulation of Ribosomes in Growing Oocytes

While it is generally accepted that ribosomal RNA is synthesized by mouse oocytes throughout their growth phase (Section IV,A and B), there is no unanimity concerning the state of ribosomes in growing and fully grown oocytes. The disagreement centers on the question of whether or not the cytoplasmic lattice arrays (also termed plaques, lamellae, or fibrillar arrays) that accumulate during oocyte growth

TABLE IV

Synthesis and Turnover of RNA during Oocyte Growth in the Mouse[a]

Class of RNA	Steady-state amount (pg)	Half-time (minute)	Rate of synthesis (pg/minute)
Stable ribosomal RNA	—	—	0.02
Stable heterogeneous RNA (<36 S)	—	—	0.01
Unstable heterogeneous RNA (<36 S)	2	20	0.08
Heterogeneous RNA (>36 S)	15	20	0.5
Total heterogeneous RNA	17	20	0.6

[a] Data taken from Bachvarova, 1981.

(Table I and Fig. 3) are actually a storage form of ribosomes. These latticelike structures are a dominant feature of the cytoplasm of both fully grown mouse oocytes and unfertilized eggs (as well as of oocytes and eggs of other rodents) but are not present at all in nongrowing oocytes and are present in diminishing numbers in implanting blastocysts (Van Blerkom and Motta, 1979).

Although described in many laboratories (e.g., Schlafke and Enders, 1967; Weakley, 1968; Calarco and Brown, 1969; Hillman and Tasca, 1969; Zamboni, 1970; Szollosi, 1972; Van Blerkom and Runner, 1976; Wassarman and Josefowicz, 1978), perhaps the most thorough description of the cytoplasmic lattices has come from examination of uranyl-acetate-stained, whole-mount preparations of mouse oocytes (Burkholder *et al.*, 1971). In such preparations the lattices appear as highly ordered aggregates of individual chains composed of particles ($\simeq$ 212 Å in diameter) that are connected by bridges ($\simeq$ 125 Å in diameter), giving a periodicity of about 300 Å to each chain ("beads on a string"). The individual chains themselves are interconnected (center-to-center distance $\simeq$ 235–300 Å), so that the lattices appear to form layers of interconnected sheets. The integrity of the lattices is disrupted by treatment with either trypsin or ribonuclease or by exposure to mild acid; the latter, perhaps, suggesting that the particles are held together by basic proteins. In some cases, particles are released from the lattices in whole-mount preparations, and these have a diameter of about 225 Å, the same diameter as eukaryotic ribosomes.

Although for the most part circumstantial in nature, other evidence has been presented that strengthens, but does not prove, the contention that the oocyte's cytoplasmic lattices are composed of ribosomes held together by proteinaceous material:

1. Electron microscopic analysis of the number of ribosomes present in growing mouse oocytes indicates that the number increases several-fold during the early and middle stages of growth (23–56 μm in diameter) but declines during the late stages of growth (> 56 μm in diameter). The total number of ribosomes begins to fall at a time when lattices begin to appear in the oocyte's cytoplasm, suggesting that ribosomes are recruited into lattices during the final stages of oocyte growth (Garcia *et al.*, 1979).

2. Comparison of the "theoretical" number of ribosomes that could be present in oocytes during their growth phase (a calculation based on the amount of ribosomal RNA present at each stage of oocyte growth) with the actual number observed (Garcia *et al.*, 1979) indicates that the theoretical number far exceeds (from two- to eightfold) the actual

number of ribosomes observed (Sternlicht and Schultz, 1981). Such calculations suggest that more than 80% of the fully grown oocyte's ribosomes could be present in cytoplasmic lattices.

3. Biochemical analyses of ribosomes extracted from mouse eggs (following lysis by freezing and thawing) suggest that only 20–25% of the total ribosome population is in polysomes. The remaining 75–80% of the ribosomes (monomers and subunits), not normally in polysomes, are unable to form high salt-stable complexes with poly(U) and factors necessary for protein synthesis (Bachvarova and DeLeon, 1977). By comparison, electron microscopic analyses of fully grown oocytes indicate that more than 90% of the recognizable free ribosomes are contained in polysomes (Garcia *et al.,* 1979). These results suggest that most of the ribosomes present in unfertilized mouse eggs are inactive in protein synthesis and must be modified in order to function in translation; such an interpretation is consistent with storage of the bulk of oocyte ribosomes in cytoplasmic lattices.

4. Biochemical analyses of ribosomes extracted from mouse eggs by lysis in a moderately hypotonic buffer indicate that 75% of the ribosome population is contained in unusually large structures that sediment at speeds of 9000 g or less and that are sensitive to freezing and thawing (used by Bachvarova and DeLeon, 1977) and to isotonic salt (Bachvarova *et al.,* 1981). These structures consist of interlacing fibrils that form a meshwork in which electron-dense particles (160–200 Å in diameter) that are sensitive to ribonuclease are abundant. The buoyant density of the fixed particles (1.33–1.38 g/cm^3) indicates that they contain about three times more protein than a typical ribosome (1.58 g/cm^3) and, consequently, are 5–15% RNA; however, exposure of the particles to Pronase increases their buoyant density so that it resembles that of ribosomes. These results are certainly consistent with the presence of a ribosomal lattice (25% ribosomes and 75% protein by weight) in mouse eggs.

Despite the evidence just described, it cannot be concluded unequivocally that the cytoplasmic lattices are, in fact, a storage form of ribosomes without more direct experimental results. For example, several arguments have recently been presented against the notion that cytoplasmic lattices are a storage form of ribosomes in mouse eggs (Pikó and Clegg, 1982). (1) The lattices have a low electron density with a selective staining procedure that results in greatly enhanced contrast of ribosomes and other nucleic-acid-containing structures. (2) The lattices are barely affected by alkali treatment that is sufficient to abolish the staining of authentic ribosomes. (3) The number of recognizable cytoplasmic ribosomes accounts for the bulk of the RNA content of mouse embryos from the one-cell to the early blastocyst stages. (4) From the periodic structure of the lattices it can be calculated that if each particle represents a ribosome the total number of stored ribosomes should be of the order of 10^9, or 4 ng of ribosomal RNA; this value is about 20 times higher than the amount of ribosomal RNA actually found. These, as well as other arguments, can be raised, and the situation certainly remains unresolved.

D. Epilogue

Results obtained in several laboratories during the past 8 years or so have provided a fairly detailed scenario for RNA synthesis during growth and meiotic maturation of mouse oocytes. The data suggest that transcription in growing oocytes occurs continuously and is more rapid than in somatic cells but does not approach the extremely high rate of transcription in vitellogenic *Xenopus* oocytes (Davidson, 1977; Anderson and Smith, 1978; Hill, 1979; Dolecki and Smith, 1979). As previously pointed out (Bachvarova, 1981), assuming that stored informational RNA has roughly the same complexity in mouse oocytes as in oocytes of nonmammalian animal species, the effective concentration of informational RNA could be achieved and maintained with considerably lower rates of synthesis. Furthermore, it is not necessary to propose extensive amplification of the mouse oocyte's ribosomal genes in order to account for the levels of ribosomal RNA synthesis observed during oocyte growth; although a fourfold amplification has been reported for oocytes from two other mammalian species (Wolgemuth *et al.*, 1979, 1980).

Recent experiments suggest that there is a dramatic reduction of stored maternal informational RNA ($\simeq$ twofold) and ribosomes by the two-cell stage of early embryogenesis in the mouse (Pikó and Clegg, 1982), in agreement with previous observations (Levey *et al.*, 1978; Sherman, 1979; Bachvarova and DeLeon, 1980), and that new transcription can be detected in the pronuclei of fertilized mouse eggs (Clegg and Pikó, 1982). Furthermore, evidence for expression of the paternal genome (i.e., for synthesis and ultilization of newly transcribed informational RNA) as early as the two-cell stage of embryogenesis in the mouse is now available (Sawicki *et al.*, 1981). Finally, between the two-cell and early blastocyst ($\simeq$ 32 cells) stages of development, the RNA content of the embryo increases about sixfold and the amount of maternal RNA is reduced to less than 10% of the total RNA (Pikó and Clegg, 1982). Therefore, a picture emerges from these and other studies which indicates a great dependence upon maternally derived informational RNA during the first 24 hours or so of embryogenesis in the mouse and a progressively declining dependence thereafter; the dependence upon maternal ribosomes probably extends to the first few cleavage divisions. This situation is substantially different from that observed with amphibian and echinoderm embryos, where reliance upon new gene expression does not occur until relatively late (insofar as cell number) in embryogenesis.

V. PROTEIN SYNTHESIS DURING OOGENESIS

More than 25 years ago it was demonstrated that oocytes contained within ovarian follicles incorporate [^{35}S]methionine into proteins following intraperitoneal injection of the radiolabeled precursor into mice (Lin, 1956). During the past 10 years or so, the availability of radiolabeled amino acids of high specific activity (e.g., [^{35}S]methionine, >500 Ci/mmol), coupled with technological advances (e.g., high-resolution two-dimensional gel electrophoresis and fluorography), has made it possible to carry out quantitative studies of protein synthesis with isolated mouse oocytes and eggs. Consequently, today it is clear that mouse oocytes synthesize and accumulate protein throughout their growth phase, thus accounting, at least in part, for the relatively high protein content of unfertilized eggs (Tables II and III).

A. Overall Patterns of Protein Synthesis

High-resolution two-dimensional gel electrophoretic analyses (O'Farrell, 1975) of proteins synthesized by growing and fully grown mouse oocytes have revealed a remarkable degree of constancy at the qualitative level (Schultz et al., 1979b; G. S. Salzmann and P. M. Wassarman, unpublished results). At least 400 discrete "spots" can be detected on fluorograms (Bonner and Laskey, 1974) of two-dimensional gels containing proteins radiolabeled with [^{35}S]Met during culture of mouse oocytes in vitro (Fig. 6). The most intensely radiolabeled proteins also appear to be the most abundant proteins in oocytes on the basis of the patterns observed with silver-stained (Oakley et al., 1980) two-dimensional gels (Fig. 7). Although changes in the overall pattern of protein synthesis can be detected during oocyte growth, most of these can be characterized as quantitative changes. In other words, apparently the same protein species are synthesized throughout oocyte growth but at different relative rates at different times in the growth

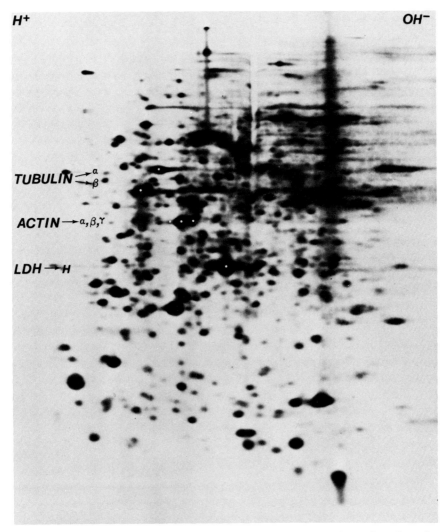

Fig. 6. A fluorogram of a high-resolution two-dimensional gel electrophoretic analysis (O'Farrell, 1975) of ^{35}S-methionine-labeled proteins following culture of fully grown mouse oocytes for 16 hours *in vitro*. White dots indicate the positions of the heart-type (H) LDH subunit, α, β, and γ actin, and α and β tubulin. For details, see Schultz *et al.*, 1979a,b and Cascio and Wassarman, 1982.

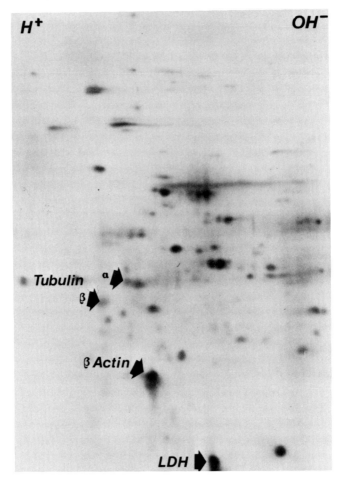

Fig. 7. A silver-stained (Oakley *et al.*, 1980), high-resolution two-dimensional gel electrophoretic analysis (O'Farrell, 1975) of proteins from isolated fully grown mouse oocytes. The positions of the heart-type (H) LDH subunit, β actin, and α and β tubulin are indicated by arrows. (Taken from unpublished results of G. S. Salzmann and P. M. Wassarman).

phase. Thus far, it has not been possible unequivocally to identify stage-specific protein markers during oocyte growth in the mouse.

Meiotic maturation of mouse oocytes is, however, accompanied by significant changes in the overall pattern of protein synthesis, as revealed by both one- and two-dimensional gel electrophoresis (Golbus and Stein, 1976; Schultz and Wassarman, 1977a,b; Schultz *et al.*,

1978b; Richter and McGaughey, 1981). Virtually all of the changes observed in protein synthesis take place subsequent to breakdown of the nucleus (GV), but they are not dependent upon the occurrence of other morphological events, such as spindle formation or polar body emission; the latter conclusion is drawn from experiments utilizing drugs (e.g., puromycin, colcemid, or cytochalasin B) that specifically block meiotic maturation *in vitro* at specific stages of nuclear progression (Wassarman *et al.*, 1976; Schultz and Wassarman, 1976, 1977b; Schultz *et al.*, 1978b). The changes in protein synthesis do not take place in oocytes that fail to undergo nuclear (GV) breakdown spontaneously or in oocytes arrested at the nuclear (GV) stage with drugs. Such data suggest that many of the changes in protein synthesis accompanying meiotic maturation may result from mixing of the oocyte's nucleoplasm and cytoplasm. While concomitant RNA and protein synthesis are not necessary for oocytes to resume meiosis and undergo nuclear (GV) breakdown, protein synthesis is necessary for a brief period following nuclear (GV) breakdown in order for maturation to proceed to metaphase I; it is possible that spindle assembly is the event that is dependent upon concomitant protein synthesis.

B. Overall Rates of Protein Synthesis

The incorporation of a radioactively labeled amino acid into cellular protein as a function of time (dI/dt) should be interpreted only as a relative rate of protein synthesis. In order to determine the absolute rate of protein synthesis (R), one must know the specific activity (SA) of the true precursor pool [$R=(dI/dt)/SA$]; in essence, this requires the determination of the specific activity of aminoacyl tRNA. While such measurements have been made with oocytes and eggs from nonmammalian animal species, they have not been practical with mice because only limited amounts of material are available. However, it has been possible to measure the sizes and specific activities of endogenous free Met pools in mouse oocytes and eggs and to use these values to determine absolute rates of protein synthesis.

Two methods have been used to determine Met pool sizes in mouse oocytes and eggs. The first is based upon the reaction of [^{3}H]fluorodinitrobenzene (FDNB) of known specific activity with the total intracellular Met pool containing a ^{35}S-labeled Met tracer (Regier and Kafatos, 1971). By measuring the ratio of ^{35}S to ^{3}H in the resulting DNP-Met, after purification by two-dimensional chromatography, the specific activities of intracellular Met pools can be calculated from $SA^{exp}/SA^{med} = (A)/(A+B)$, where A (moles) = Met taken up into the intracellular pool, B (moles) = size of the endogenous Met pool, SA^{exp} (dpm/mole) = specific activity of the intracellular Met, and SA^{med} (dpm/mole) = specific activity of Met in the culture medium. The second method used to determine endogenous Met pool sizes in mouse oocytes and eggs depends upon differential expansion of the Met pool, such that apparent rates of incorporation are altered (dI/dt) while absolute rates (R) remain the same (Ecker, 1972). Under two different sets of conditions, 1 and 2, insofar as expansion of the Met pool is concerned, $(dI_1/dt)/[L_1/(P+G_1)]=(dI_2/dt)/[L_2/(P+G_2)]$, where L (dpm) = [^{35}S]Met in the acid-soluble fraction, P (moles) = size of the endogenous Met pool, and G (moles) = Met taken up into the intracellular pool. Thus, measurement of dI/dt, L, and G at two different Met concentrations (conditions 1 and 2), permits solving for P; in practice, these measurements are made at several points over a wide range of Met concentrations. It should be noted that the latter method measures the size of the "kinetic" precursor pool, whereas the FDNB method measures the size of the total precursor pool.

1. Oocyte Growth

In order to determine absolute rates of total protein synthesis during oocyte growth and meiotic maturation (i.e., conversion of fully grown oocytes into unfertilized eggs), various procedures (e.g., Rafferty, 1970; Mangia and Epstein, 1975; Eppig, 1977a,b; Schultz et al., 1979b) have been used to collect oocytes from juvenile (3–21 days old) and adult (>21 days old) female mice for culture under in vitro conditions. It has only been within the past 10 years that procedures have been devised to isolate and culture growing oocytes from juvenile mice (Szybec, 1972; Mangia and Epstein, 1975; Sorensen and Wassarman, 1976; Schultz and Wassarman, 1977a; Eppig, 1977a,b; Bachvarova et al., 1981) and, since the size of the oocytes recovered increases with the age of the donor, this has proved to be an important methodological advance. Mouse oocytes ranging from about 12 to 80 µm in diameter can be obtained from ovaries of mice 3 to 21 days old, with the size of the oocytes directly related to the age of the mice. At any given age, the diameter of the oocytes recovered will vary by about ±10%, thus providing relatively homogeneous pools of growing oocytes, at least with respect to size. One indicator of the viability of such cells in vitro (aside from trypan blue dye exclusion) is the observation that oocytes less than about 60 µm in diameter remain in the nuclear (GV) stage during culture, whereas those greater than 60 µm resume meiosis, undergo nuclear germinal vesicle breakdown (GVBD) and arrest at metaphase II in an apparently normal manner (Sorensen and Wassarman, 1976; Schultz and Wassarman, 1977a). In fact, under certain conditions mouse oocytes will actually continue to "grow" *in vitro* (Eppig, 1977a,b; Baran and Bachvarova, 1977; Eppig, 1979; Bachvarova *et al.*, 1981). These conditions include the presence of granulosa cells surrounding the growing oocyte, suggesting that intercellular communication via gap junctions may play a role in oocyte growth (Anderson and Albertini, 1976; Gilula *et al.*, 1978; Heller and Schultz, 1980; Moor *et al.*, 1980; Heller *et al.*, 1981; Brower and Schultz, 1982).

The sizes of endogenous Met pools and absolute rates of protein synthesis in growing oocytes, fully grown oocytes, and unfertilized eggs from mice have been determined using both the FDNB and kinetic methods described above (Schultz *et al.*, 1978a, 1979a,b; Wassarman *et al.*, 1979, 1981). The results of these experiments are summarized in Figs. 8 and 9 and Table V. The FDNB and kinetic methods give vir-

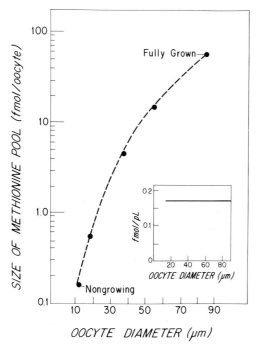

Fig. 8. The relationship between diameters of growing mouse oocytes and sizes of intracellular methionine pools. The closed circles refer to the experimentally determined values for methionine pool sizes. The broken line is a theoretical curve constructed by assuming a simple linear relationship between methionine pool size and oocyte volume, using a value of 56 fmole of methionine per oocyte for the fully grown oocyte. Inset: Data converted to femtomoles of methionine per picoliter as a function of oocyte diameter. For details, see Schultz *et al.*, 1979b.

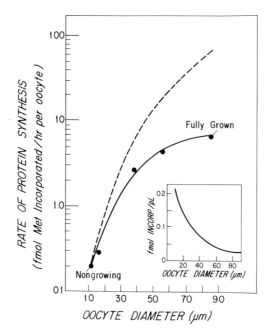

Fig. 9. The relationship between diameters of growing mouse oocytes and absolute rates of protein synthesis. The closed circles refer to the experimentally determined values for absolute rates of protein synthesis. The broken line is a theoretical curve constructed by assuming a simple linear relationship between absolute rates of protein synthesis and oocyte volume, using a value of 41.8 pg/hour per oocyte for the fully grown oocyte. Inset: Data converted to femtomoles of methionine incorporated per picoliter as a function of oocyte diameter. For details, see Schultz *et al.*, 1979b.

tually the same values for endogenous Met pool sizes during oocyte growth, strongly suggesting that the entire Met pool, not just a smaller "compartment" of the pool, serves as precursor for protein synthesis. As the oocyte undergoes about a 350-fold increase in volume during its growth phase (from 12 to 85 μm in diameter), a corresponding increase also occurs in the size of the oocyte's endogenous Met pool (from 0.16 to 56 fmol). Therefore, each doubling of oocyte volume is accompanied by a doubling of the size of the Met pool, such that the concentration of intracellular free Met remains constant at about 170 μM throughout oocyte growth (Fig. 8 and Table V). On the other hand, while the absolute rate of protein synthesis increases during oocyte growth, from 1.1 to 41.8 pg/hour per oocyte, the increase is only about 38-fold as compared to the 350-fold increase in oocyte volume. Consequently, the absolute rate of protein synthesis, expressed on a volume (per picoliter) basis, actually decreases during oocyte growth (Fig. 9 and Table V), so

TABLE V

Absolute Rates of Protein Synthesis and Sizes of Methionine Pools during Oogenesis in the Mouse[a]

Stage	Pool size (fmole Met/cell)	Absolute rate (pg/hr per cell)
Nongrowing oocyte	0.16 ± 0.1	1.10 ± 0.4
Growing oocyte		
≈15–20 μm	0.55 ± 0.2	1.49 ± 0.7
≈35–45 μm	4.80 ± 1.9	13.2 ± 5.4
≈50–60 μm	13.3 ± 6.0	27.5 ± 5.5
Fully grown oocyte	56.0 ± 19	41.8 ± 5.5
Unfertilized egg	74.0 ± 12	33.0 ± 2.2

[a] Data taken from Schultz et al., 1978, 1979a,b.

that it takes about 10 pl of cytoplasm from a fully grown oocyte to synthesize as much protein as 1 pl from a nongrowing oocyte. However, this comparison may be somewhat misleading in that it is difficult to assess the actual amount of "synthetically active" cytoplasm in growing and fully grown mouse oocytes. For example, it is estimated that 90% of the cytoplasmic volume of amphibian oocytes consists of yolk platelets, leaving only about 10% as "active" cytoplasm.* Since the cytoplasm of growing mouse oocytes becomes progressively more densely populated with organelles and inclusions, perhaps including a "yolklike" component, it is very unlikely that the amount of "synthetically active" cytoplasm increases 350-fold during oocyte growth. Such a situation would explain why the absolute rate of protein synthesis does not appear to keep pace with volume during oocyte growth (Fig. 9).

Less than 60% of the protein present in fully grown mouse oocytes can be accounted for by protein synthesis during oocyte growth (Schultz et al., 1979b; Wassarman et al., 1981). While it is possible that this discrepancy results from errors in one or more of the measurements used in the calculation (e.g., absolute rates of synthesis, timing of growth, total protein content, etc.), it may reflect the presence of a "yolklike" component in mouse oocytes that is synthesized elsewhere in the organism and taken up into the oocytes by endocytosis. The latter situation would be analogous to the process of yolk accumulation

* In fact, when this is taken into consideration, the absolute rate of protein synthesis in fully grown mouse oocytes, 0.17 pg/hour per picoliter, compares quite favorably with that reported for amphibian oocytes, 0.34 pg/hour per picoliter (Smith, 1975; Schultz et al., 1978a).

in the amphibian, where as much as 80% of the protein in fully grown oocytes is associated with yolk platelets and this protein is synthesized, not by the oocyte, but by the liver (Wallace, 1972). A similar situation is found in insects; although the nurse cells furnish the oocyte with a significant proportion of macromolecules, such as protein and RNA (Bier, 1963), the oocyte possesses receptors involved in the selective pinocytotic uptake of specific proteins present in the blood of the female (Telfer, 1960). While it has been suggested from morphological observations that mammalian oocytes contain a "yolklike" component (Szollosi, 1972), there is no clear biochemical evidence that either supports or refutes this suggestion. However, the presence of a mammalian yolk could resolve a paradox; for, during early mammalian embryogenesis, while the absolute rate of protein synthesis increases and the rate of degradation of newly synthesized protein does not change dramatically (Brinster *et al.*, 1976; Schultz *et al.*, 1979a,b), the protein content of the mouse embryo actually decreases substantially (Brinster, 1967). Degradation of a yolk component during early embryogenesis could account for these findings.

A number of studies has shown that mouse oocytes can selectively take up proteins from the blood, and it has been suggested that with mammalian oocytes, endocytosis may serve as a mechanism for internalizing nutritive substances (e.g., Anderson, 1972). The ovarian localization of bovine plasma albumin, bovine plasma globulin, rabbit plasma globulin, and mouse autologous serum antigens injected into mice has been evaluated by immunofluorescent microscopy (Glass, 1961, 1966). It was found that, although bovine plasma albumin and autologous serum antigens could be located within the oocyte, bovine and rabbit plasma globulin could not be detected there. Subsequent studies revealed that albumin was taken up by oocytes throughout their growth phase, although the extent of uptake depended upon the stage of ooctye growth; small oocytes invested with an incomplete layer of granulosa cells and oocytes enclosed in follicles containing an antrum manifested the highest degree of uptake (Glass and Cons, 1968). Therefore, mouse oocytes at least have the capacity to accumulate a yolk component (and/or other proteins) from the blood. It remains to be determined whether or not a specific protein(s) taken up by the growing oocyte serves a nutritional function during early embryogenesis.

2. Meiotic Maturation

During meiotic maturation of mouse oocytes there is a significant decrease in the absolute rate of protein synthesis (Schultz *et al.*, 1978a, 1979a; Wassarman *et al.*, 1979, 1981). As oocytes progress from dictyate of the first meiotic prophase to metaphase II, the absolute rate of protein synthesis decreases by about 20%, from 41.8 to 33.0 pg/hour per cell (Table V). It is possible that this modest decrease in protein synthesis during meiotic maturation is attributable to degradation and/or modification of informational RNA, since the rate of RNA synthesis appears to decrease dramatically following nuclear (GV) breakdown(Wassarman and Letourneau, 1976; Rodman and Bachvarova, 1976). The decline in both RNA and protein synthesis seen during meiotic maturation may, in fact, be analogous to that observed with various types of somatic cells during the mitotic phase of the cell cycle (Mitchison, 1971; Prescott, 1976); in both instances, chromosomes are present in a highly condensed configuration and mixing of nucleoplasm and cytoplasm has occurred. Furthermore, just as fertilization results in an increase in the rate of protein synthesis by mouse eggs, emergence of somatic cells from mitosis results in a restoration of higher rates of protein synthesis.

C. Synthesis of Specific Proteins

At least three different experimental approaches have been employed to identify specific proteins and to study their synthesis during oogenesis in the mouse. (1) Immunoprecipitation of metabolically radiolabeled oocyte or egg proteins with antisera directed against a specific mouse protein (e.g., lactate dehydrogenase). (2) High-resolution two-dimensional gel electrophoresis of metabolically radiolabeled oocyte or egg proteins in the presence of a protein purified from mouse tissue. Coelectrophoresis (i.e., identical isoelectric points and molecular weights) of a radiolabeled "spot" (detected by fluorography) with the purified protein "spot" (detected by staining) is taken, along with other criteria, as proof of the identity of the oocyte and/or egg protein (e.g., tubulin and actin). (3) Use of inhibitors that specifically prevent synthesis of particular proteins, while allowing the synthesis of other proteins (e.g., mitochondrial proteins) to continue. When these approaches are used in combination with a knowledge of the absolute rates of total protein synthesis during oogenesis, the rates of synthesis of specific proteins can be assessed in a reliable manner.

1. Tubulin

Tubulin comprises a relatively large amount of the total protein in oocytes and eggs of nonmammalian animal species; values ranging from about 0.5 to 3% of the total protein content have been reported (Miller and Epel, 1973; Pestell, 1975; Raff et al., 1975; Raff, 1977; Loyd *et al.*, 1981). Tubulin accumulates continuously during oocyte growth in these nonmammalian species, and it appears likely that tubulin is a good example of a protein that is "stockpiled" during oogenesis for utilization during early embryogenesis (e.g., Bibring and Baxandall, 1977).

The α and β subunits of tubulin are synthesized throughout oocyte growth and meiotic maturation in the mouse (Fig. 10) and are among the most abundant proteins in mouse oocytes and eggs (Schultz *et al.*, 1979a,b). The absolute rate of tubulin synthesis increases from 0.4 to 0.6 pg/hour per oocyte as oocytes grow from 40 to 85 μm in diameter; however, the percentage of total protein synthesis devoted to tubulin actually declines somewhat during this period, from 2.0 to 1.5% (Table VI). During meiotic maturation the absolute rate of tubulin synthesis declines from 0.60 pg/hour per oocyte to 0.36 pg/hour per unfertilized egg, a 40% decrease in the rate of tubulin synthesis compared with a 21% decrease in the rate of total protein synthesis during the same period. Furthermore, although tubulin subunits are present in equimolar amounts in microtubules, the ratio of the rate of synthesis of the β subunit to that of the α subunit is significantly greater than 1.0 at all stages of oocyte growth and meiotic maturation.

From measurements of the absolute rates of tubulin synthesis in mouse oocytes, it can be estimated that the unfertilized egg contains from 250 to 300 pg of tubulin. This represents about 50 times more tubulin than that found in various types of somatic cells, but is only about two times the amount found in sea urchin eggs and about 1000 times less than that found in amphibian eggs. These comparisons indicate that the quantity of tubulin is related to cell size, such that the concentration of tubulin is maintained within a relatively narrow range of values. Presumably, partitioning of the mouse egg's store of tubulin among the blastomeres of preimplantation embryos restores

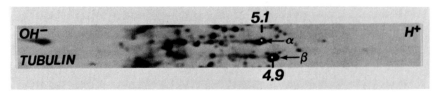

Fig. 10. A portion of a fluorogram of a high-resolution two-dimensional gel electrophoretic analysis of [35S]methionine-labeled proteins following culture of growing mouse oocytes for 16 hours *in vitro*. Shown is the region in which newly synthesized α and β tubulin is resolved with isoelectric points of 5.1 and 4.9, respectively. For details, see Schultz *et al.*, 1979a,b.

TABLE VI

Synthesis of Tubulin and Actin during Oogenesis in the Mouse

	Total protein synthesis (%)		Absolute rate (pg/hr per cell)	
Stage	Tubulin[a]	Actin[b]	Tubulin[a]	Actin[b]
Growing oocyte				
≈40–50 μm	2.0	0.9	0.40	0.20
Fully grown oocyte	1.5	0.3	0.60	0.10
Unfertilized egg	1.1	0.2	0.36	0.06

[a] Data taken from Schultz *et al.*, 1979a,b.
[b] Unpublished results of G. S. Salzmann, R. J. Roller, and P. M. Wassarman.

the amount per cell to somatic cell values. For, although tubulin continues to be synthesized during early cleavage (Abreu and Brinster, 1978; Schultz *et al.*, 1979a), its contribution to the total tubulin pool inherited from the egg is relatively small (≈ 20%).

2. Actin

Actin is involved in a wide variety of biological processes, including cell division, cell motility, and muscle contraction; consequently, it is a relatively abundant protein (≈ 2–8% of total cellular protein) found in virtually all eukaryotic cells (Pollard and Weihing, 1974; Inoué and Stephens, 1975; Goldman *et al.*, 1976; Clarke and Spudich, 1977; Pollard, 1981; Firtel, 1981; Fulton, 1981). Three different forms of actin, α, β, and γ, have been distinguished in mammalian cells by high-resolution two-dimensional gel electrophoresis, with α actin(s) characteristic of muscle (skeletal, cardiac, and smooth muscle actins) and β and γ actins (cytoplasmic) characteristic of cytoskeleton. The muscle actins appear to be more closely related to one another than to the cytoplasmic actins.

Recently, actin synthesis has been examined during the course of oocyte growth and meiotic maturation in the mouse (G. S. Salzmann, R. J. Roller, and P. M. Wassarman, unpublished results). It was found that actin is synthesized throughout these stages of oogenesis in the mouse (Fig. 11), representing, on average, more than 0.8% of total protein synthesis in growing and fully grown oocytes and about 0.15% in unfertilized eggs (Table VI). The distribution of synthesis (percentage of total) among α, β, and γ actin during oocyte growth is approximately 5, 80, and 15%, respectively; on the other hand, in unfertilized

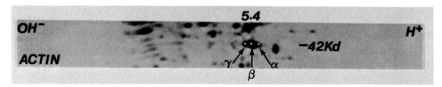

Fig. 11. A portion of a fluorogram of a high-resolution two-dimensional gel electrophoretic analysis of [^{35}S]methionine-labeled proteins following culture of growing mouse oocytes for 16 hours *in vitro*. Shown is the region in which newly synthesized α, β, and γ actin is resolved at 42 kilodaltons. Taken from unpublished results of G. S. Salzmann, R. J. Roller, and P. M. Wassarman.

eggs the distribution changes dramatically to 20, 20, and 60% for α, β, and γ actin, respectively.

The percentage of total protein synthesis devoted to actin synthesis in fully grown mouse oocytes (0.3%) is very similar to the value reported for *Xenopus* oocytes (Sturgess *et al.*, 1980); in both cases, β and γ actins are among the most abundant newly synthesized proteins in oocytes. The decrease in actin synthesis in unfertilized mouse eggs, relative to fully grown oocytes, is also consistent with the situation in *Xenopus*. Therefore, as in the case of tubulin, the fertilized egg inherits a large maternal pool of actin which is augmented to a small extent by continued actin synthesis during early cleavage (Abreu and Brinster, 1978; G. S. Salzmann, R. J. Roller, and P. M. Wassarman, unpublished results).

3. Lactate Dehydrogenase

Fully grown mouse oocytes exhibit very high levels of lactate dehydrogenase (LDH) activity, with virtually all of the activity attributable to the "heart-type" enzyme, LDH-H$_4$ (Auerbach and Brinster, 1968; Mangia and Epstein, 1975; Mangia *et al.*, 1976; Cascio and Wassarman, 1982). Electrophoretic comparisons of the LDH isozymes present in mouse heart, muscle, and kidney, with those present in growing and fully grown oocytes, demonstrate clearly that LDH-H$_4$ is the major isozyme present in mouse oocytes at all stages of growth (Fig. 12).

Use of an antiserum directed specifically against mouse LDH-H$_4$ (Spielmann *et al.*, 1974) to precipitate radiolabeled proteins, has permitted estimates of the relative rates of LDH synthesis (percentage of total protein synthesis) to be made during oocyte growth and meiotic maturation (Mangia *et al.*, 1976). These values range from about 3.8 to 5% during oocyte growth, and 0.75 to 1.6% following meiotic maturation. On the other hand, while recent experiments confirm that LDH

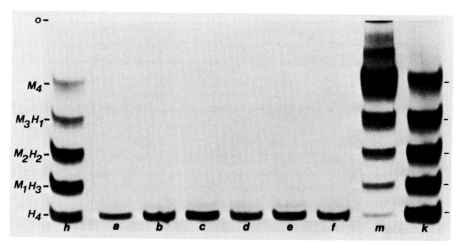

Fig. 12. An electrophoretic analysis of lactate dehydrogenase isozymes present in mouse tissues and growing oocytes. Shown are LDH isozyme patterns for growing oocytes 35, 45, 55, 61, and 77 μm in diameter (a–e, respectively); fully grown oocytes (f); heart (h); muscle (m); and kidney (k). The positions of pure muscle-type (M_4), heart-type (H_4), and three heteropolymers (M_3H_1, M_2H_2, M_1H_3) of LDH are indicated. o, Origin of gel. For details, see Cascio and Wassarman, 1982.

is, indeed, synthesized at a high rate during oocyte growth (Fig. 13), as a percentage of total protein synthesis it never exceeds 2% (Cascio and Wassarman, 1982). These experiments indicate that the absolute rate of LDH synthesis increases from 0.1 to 0.7 pg/hour per oocyte during oocyte growth (30–85 μm in diameter), and falls to about 0.1 pg/hour in unfertilized eggs. Using these data, one can estimate that the fully grown mouse oocyte contains more than 200 pg of LDH.

A comparison of levels of LDH in various mouse cell types (Nadal-Ginard, 1978) and in mouse oocytes (Table VII) indicates that, on a

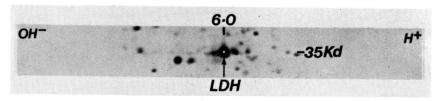

Fig. 13. A portion of a fluorogram of a high-resolution two-dimensional gel electrohoretic analysis of [35S]methionine-labeled proteins following culture of growing mouse oocytes for 16 hours *in vitro*. Shown is the region in which newly synthesized heart-type (H) LDH subunit (indicated by a white dot) is resolved at 35 kilodaltons. For details, see Cascio and Wassarman, 1982.

TABLE VII

Synthesis and Accumulation of Lactate Dehydrogenase in Mouse Cells

Cell type	Rate of LDH synthesis (molecules/cell per minute)	LDH content (molecules/cell)
Heart[a]	3.7×10^3	1.1×10^8
Muscle[a]	4.0×10^3	3.6×10^8
Liver[a]	4.4×10^3 (8.8×10^{12})[c]	3.9×10^7 (7.8×10^6)[c]
Kidney[a]	3.1×10^3	3.9×10^7
Fully grown oocyte[b]	4.8×10^4 (1.5×10^2)[c]	8.5×10^8 (2.7×10^6)[c]

[a] Calculated from the data of Nadal-Ginard, 1978.
[b] Calculated from the data of Cascio and Wassarman, 1982.
[c] Values in parentheses expressed on a per picoliter basis.

cellular basis, fully grown oocytes contain from 2 to 20 times more LDH than other cell types; on a volume (per picoliter) basis, however, oocytes contain less LDH (2.7×10^6 molecules/pl) than other cell types (e.g., liver; 7.8×10^6 molecules/pl). Similarly, while the overall rate of LDH synthesis is about 10 times higher in oocytes than in other mouse cells, on a volume (per picoliter) basis, LDH synthesis in oocytes (1.5×10^2 molecules/pl per minute) is significantly lower than in other cell types (e.g., liver; 8.8×10^2 molecules/pl per minute).

There is a significant decrease in the rate of LDH synthesis in unfertilized eggs (sevenfold) and one-cell embryos (20-fold), as compared to fully grown oocytes (Cascio and Wassarman, 1982). Results of recent experiments involving *in vitro* translation of oocyte, egg, and embryo RNA in a cell-free reticulocyte lysate system suggest that the decrease in rates of synthesis of LDH following meiotic maturation is attributable to decreased levels of LDH messenger RNA (Cascio and Wassarman, 1982, and unpublished results). It is not clear as yet whether or not the residual synthesis of LDH following meiotic maturation utilizes maternally inherited or newly transcribed LDH messenger RNA.

4. Histones

Histone synthesis has been studied extensively during early development of a variety of nonmammalian animal species (Davidson, 1977). Due to a very rapid rate of cell division, histones are required in relatively large amounts during early development in order to organize newly replicated DNA into nucleosomes. It has been shown that, in certain cases, this requirement is partially satisfied by the synthesis and storage of histones during oogenesis (Adamson and Woodland,

1974). For example, unfertilized *Xenopus* eggs contain a pool of histones sufficient to support early development to a late blastula stage consisting of about 20,000 cells (Woodland and Adamson, 1977). A significant portion of this pool is attributable to histones synthesized following conversion of oocytes to eggs (meiotic maturation), at which time the rate of histone synthesis increases about 20-fold such that it represents as much as 10% of total protein synthesis. It is probable that the increased rate of histone synthesis in unfertilized amphibian eggs is due to the mobilization of a large oogenetic store of histone messenger RNA, rather than to a change in the efficiency of translation (Adamson and Woodland, 1977).

Recently, the synthesis of histone H4, one of the four types of nucleosomal "core" histones (McGhee and Felsenfeld, 1980), has been examined in growing and fully grown mouse oocytes and unfertilized eggs (Wassarman and Mrozak, 1981). It was found that histone H4 is synthesized at all stages of oogenesis examined and accounts for about 0.07, 0.05, and 0.04% of total protein synthesis in growing oocytes ($\simeq$ 60 μm), fully grown oocytes, and unfertilized eggs, respectively; these values correspond to absolute rates of synthesis of 38.4 (growing oocyte), 42.8 (fully grown oocyte), and 26.4 (unfertilized egg) fg/hour per oocyte or egg. Therefore, as in amphibian oocytes, histone synthesis takes place in mammalian oocytes in the absence of cell division and DNA replication.

By assuming that the other nucleosomal "core" histones (H2A, H2B, and H3) are synthesized at the same rate as histone H4 during oogenesis in the mouse, a comparison can be made with measurements of histone synthesis during oogenesis in the amphibian (Adamson and Woodland, 1974, 1977; Shih *et al.*, 1980). Accordingly, histone synthesis in mouse and *Xenopus* oocytes represents about the same percentage of total protein synthesis, from 0.2 to 0.3% and from 0.3 to 1.0%, respectively. However, since there is about a 1000-fold difference in the absolute rates of total protein synthesis in mouse and amphibian oocytes (Smith, 1975; Schultz *et al.*, 1978a), only about 60 pg of histone is made in mouse oocytes, as compared to 140 ng in the amphibian. Since the nucleus of a mouse somatic cell contains about 6 pg of chromosomal DNA, and chromatin contains equal masses of DNA and histone, it can be estimated that only enough histone is synthesized during oogenesis in the mouse to support the first few cleavage divisions. This differs considerably from the situation in the amphibian, where it is estimated that the unfertilized egg contains a pool of histone sufficient to support early development to a late blastula stage consisting of about 20,000 cells (Woodland and Adamson, 1977). Finally, also unlike the situation in amphibians where histone synthesis increases 20-fold during meiotic maturation (Adamson and Woodland, 1977), the rate of histone synthesis actually declines during maturation of mouse oocytes; histone synthesis in unfertilized mouse eggs takes place at about one-half the rate measured in fully grown oocytes. Results of recent experiments indicate that histone synthesis continues during early embryogenesis in the mouse, at a rate that is of the order of that required for nuclear replication (Kaye and Wales, 1981).

5. Ribosomal Proteins

Eukaryotic ribosomes (80 S) contain a total of at least 70 unique proteins, 30 as part of the small ribosomal subunit (40 S) and 40 associated with the large subunit (60 S). It has been estimated that most, if not all, of these proteins are present in ribosomes in equimolar amounts. In general, it has been found that the synthesis of preribosomal RNA (45 S) is not dependent upon concomitant ribosomal protein synthesis and, similarly, that the synthesis of ribosomal proteins is independent of ribosomal RNA synthesis (Nomura et al., 1974; Wool, 1979; Chambliss et al., 1980).

In the amphibian Xenopus laevis, as much as 30% of a growing oocyte's total protein synthesis can be accounted for as ribosomal protein synthesis during midoogenesis (Hallberg and Smith, 1975) when ribosomal RNA synthesis has reached a maximum rate. Although fully grown Xenopus oocytes continue to synthesize ribosomal RNA at substantial rates, only about 1% of total protein synthesis in these oocytes is devoted to ribosomal proteins. Therefore, as a result of continuous synthesis throughout oogenesis, it can be estimated that the fully grown amphibian oocyte, just prior to ovulation, contains about 4 μg of ribosomal protein, accounting for 16% or more of the total non-yolk protein of the oocyte (Hallberg and Smith, 1975).

Ribosomal protein synthesis has been assessed during oogenesis in the mouse by determination of the absolute rates of synthesis of 12 different ribosomal proteins (11 associated with the 60 S and one with the 40 S subunits; molecular weights from 20,500 to 56,000) in growing and fully grown mouse oocytes and unfertilized eggs (LaMarca and Wassarman, 1979). The rates of synthesis of these 12 proteins in growing oocytes (50–60 μm in diamter) represent from 0.005 to 0.054% of the rate of total protein synthesis; these values correspond to absolute rates of synthesis from 1.4 to 15.4 fg/hour per oocyte (0.5 to 4.4 × 10^{-19} moles/hour per oocyte). These proteins are also synthesized at different rates in fully grown oocytes with their synthesis accounting for 0.04 to 0.71% of the rate of total protein synthesis; these values correspond to absolute rates of synthesis from 1.6 to 30.4 fg/hour per oocyte (0.6 to 8.7 $\times 10^{-19}$ moles/hour per oocyte). Furthermore, despite the termination of ribosomal RNA synthesis, each of the 12 ribosomal proteins continues to be synthesized in unfertilized mouse eggs; however, in nearly every case at a reduced rate (from 0.7 to 16.2 fg/hour per egg or 0.3 to 4.9 $\times 10^{-19}$ moles/hour per egg) as compared to fully grown oocytes.

At least three conclusions can be drawn from the results just described. (1) The synthesis of ribosomal proteins takes place throughout the period of oocyte growth, as well as during meiotic maturation. (2) The synthesis of different ribosomal proteins in growing and fully grown oocytes and in unfertilized eggs is not under tight coordinate control, even though the proteins are present in ribosomes in equimolar amounts. (3) Although the different ribosomal proteins are synthesized at greater rates in fully grown than in growing oocytes, in both cases their synthesis represents about 0.25% of the rate of total protein synthesis (0.19% in unfertilized eggs).

Since eukaryotic ribosomes contain 70 unique proteins, it can be estimated (assuming that the 12 ribosomal proteins examined above are representative of the total complement) that synthesis of ribosomal proteins accounts for about 1.5% of total protein synthesis during oocyte growth and 1.1% in unfertilized eggs. Since there is negligible turnover of newly synthesized protein during oocyte growth, it can also be estimated that fully grown mouse oocytes, just prior to ovulation, contain about 0.2 ng of ribosomal proteins as compared to the 4 μg in *Xenopus* oocytes. When one considers that fully grown *Xenopus* oocytes are about 4000 times larger (volume) than mouse oocytes, the concentrations of ribosomal proteins in oocytes of the two species are actually quite similar (within a factor of 5); this conclusion is consistent with estimates made of the concentrations of ribosomal RNA in *Xenopus* and mouse oocytes. It should be noted that ribosomal proteins continue to be synthesized during early embryogenesis in the mouse and that there is about an 11-fold increase in the rate of synthesis of ribosomal proteins between the 1- and 8-cell stages of development (LaMarca and Wassarman, 1979), when the rate of ribosomal RNA synthesis and ribosome content increase markedly (Clegg and Pikó, 1977; Pikó and Clegg, 1982).

6. Mitochondrial Proteins

The eggs of a variety of animal species contain a large store of mitochondria. For example, unfertilized eggs of amphibians and mice contain approximately 10^8 and 10^5 mitochondrial DNA molecules, respectively (Chase and Dawid, 1972; Pikó and Matsumoto, 1976). Furthermore, several lines of evidence indicate that mitochondrial DNA replication either does not occur at all or takes place at a very low level during early embryogenesis (Pikó, 1970; Dawid, 1972; Chase and Dawid, 1972; Matsumoto *et al.*, 1974; Renaldi *et al.*, 1979). This, as well as other evidence, strongly suggests that the store of mitochondria present in unfertilized eggs is distributed among and utilized by the blastomeres of early embryos. The results of experiments carried out with *Neurospora* and amphibians indicate further that mitochondria are derived solely from the female gamete and, therefore, represent an example of extrachromosomal inheritance (Preer, 1971; Dawid and Blackler, 1972).

The number of mitochondria found in the mouse oocyte's cytoplasm increases significantly during oocyte growth (Tables I and III). In addition, extensive changes in mitochondrial morphology occur as mouse oocytes grow (Table I and Fig. 2). While elongated mitochondria with transverse cristae are present during early stages of growth, small, round mitochondria with concentrically arranged cristae predominate during the middle and late stages of growth (Wischnitzer, 1967; Wassarman and Josefowicz, 1978). Consequently, the morphology of mitochondria in fully grown mouse oocytes and unfertilized eggs is radically different from that of mitochondria in nongrowing oocytes. There is a gradual return to elongated mitochondria during early embryogenesis in the mouse, presumably the result of transformation of preexisting round mitochondria (Hillman and Tasca, 1969; Calarco and Brown, 1969; Stern *et al.*, 1971; Pikó and Chase, 1973).

It is known that mitochondrial DNA codes for mitochondrial rRNA, mitochondrial tRNAs, and several mitochondrial inner membrane proteins (Schatz and Mason, 1974; Tzagoloff *et al.*, 1979). When various cell types (including HeLa, yeast, *Neurospora,* and BHK cells) are radiolabeled with amino acids in the presence of inhibitors of cytoplasmic protein synthesis (e.g., cycloheximide or emetine), a number of prominent bands are seen in autoradiograms of gels of detergent-solubilized mitochondria. These bands appear to correspond to the three largest subunits of cytochrome c oxidase, one of the subunits of coenzyme Q-cytochrome c reductase, from two–four of the subunits of the oligomycin-sensitive ATPase, and, perhaps, a polypeptide associated with mitochondrial ribosomes (Schatz and Mason, 1974; Borst, 1977; O'Brien, 1977; Tzagolff *et al.*, 1979). Less than 15% of the protein mass of mitochondria is attributable to proteins encoded by the mitochondrial genome and from 1 to 2% of total protein synthesis is usually accounted for by mitochondrial protein synthesis.

In order to determine whether or not proteins encoded by the mitochondrial genome are synthesized during oocyte growth in the mouse, a period during which mitochondria undergo extensive morphological alterations (see discussion above), one- and two-dimensional gel electrophoretic patterns of proteins radiolabeled with [^{35}S]Met in the presence or absence of emetine and/or chloramphenicol have been examined (Cascio and Wassarman, 1981). While emetine is an inhibitor of cytoplasmic protein synthesis, chloramphenicol is an effective inhibitor of mitochondrial, but not cytoplasmic, protein synthesis. The results of these experiments demonstrate that, in the mouse, growing and fully grown oocytes, eight-cell compacted embryos, and follicle cells all synthesize proteins encoded by the mitochondrial genome. Five major radiolabeled bands, designated α, β, γ, δ, and ϵ, are routinely observed with oocytes, embryos, and follicle cells cultured in the presence of emetine alone, but not in the presence of both emetine and chloramphenicol; the molecular weights of these polypeptides correspond to those of mitochondrial proteins identified in a variety of other eukaryotic cells (Fig. 14). Furthermore, mitochondrial protein synthesis represents from 1 to 2% of total protein synthesis during oocyte growth, also in agreement with estimates made with various other eukaryotic cells (Hawley and Greenwalt, 1970; Brega and Baglioni, 1971; England and Attardi, 1974; Jeffreys and Craig, 1976), including mouse blastocysts (Pikó and Chase, 1973). These results suggest that the morphological transformations that mitochondria undergo during oocyte growth are not attributable to the turning on and off of mitochondrial gene expression during oocyte growth.

7. Zona Pellucida Glycoproteins

The zona pellucida is a relatively thick, translucent, acellular coat that surrounds the plasma membrane of fully grown mammalian oocytes and performs a variety of vital biological functions during early development. The zona pellucida is laid down during growth of the ovarian follicle, remains throughout preimplantation development, and is finally shed as the blastocyst readies for implantation. Several lines of evidence suggest that the zona pellucida possesses a receptor for sperm, that it acts as a barrier to sperm penetration after fertilization, and that its presence is necessary for early development *in vivo* (Austin and Short, 1972; Gwatkin, 1977; Jones, 1978). Numerous studies have been carried out in order to identify the cellular site(s) of origin of the zona pellucida and, based primarily upon morphological and autoradiographic observations, the growing oocyte itself and/or

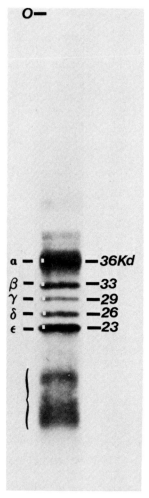

Fig. 14. A fluorogram of a one-dimensional gel electrophoretic analysis of [³⁵S]me-thionine-labeled proteins following culture of fully grown mouse oocytes for 12 hours *in vitro* in the presence of emetine. White dots indicate the positions of mitochondrial proteins α–ε, Low-molecular-weight material is indicated by a bracket. For details, see Cascio and Wassarman, 1981. o, Origin of gel.

follicle cells have been implicated as the site(s) of synthesis of the zona pellucida's components (e.g., Chiquoine, 1960; Kang, 1974; Haddad and Nagai, 1977).

Recently, it has been possible to identify the cellular site of synthesis of the zona pellucida in the mouse. The mouse oocyte's zona pellucida consists of three different glycoproteins, ZP1, ZP2, and ZP3, having apparent molecular weights of 200,000, 120,000, and 83,000, respectively; ZP2 apparently serves a structural role in the zona pellucida, whereas ZP3 acts as a sperm receptor and inducer of the acrosome reaction (Bleil and Wassarman, 1980a,b; Bleil *et al.*, 1981; Wassarman and Bleil, 1982; Wassarman, 1982). Characterization of zona pellucida components ZP1–3 has permitted studies of their synthesis in denuded (i.e., without surrounding follicle cells) and follicle-enclosed mouse oocytes at various stages of growth (Bleil and Wassarman, 1980c, Wassarman *et al.*, 1981; Wassarman and Bleil, 1982; Greve *et al.*, 1982; J. M. Greve, G. S. Salzmann, R. J. Roller, and P. M. Wassarman, unpublished results). Using either isolated oocytes or intact follicles cultured *in vitro,* about 1.5% of [^{35}S]Met and as much as 45% of [^{3}H]fucose incorporated into protein is found associated with the zonae pellucidae. Electrophoretic analyses of the radiolabeled proteins present in oocytes, zonae pellucidae, and follicle cells reveal that denuded oocytes synthesize and secrete all three zona pellucida glycoproteins; no evidence has been obtained to suggest that follicle cells synthesize these glycoproteins. Denuded oocytes ranging in diameter from about 40 to 70 μm incorporate both [^{35}S]Met and [^{3}H]fucose into zona pellucida glycoproteins (ZP1–3) during culture *in vitro,* whereas zonae pellucidae removed from fully grown oocytes (80–85 μm) are radiolabeled to a much lesser extent (Fig. 15). In fact, more than 90% of the [^{3}H]fucose incorporated into oocyte glycoproteins is found in ZP1–3, suggesting that zona pellucida glycoproteins are the major class of proteins glycosylated during oocyte growth. These and other results (Bousquet *et al.*, 1981) provide strong biochemical evidence supporting the idea that the zona pellucida components originate from the growing oocyte itself, rather than from the surrounding follicle cells. Estimates of the rates of synthesis of zona pellucida glycoproteins in growing mouse oocytes indicate that more than 10% of the oocyte's total protein synthesis is represented by ZP1–3; this is probably a conservative estimate and more accurate measurements will undoubtedly result in a significantly higher value.

D. Epilogue

Protein accumulates in mouse oocytes throughout their growth phase, resulting ultimately in about 25 ng of protein (exclusive of the zona pellucida) per fully grown oocyte. It is now clear that the overall rate of protein synthesis increases substantially ($\simeq$ 40-fold) during growth of mouse oocytes, while the overall spectrum of polypeptides synthesized remains fairly constant. On the other hand, it is possible

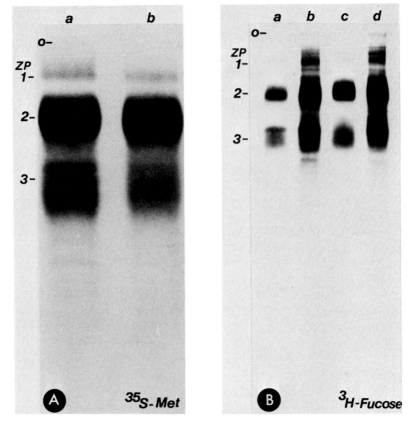

Fig. 15. Fluorograms of one-dimensional gel electrophoretic analyses of [35S]methionine (A) and [3H]fucose (B) labeled zonae pellucidae following culture of growing mouse oocytes for 12 hours *in vitro*. (A) Solubilized zonae pellucidae from denuded oocytes 58 (a) and 68 (b) μm in diameter. (B) solubilized zonae pellucidae from denuded (a) and follicle-enclosed (c) growing oocytes, and the corresponding zona pellucida-free oocytes (b and d). For details, see Bleil and Wassarman (1980c) and Wassarman and Bleil (1982). o, Origin of gel.

that some of the oocyte's protein store may not be synthesized by the growing oocyte itself, but may be taken up by endocytosis in a manner analogous to yolk accumulation by oocytes from a number of nonmammalian animal species. Degradation of a "yolklike" component during early embryogenesis could account for the dramatic decrease in protein content and the rise in amino acid pool sizes during this period of development.

Biochemical analyses of the synthesis of specific proteins during oocyte growth have revealed several examples of proteins that repre-

TABLE VIII

Synthesis of Specific Proteins during Oocyte Growth in the Mouse

Item	Total protein synthesis (%)
Tubulin (α and β)	$\simeq 1.5$
Actin (α, β, and γ)	$\simeq 1.0$
Lactate dehydrogenase (H_4)	$\simeq 1.5$
Histones (H2A, H2B, H3, and H4)	$\simeq 0.25$
Ribosomal proteins (70)	$\simeq 1.5$
Mitochondrial proteins	$\simeq 2$
Zona pellucida glycoproteins (ZP1–3)	>10

sent relatively high percentages of total protein synthesis during this period of development (Table VIII). From these data, it is clear that the fertilized mouse egg inherits large pools of tubulin, actin, and lactate dehydrogenase, as well as unusually large numbers of ribosomes and mitochondria, from the oocyte. Furthermore, during its growth phase the oocyte synthesizes and secretes the three glycoproteins that constitute the zona pellucida; one of these glycoproteins, ZP3, functions as a sperm receptor at fertilization.

Although the synthesis of tubulin and actin continues during the early cleavage stages, the mass of these proteins made during this period is relatively small compared to that contributed by the unfertilized egg; this is particularly apparent when synthesis is considered on a per cell, rather than on a per embryo, basis. For example, about 250 pg of tubulin is present in unfertilized eggs and, if partitioned equally, could result in about 30 pg per blastomere of the eight-cell embryo. On the other hand, during the period of development from the one- to eight-cell stage ($\simeq 60$ hours) only an additional 6 pg or so of newly synthesized tubulin would be added to the tubulin pool of each blastomere (i.e., $\simeq 20\%$ of the total); a similar case can be made for actin and, of course, for lactate dehydrogenase whose synthesis is barely detectable during early cleavage.

VI. SUMMARY

The process of oogenesis has traditionally been of great interest to scientists since, for more than a century, it has been recognized that the unfertilized egg contains a reserve of developmental potential upon which the progress of early embryogenesis depends (Wilson, 1925; Davidson, 1977). However, only within the past decade or so has research on mammalian development begun directly to address questions concerning the precise nature of the macromolecular reserves of unfertilized mammalian eggs. Consequently, the gap in our knowledge about oogenesis and early embryogenesis in mammals, as compared to nonmammalian animal species, has been significantly narrowed. It is likely that this trend will continue.

It should be clear from the experimental evidence presented here that, in the mammal, as in nonmammalian animal species, "embryogenesis really begins during oogenesis" (Wilson, 1925). The initiation of oocyte growth represents the setting into motion of a complex program designed to ensure the successful completion of meiosis, fertilization, cleavage divisions, and cellular differentiation. It is now clear that the one-cell mammalian embryo does, indeed, inherit a relatively extensive maternal reserve of macromolecules and organelles that, to varying degrees, supports the nutritional, synthetic, energetic, and regulatory requirements of the early embryo. The results of future research on mammalian oogenesis should provide us with new insight into the nature, establishment, and utilization of this maternal reserve.

ACKNOWLEDGMENTS

I am grateful to the National Institute of Child Health and Human Development, the National Science Foundation, and the Rockefeller Foundation for supporting the research carried out in our laboratory that is described here. My colleagues who have contributed to this research include Dr. Jeffrey Bleil, Ms. Stephanie Cascio, Dr. Jeffrey Greve, Ms. Wendy Josefowicz, Dr. Michael LaMarca, Ms. Gail Letourneau, Ms. Suzanne Mrozak, Mr. Richard Roller, Mr. George Salzmann, Dr. Richard Schultz, and Dr. Ralph Sorensen. Finally, I thank Dr. Melvin DePamphilis and the members of his laboratory for invaluable discussions of our research over the years on Wednesday mornings.

REFERENCES

Abreu, S. L., and Brinster, R. L. (1978). Synthesis of tubulin and actin during the preimplantation development of the mouse. *Exp. Cell Res.* **114,** 135–141.

Adamson, E. D., and Woodland, H. R. (1974). Histone synthesis in early amphibian development: Histone and DNA synthesis are not coordinated. *J. Mol. Biol.* **88,** 263–285.

Adamson, E. D., and Woodland, H. R. (1977). Changes in the rate of histone synthesis during oocyte maturation and very early development of *Xenopus laevis. Dev. Biol.* **57,** 136–149.

Anderson, D. M., and Smith, L. D. (1978). Patterns of synthesis and accumulation of heterogeneous RNA in lampbrush stage oocytes of *Xenopus laevis. Dev. Biol.* **67,** 274–285.

Anderson, E. (1972). The localization of acid phosphatase and the uptake of horseradish peroxidase in the oocytes and follicle cells of mammals. *In* "Oogenesis" (J. D. Biggers and A. W. Schuetz, eds.), pp. 87–117. Univ. Park Press, Baltimore, Maryland.

Anderson, E., and Albertini, D. F. (1976). Gap junctions between the oocyte and companion follicle cells in the mammalian ovary. *J. Cell Biol.* **71**, 680–686.

Auerbach, S., and Brinster, R. L. (1968). Lactate dehydrogenase isozymes in mouse blastocyst culture. *Exp. Cell Res.* **53**, 313–315.

Austin, C. R., and Short, R. V. (1972). "Reproduction in Mammals," Vol. 2. Cambridge Univ. Press, London and New York.

Bachvarova, R. (1974). Incorporation of tritiated adenosine into mouse ovum RNA. *Dev. Biol.* **10**, 52–58.

Bachvarova, R. (1981). Synthesis, turnover and stability of heterogeneous RNA in growing mouse oocytes. *Dev. Biol.* **86**, 384–392.

Bachvarova, R., and DeLeon, V. (1977). Stored and polysomal ribosomes of mouse ova. *Dev. Biol.* **58**, 248–254.

Bachvarova, R., and DeLeon, V. (1980). Polyadenylated RNA of mouse ova and loss of maternal RNA in early development. *Dev. Biol.* **74**, 1–8.

Bachvarova, R., DeLeon, V., and Spiegelman, I. (1981). Mouse egg ribosomes: Biochemical evidence for storage in lattices. *J. Embryol. Exp. Morphol.* **62**, 153–164.

Baran, M. M., and Bachvarova, R. (1977). *In vitro* culture of growing mouse oocytes. *J. Exp. Zool.* **202**, 283–289.

Bibring, T., and Baxandall, J. (1977). Tubulin synthesis in sea urchin embryos: Almost all tubulin of the first cleavage mitotic apparatus derives from the unfertilized egg. *Dev. Biol.* **55**, 191–195.

Bier, K. (1963). Synthese, interzellulärer Transport, und abbua von Ribonukleinsäure in Ovar der Stubenfliege *Musca domestica*. *J. Cell Biol.* **16**, 436–448.

Biggers, J. D., and Schuetz, A. W., eds. (1972). "Oogenesis." Univ. Park Press, Baltimore, Maryland.

Bleil, J. D., and Wassarman, P. M. (1980a). Mammalian sperm-egg interaction: Identification of a glycoprotein in mouse egg zonae pellucidae possessing receptor activity for sperm. *Cell* **20**, 873–882.

Bleil, J. D., and Wassarman, P. M. (1980b). Structure and function of the zona pellucida: Identification and characterization of the proteins of the mouse oocyte's zona pellucida. *Dev. Biol.* **76**, 185–202.

Bleil, J. D., and Wassarman, P. M. (1980c). Synthesis of zona pellucida proteins by denuded and follicle-enclosed mouse oocytes during culture *in vitro*. *Proc. Natl. Acad. Sci. U.S.A.* **77**, 1029–1033.

Bleil, J. D., Beall, C. F., and Wassarman, P. M. (1981). Mammalian sperm-egg interaction: Fertilization of mouse eggs triggers modification of the major zona pellucida glycoprotein, ZP2. *Dev. Biol.* **86**, 189–197.

Bloom, A. M., and Mukherjee, B. B. (1972). RNA synthesis in maturing mouse oocytes. *Exp. Cell Res.* **74**, 577–582.

Bonner, W. M., and Laskey, R. A. (1974). A film detection method for tritium labelled protein and nucleic acids in polyacrylamide gels. *Eur. J. Biochem.* **46**, 83–88.

Borst, P. (1977). Structure and function of mitochondrial DNA. *In* "International Cell Biology" (B. R. Brinkley and K. R. Porter, eds.), pp. 256–263. Rockefeller Univ. Press, New York.

Bousquet, D. Le'veillé, M. C., Roberts, K. D., Chapdelaine, A., and Bleau, G. (1981). *J. Exp. Zool.* **215**, 215–218.

Brega, A., and Baglioni, C. (1971). A study of mitochondrial protein synthesis in intact HeLa cells. *Eur. J. Biochem.* **22**, 415–422.

Brinster, R. L. (1967). Protein content of the mouse embryo during the first five days of development. *J. Reprod. Fertil.* **10**, 227–240.

Brinster, R. L., wiebold, J. L., and Brunner, S. (1976). Protein metabolism in pre-implanted mouse ova. *Dev. Biol.* **51**, 215–224.

Brower, P. T., and Schultz, R. M. (1982). Intercellular communication between granulosa cells and mouse oocytes: Existence and possible nutritional role during oocyte growth. *Dev. Biol.* **90**, 144–153.

Brower, P. T., Gizang, E., Boreen, S. M., and Schultz, R. M. (1981). Biochemical studies of mammalian oogenesis: Synthesis and stability of various classes of RNA during growth of the mouse oocyte *in vitro*. *Dev. Biol.* **86**, 373–383.

Burkholder, G. D., Comings, D. E., and Okada, T. A. (1971). A storage form of ribosomes in mouse oocytes. *Exp. Cell Res.* **69**, 361–371.

Calarco, P. G., and Brown, E. H. (1969). An ultrastructural and cytological study of preimplantation development of the mouse. *J. Exp. Zool.* **171**, 253–283.

Cascio, S. M., and Wassarman, P. M. (1981). Program of early development in the mammal: Synthesis of mitochondrial proteins during oogenesis and early embryogenesis in the mouse. *Dev. Biol.* **83**, 166–172.

Cascio, S. M., and Wassarman, P. M. (1982). Program of early development in the mammal: Post-transcriptional control of a class of proteins synthesized by mouse oocytes and early embryos. *Dev. Biol.* **89**, 397–408.

Chambliss, G., Craven, G. R., Davies, J., Davis, K., Kahan, L., and Nomura, M. (1980). "Ribosomes: Structure, Function, and Genetics." Univ. Park Press, Baltimore, Maryland.

Chase, J. W., and Dawid, I. B. (1972). Biogenesis of mitochondria during *Xenopus laevis* development. *Dev. Biol.* **27**, 504–518.

Chiquoine, A. D. (1960). The development of the zona pellucida of the mammalian ovum. *Am. J. Anat.* **106**, 149–170.

Chouinard, L. A. (1971). A light- and electron-microscope study of the nucleolus during growth of the oocyte in the prepubertal mouse. *J. Cell Sci.* **9**, 637–663.

Clarke, M., and Spudich, J. (1977). Non-muscle contractile proteins: The role of actin and myosin in cell motility and shape determination. *Annu. Rev. Biochem.* **46**, 497–822.

Clegg, K. B., and Pikó, L. (1977). Size and specific activity of the UTP pool and overall rates of RNA synthesis in early mouse embryos. *Dev. Biol.* **58**, 76–95.

Davidson, E. H. (1977). "Gene Activity in Early Development," 2nd ed. Academic Press, New York.

Dawid, I. B. (1972). Cytoplasmic DNA. *In* "Oogenesis" (J. D. Biggers and A. W. Schuetz, eds.), pp. 215–226. Univ. Park Press, Baltimore, Maryland.

Dawid, I. B., and Blackler, A. W. (1972). Maternal and cytoplasmic inheritance of mitochondrial DNA in *Xenopus*. *Dev. Biol.* **29**, 152–161.

Dolecki, G. J., and Smith, L. D. (1979). Poly(A)⁺ RNA metabolism during oogenesis in *Xenopus laevis*. *Dev. Biol.* **69**, 217–236.

Ecker, R. E. (1972). The regulation of protein synthesis in anucleate frog oocytes. *In* "Biology and Radiobiology of Anucleate Systems" (S. Bonotto, R. Goutier, R. Kirchmann, and J. R. Maisin, eds.), Vol. 1, pp. 165–179. Academic Press, New York.

England, J. M., and Attardi, G. (1974). Expression of the mitochondrial genome in HeLa cells. XXI. Mitochondrial protein synthesis during the cell cycle. *J. Mol. Biol.* **85**, 433–444.

Eppig, J. J. (1977a). Analysis of mouse oogenesis *in vitro:* Oocyte isolation and utilization of exogenous energy sources by growing oocytes. *J. Exp. Zool.* **198,** 375–382.

Eppig, J. J. (1977b). Mouse oocyte development *in vitro* with various culture systems. *Dev. Biol.* **60,** 371–388.

Eppig, J. J. (1979). A comparison between oocyte growth in coculture with granulosa cells and oocytes with granulosa cells-oocyte junctional contact maintained. *J. Exp. Zool.* **209,** 345–353.

Firtel, R. A. (1981). Multigene families encoding actin and tubulin. *Cell* **24,** 6–7.

Fulton, A. B. (1981). How do eukaryotic cells construct their cytoarchitecture? *Cell* **24,** 4–5.

Garcia, R. B., Pereyra-Alfonso, S., and Sotelo, J. R. (1979). Protein-synthesizing machinery in the growing oocyte of the cyclic mouse. *Differentiation* **14,** 101–106.

Gilula, N. B., Epstein, M. L., and Beers, W. H. (1978). Cell-to-cell communication and ovulation. A study of the cumulus-oocyte complex. *J. Cell Biol.* **78,** 58–75.

Glass, L. E. (1961). Localization of autologous and heterologous serum antigens in the mouse ovary. *Dev. Biol.* **3,** 797–804.

Glass, L. E. (1966). Serum antigen transfer in the mouse ovary: Dissimilar localization of bovine albumin and globin. *Fertil. Steril.* **17,** 226–233.

Glass, L. E., and Cons, J. M. (1968). Stage-dependent transfer of systematically injected foreign protein antigen and radiolabel into mouse ovarian follicles. *Anat. Rec.* **162,** 139–156.

Golbus, M. S., and Stein, M. P. (1976). Qualitative patterns of protein synthesis in mouse oocyte. *J. Exp. Zool.* **198,** 337–342.

Goldman, R., Pollard, T., and Rosenbaum, J. (1976). "Cell Motility." Cold Spring Harbor Lab., Cold Spring Harbor, New York.

Greve, J. M., Salzmann, G. S., Roller, R. J., and Wassarman, P. M. (1982). Biosynthesis of the major zona pellucida glycoprotein secreted by oocytes during mammalian oogenesis. *Cell* **31,** 749–759.

Gwatkin, R. B. L. (1977). "Fertilization Mechanisms in Man and Mammals." Plenum, New York.

Haddad, A., and Nagai, E. T. (1977). Radioautographic study of glycoprotein biosynthesis and renewal in the ovarian follicles of mice and the origin of the zona pellucida. *Cell Tissue Res.* **177,** 347–369.

Hallberg, R. L., and Smith, D. C. (1975). Ribosomal protein synthesis in *Xenopus laevis* oocytes. *Dev. Biol.* **42,** 40–52.

Hawley, E. S., and Greenwalt, J. W. (1970). An assessment of *in vivo* mitochondrial protein synthesis in *Neurospora crassa.* *J. Biol. Chem.* **245,** 3574–3583.

Heller, D. T., and Schultz, R. M. (1980). Ribonucleoside metabolism by mouse oocytes: Metabolic cooperativity between the fully-grown oocyte and cumulus cells. *J. Exp. Zool.* **214,** 355–364.

Heller, D. T., Cahill, D. M., and Schultz, R. M. (1981). Biochemical studies of mammalian oogenesis: Metabolic cooperativity between granulosa cells and growing mouse oocytes. *Dev. Biol.* **84,** 455–464.

Hill, R. S. (1979). A quantitative electron-microscope analysis of chromatin from *Xenopus laevis* lampbrush chromosomes. *J. Cell Sci.* **40,** 145–169.

Hillman, N., and Tasca, R. J. (1969). Ultrastructural and autoradiographic studies of mouse cleavage stages. *Am. J. Anat.* **126,** 151–174.

Inoue, S., and Stephens, R. E. (1975). "Molecules and Cell Movement." Raven Press, New York.

Jahn, C. L., Baran, M. M., and Bachvarova, R. (1976). Stability of RNA synthesized by the mouse oocyte during its major growth phase. *J. Exp. Zool.* **197,** 161–172.

Jeffreys, A. J., and Craig, I. W. (1976). Analysis of proteins synthesized in mitochondria of cultured mammalian cells. *Eur. J. Biochem.* **68**, 301–311.

Jones, R. E. (1978). "The Vertebrate Ovary." Plenum, New York.

Kang, Y. (1974). Development of the zona pellucida in the rat oocyte. *Am. J. Anat.* **139**, 535–566.

Kaye, P. L., and Wales, R. G. (1981). Histone synthesis in preimplantation mouse embryos. *J. Exp. Zool.* **216**, 453–459.

LaMarca, M. J., and Wassarman, P. M. (1979). Program of early development in the mammal: Changes in absolute rates of synthesis of ribosomal proteins during oogenesis and early embryogenesis in the mouse. *Dev. Biol.* **73**, 103–119.

Levey, I. L., Stull, G. B., and Brinster, R. L. (1978). Poly(A) and synthesis of polyadenylated RNA in the preimplantation mouse embryo. *Dev. Biol.* **64**, 140–148.

Lin, T. P. (1956). DL-Methionine (Sulphur-35) for labelling unfertilized mouse eggs in transplantation. *Nature (London)* **178**, 1175–1176.

Lowenstein, J. E., and Cohen, A. I. (1964). Dry mass, lipid content, and protein content of the intact and zona-free mouse ovum. *J. Embryol. Exp. Morphol.* **12**, 113–121.

Loyd, J. E., Raff, E. C., and Raff, R. A. (1981). Site and timing of synthesis of tubulin and other proteins during oogenesis in *Drosophila melanogaster*. *Dev. Biol.* **86**, 272–284.

McGhee, J. D., and Felsenfeld, G. (1980). Nucleosome structure. *Annu. Rev. Biochem.* **49**, 1115–1156.

Mangia, F., and Epstein, C. J. (1975). Biochemical studies of growing mouse oocytes: Preparation of oocytes and analysis of glucose-6-phosphate dehydrogenase and lactate dehydrogenase activities. *Dev. Biol.* **45**, 211–220.

Mangia, F., Erickson, R. P., and Epstein, C. J. (1976). Synthesis of LDH-1 during mammalian oogenesis and early development. *Dev. Biol.* **54**, 146–150.

Matsumoto, L., Kasamatsu, H., Pikó, L., and Vinograd, L. (1974). Mitochondrial DNA replication in sea urchin oocytes. *J. Cell Biol.* **63**, 146–159.

Miller, J. H., and Epel, D. (1973). Studies of oogenesis in *Urechis caupo*. II. Accumulation during oogenesis of carbohydrate, RNA, microtubule protein and soluble mitochondrial and lysosomal enzymes. *Dev. Biol.* **32**, 331–344.

Mitchison, J. M. (1971). "The Biology of the Cell Cycle." Cambridge Univ. Press, London and New York.

Moore, G. P. M., and Lintern-Moore, S. (1974). A correlation between growth and RNA synthesis in the mouse oocyte. *J. Reprod. Fertil.* **39**, 163–166.

Moore, G. P. M., and Lintern-Moore, S. (1978). Transcription of the mouse oocyte genome. *Biol. Reprod.* **17**, 865–870.

Moore, G. P. M., Lintern-Moore, S., Peters, H., and Faber, M. (1974). RNA synthesis in the mouse oocyte. *J. Cell Biol.* **60**, 416–422.

Moore, R. M., Smith, M. W., and Dawson, R. M. C. (1980). Measurement of intercellular coupling between oocytes and cumulus cells using intracellular markers. *Exp. Cell Res.* **126**, 15–29.

Nadal-Ginard, B. (1978). Regulation of lactate dehydrogenase levels in the mouse. *J. Biol. Chem.* **253**, 170–177.

Nomura, M., Tissières, A., and Lengyel, P. (1974). "Ribosomes." Cold Spring Harbor Lab., Cold Spring Harbor, New York.

Oakberg, E. F. (1967). ^{3}H-Uridine labeling of mouse oocytes. *Arch. Anat. Microsc. Morphol. Exp.* **56**, Suppl. 3–4, 171–184.

Oakberg, E. F. (1968). Relationship between stage of follicle development and RNA synthesis in the mouse oocyte. *Mutat. Res.* **6**, 155–165.

Oakley, B. R., Kirsch, D. R., and Morris, N. R. (1980). A simplified ultrasensitive silver stain for detecting proteins in polyacrylamide gels. *Anal. Biochem.* **105,** 361–363.

O'Brien, T. W. (1977). Transcription and translation in mitochondria. *In* "International Cell Biology" (B. R. Brinkley and K. R. Porter, eds.), pp. 245–255. Rockefeller Univ. Press, New York.

O'Farrell, P. H. (1975). High resolution two-dimensional electrophoresis of proteins. *J. Biol. Chem.* **250,** 4007–4021.

Olds, P. J., Stern, S., and Biggers, J. D. (1973). Chemical estimates of the RNA and DNA contents of the early mouse embryo. *J. Exp. Zool.* **186,** 39–46.

Palombi, F., and Viron, A. (1977). Nuclear cytochemistry of mouse oogenesis. I. Changes in extranucleolar ribonucleoprotein components through meiotic prophase. *J. Ultrastruct. Res.* **61,** 10–20.

Parkes, A. S., ed. (1956). "Marshall's Physiology of Reproduction," Vol. 1. Longmans, Green, New York.

Pederson, T. (1969). Follicle growth in the immature mouse ovary. *Acta Endocrinol. (Copenhagen)* **62,** 117–132.

Pederson, T. (1970). Follicle kinetics in the ovary of the cyclic mouse. *Acta Endocrinal. (Copenhagen)* **64,** 304–323.

Pestell, R. Q. W. (1975). Microtubule protein synthesis during oogenesis and early embryogenesis in *Xenopus laevis. Biochem. J.* **145,** 527–534.

Pikó, L. (1970). Synthesis of macromolecules in early mouse embryos cultured *in vitro:* RNA, DNA, and a polysaccharide component. *Dev. Biol.* **21,** 257–279.

Pikó, L., and Chase, D. G. (1973). Role of the mitochondrial genome during early development in mice: Effects of ethidium bromide and chloramphenicol. *J. Cell Biol.* **58,** 357–378.

Pikó, L., and Clegg, K. B. (1982). Quantitative changes in total RNA, total poly(A), and ribosomes in early mouse embryos. *Dev. Biol.* **89,** 362–378.

Pikó, L., and Matsumoto, L. (1976). Number of mitochondria and some properties of mitochondrial DNA in the mouse egg. *Dev. Biol.* **49,** 1–10.

Pollard, T. D. (1981). Cytoplasmic contractile proteins. *J. Cell Biol.* **91,** 156S–165S.

Pollard, T. D., and Weihing, R. R. (1974). Actin and myosin and cell movement. *CRC Crit. Rev. Biochem.* **2,** 1–65.

Preer, J. R. (1971). Extrachromosomal inheritance: Hereditary symbionts, mitochondria, and chloroplasts. *Annu. Rev. Genet.* **5,** 361–396.

Prescott, D. M. (1976). "Reproduction of Eukaryotic Cells." Academic Press, New York.

Raff, E. C. (1977). Microtubule proteins in axolotl eggs and developing embryos. *Dev. Biol.* **58,** 56–75.

Raff, R. A., Brandis, J. W., Green, L. H., Kaumeyer, J. D., and Raff, E. C. (1975). Microtubule protein pools in early development. *Ann. N.Y. Acad. Sci.* **253,** 304–317.

Rafferty, K. A. (1970). "Methods in Experimental Embryology of the Mouse." Johns Hopkins Press, Baltimore, Maryland.

Reiger, J. C., and Kafatos, F. C. (1971). Microtechnique for determining the specific activity of radioactive intracellular leucine and applications to *in vivo* studies of protein synthesis. *J. Biol. Chem.* **246,** 6480–6488.

Renaldi, A. M., DeLeo, G., Arzone, A., Salcher, I., Storace, A., and Mutolo, V. (1979). Biochemical and electron microscopic evidence that cell nucleus negatively controls mitochondrial genomic activity in early sea urchin development. *Proc. Natl. Acad. Sci. U.S.A.* **76,** 1916–1920.

Richter, J. D., and McGaughey, R. W. (1981). Patterns of polypeptide synthesis in mouse oocytes during germinal vesicle breakdown and during maintenance of the germinal vesicle stage by dibutyryl cyclic AMP. *Dev. Biol.* **83,** 188–192.

Rodman, T. C., and Bachvarova, R. (1976). RNA synthesis in preovulatory mouse oocytes. *J. Cell Biol.* **70,** 251–257.

Sawicki, J. A., Magnuson, T., and Epstein, C. J. (1981). Evidence for expression of the paternal genome in the two-cell mouse embryo. *Nature (London)* **294,** 450–451.

Schatz, G., and Mason, T. L. (1974). The biosynthesis of mitochondrial proteins. *Annu. Rev. Biochem.* **43,** 51–87.

Schlafke, S., and Enders, A. C. (1967). Cytological changes during cleavage and blastocyst formation in the rat. *J. Anat.* **102,** 13–32.

Schultz, R. M., and Wassarman, P. M. (1977a). Biochemical studies of mammalian oogenesis: Protein synthesis during oocyte growth and meiotic maturation in the mouse. *J. Cell Sci.* **24,** 167–194.

Schultz, R. M., and Wassarman, P. M. (1977b). Specific changes in the pattern of protein synthesis during meiotic maturation of mammalian oocytes *in vitro. Proc. Natl. Acad. Sci. U.S.A.* **74,** 538–541.

Schultz, R. M., and Wassarman, P. M. (1980). Efficient extraction and quantitative determination of nanogram amounts of cellular RNA. *Anal. Biochem.* **104,** 328–334.

Schultz, R. M., LaMarca, M. J., and Wassarman, P. M. (1978a). Absolute rates of protein synthesis during meiotic maturation of mammalian oocytes *in vitro. Proc. Natl. Acad. Sci. U.S.A.* **75,** 4160–4164.

Schultz, R. M., Letourneau, G. E., and Wassarman, P. M. (1978b). Meiotic maturation of mouse oocytes *in vitro:* Protein synthesis in nucleate and anucleate oocyte fragments. *J. Cell Sci.* **30,** 251–264.

Schultz, R. M., Letourneau, G. E., and Wassarman, P. M. (1979a). Program of early development in the mammal: Changes in patterns and absolute rates of tubulin and total protein synthesis during oogenesis and early embryogenesis in the mouse. *Dev. Biol.* **68,** 341–359.

Schultz, R. M., Letourneau, G. E., and Wassarman, P. M. (1979b). Program of early development in the mammal: Changes in the patterns and absolute rates of tubulin and total protein synthesis during oocyte growth in the mouse. *Dev. Biol.* **73,** 120–133.

Sellens, M. H., Stein, S., and Sherman, M. I. (1981). Protein and free amino acid content in preimplantation mouse embryos and in blastocysts under various culture conditions. *J. Reprod. Fertil.* **61,** 307–315.

Sherman, M. I. (1979). Developmental biochemistry of preimplantation mammalian embryos. *Annu. Rev. Biochem.* **48,** 443–470.

Shih, R. J., Smith, L. D., and Keem, K. (1980). Rates of histone synthesis during early development of *Rana pipiens. Dev. Biol.* **75,** 329–342.

Smith, L. D. (1975). Molecular events during oocyte maturation. *In* "Biochemistry of Animal Development" (R. Weber, ed.), Vol. 3, pp. 1–46. Academic Press, New York.

Sorensen, R., and Wassarman, P. M. (1976). Relationship between growth and meiotic maturation of the mouse oocyte. *Dev. Biol.* **50,** 531–536.

Spielmann, H., Erickson, R. P., and Epstein, C. J. (1974). The production of antibodies against mammalian LDH-1. *Anal. Biochem.* **59,** 462–467.

Stern, S., Biggers, J. D., and Anderson, E. (1971). Mitochondria and early development of the mouse. *J. Exp. Zool.* **176,** 179–192.

Sternlicht, A. L., and Schultz, R. M. (1981). Biochemical studies of mammalian oogenesis: Kinetics of accumulation of total and poly(A)-containing RNA during growth of the mouse oocyte. *J. Exp. Zool.* **215,** 191–200.

Sturgess, E. A., Ballantine, J. E. M., Woodland, H. R., Mohun, P. R., Lane, C. D., and Dimitriadis, G. J. (1980). Actin synthesis during the early development of *Xenopus laevis*. *J. Embryol. Exp. Morphol.* **58**, 303–320.

Szollosi, D. (1972). Changes in some cell organelles during oogenesis in mammals. In "Oogenesis" (J. D. Biggers and A. W. Schuetz, eds.), pp. 47–64. Univ. Park Press, Baltimore, Maryland.

Szybek, K. (1972). *In vitro* maturation of oocytes from sexually immature mice. *J. Endocrinol.* **54**, 527–58.

Telfer, W. H. (1960). The selective accumulation of blood proteins by the oocytes of saturniie moths. *Biol. Bull. (Woods Hole, Mass.)* **118**, 338–351.

Tzagoloff, A., Macino, G., and Sebald, W. (1979). Mitochondrial genes and translation products. *Annu. Rev. Biochem.* **48**, 419–441.

Van Blerkom, J., and Motta, P. (1979). "The Cellular Basis of Mammalian Reproduction." Urban & Schwarzenberg, Baltimore-Munich.

Van Blerkom, J., and Runner, M. N. (1976). The fine structural development of preimplantation mouse parthenotes. *J. Exp. Zool.* **196**, 113–123.

Wallace, R. A. (1972). The role of protein uptake in vertebrate oocyte growth and yolk formation. In "Oogenesis" (J. D. Biggers and A. W. Schuetz, eds.), pp. 339–359. Univ. Park Press, Baltimore, Maryland.

Wassarman, P. M. (1982). Fertilization. In "Cell Interactions and Development: Molecular Mechanisms" (K. Yamada, ed.), pp. 1–27. Wiley, New York.

Wassarman, P. M., and Bleil, J. D. (1982). The role of zona pellucida glycoproteins as regulators of sperm-egg interactions in the mouse. In "Cellular Recognition" (L. Glaser, W. Frazier, and D. Gottlieb, eds.). Alan R. Liss, Inc., New York (in press).

Wassarman, P. M., and Fujiwara, K. (1978). Immunofluorescent anti-tubuliun staining of spindles during meiotic maturation of mouse oocytes *in vitro*. *J. Cell Sci.* **29**, 171–188.

Wassarman, P. M., and Josefowicz, W. J. (1978). Oocyte development in the mouse: An ultrastructural comparison of oocytes isolated at various stages of growth and meiotic competence. *J. Morphol.* **156**, 209–236.

Wassarman, P. M., Josefowicz, W. J., and Letourneau, G. E. (1976). Meiotic maturation of mouse oocytes in vitro: Inhibition of maturation at specific stages of nuclear progression. *J. Cell Sci.* **22**, 531–541.

Wassarman, P. M., and Letourneau, G. E. (1976). RNA synthesis in fully-grown mouse oocytes. *Nature (London)* **261**, 73–74.

Wassarman, P. M., and Mrozak, S. C. (1981). Program of early development in the mammal: Synthesis and intracellular migration of histone H4 during oogenesis in the mouse. *Dev. Biol.* **84**, 364–371.

Wassarman, P. M., Schultz, R. M., Letourneau, G. E., LaMarca, M. J., and Bleil, J. D. (1979). Meiotic maturation of mouse oocytes *in vitro*. In "Ovarian Follicular and Corpus Luteum Function" (C. P. Channing, J. Marsh, and W. D. Sadler, eds.), pp. 251–268. Plenum, New York.

Wassarman, P. M., Bleil, J. D., Cascio, S. M., LaMarca, M. J., Letourneau, G. E., Mrozak, S. C., and Schultz, R. M. (1981). Programming of gene expression during mammalian oogenesis. In "Bioregulators of Reproduction" (G. Jagiello and H. J. Vogel, eds.), pp. 119–150. Academic Press, New York.

Weakley, B. S. (1968). Comparison of cytoplasmic lamellae and membranous elements in the oocytes of five mammalian species. *Z. Zellforsch. Mikrosk. Anat.* **85**, 109–123.

Wilson, E. B. (1925). "The Cell in Development and Heredity." Macmillan, New York.

Wischnitzer, S. (1967). Intramitochondrial transformations during oocyte maturation in the mouse. *J. Morphol.* **121**, 29–46.

Wolgemuth, D. J., Jagiello, G. M., and Henderson, A. S. (1979). Quantitation of riboso-
    mal genes in fetal human oocyte nuclei using rRNA:DNA hybridization *in situ*.
    Exp. Cell Res. **118,** 181–190.
Wolgemuth, D. J., Jagiello, G. M., and Henderson, A. S. (1980). Baboon late diplotene
    oocytes contain micronuclei and a low level of extra rRNA templates. *Dev. Biol.* **78,**
    598–604.
Woodland, H. R., and Adamson, E. D. (1977). The synthesis and storage of histones
    during the oogenesis of *Xenopus laevis. Dev. Biol.* **57,** 118–135.
Wool, I. G. (1979). The structure and function of eukaryotic ribosomes. *Annu. Rev.
    Biochem.* **48,** 719–754.
Zamboni, L. (1970). Ultrastructure of mammalian oocytes and ova. *Biol. Reprod., Suppl.*
    2, 44–63.
Zuckerman, S., ed. (1962). "The Ovary," Vol. 1. Academic Press, New York.
Zuckerman, S., and Weir, B. J., eds. (1977). "The Ovary," 2nd ed., Vol. 1. Academic
    Press, New York.

2

The Mammalian Spermatozoon: Structure and Temporal Assembly

ANTHONY R. BELLVÉ AND DEBORAH A. O'BRIEN

Mechanism and Control of Animal Fertilization
Copyright © 1983 by Academic Press, Inc.
All rights of reproduction in any form reserved.
ISBN 0-12-328520-8

I. INTRODUCTION

The spermatozoon, an intricate and highly polarized cell, has evolved structurally and functionally to ensure efficient transmission of the paternal genome to the oocyte at fertilization. To facilitate this transfer of DNA, primordial germ cells undergo extensive growth and differentiation. Progenitor cells proliferate to provide adequate numbers of sperm at the site of fertilization. Synaptonemal complexes assemble between pairing homologous chromosomes to enable recombination of DNA sequences and hence promote genetic diversity. The nucleus transforms to condense and protect its unique, haploid assortment of genes. Motility is acquired by each cell following formation of the tail with its complement of mitochondria. An acrosome forming over the apical pole of the nucleus is packaged with a variety of hydrolytic enzymes that later allow the sperm to penetrate the investments of the egg. These various structures of the sperm cell are assembled during meiosis, spermiogenesis, and epididymal maturation, their biogenesis involving an precise temporal integration of transcriptional and translational events (for reviews, see Bellvé, 1979, 1982).

II. MOLECULAR ORGANIZATION OF MAMMALIAN SPERMATOZOA

Mammalian sperm are topographically organized into distinct head and tail segments (Fig. 1). The head consists of the condensed nucleus and the overlying acrosome, both of which are required to transmit the haploid genome at fertilization. The tail, containing the axoneme, mitochondria, and structural elements, is responsible for the cell's motility.

A. Molecular Structure of the Sperm Head

Mammalian sperm nuclei are more condensed and elongated than those of somatic cells and have shapes that are characteristic for each species. The chromatin generally is uniform in density but may contain occasional small clear areas (Fawcett, 1975a). The human sperm nucleus, an exception, frequently contains larger clear spaces, often termed nuclear vacuoles even though they are not membrane-limited (Bedford et al., 1973). This species also exhibits regional differences in the degree of chromatin condensation (Zamboni et al., 1971; Bedford et al., 1973).

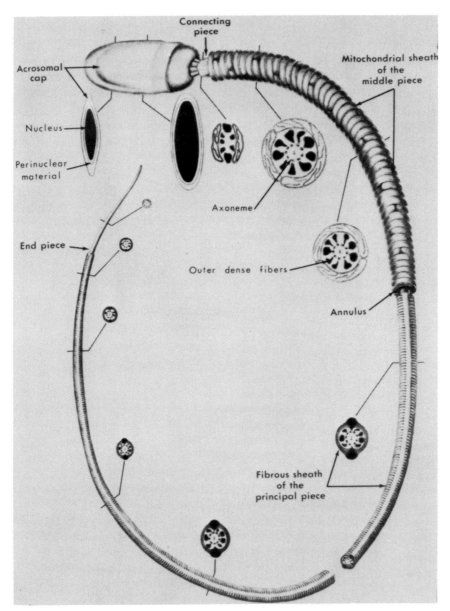

Fig. 1. Schematic diagram of the mammalian spermatozoon depicting the principal elements of this polarized cell. The dense chromatin is surrounded and protected by the nuclear envelope and perinuclear theca. Capping the anterior pole of the nucleus is the acrosome with its constituent enzymes. The prominent tail contains the centrally located axoneme with its associated outer dense fibers. Mitochondria form a double helical gyre around the midpiece, while the fibrous sheath envelops the principal piece of the tail. (Reproduced from Bloom and Fawcett, 1975, by permission of the publisher, W. B. Saunders Company.)

The arrangement of chromatin within sperm nuclei has not been defined adequately. Chromatin in the sperm nucleus of the domestic fowl appears to be oriented randomly (Walker, 1971). In many invertebrates the chromosomes may be organized with their DNA fibers oriented parallel to the long axis of the sperm, although they may be secondarily coiled (Inoué and Sato, 1962; Mello and Vidal, 1973). Likewise, mammalian sperm have highly ordered chromatin. Freeze-fracture studies of sperm from several mammalian species reveal chromatin fibers arranged in a stacked lamellar pattern (Koehler, 1966, 1970; Fléchon, 1974; Friend and Fawcett, 1974) that is consistent with the platelike substructure observed in bull sperm by form birefringence (Bendet and Bearden, 1972). Several physical parameters suggest the DNA molecules of stallion sperm also occur in highly ordered structures that are aligned in parallel planes (Sipski and Wagner, 1977). By contrast, human and mouse sperm may be exceptions among the mammals, since morphological evidence indicates their nucleoprotein is packed in a fibrogranular pattern (Koehler, 1972; Bellvé, 1982).

The dense conformation of the mature sperm nucleus obviates meaningful morphological studies on the nature of chromatin structure *in situ*. Consequently, most investigators have utilized sulfhydryl reducing agents, proteases, and/or chemical denaturants to disperse the chromatin for observation. The chromatin of both human and bull sperm, on exposure to alkaline thioglycolate and critical point drying, exhibits an irregular network of fibers with diameters ranging from 14 to 24 nm (Lung, 1968, 1972). These fibers may be dispersed further by treatment with dithiothreitol (DTT) and Sarkosyl, an ionic detergent, to yield a mesh of 2 to 3 nm fibrils interconnecting larger spherical and cordlike bodies (Evenson *et al.*, 1978). The 2–3 nm fibrils could represent naked DNA strands. However, these denaturing conditions may not reveal chromatin in its "native" configuration, particularly since protamines are precipitated by reagents such as SDS and Sarkosyl.

Recent efforts have focused on using DTT and $Ca^{2+} \cdot Mg^{2+}$ (3:2 molar ratio) as a nondenaturing protocol for dispersing the nucleoprotein (Bellvé, 1982). When used in combination, these two divalent cations preferentially displace protamine from the mouse sperm nucleus in a concentration-dependent manner (Hirtzer and Bellvé, 1979). These nuclei, when examined by phase-contrast microscopy, appear to retain their regular size and shape, even though the displaced protamines comprise more than 90% of total nuclear protein. However, after exposure to ethidium bromide, a DNA-intercalating fluorochrome, the protamine-depleted nuclei exhibit a clearly defined halo of DNA fibers (Bellvé, 1982). The nuclear structure consists of intermeshed bundles of coarse chromatin fibers with a branching network of finer fibrils (Fig. 2). A meshwork of these finer fibrils also penetrates perforations in the distended perinuclear theca to form the enveloping halo of DNA. Significantly, the structure of the nuclear material is comparable to that of condensing chromatin in spermatids (cf. Loir and Courtens, 1979). There is no indication of the large, spherical "chromatin bodies" that are seen following treatment of human (Evenson *et al.*, 1978) and

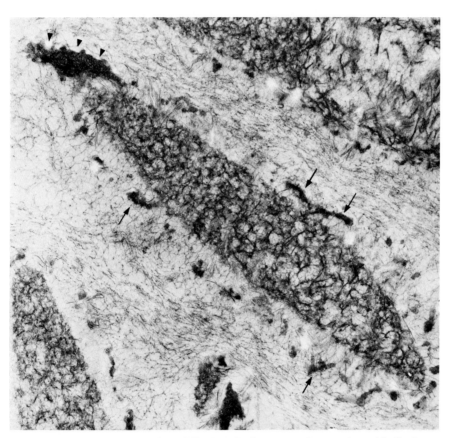

Fig. 2. Mouse sperm nucleus following displacement of protamine with divalent cations. Nuclei were incubated with DTT and PMSF for 30 minutes and then exposed to 250 mM Ca^{2+} · Mg^{2+} (3:2 molar ratio). This protocol is effective in displacing the type-2 protamine. It also partially disperses the dense chromatin to reveal coarse fibro-granular structures interconnected by a meshwork of finer, branching fibrils. A similar fibrillar network appears to spill through perforations in the perinuclear material to form a cloud of DNA surrounding the nucleus. Arrow heads, perforatorium; arrows, perinuclear theca (×32,000).

mouse sperm nuclei with Sarkosyl. The latter bodies may reflect an artifactual aggregation of the nucleoprotamine polymers. Since the progressive displacement of protamines by the divalent cations appears to generate native structures, this protocol may be valuable for elucidating the role of protamines in the condensation of chromatin.

The extreme condensation and unusual shapes of sperm nuclei have been attributed to the presence of unique chromosomal proteins. In many vertebrate and invertebrate species, somatic histones are replaced during spermatogenesis by protamines or by unique species of histones (for review, see Bellvé, 1979). Protamines, first identified and characterized in fish by Miescher (1878) and Kossel (1928), now have been isolated from the sperm of several mammals (Coelingh et al., 1972; Kistler et al., 1973, 1976; Monfoort et al., 1973; Bellvé et al., 1975; Kolk and Samuel, 1975; Calvin, 1976a; Balhorn et al., 1977). These proteins are smaller and more basic than histones and have distinct primary structures. Although not phylogenetically conserved, the various mammalian protamines contain some common structural determinants. Partial sequence analyses of protamine from the bull (Coelingh et al., 1972), the stallion, boar, and ram (Monfoort et al., 1973), the rat (Kistler et al., 1976) and the human (Kolk and Samuel, 1975; Gaastra et al., 1978) suggest the immediate amino-terminal region may be quite invariant. As for the fish protamines, the number and position of the arginyl domains may be another common feature of mammalian protamines. But, since no eutherian protamine other than the bull protein has yet been sequenced in entirety, this would be a premature conclusion. Moreover, while most mammalian sperm contain only a single protamine species, mouse (Bellvé et al., 1975; Balhorn et al., 1977) and human sperm nuclei (Kolk and Samuel, 1975) each contain two distinct arginine-rich protamines: a typical type 1 protamine and the predominant type 2 protamine that has a high histidine content (Kolk and Samuel, 1975; Bellvé and Carraway, 1978; Bellvé, 1979). Thus, any model of protamine–DNA interactions must allow for the possibility of the type 2 protamines having very unique primary structures.

The interaction of protamines with DNA has been examined with a variety of physical, biochemical, and morphological techniques. Studies of nonmammalian sperm nuclei and reconstituted DNA-protamine complexes suggest protamines stabilize DNA in a modified β^* conformation that resists structural transitions (Feughelman et al., 1955; Suau and Subirana, 1977; Warrant and Kim, 1978). Furthermore, arginine-rich protamines from several aquatic species are equally effective in stabilizing DNA (Suau and Subirana, 1977). Based on these data, several models of nucleoprotamine organization have been proposed.

One model depicts protamine in an extended form, winding along the minor groove of the DNA double helix, with successive arginyl groups interacting alternately with the phosphate groups of the two DNA strands (Feughelman *et al.*, 1955; Suau and Subirana, 1977). In the case of mammalian protamines the more conserved amino-terminal extension may fold back and interact with an inner domain of the peptide as depicted in Balhorn's (1982) elegant model (Fig. 3A). The variable carboxyl-terminal region containing several cysteinyl and tyrosinyl groups (Monfoort *et al.*, 1973) could interact with another protamine molecule overlapping in the same minor groove (Fig. 3B and 4A). The close alignment of cysteinyl groups probably facilitates formation of the intermolecular disulfide bonds that are prevalent in mammalian sperm chromatin. Alternatively, the carboxyl-terminus, which also frequently contains several arginyl groups (Monfoort *et al.*, 1973), may interact with an adjacent DNA double helix to ensure close, parallel packaging of the chromatin strands. Covalent disulfide linkages presumably must occur between protamine molecules existing on apposed DNA helices to render the chromatin resistant to dispersion by high salt, urea, and guanidine hydrochloride.

While this model allows for an orderly condensation of sperm chromatin, it is not compatible with all of the available evidence. Studies using laser Raman spectroscopy (Mansy *et al.*, 1976) provide evidence which suggests that these proteins are located in the major groove of the double helix. Kinetic analysis of DNA methylation also indicates that the interaction of protamine with DNA perferentially shields ($\sim$ 15%) the N-7 of guanine in the major groove from methylation, rather than the N-3 of adenine in the minor groove (Mirzabekov *et al.*, 1977). According to one interpretation, this observation is inconsistent with protamine binding within the minor groove of the DNA double helix. However, the reduced accessibility of this guanine group to the methylating agent simply may reflect its interaction with a protamine molecule located in the minor groove of an adjacent and closely interlocking DNA strand (Fig. 4B). Thus, the data can be interpreted to favor protamine binding in either the minor or the major groove.

A second model, proposed by Warrant and Kim (1978), suggests protamine exists in an α-helical configuration, forming a segmented cylinder that could occupy either the major or the minor groove of the DNA double helix. Bull protamine may contain two α-helical domains, one extending from amino acids 13 to 28 and the other from positions 31 to 36, with the intervening -Phe-Gly- sequence providing a flexible

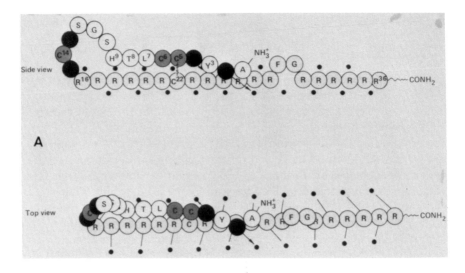

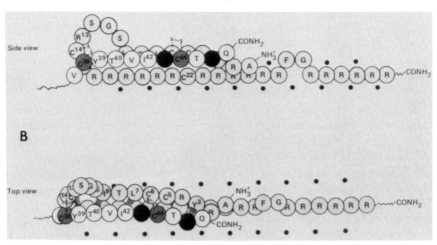

Fig. 3. A model depicting the interaction of bull protamine with DNA. (A) The N-terminal sequence of the type-1 protamine is shown with the three arginyl domains (R) in the minor groove, interacting (bars) with the phosphate groups (small solid circles) along a single turn in the DNA double helix. The N-terminal segment may be turned back on the molecule, thereby allowing a covalent disulfide bond to form between cysteinyl groups 5 and 22. (B) The cysteine at position 14 may form a disulfide bond with cysteine 38 in the overlapping C-terminus of an adjacent protamine molecule. Likewise, a third disulfide bridge may form between cysteine 6 of the N-terminal region with cysteine 44 in the C-terminal region of the overlapping protamine. This C-terminal segment of the adjacent molecule may be aligned initially by intermolecular hydrogen and hydrophobic bonds (parallel bars). The disulfide interaction would lock overlapping protamine molecules around the DNA. Amino acid nomenclature: A, alanine; C, cysteine; F, phenylalanine; G, glycine; H, histidine; I, isoleucine; L, leucine; Q, glutamine; R, arginine; S, serine; T, threonine; V, valine; Y, tyrosine. (Reproduced from Balhorn, 1982, by permission of the editor, *Journal of Cell Biology*).

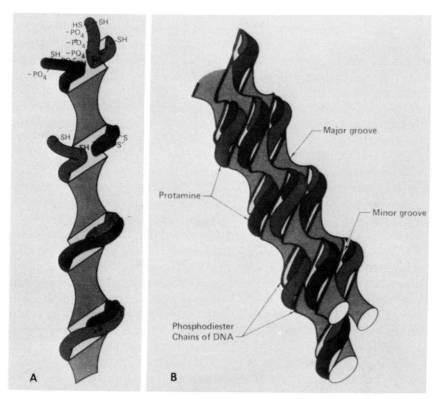

Fig. 4. Schematic presentations of overlapping protamine molecules interacting with DNA in the minor groove (A), and the parallel packing of nucleoprotamine polymers (B). (A) Phosphorylated protamine binds to the DNA with the arginyl domain completing a single turn around the double helix. Following dephosphorylation of the serine and threonine groups, the N-terminal segment may fold back to form cystinyl cross-links. Similarly, this N-terminal sequence may form disulfide bonds with the cysteinyl groups located in the C-terminal sequence of an overlapping protamine molecule (cf. Fig. 3B). (B) The nucleoprotamine complexes, with the phosphodiester backbone completely neutralized, now align with the protamine protruding from the minor groove of one DNA strand fitting into the major groove of a parallel strand. This interaction may be stabilized by hydrogen bonding of the C-terminal arginyl groups inside the major groove. Alternatively, the flexible phenylalanyl-glycyl joint at positions 29 and 30 may allow the third arginyl domain to interact with the minor groove of an adjacent DNA strand. This could allow the formation of intermolecular disulfide bonds to lock adjacent DNA strands together, thereby rendering the chromatin resistant to dissociation by guanidine hydrochloride in the absence of DTT. (Reproduced from Balhorn, 1982, by permission of the editor, *Journal of Cell Biology*).

joint. This mode of interaction also could enable the protamine molecule to interact across adjacent DNA double helices, thus facilitating an orderly condensation and covalent crosslinking of chromatin strands. Alternatively, the two α-helical domains may lie completely within the major groove of the same DNA double helix and the amino- and carboxyl-termini effect the interstrand cross links. This model, based on X-ray diffraction and circular dichroism studies of protamine–tRNA complexes, is attractive but may not be applicable to DNA-protamine interactions (Bradbury *et al.*, 1962). In the shorter α-helical form, the total protamine length may be sufficient to bind only half the total length of the haploid DNA.

These two models suggest that smooth branching chromatin fibers probably are formed by the parallel packing of nucleoprotamine strands, with the protruding backbone of the protamine molecule fitting into the major groove of an adjacent DNA double helix (Fig. 4B) (Suau and Subirana, 1977; Bode and Leseman, 1977; Kierszenbaum and Tres, 1978; Balhorn, 1982). This concept of nucleoprotamine conformation is not compatible with the existence of nucleosomes in sperm chromatin. Yet, several morphological studies report observing nucleosomelike structures (12–15 nm) in the chromatin of dogfish, bull, man (Gusse and Chevaillier, 1980), and ram sperm (Tsanev and Avramova, 1981). In this regard, it is interesting to note that protease digestion of sperm chromatin from several mammalian species produces distinct limit fragments of the protamines (Marushige and Marushige, 1974; Zirkin *et al.*, 1980). These proteolytic products are reminiscent of the polypeptides remaining after enzymatic hydrolysis of somatic nucleosomes. In this case the accessible amino-terminal regions of histones 2A, 2B, 3, and 4 are digested, while the greater portion of each protein is protected by the tertiary structure of the nucleosome (Weintraub, 1975). The principal question, of course, is whether the enzyme cleavage sites along the primary sequence of the respective protamines can be used to distinguish between the hypothetical models of protamine–DNA interactions. Cross-linking studies using bifunctional reagents also may yield valuable information on protamine–protamine interactions. Such studies are needed to clarify current concepts of nucleoprotamine organization in mammalian sperm.

The nonprotamine chromosomal proteins (NPCPs) of sperm nuclei are limited in quantity and number. Early research on fish sperm nuclei identified a class of tryptophan-rich, nonbasic proteins that comprise 15 to 40% of sperm dry weight (Stedman and Stedman, 1947; for review, see Mann, 1964). Mammalian sperm NPCPs have either been undetected (Platz *et al.*, 1975; Balhorn *et al.*, 1977) or detected only in low quantities and in limited complexity (Bellvé *et al.*, 1975; Kolk and Samuel, 1975; O'Brien and Bellvé, 1980a). These proteins may include structural components of the sperm nucleus, such as residual histones (Kolk and Samuel, 1975; Puwaravutipanich and Panyim, 1975; Pongsawasdi and Svasti, 1976; O'Brien and Bellvé, 1980a) and constituents of the perinuclear theca (O'Brien and Bellvé, 1980a; Bellvé, 1982). They also may include the enzymes DNA polymerase (Philippe and Chevaillier, 1976; Witkin *et al.*, 1977), RNA polymerase (Fuster *et al.*, 1977) and a possible chromatin-bound protease (Marushige and Marushige, 1975).

The nuclear envelope of mammalian sperm, which surrounds and is applied closely to the dense chromatin, has several unusual structural features. It consists of two membranes spaced 7 to 10 nm apart (Fawcett, 1975a), each having distinct patterns of intramembranous particles (Stackpole and Devorkin, 1974). Near the caudal pole of the sperm head, the nuclear membranes and the plasma membrane fuse to form the posterior ring (Friend and Fawcett, 1974), which apparently acts as a seal to separate the head and tail compartments (Koehler, 1970, 1972). Below the posterior ring, the nuclear envelope assumes a more typical appearance as the two membranes, now separated by 40 to 60 nm, extend into the neck region away from the condensed chromatin (Wooding and O'Donnell, 1971; Zamboni *et al.*, 1971; Fawcett, 1975a). This latter area of "redundant envelope" contains nuclear pores (Koehler, 1970, 1972; Pedersen, 1972a; Friend and Fawcett, 1974) arranged in a close, hexagonal pattern (Pedersen, 1972a; Phillips, 1975a; Mortimer and Thompson, 1976; Friend, 1982). It has not yet been determined whether this region of redundant nuclear envelope is functional in mature sperm (Wooding and O'Donnell, 1971; Zamboni *et al.*, 1971) or simply reflects the marked reduction in nuclear volume that occurs during spermiogenesis (Fawcett, 1965).

The implantation fossa, the attachment site of the tail, lies in a recess at the base of the nucleus. In this region nuclear pores again are absent (Friend and Fawcett, 1974) and the two membranes of the nuclear envelope are apposed closely (6–7 nm) (Pedersen, 1972a). Regular periodic densities traverse this narrow cleft, perhaps serving to reinforce the nuclear envelope in the region adjacent to the motile tail (Pedersen, 1972b; Stackpole and Devorkin, 1974).

B. Structure and Function of the Perinuclear Theca

The perinuclear theca lies in the subacrosomal space closely apposed to the nucleus. It consists of two distinct structures, the perinuclear material (PNM) and the postacrosomal dense lamina (PDL). The PNM forms an amorphous layer covering almost the entire nucleus (Jones, 1971; Courtens *et al.*, 1976). The PDL envelops only the caudal pole of the nucleus and appears to be structurally contiguous with the subjacent PNM (Lalli and Clermont, 1981). Both of these structures are resistant to detergent extraction, but can be solubilized in the presence of disulfide reducing agents (Koehler, 1973; Bedford and Calvin, 1974b).

In most mammalian species the PNM usually forms a thin envelope covering the entire nucleus above the posterior ring. More pronounced thickenings occur in the apical region of the nucleus and at the equatorial segment's anterior border (Nicander and Bane, 1966; Bernstein and Teichman, 1972; Courtens *et al.*, 1976). In rodent sperm the PNM forms the perforatorium, a prominent pyrimidal structure attached to the anterior tip of the nucleus (Clermont *et al.*, 1955; Austin and Bishop, 1958a). This rigid apical structure formerly was thought to play either a mechanical (Yanagimachi and Noda, 1970a) or an enzymatic (Austin and Bishop, 1958b) role in fertilization.

The PDL, enveloping the caudal region of the nucleus, immediately underlies and runs parallel to the plasmalemma at a distance of 15 to 20 nm until terminating at the posterior ring (Fawcett, 1975a). The PDL has received considerable attention, since it lies immediately subjacent to the region of sperm membrane that first fuses with the egg (Pikó, 1969; Stefanini *et al.*, 1969; Yanagimachi and Noda, 1970a,b; Lalli and Clermont, 1981). Two distinct regions can be discerned in the dense lamina of the bull (Koehler, 1966), rabbit (Koehler, 1970), and human (Koehler, 1972; Pedersen, 1972a,b). In the anterior region regular periodic densities, 12 nm apart, extend from the PDL toward the overlying plasma membrane (Wooding and O'Donnell, 1971; Zamboni *et al.*, 1971; Pedersen, 1972a,b). These densities are oriented circumferentially in man but longitudinally in the Macaca monkey and perhaps the bull (Pedersen, 1972a). Surface replicas of membrane-free rodent sperm suggest that these periodic structures represent evenly spaced ridges on the PDL (Phillips, 1975a). In several species the posterior region of the dense lamina is characterized by basal striations, obliquely oriented cords terminating at the posterior ring (Koehler, 1966, 1970, 1972; Pedersen, 1972a,b). The function of these structures presently is unknown.

The perinuclear theca can be isolated as an integral element of the sperm nuclear matrix. Exposure of mouse sperm nuclei to ~ 200 mM $Ca^{2+} \cdot Mg^{2+}$ (3:2 ratio), DTT, and DNase I (~ 100 µg/ml) displaces protamine and hydrolyzes the DNA (Hirtzer and Bellvé, 1979). This protocol leaves a nuclear component that conforms to the original size and shape of the sperm nucleus (Fig. 5). In some respects the structure resembles the nuclear matrix of somatic cells, which consists of the pore-lamina complex, an internal fibrous matrix, remnant nucleoli, and interchromatinic material (Berezny, 1979; Shaper et al., 1979; Agutter and Richardson, 1980; Franke et al., 1981). The sperm nuclear matrix, which may provide structural integrity to the nucleus, consists of a clearly defined perinuclear theca and an internal network of fibrous material. However, it differs in many other respects. First, the perinuclear theca component of the nuclear matrix is located external rather than immediately internal to the nuclear envelope. Second, annular pores are absent; presumably those pores localized in the redundant region of the nuclear envelope are removed during the isolation procedure. Third, there is no evidence of remnant nucleolar structures. Finally, the sperm nuclear matrix comprises a diverse population of polypeptides with M_r's ranging from ~8,000 to 80,000, with major bands evident at 25,000, 16,500, 15,000, and 13,000 daltons (Bellvé, 1982). The triplet of acidic proteins, M_r's 65,000–75,000, that are prominent constituents of the somatic nuclear matrix (Franke et al., 1981) are not detected among the proteins of the sperm perinuclear theca.

The distinct structural features of the sperm perinuclear theca suggest that it may serve unusual functions. However, there only is limited information available concerning the identity and function of the thecal constituents. Cytochemical studies indicate that the PDL has an affinity for silver (Krimer and Esponda, 1978) and phosphotungstic acid (Nicander and Bane, 1966), suggesting it is composed of basic proteins. Similar observations indicate that the PNM may contain lysine-rich proteins (Courtens et al., 1976). The perforatorium isolated from rat sperm reportedly consists of a single cysteine-rich protein of M_r ~13,000 (Olson et al., 1976b), suggesting that the native structure is highly polymerized and stabilized by intermolecular covalent bonds. It is not known whether this protein also is located in the PNM posterior to the perforatorium. Acid phosphatase activity (Teichman and Bernstein, 1971) and possibly choline plasmalogen (Teichman et al., 1972, 1974) have been detected in the postacrosomal perinuclear region of several mammalian species.

Significantly, several studies have detected actin in the postacrosomal region by using antibody probes, heavy meromyosin (Campanella et al., 1979; Baccetti et al., 1980), and DNase I binding (Tamblyn, 1980). Ultrastructural studies suggest that this actin, and perhaps myosin, is localized primarily in the perinuclear theca (Baccetti et al., 1980). These observations must be considered with caution, however,

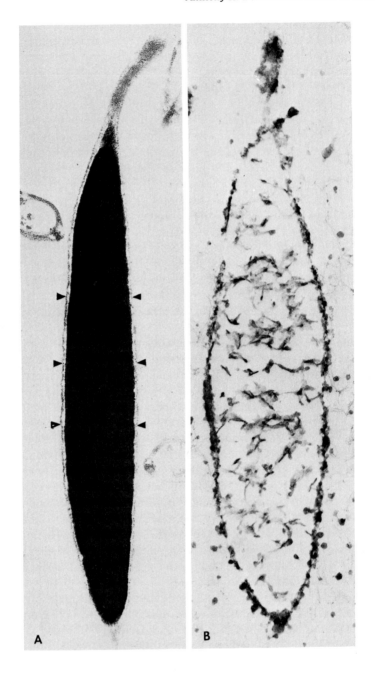

since they have not been confirmed by biochemical investigations (Franke *et al.*, 1978; Strauch *et al.*, 1980). The existence of actin in this postacrosomal region would have considerable implications. Actin filaments enveloping and traversing the nucleus could promote changes in nuclear shape during spermiogenesis, determine the directional vector of sperm motility, and facilitate sperm penetration at fertilization. Thus, the question of whether actin is present in the perinuclear theca is of fundamental importance to the elucidation of sperm function.

C. The Acrosome and Its Constituent Enzymes

The acrosome, varying considerably in size and shape among species, is a membrane-delimited structure capping the anterior pole of the sperm nucleus (Fawcett, 1958; Fawcett and Phillips, 1969a). In most mammals the acrosome is a continuous organelle, although in rats and mice there is a small, separate vesicle located adjacent to the ventral surface of the perforatorium (Pikó, 1969; Lalli and Clermont, 1981).

The acrosome plays an active role in fertilization. Following Swyer's (1947) demonstration of hyaluronidase in sperm, it was suggested that this enzyme may be sequestered in the acrosome and released at fertilization to disperse the hyaluronic acid matrix of the cumulus cells enveloping the oocyte (Schrader and Leuchtenberger, 1951). This hypothesis was supported by Austin and Bishop (1958b) who noted the acrosome being lost from sperm just prior to fertilization. This "acrosome reaction" is an exocytotic process in which the outer acrosomal membrane and plasmalemma fuse to form numerous small vesicles (Bedford, 1968, 1972; Franklin *et al.*, 1970; Yanagimachi and Noda, 1970a). The inner acrosomal membrane and the equatorial segment of the acrosome persist during this vesiculation process. While some hyaluronidase remains associated with the dispersed vesicles, most of the enzyme can be recovered in soluble form from the surrounding

---

Fig. 5. Electron micrograph of a mouse sperm nucleus and its associated perinuclear theca and matrix. (A) Nuclei are prepared by a brief exposure of spermatozoa to 1% SDS, followed by sucrose density gradient centrifugation (Bellvé *et al.*, 1975). This protocol decapitates the sperm and removes the acrosome and nuclear envelope from the nucleus. The perinuclear theca (arrow heads) remains closely associated with the dense nucleus. (B) When these nuclei are exposed to 50 mM DTT, $\sim$ 190 mM Ca^{2+} · Mg^{2+} (3:2 molar ratio), and 100 μg DNase/ml, the protamines and DNA are removed. This protocol leaves the perinuclear theca and a coarse network of internal fibers relatively intact. This matrix structure approximates the conformation and size of the original nucleus.

milieu (Primakoff *et al.*, 1980a) and therefore would be available for dissociating the cumulus oophorous and corona radiata.

A variety of other hydrolytic enzymes have been identified as acrosomal constituents (McRorie and Williams, 1974). These include acid phosphatase, arylsulfatase, β-*N*-acetylglucosaminidase, phospholipase A, and protease activities (Srivastava *et al.*, 1965; Stambaugh and Buckley, 1970; Allison and Hartree, 1970). The localization of hyaluronidase and a specific protease in the acrosome has been confirmed with immunohistochemical techniques (Gould and Bernstein, 1975; Morton, 1975; Garner and Easton, 1977; Allison and Hartree, 1970). These findings, plus similar staining characteristics and a common Golgi origin, led Allison and Hartree (1970) to suggest that the acrosome is a "specialized" lysosome. This contention should be considered with caution, however. The acrosome reaction has an obligatory requirement for Ca^{2+}, is stimulated by an influx of K^+, and appears to need an active Na^+, K^+-ATPase (Mrsny and Meizel, 1981). These features are similar to those of secretory exocytosis, suggesting that the acrosome may be a specialized zymogen granule (Friend, 1977). Furthermore, the acrosome has characteristics distinguishing it from typical lysosomes. For instance, alkaline phosphatases (Gordon *et al.*, 1978) and proteases with widely divergent pH optima (Yanagimachi and Teichman, 1972; Zaneveld *et al.*, 1972a; Bernstein and Teichman, 1973) have been identified in the acrosome. Also, the acid phosphatase originally ascribed to the acrosome may be localized primarily in the subacrosomal and postacrosomal regions of rabbit and bull sperm (Teichman and Bernstein, 1971). However, Gonzales and Meizel (1973) have identified multiple forms of acid phosphatase in rabbit sperm, two of which may be acrosomal.

Hyaluronidase isolated from testis or spermatozoa is an isoenzymic form distinct from lysosomal hyaluronidase (Zaneveld *et al.*, 1973; Yang and Srivastava, 1974). This enzyme has not been characterized completely, but appears to have four subunits (Khorlin *et al.*, 1973) and a low pH optimum (Yang and Srivastava, 1974). Acrosin, another acrosomal constituent, is a unique serine protease of mammalian sperm (Polakoski and Parrish, 1977; Tobias and Schumacher, 1977; Brown and Harrison, 1978; Mukerji and Meizel, 1979). Although interspecific differences do occur, the various acrosins share similar properties (for review, see McRorie and Williams, 1974; Stambaugh, 1978; Meizel, 1978). Like trypsin, acrosin shows optimal activity at pH 8 and can hydrolyze synthetic trypsin substrates (Stambaugh and Buckley, 1969). Yet this enzyme has properties distinguishing it from trypsin, including a higher M_r and unique substrate and inhibitor specificities (Zaneveld *et al.*, 1971, 1972a; Polakoski *et al.*, 1972). Acrosin exists within the acrosome as an inactive zymogen precursor, proacrosin (Meizel, 1972; Mukerji and Meizel, 1975; Polakoski and Parrish, 1977; Tobias and Schumacher, 1977; Brown and Harrison, 1978; Mukerji and Meizel, 1979), which may be inactivated and stabilized by local concentrations of specific inhibitors (Zaneveld *et al.*, 1972b; Fink *et al.*, 1973; Brown and Hartree, 1975; Goodpasture *et al.*, 1980). The enzyme may occur in multiple, enzymatically active forms, some of which could be membrane-bound (for review, see Parrish and Polakoski, 1979). Although it has been postulated that acrosin enables sperm to penetrate the zona pellucida (Stambaugh and Buckley, 1969), the supporting evidence is not conclusive (cf. Hartree, 1977; Shams-Borhan *et al.*, 1979).

A variety of additional enzymes detected in mammalian sperm may be localized within the acrosome. Several of these have proteolytic activity including arylaminidase (Meizel and Cotham, 1972), acrolysin (McRorie *et al.*, 1976), collagenase-like peptidase (Koren and Milković, 1973), and a cathepsin D-like protease (Erickson and Martin, 1974). Other potential acrosomal enzymes include neuraminidase (Srivastava *et al.*, 1970), arylsulfatase (Seiguer and Castro, 1972), and nonspecific esterases (Bryan and Unnithan, 1972). Interestingly, the overlying plasma membrane and/or outer acrosomal membrane of hamster sperm probably contains a Mg^{2+}-ATPase porton pump for maintenance of the acidic pH of the acrosome (Working and Meizel, 1981, 1982).

Acrosomal enzymes may be packaged in an organized pattern, particularly in the guinea pig and chinchilla (Fawcett and Hollenberg, 1963; Fawcett and Phillips, 1969a). Periodic structures including crystalline arrays (Friend and Fawcett, 1974; Fléchon, 1975) and parallel striations (Phillips, 1972a) occur in discrete regions. The delimiting membranes of the acrosome also contain unusual particles tightly packed in paracrystalline arrangements (Koehler, 1972; Friend and Fawcett, 1974; Stackpole and Devorkin, 1974; Phillips, 1975a). Furthermore, these particles vary in size and are distributed in different regions of the acrosomal membranes (Plattner, 1971; Stackpole and Devorkin, 1974; Phillips, 1977a). Cytochemical studies suggest a specific alkaline phosphatase is localized within the outer acrosomal membrane (Gordon *et al.*, 1978). While some acrosomal enzymes, such as hyaluronidase, are easily removed, others require more rigorous extraction procedures. On this basis acrosin (Brown and Hartree, 1974;

Srivastava *et al.*, 1974) and neuraminidase (Srivastava and Abou-Issa, 1977) appear to integral constituents of the inner acrosomal membrane of the equatorial region (cf. Shams-Borhan *et al.*, 1979).

D. Organization of the Sperm Tail

The mammalian sperm tail has four discrete segments: the neck, midpiece, principal piece, and end piece (Fig. 1). The neck is a short, morphologically complex region located immediately posterior to the sperm head. Extending further distally is the thicker midpiece, which is characterized by the helically arranged mitochondria surrounding the axoneme and outer dense fibers. This segment terminates at the annulus, a dense ring-shaped structure that is fused to the plasma membrane. The principal piece, the longest segment of the sperm tail, also contains the axoneme and outer dense fibers. In this segment, however, the mitochondrial helix is replaced by the fibrous sheath (Fig. 1). The most distal segment, the end piece, contains less-developed regions of fibrous sheath and the axoneme, in which the typical orientation of the microtubules is altered (Phillips, 1975b).

1. The Neck Region

The basal plate lines the implantation fossa and joins the nucleus to the flagellar neck. This dense attachment structure stains heavily with phosphotungstic acid, indicative of basic proteins (Nicander and Bane, 1962). Between the basal plate and remaining neck structures is a narrow clear zone, traversed by thin filaments which appear to attach the basal plate to the connecting piece.

Ultrastructural studies of the neck region have led to some controversy concerning the morphology of the connecting piece (Fawcett and Phillips, 1969b; Zamboni and Stefanini, 1971). At the distal end of the neck, the connecting piece is composed of nine segmented or striated columns. These columns are oriented longitudinally and are composed of alternating dense and light bands. High resolution micrographs of these columns reveal a regular periodicity similar to that seen in ciliary rootlets and other centriole-related structures (Fawcett and Phillips, 1969b; Phillips, 1975b). Fawcett and Phillips (1969b) suggest that these structures stabilize the base of the motility apparatus. In several rodent species, including the mouse, the segmented columns gradually merge and connect with the proximal articular region of the connecting piece, the capitulum (Fawcett and Phillips, 1969b). In contrast, Zamboni and Stefanini (1971) did not observe an anterior fusion of the segmented columns in mature spermatozoa of the rabbit, man, and monkey, and suggest that the capitulum disappears during spermiogenesis. Perhaps the differences noted in these two studies reflect species variations.

Other structures within the neck region include the redundant portion of the nuclear envelope, one or two mitochondria projecting anteriorly from the midpiece, the initial segments of the outer dense fibers, and the anterior extension of the axonemal central pair microtubules (Fawcett, 1975a). In the distal region of the neck, the nine segmented columns are each attached firmly to the anterior end of an outer dense fiber (Fawcett and Phillips, 1969a,b; Phillips, 1975b; Zamboni and Stefanini, 1971). The central pair of microtubules extends from the axoneme proper through the central cavity of the connecting piece to the surface of the proximal centriole (Fawcett and Phillips, 1969b; Zamboni and Stefanini, 1971). In most mammalian species the proximal centriole, oriented between 45° and 90° to the flagellar axis, persists in mature sperm (Nicander and Bane, 1962; Fawcett, 1965; Illisson, 1966; Zamboni and Stefanini, 1971; Pedersen, 1972b). This structure may be functional only during earlier stages of tail differentiation, however, since it has not been observed in motile rat sperm (Woolley and Fawcett, 1973).

Biochemical information on the neck region is scant. The basal plate and connecting piece can be solubilized with detergent only in the presence of DTT (Bedford and Calvin, 1974a; Bellvé et al., 1975), suggesting that both structures are stabilized by intermolecular disulfide bonds.

2. Axonemal Elements

The axoneme is responsible for sperm motility. Like cilia and flagella of all species (Fawcett and Porter, 1954), the sperm axoneme has a typical 9 + 2 radial symmetry with nine peripherally arranged doublet microtubules, each possessing two arms, and two central microtubules with a surrounding sheath (Fawcett, 1975a; Amos et al., 1976; Baccetti and Afzelius, 1976; Linck et al., 1981). The peripheral doublets are interconnected by nexin bridges and are joined to the central sheath by nine spokes or radial links. Each peripheral doublet is composed of a circular A tubule attached to a larger C-shaped B tubule. Tubule A is composed of 13 parallel protofilaments, while either 10 or 11 similar protofilaments form subfiber B. Each A tubule has two projections or arms which extend toward the B tubule of the next peripheral doublet. Other interconnections between the microtubules also arise from the A tubule, including the nexin bridges and the radial links. The C_1 and C_2 central microtubules, each of which is circular in cross section and is composed of 13 protofilaments, also are connected by bridges. The central sheath, often interpreted as a helically wound filament, is composed of paired rows of projections which are attached to each of the central tubules. Olson and Linck (1977) have confirmed that structural elements of rat sperm axonemes exhibit polarities and spatial periodicities typical of simpler cilia and flagella. These investigators also have described barb-shaped structures attached to the C_2 central tubule that may interact with the radial links.

The axonemal microtubules are primarily composed of α- and β-tubulin, two proteins having distinct amino acid compositions and M_rs of ~56,000 and 54,500 daltons, respectively (Stephens, 1970a; Fine, 1971; Bryan and Wilson, 1971). Microheterogeneity within these two subclasses can be observed following isoelectric focusing and high resolution SDS-polyacrylamide gel electrophoresis (Feit et al., 1971; Witman et al., 1972). Based on peptide mapping and sequencing data, Luduena and Woodward (1973) have demonstrated that α- and β-tubulins are both phylogenetically conserved. Although the molecular organization of the tubulins within the axonemal microtubules has not been completely resolved, Stephens (1974) has proposed a model for microtubule substructure. In this model tubulin heterodimers, each composed of one α- and one β-subunit, are arranged vertically in each protofilament with a head-to-tail association, while heterodimers in adjacent protofilaments are staggered to form a helical array (see also Linck and Langevin, 1981; Linck et al., 1981).

Dynein, a class of flagellar ATPases, is involved in the generation of axonemal movement. This protein, first isolated by Gibbons and Rowe (1965), exists in multiple components with M_r's $\geq 300,000$ (Linck, 1973; Gibbons et al., 1976; Gibbons, 1981). Dynein is specific for ATP and requires divalent cations for enzymatic activity (Gibbons, 1966; Ogawa and Mohri, 1972). The major flagellar ATPase, dynein 1, can exist in multiple forms (Gibbons et al., 1976; Gibbons, 1981) and is localized primarily in the outer arms projecting from the A tubule of the peripheral doublets (Ogawa et al., 1977, 1982).

Other proteins of isolated axonemes have been characterized by SDS polyacrylamide gel electrophoresis. The most prominent of these is nexin, M_r 165,000, a protein localized in the nexin bridges (Stephens, 1970b). More recent studies using two-dimensional polyacrylamide gel electrophoresis have identified > 100 polypeptides present in the axonemal structures of Chlamydomonas (Piperno et al., 1977; Adams et al., 1981; Huang et al., 1982; Brokaw et al., 1982). Mutants expressing a variety of motility dysfunctions are proving invaluable for dissection of the structure-function relationships of flagellar components. Although comparable genetic studies are not feasible in mammals, a considerable amount of information could be obtained by utilization of monoclonal antibody probes against specific flagellar constituents in conjunction with biochemical and morphological techniques.

The concept of flagellar motion being generated by the differential sliding of the peripheral doublets is accepted generally (Afzelius, 1959). This sliding microtubule model is supported by Satir (1965, 1968) who first demonstrated the fixed length of the respective doublets and their relative displacement during ciliary motion. It since has been confirmed more definitively by the observation that addition of ATP to trypsin-treated axonemes promotes active sliding between the peripheral doublets, as demonstrated with sea urchin (Summers and Gibbons, 1971) and bull sperm (Summers, 1974; Lindemann and Gibbons, 1975). This sliding motion apparently is promoted by the dynein arms, which form transient cross bridges between adjacent microtubule doublets (Gibbons et al., 1976). The mechanisms responsible for converting the interdoublet sliding into flagellar bending has not been well defined, although interactions between the radial spokes and the sheath of the central pair have been implicated (Warner, 1976; Olson and Linck, 1977). Recent studies of suppressor mutations in *Chlamydomonas* lacking functional radial spoke heads demonstrate that these structures may be responsible for converting the symmetric flagellar beat into an efficient asymmetric beat (Brokaw et al., 1982). Presumably, the radial spoke system, perhaps in concert with the outer dense fibers, also may modulate flagellar beat in mammalian sperm.

3. Flagella Accessory Structures

Mammalian sperm tails have elaborate structural elements (Fig. 1). These include the basal plate, connecting piece, outer dense fibers, outer mitochondrial membranes, and the fibrous sheath. These structures can be isolated as an integral unit following exposure of mouse sperm to 1% SDS (Bellvé et al., 1975; O'Brien and Bellvé, 1980a). This tail element, when subjected to two-dimensional polyacrylamide gel electrophoresis, displays a limited diversity of polypeptide species ($<$ 29) with M_r's ranging from 10,000 to 75,000 and p_I's of 4.0 to 7.0 following carboxymethylation (Bradley et al., 1981). Five of these protein spots have identical M_r's to other proteins and differ in their isoelectric points by only a single unit charge, suggesting that they may be variant polypeptides or represent posttranslational modifications. Thus, these structural tail elements may comprise only 25 polypeptide species. Interestingly, such posttranslational modifications as phosphorylation, acetylation, methylation, glycosylation, and ADP ribosylation usually reflect different functional states of native polypeptides.

The outer dense fibers and the fibrous sheath are the most prominent components of the sperm tail. Both structures are stabilized by covalent disulfide bonds and are interlocked with the axoneme to form a single functional unit (Olson et al., 1976a; Olson and Linck, 1977). In comparative studies, Phillips (1972b) has observed a correlation between the size of the outer dense fibers and the radius of curvature for beating flagella. This suggests that the outer dense fibers, and perhaps the fibrous sheath, may serve to stiffen the sperm tail, thereby modifying flagellar beat and facilitating forward movement through the viscous genital secretions.

The basic ultrastructural features of the outer dense fibers are comparable among mammals, although they may vary in size and length (Fawcett, 1970, 1975a). Each of the nine outer dense fibers is located adjacent to one of the peripheral doublets of the axoneme, thereby forming the 9 + 9 + 2 cross-sectional pattern characteristic of mammalian sperm (Fig. 1). In the neck region, each outer dense fiber is attached to one of the segmented columns. The fibers taper as they extend caudally and terminate at different levels along the principal piece (Telkka et al., 1961). Fibers 1, 5, and 6 generally are larger and longer than the others. A thin cortical region of each fiber can be distinguished by its reduced electron density and unique staining properties (Gordon and Bensch, 1968; Fawcett, 1975a; Olson and Sammons, 1980). The outer dense fibers are cross-striated with a regular periodicity more complex in the cortex than the fiber interior (Pedersen, 1972b; Woolley, 1970; Baccetti et al., 1973; Olson et al., 1977). The striated pattern may result from the lateral packing of protofibrillike subunits (Baccetti et al., 1976b; Olson and Sammons, 1980).

Recently, the outer dense fibers from three mammalian species were isolated and partially characterized (Baccetti et al., 1973, 1976a; Price, 1973; Calvin, 1976b; Olson et al., 1976a; Olson, 1979). Their protein constituents when resolved by SDS-PAGE, reveal similar profiles among species. In the rat, bull, and man, the outer dense fibers consist primarily of five proteins, M_r's ~ 14,000, 28,000, 38,000, 44,000, and 87,000. The three smaller proteins are rich in cysteine, leucine, proline, and serine (Olson and Sammons, 1980). The lysine-rich, 87,000-dalton component probably is localized in the outer cortex of the fibers. A large proportion of the zinc in isolated tails is associated with the outer dense fibers (Calvin et al., 1975; Baccetti et al., 1976a,b), possibly in ligand conformation with the cysteinyl groups of the 38,000- and

41,000-dalton proteins (Calvin, 1979). Two reports suggest that these fibers are rich in triglycerides and perhaps carbohydrate (Baccetti *et al.*, 1973; Price, 1973).

The fibrous sheath is a prominent segmented cylinder denoting the proximal and distal limits of the principal piece. It is composed of two longitudinal columns located on opposite sides of the axoneme, and a series of closely spaced, semicircular ribs that fuse with the longitudinal columns (Fawcett, 1970, 1975a). In the mouse and some other mammals, the ribs branch and fuse extensively, forming an irregular network of broad circumferential bands (Fawcett, 1970). The circumferential orientation of the ribs may facilitate planar bending of the motile sperm tail (Phillips, 1975b). Both elements of the fibrous sheath appear to have a filamentous substructure, although the polymer subunits of the longitudinal columns are larger and packed more loosely than those of the ribs. At the proximal end of the fibrous sheath, the longitudinal columns are attached to outer dense fibers 3 and 8. Distal to the termini of these two dense fibers, the longitudinal columns are attached to small ridges which project from the corresponding axonemal doublets. The fibrous sheath of rat sperm, when isolated as a discrete structural entity, is composed primarily of a single protein, M_r 80,000 (Olson *et al.*, 1976a; Olson, 1979).

4. The Helical Mitochondria

Sperm mitochondria are arranged in the tail midpiece, end-to-end in a helical array around the outer dense fibers. There is wide variation among mammals in the form of the mitochondrial helix (Phillips, 1977b) and in the midpiece length (Fawcett, 1975a). In the mouse, the midpiece is ~21 μm in length and is composed of ~89 mitochondrial gyres arranged in a double helix, although some regions of triple helix also are evident (Phillips, 1977b). Except in a few species, the mitochondria are of unequal length so junctions between them occur randomly along the helical gyre.

Mitochondria in mammalian sperm, like those in somatic cells, have identifiable outer and inner membranes and an internal matrix (Favard and André, 1970; Fawcett, 1975a). However, they also exhibit unusual ultrastructural features, including peculiar specializations on the outer membrane (Friend and Heuser, 1981), a dense matrix, and longitudinally arranged cristae (Fawcett, 1970; Phillips, 1975b). The outer mitochondrial surface of guinea pig sperm exhibits remarkable particulate structures existing in orderly arrays (Friend and Heuser, 1981). The convex surface facing the plasmalemma contains randomly dispersed rods each composed of two to four 7- to 8-nm particles, spaced

2 nm apart. By contrast, the concave surface apposing the outer dense fibers has similar rod structures organized in parallel to form stepladder configurations, 8 nm apart, which course across the surface at 45° to the mitochondrial axis. These highly organized particles may be enzymes having crucial roles in cell metabolism and/or motility.

The outer membrane of sperm mitochondria is particularly resistant to disruption and solubilization. This membrane retains its size and helical shape even following exposure to hypotonic solutions (Keyhani and Storey, 1973), Triton X-100 (Wooding, 1973), or SDS (Bedford and Calvin, 1974a; Bellvé et al., 1975). It is composed predominently of three polypeptides: M_r's 20,000, 29,000, and 31,000, with the first containing strikingly high molar ratios of cysteine and proline (Pallini et al., 1979). Thus, the unusual structural stability may, in part, be due to intermolecular disulfide bonds, although the outer mitochondrial membranes retain their shape even after incubation with 10 mM DTT (Bartoov and Messer, 1976). This structural resistance also may depend on the existence of intermolecular cysteinyl-selenium ligands (Pallini and Bacci, 1979) and strong hydrophobic interactions.

The peculiar structural properties of the mitochondria have facilitated their isolation from ram and bull spermatozoa (Bartoov and Messer, 1976; Hrudka, 1978; Pallini et al., 1979). These isolated mitochondria appear to retain normal structural integrity (Pallini, 1979) and may be useful for assessment of their metabolic properties.

Several findings suggest that sperm mitochondria have typical metabolic capabilities. Thus, sperm contain enzymes capable of aerobically metabolizing glycolysable sugars, glycerol, sorbitol, lactate, pyruvate, acetate, other fatty acids, and several amino acids (Mann and Lutwak-Mann, 1981). The cytochromes, including the testis-specific cytochrome c_t (Wheat et al., 1977), and several enzymes of the Krebs cycle have been localized to sperm midpieces or isolated mitochondria (see Mohri et al., 1965; Bartoov and Messer, 1976; Pallini, 1979). Sperm mitochondria contain appropriate polymerases (Hecht, 1974; Fuster et al., 1977) and are capable of DNA and RNA synthesis (Premkumar and Bhargava, 1972, 1973). Finally, ram sperm mitochondria contain circular DNA with physical and chemical properties typical of somatic cells (Fisher et al., 1977).

One feature distinguishing sperm mitochondria from those found in somatic cells is their ability to oxidize lactate directly (Storey and Kayne, 1977). Indirect pathways, such as the malate/aspartate shuttle, are utilized to transfer NADH-reducing equivalents from the cytosol to the mitochondria in somatic tissues. By contrast, a portion of the sperm lactate dehydrogenase (LDH-C_4) may be localized within mitochondria (Montamat and Blanco, 1976; Storey and Kayne, 1977, 1978; Van Dop et al., 1977; Hutson et al., 1977). The sperm-specific LDH-C_4 isoenzyme ($M_r \sim 34,000$) has been purified and, following crystallization, its structure has been resolved to a resolution of 2.9 Å (Musick and Rossmann, 1979). This isoenzyme has a broad specificity for α-hydroxy acids and can oxidize lactate to pyruvate, thereby allowing further energy production via the Krebs cycle (Mita and Hall, 1982; cf. Storey and Kayne, 1977, 1978).

E. Regional Topography of the Sperm Plasma Membrane

The highly polarized spermatozoon is enveloped by a plasmalemma exhibiting distinct functional domains. Thus, the plasma membrane covering the anterior head region participates in the acrosome reaction, while the postacrosomal surface is considered responsible for the initial fusion of male and female gametes.

Freeze-fracture studies of eutherian sperm reveal regional differences in the size, distribution, and relative density of intramembranous particles (Fléchon, 1974; Friend and Fawcett, 1974; Stackpole and Devorkin, 1974; Olson et al., 1977). Particle organization ranging from random arrays to crystalline domains varies considerably among species (Friend and Fawcett, 1974; Fawcett, 1975a; Suzuki, 1981). Surface replicas of rodent sperm also reveal regional specializations of the plasma membrane, including arrays of small tubules and vesicles localized over the acrosome (Phillips, 1975a). Similarly, the glycocalyx coat is distributed asymmetrically on the surface of cauda and ejaculated rabbit sperm (Fléchon, 1975), and has distinct ultrastructural regions in the guinea pig (Friend and Fawcett, 1974). One feature common to mammalian sperm is the zipper, a linear array of particles coursing down the principal piece in the plasma membrane overlying outer dense fiber 1 (Friend and Heuser, 1981). Fawcett (1975a) suggests that the zipper may attach the plasma membrane to the subjacent ribs of the fibrous sheath, thereby facilitating coordinated locomotion.

Surface constituents are topographically regionalized in the sperm plasma membrane. Distinct surface domains are evident following the binding of lectins (Edelman and Millette, 1971; Gordon et al., 1974; Nicolson and Yanagamachi, 1972, 1974; Schwartz and Koehler, 1979; for reviews, see Koehler, 1978, 1981) and heterologous antibodies (Koehler and Perkins, 1974; Koehler, 1975; Millette and Bellvé, 1977, 1980; Tung et al., 1982). These molecular probes show species-specific distributions (Koehler, 1981), suggesting that many surface constituents are not phylogenetically conserved. Furthermore, the lateral mobility of lectin and antibody receptors within the plasma membrane appears to be restricted in sperm (Koehler, 1975; O'Rand, 1977), particularly in regions other than the postacrosomal surface of the head (Nicolson and Yanagimachi, 1974). Restricted mobility of surface constituents may be due to their lateral association with other integral or peripheral surface components or to their interactions with subsurface cytoskeletal elements (Nicolson, 1982).

Sperm membrane lipids also may be localized in discrete domains. Filipin, a probe for membrane cholesterol, forms complexes preferentially in regions of the plasmalemma overlying the acrosome of the guinea pig sperm (Elias *et al.*, 1979). Similarly, the localized interaction of polymyxin with fusogenic membrane regions over the acrosome and cytoplasmic droplet suggests high local concentrations of anionic lipids (Bearer and Friend, 1982). Such lipid domains may facilitate the membrane events attending capacitation and the acrosome reaction.

Several surface antigens on spermatogenic cells have been characterized by immunological, genetic, and biochemical procedures. These determinants include histocompatibility antigens (Erickson *et al.*, 1977), H-Y antigen (Goldberg *et al.*, 1971), antigens specified by the T-locus (Bennett *et al.*, 1972; Yanagisawa *et al.*, 1974), F9 and related teratoma antigens (Artzt *et al.*, 1973, 1974), and antigens shared by spermatozoa and neonatal cerebellum (Schachner *et al.*, 1975; Seeds, 1975). At least two of these antigens are distributed regionally on the sperm surface. An antigen shared with teratocarcinoma cells is confined to the postacrosomal surface in both human and mouse sperm (Fellous *et al.*, 1974), while mouse H-Y antigen is localized primarily over the acrosomal cap (Koo *et al.*, 1973). It can be questioned as to whether H-Y antigen is in fact an integral surface constituent and functionally important on spermatozoa. This particular antigen could simply be adsorbed to the cell surface prior to spermiation, along with other known Sertoli cell products (cf. Franke *et al.*, 1978; Phillips, 1980).

Autoantigenic surface constituents have been identified on spermatozoa in the rabbit (O'Rand and Porter, 1979) and guinea pig (Tung *et al.*, 1979, 1980). RSA-1, a plasma membrane antigen on rabbit sperm, is a sialoglycoprotein ($M_r \sim 13{,}000$) that binds *Ricinis communis* I lectin (O'Rand and Porter, 1979; O'Rand and Romrell, 1980b). Initial biochemical characterizations of guinea pig surface autoantigens reveal multiple determinants with M_r's ranging between 19,000 and 69,000 (Teuscher *et al.*, 1982). In addition, these investigators have identified an unusual antigen ($M_r \sim 6000$) on acrosome-reacted sperm that may be a glycolipid. Similarly, immunoprecipitation techniques using heterologous antisera have defined several surface determinants on mouse sperm (Herr and Eddy, 1980).

Recent investigations have utilized monoclonal antibody probes directed against specific surface determinants of guinea pig (Myles *et al.*, 1981) and mouse spermatozoa (Feuchter *et al.*, 1981). The hybridoma technology permits the isolation of clonally derived cell lines, each producing antibody that recognizes a single antigenic determinant. Four monoclonal antibodies elicited against mouse spermatozoa have been shown to bind to distinct zones on the cell surface, three to discrete regions on the head and one to the tail (Feuchter *et al.*, 1981). These particular autoantigens are not detected on the cell surface until the maturing spermatozoa reach the corpus epididymis. Similarly, xenogeneic monoclonal antibodies have been isolated after immunization of mice with membrane vesicles released from guinea pig spermatozoa during the A23187 ionophore-induced acrosome reaction (Primakoff *et al.*, 1980a). The cell fusion produced 116 hybridoma cell lines, each secreting antibody that binds to a polarized domain on the sperm cell surface (Myles *et al.*, 1980, 1981; Primakoff *et al.*, 1980b). The patterns obtained with four of these monoclonal antibodies are shown in Figs 6 and 7. Three of the monoclonal antibodies immunoprecipitate ^{125}I-labeled proteins having M_r's of ~42,000 (whole

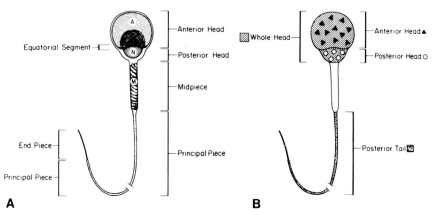

Fig. 6. Schematic diagram of the guinea pig spermatozoon showing the principal structures and surface domains of this polarized cell. (A) The major components of the sperm cell are shown, including the acrosome (A), nucleus (N), and mitochondria (M) (cf. Fig. 1). (B) Four monoclonal antibodies prepared against constituents of acrosomic vesicles bind to distinct topographic domains on the cell surface. Regions recognized by these antibodies include the anterior head, posterior head, whole head, and tail. (Reproduced from Myles *et al.*, 1981, by permission of the editor, *Cell*.)

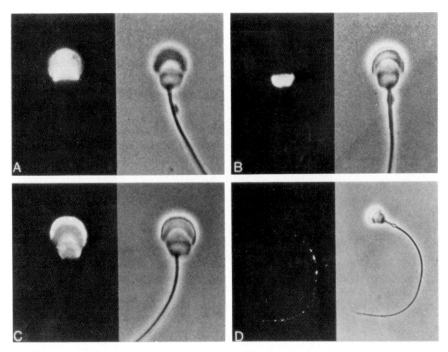

Fig. 7. Binding patterns of the respective monoclonal antibodies to the guinea pig cell surface. The sperm were fixed in 0.5% paraformaldehyde and then incubated with antibody. Photomicrographs show antibody binding by indirect immunofluorescence and the corresponding phase-contrast image. Antibodies recognize protein constituents on the anterior head (M_r 52,000), posterior head (M_r 60,000), whole head (M_r 42,000), and posterior tail (Fig. 7A-C, ×1300; Fig. 7D, ×620). (Reproduced from Myles *et al.*, 1981, by permission of the editor, *Cell*.)

head), 52,000 (anterior head), and 60,000 (posterior head). The discrete localization of these components to membrane domains within the acrosomal and postacrosomal regions suggests that they may have functions during capacitation, the acrosome reaction, or fertilization.

III. BIOGENESIS OF THE SPERMATOZOON

Since Leeuwenhoek (1680) first observed sperm cells "coming to life" in the rat testis, much has been documented concerning their origin and biogenesis (for review, see Bellvé, 1979). Primordial germ cells, originating at an extraembryonic site in fetal life, migrate to the genital anlagen and proliferate to yield the stem cells of the neonatal seminiferous epithelium (Eddy *et al.*, 1981). Later during prepubertal development these cells, and their congeners in the adult, undergo a series of divisions to renew the original stem cell and to form the lineage of differentiating spermatogonia (Fig. 8). This mitotic sequence yields preleptotene spermatocytes which undergo a final phase of DNA synthesis and then, without dividing, enter meiosis. Meiotic

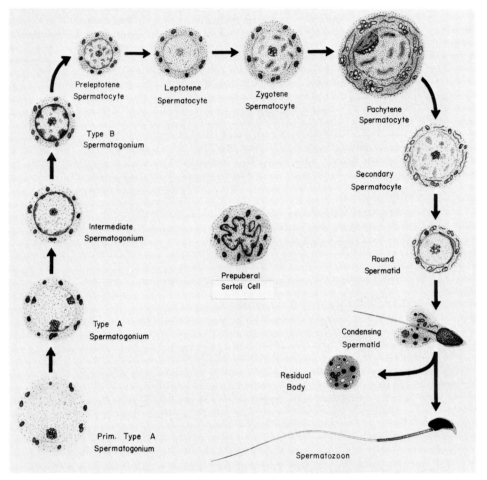

Fig. 8. Schematic diagram depicting the sequence of differentiation that occurs during mouse spermatogenesis. The volumes and characteristic morphology of the respective cell types are presented. This process occurs in three phases: spermatogonia proliferate by a series of mitotic divisions (ascending axis), spermatocytes undergo cytological differentiation during meiotic prophase (horizontal axis), and then proceed through two reduction divisions to yield the haploid spermatids. The latter cells pass through a complex phase of differentiation which culminates in the production of spermatozoa (descending axis). (Reproduced from Bellvé *et al.*, 1977a, by permission of the editor, *Journal of Cell Biology*.)

prophase is characterized by a complex series of chromosomal rear-
rangements including the progressive synapsis of homologous chromosomes by synaptonemal complexes (Westergaard and von Wettstein,
1972), genetic recombination (Henderson, 1970), and premature condensation of the sex chromosomes (Solari, 1974). In mouse spermatocytes the multiple nucleoli coalesce to form a single body that
associates with the X-Y heterochromatin. The lampbrush chromosomes pass through a diffuse diplotene stage in mouse and Rhesus
monkey spermatocytes (Kierszenbaum and Tres, 1974a,b; for review,
see Bellvé, 1979). During the period of meiotic prophase, which lasts
12.5 to 13 days in the mouse and 20 days in the human, the spermatocyte increases $\sim$ 12-fold in volume. Both ribosomal and unique
gene sequences are transcribed extensively to provide proteins essential for further differentiation of the germ cell. Following the two meiotic reduction divisions, which allow random segregation of the homologous chromosomes, the haploid spermatids undergo a marked
morphological transformation. Throughout spermiogenesis the cells
gradually acquire the distinctive polar architecture of the mature
sperm (Fig. 8). Further maturational changes also occur after spermiation while the cells are in transit through the excurrent ducts to their
storage site in the cauda epididymides.

A. The Dynamics of Nuclear Reorganization during Spermiogenesis

During mammalian spermiogenesis the nucleus gradually condenses and assumes a shape characteristic of each species (Fig. 8)
(Fawcett et al., 1971). During the initial phase (steps 1–3) of mouse
spermiogenesis the nucleus is spherical and contains a central density
(Dooher and Bennett, 1973), sometimes identified as a nucleolus although it incorporates only minimal amounts of [^{3}H]uridine (Kierszenbaum and Tres, 1975). Subjacent to the attached proacrosomal granule, the nuclear membranes become apposed closely and dense heterochromatin forms on the inner surface of the envelope. During the cap
phase (steps 4–7) the nucleus initially flattens beneath the forming
acrosome and then later assumes an oval shape.

At the onset of the acrosome phase, the distinctly polarized nucleus
rotates, directing the acrosomal pole toward the basement membrane
of the seminiferous tubule. Alterations in nuclear shape, including
elongation, lateral flattening, and development of the apical curvature, are initiated during this latter phase. First, the "nucleoluslike
body" disappears and numerous chromatin densities form along the
inner margin of the nuclear envelope. The nucleosome substructure is

lost as the chromatin fibrils gradually become smooth in contour and aggregate to form branching fiber bundles 2.7 to 38 nm in diameter (Kierszenbaum and Tres, 1975; Loir and Courtens, 1979). The chromatin gradually assumes a fibrillar appearance except for a thin peripheral zone, and dense material accumulates on the inner nuclear membrane adjacent to the implantation fossa (Loir and Courtens, 1979). The manchette, an array of microtubules, forms transiently around the caudal pole of the nucleus. During the final phase of mouse spermiogenesis (steps 12–16), the chromatin condenses, initially at the anterior pole of the nucleus and proceeding from the center to the periphery. Eventually, the nucleus becomes uniformly dense except in the small region enclosed by the redundant nuclear envelope.

During the final maturation phase of rat spermatids (steps 15–19), the partially condensed nucleus continues to be molded into a more pronounced falciform shape (see Fig. 9) (Lalli and Clermont, 1981). While the apical regions of the nucleus become increasingly curved, the chromatin condenses further, first assuming a granulofilamentous appearance and then acquiring a uniform density. Chromatin in the most caudal zone of the nucleus near the implantation fossa, still variable in texture at step 17, is the last region to achieve full condensation at the end of step 18 (Lalli and Clermont, 1981). As the condensation of chromatin proceeds the nucleus diminishes in volume, leaving redundant areas of nuclear envelope folded along the ventral spur. Portions of this excess envelope undergo dissolution to yield whorls of membrane that accumulate among the regions of redundant envelope enfolded near the implantation fossa.

B. Determinants of Sperm Nuclear Shape

The determinants of nuclear shape have been subjected to considerable study. Some studies implicate microtubules as extrinsic elements responsible for molding the nucleus in nonmammalian species (McIntosh and Porter, 1967). In mammalian spermatids a microtubular complex, the manchette, transiently appears around the caudal region of the nucleus. However, after assessing available evidence, Fawcett *et al.* (1971) concluded that while microtubules may have a role in redistributing the cytoplasm, they probably are not directly responsible for changes in nuclear shape. Instead they suggested the pattern of chromatin condensation acts as an intrinsic determinant of nuclear conformation. Microtubules may play a secondary role, either by structurally reinforcing the differentiating nucleus (Rattner and Brinkley, 1972) or by establishing the axis of elongation (Dooher and Bennett, 1977).

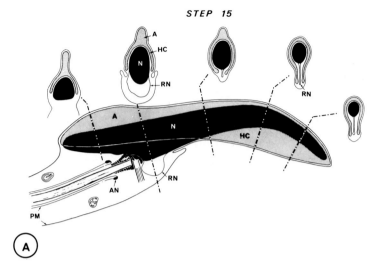

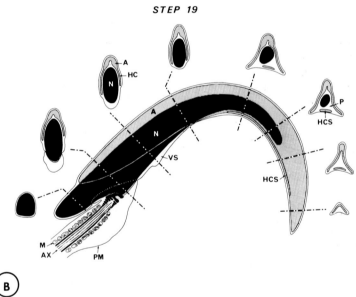

Fig. 9. Schematic diagrams of the sperm head at steps 15 and 19 of the maturation phase of rat spermiogenesis. The head structure is shown in sagittal section, with several demarcated cross views. During this phase the nucleus undergoes further condensation and develops a pronounced falciform curvature. The acrosome, which covers most of the nuclear surface at step 15, is displaced forward during steps 18 and 19. The perinuclear theca also develops further during this phase, but is not shown. A, acrosome; AN, annulus; AX, axoneme; HC, head cap; HCS, separated head-cap segment; M, mitochondria; N, nucleus; P, perforatorium; PM, plasma membrane; RN, redundant nuclear envelope; VS, ventral spur. (Reproduced from Lalli and Clermont, 1981, by permission of the editor, *American Journal of Anatomy*.)

The protamines, the species-specific proteins associated with the condensed chromatin, have been implicated as the intrinsic determinants of sperm nuclear shape (Fawcett *et al.*, 1971). Recent studies, however, do not support this contention. There appears to be no correlation between nuclear conformation and the type of protamine present in different mammalian species (Bellvé, 1979). Thus, the nuclei of mouse and human spermatozoa have similar complements of type 1 and type 2 protamine but have falciform and globular shapes, respectively. Rat spermatozoa are falciform in shape but completely lack the histidine-rich type 2 protamine that is the major polypeptide constituent of the mouse sperm nucleus (Bellvé, 1982). A similar argument can be extended to the rat and guinea pig sperm nucleus, which contain analogous type 1 protamines and yet are very dissimilar in shape.

The perinuclear theca may act as an extrinsic determinant of nuclear shape. This matrix structure, when isolated from the mouse sperm nucleus, retains the original nuclear configuration even after protamine and DNA are removed (Fig. 5B). This structure may contain actin and myosin which could provide the mechanistic force needed to transform nuclear shape. Actin has been localized to the postacrosomal region of the sperm nucleus of several mammalian species (Clarke and Yanagimachi, 1978; Tamblyn, 1980), primarily within the perforatorium and postacrosomal regions of the perinuclear theca (Campanella *et al.*, 1979; Baccetti *et al.*, 1980; cf. Strauch *et al.*, 1980). These observations, however, need to be confirmed by more definitive studies. With this reservation in mind, it is reasonable to speculate that cables of actin filaments envelop the spermatid nucleus, perhaps traversing the nucleus and contiguous with the intranuclear matrix. These filaments may act in concert to mold the nucleus into its predetermined shape. This process could be guided extrinsically by the microtubular manchette during the early phases of nuclear reorganization and would be facilitated further by the selective elimination of many NPCPs and by the deposition of protamines. The continued deposition of protein constituents of the perinuclear theca would allow the structure to conform to the changing nuclear shape. Moreover, at late spermiogenesis these polypeptides could crosslink by forming intra- and intermolecular covalent disulfide bonds, thereby stabilizing nuclear shape.

The major constituents of the perinuclear theca, the nonprotamine nuclear proteins, are synthesized primarily during spermiogenesis coincident with the period of nuclear transformation (O'Brien and Bellvé, 1980b). Perinuclear material (PNM), the anlage of the perinuclear theca, first appears in early spermatids between the forming acrosomal granule and the nuclear envelope. The structure extends peripherally over the anterior pole of the nucleus during spermiogenesis, just preceding the leading edge of the forming acrosome (Courtens *et al.*, 1976). Later the subacrosomal space widens further, allowing the deposition of additional material and the extension of the PNM into the postacrosomal region (Lalli and Clermont, 1981). In myomorph rodents, during late spermiogenesis, the apical portion of the PNM is modified to form the perforatorium (Lalli and Clermont, 1981). The other component of the perinuclear theca, the postacrosomal dense lamina (PDL), first appears in elongating spermatids, at the time the PNM extends into the postacrosomal region (Courtens *et al.*, 1976; Lalli and Clermont, 1981).

C. The Golgi Apparatus and the Developing Acrosomic System

The Golgi complex plays an important, central role in spermiogenesis. This complex organelle migrates toward the apical pole of the nucleus during step 2 of spermiogenesis. When proximal to the nucleus, the Golgi body assumes a hemispherical shape while orienting its concave surface toward the nucleus (Burgos and Fawcett, 1955; Sandoz, 1970; Susi *et al.*, 1971). The convex cytoplasmic face (cis face) is delimited by a single, discontinuous layer of flattened cisternae of the endoplasmic reticulum (Figs. 10A,B). Immediately internal to the cis face lies a cortical layer of complex, anastomosing tubules and small vesicles (Hermo *et al.*, 1979, 1980). The vesicles appear to be released from the tubular network and pass to the outer face of the 6 to 12 parallel saccules forming the body of the Golgi complex. Extensively interconnected by small cisternae, these saccules are actively involved in the posttranslational modification of glycoproteins, deleting dolichol-derived mannose units and adding appropriate sugar and sialic acid groups as the parent molecules are processed through the successive saccules (for review, see Farquhar and Palade, 1981).

These Golgi saccules are polarized functionally, with the successive cisternae containing different enzyme complexes. Only the second through fifth saccules from the cis face show reasonable levels of nicotinamide adenine dinucleotide phosphatase activity (NADPase), whereas thiamine pyrophosphatase activity (TPPase) is detectable almost exclusively in the innermost two saccules at the trans face (Fig. 10A, B) (Clermont *et al.*, 1981). By contrast, cytidine monophosphatase activity (CMPase) is localized in the rigid lamellae (GERL), their associated buds, and the forming acrosomic system. This regionalization of Golgi functions presumably has significant implications for the pro-

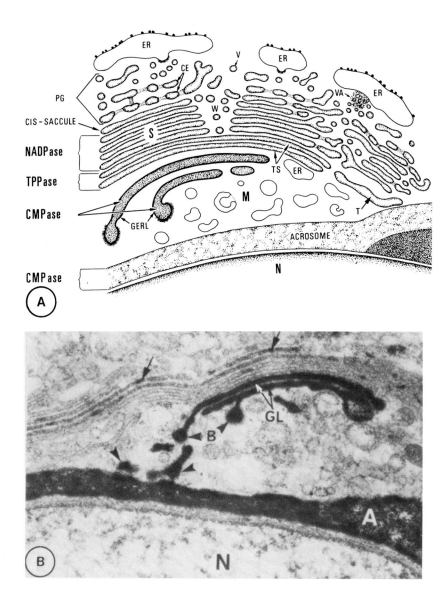

Fig. 10. Diagrammatic representation and a corresponding electron micrograph demonstrating regional localization of enzyme activities within the Golgi complex of the rat spermatid. (A) The polar organization of the Golgi complex is shown by the discrete localization of NADPase in the outer saccules at the cis face, TPPase in the inner trans saccules, and CMPase within the GERL structures and in the forming acrosome. GERL, rigid lamellae; T, membranous tubules interconnecting saccules; W, well; S, saccules; VA, vesicular aggregates; PG, peripheral Golgi region; TS, trans saccules; M, medulla; N, nucleus; CE, osmiophilic element at the cis face. (B) Electron micrograph of the spermatid (step 7) Golgi complex showing cytidine monophosphatase activity (CMPase) in the innermost trans saccules, the GERL (GL) region and associate buds (B), and the adjacent acrosomic system (A) overlying the nucleus (N) (×40,000). (Reproduced after Clermont *et al.*, 1981, by permission of the editor, *The Anatomical Record*.)

cessing of glycoproteins which are en route to other cellular organelles, the plasma membrane, and the acrosomic system of the developing spermatid.

Mammalian spermiogenesis occurs in four principal phases: the Golgi, cap, acrosome, and maturation phases of acrosome development (Leblond and Clermont, 1952). In the Golgi phase spermatids, carbohydrate-rich, granular vesicles emanate from the Golgi complex and coalesce to form the proacrosomal vesicle. This large vesicle attaches to the small zone of modified nuclear envelope at the anterior pole of the nucleus (see also Sandoz, 1970). During the cap phase the acrosomal system spreads laterally, gradually enveloping the anterior pole of the nucleus as it acquires additional material from the small vesicles forming at the nearby Golgi apparatus (Susi *et al.*, 1971; Hermo *et al.*, 1979, 1980).

Early in the acrosome phase the spermatid reorients to direct the acrosome toward the basement membrane of the seminiferous epithelium. The acrosome, now uniformly dense, extends caudally over the dorsal pole of the elongating nucleus, as the cytoplasm is displaced gradually toward the developing tail segment. During this phase small vesicles originating directly from the endoplasmic reticulum continue to fuse with the acrosome (Fawcett, 1975b). Some protein constituents, at least in the guinea pig, may be inserted cotranslationally into the acrosome from membrane-associated polyribosomes (Mollenhauer and Morré, 1978). During the maturation phase (mouse, steps 12–16; rat, steps 15–19), while the equatorial segment is forming, the shaping of the acrosome and nucleus continues (Fawcett and Phillips, 1969a; Lalli and Clermont, 1981). By the end of the maturation period, the rat acrosome is crescent-shaped, having a prominent apical segment and a relatively short equatorial segment (Fig. 9).

D. Assembly of the Tail Structures

Development of the tail begins early in spermiogenesis when the centrioles migrate to the equatorial pole opposite the forming acrosome (Fawcett and Phillips, 1969b, 1970; Dooher and Bennett, 1973). There the distal centriole orients perpendicular to the cell surface and rapidly enucleates the axoneme. Elongation of the flagellum continues, apparently by the polymerization of tubulin and associated proteins at the distal ends of the microtubules. The structural elements of the neck region also begin to form during early spermiogenesis. The capitulum anlage, a curved sheet of dense material, forms above the proximal centriole. Periodic densities appearing along the wall of the distal centriole form the first elements of the segmented columns. Later (mouse, step 5) the centrioles migrate to the implantation fossa near the caudal nuclear pole. Thereafter, the connecting piece forms in a precise sequence. Dense material accumulates between the triplet tubules of the proximal centriole, with anterior extensions fusing to form the capitulum. Lateral and caudal extensions then appear clockwise forming the anterior ends of the segmented columns. Similar matrix material accumulates at the distal centriole and assembles to yield the posterior portions of the segmented columns which progressively disrupt centriolar structure.

With the onset of the acrosome phase and the appearance of the annulus, the anlagen of the outer dense fibers appear as ridgelike projections on the A tubules. These polymerize throughout the length of the axoneme in a proximal to distal direction (Irons and Clermont, 1982). Later, during steps 15 and 16, additional material accumulates along the entire length of the dense fibers, with the rate varying in a proximal-distal gradient. The fibers continue to grow until they reach their mature size at step 19 when they separate from the microtubule doublets throughout their entire length, except at the distal termini. Anteriorly, the dense fibers remain fused with the segmented columns of the connecting piece.

Elements of the fibrous sheath first are evident after mouse spermatids rotate and project their tail rudiments into the lumen of the seminiferous tubule (Fawcett and Phillips, 1970). Clermont and Rambourg (1978) noted fibrous sheath construction commencing in the rat early in the maturation phase, with assembly occurring in a distal–proximal direction. Generally, the longitudinal columns of the sheath assemble a short time before the circumferential ribs, which gradually thicken and fuse to form the irregular spacing pattern seen in mature sperm.

E. Biogenesis of Mitochondria and Their Intercalation into the Midpiece

During mammalian spermatogenesis the mitochondria undergo marked alterations in internal structure (André, 1962; Fawcett, 1970). Spermatogonia have typical mitochondria with cristae oriented perpendicular to the outer membrane. In spermatocytes the cristae assume irregular forms, while elongating and orienting parallel to the outer mitochondrial membrane. The internal matrix increases in density and the intracristal spaces expand considerably (Fawcett, 1970; De Martino et al., 1979). These mitochondria often are associated in clusters with intervening granular material (Fawcett, 1972) that later may become part of the chromatoid body (Fawcett et al., 1970; Fawcett, 1972; Russell and Frank, 1978).

During early spermiogenesis the mitochondria initially migrate to the periphery of the cell (André, 1962; Kaya and Harrison, 1976) but then later may distribute throughout the cytoplasm (Gardner, 1966). During steps 15 and 16 of mouse spermiogenesis, after the manchette disassembles and the annulus migrates caudally, the mitochondria gather adjacent to the midpiece region and then join end-to-end to form a helical gyre peripheral to the outer dense fibers (Woolley, 1970, Fawcett et al., 1971; Dooher and Bennett, 1973; De Martino et al., 1979). Those mitochondria not incorporated into the midpiece region soon are discarded within the residual body (Smith and Lacy, 1959; Sandoz, 1970).

There is only limited information available concerning the metabolic functions of the mitochondria of spermatogenic cells. The condensed mitochondria of isolated rat spermatogenic cells (primarily spermatocytes and spermatids) are capable of oxidative phosphorylation (De Martino et al., 1979). However, rat spermatids preferentially utilize lactate rather than glucose as an energy source (Mita and Hall, 1982). The findings of the latter authors suggest that exogenous lactate is oxidized by lactate dehydrogenase, then by pyruvate dehydrogenase and the Krebs cycle enzymes. Since the LDH-C$_4$ (LDH-X) isoenzyme is located partially in the mitochondria of spermatocytes and spermatids (Montamat and Blanco, 1976; Meistrich et al., 1977), the NADH produced can readily be utilized for the production of ATP. Significantly, germ cells incubated in the presence of lactate substantially increase their rate of O$_2$ consumption (Jutte et al., 1981) and protein synthesis (Nakamura et al., 1981). The high concentration (0.67 mM) of lactate in seminiferous tubule fluid (Evans and Setchell, 1978) is produced by Sertoli cells (Robinson and Fritz, 1981). Collectively, these observations provide the first definitive evidence for a sustentacular role of Sertoli cells in mammalian spermatogenesis.

F. Topographical Reorganization of the Cell Surface

During the course of spermatogenesis the plasma membrane undergoes a major transformation as it acquires a variety of novel constituents and organizes them into the discrete regional domains that exist on the mature spermatozoon (Millette and Bellvé, 1980; for reviews, see Bellvé, 1979, 1982). One unique aspect of spermatogenesis is the appearance of a peculiar sulfatoxylgalactosyl glycerolipid at the cell surface of spermatocytes (Kornblatt, 1979). This novel surface constituent is present throughout spermiogenesis and persists in the plasma membrane of spermatozoa (Klugerman and Kornblatt, 1980; Lingwood and Schachter, 1981). Whether this novel sulfatoxylgalactosyl glycerolipid is regionally localized in the plasma membrane is not known. Bechtol *et al.* (1979), using monoclonal antibodies, identified two undefined antigens, presumably on the cell surface of mouse spermatogenic cells. Both antigens appear during testicular development and have not been detected in significant quantities on spermatozoa. Several differentiation antigens first appear on pachytene spermatocytes and continue to be expressed during the subsequent ontogeny of the germ cell. These cell surface antigenic determinants have been detected in spermatocytes, spermatids, residual bodies, and spermatozoa of the rabbit (O'Rand and Romrell,1977), the mouse (Millette and Bellvé, 1977), and the rat (Tung and Fritz, 1978). The complexity of determinants being recognized by these xenogeneic and isogeneic polyclonal antibodies has not been determined. Presumably, multiple surface determinants are being recognized since four different antibody preparations exhibited distinct binding patterns on the surface of mature mouse spermatozoa (Millette and Bellvé, 1977).

Additional surface components are first expressed at later stages of spermatogenesis. Autoantigen T, a surface component of guinea pig germ cells, is not detected on primary spermatocytes and "Golgi phase" spermatids (Radu and Voisin, 1975; Le Bouteiller *et al.,* 1979). Other autoantigens, both guinea pig and rabbit, may not arise until the acrosome phase of spermiogenesis (Tung *et al.,* 1979; O'Rand and Romrell, 1980a). Certain alloantigenic components are detectable initially in low numbers on pachytene spermatocytes and early spermatids but then at substantially increasing numbers during the later phases of spermiogenesis (Romrell and O'Rand, 1978; O'Rand and Romrell, 1980a). These different temporal patterns presumably reflect the sequential insertion of multiple components into the cell surface as spermatogenesis proceeds.

The recent development of techniques for obtaining purified plasma membranes (Millette *et al.,* 1980) from discrete classes of isolated mouse spermatogenic cells (Romrell *et al.,* 1976; Bellvé *et al.,* 1977a,b) provides a definitive approach for identifying new membrane constituents. Using this approach Millette and Moulding (1981) identified by two-dimensional polyacrylamide gel electrophoresis two cell surface components, denoted as Pa and Pb, that exist only on pachytene spermatocytes. Another four, RSa–d, are restricted to round spermatids (steps 1–8). A considerable number of other constituents are common to the surfaces of both cell types. This particular study did not report whether any of these plasma membrane components also exist on mature sperm or on cells prior to pachynema. Another cell surface component, $M_r \sim 28,000$, has been detected on the surface of pachytene spermatocytes, spermatids, and spermatozoa of the mouse with a monoclonal antibody (Gaunt, 1982). Unlike many other germ cell antigens this component is present on the surface of rat, rabbit, vole, and guinea pig spermatozoa and, therefore, may be conserved across species.

Surface constituents of mature spermatozoa are segregated into distinct topographical domains, where severe constraints are imposed on their lateral mobility. By contrast, at earlier stages of spermatogenesis, surface antigens are distributed diffusely in the cell plasma membrane and are able to form patches and caps in the presence of multivalent ligands (Millette, 1977; Romrell and O'Rand, 1978; Tung et al., 1979). These different properties suggest that mechanisms must operate to partition surface components into discrete domains during spermiogenesis. Regionalization of the cell surface could occur by several mechanisms. First, plasma membrane constituents may be partitioned selectively onto the surface of the residual body during spermiation, thereby being excluded from participating in the further differentiation of the spermatozoon. Certain antigens present on the surface of spermatogonia, spermatocytes, and spermatids appear to be partitioned onto the residual body in this manner (Millette and Bellvé, 1980). Second, some membrane antigens could be masked due to posttranslational modifications, steric hindrance, or a conformational change. Components may also be lost from the cell surface, perhaps internalized and subjected to proteolysis. Certain iso- and alloantigens may fall into this latter category (Tung and Fritz, 1978; Romrell et al., 1982). Third, other membrane constituents may be translocated laterally from certain regions by steric exclusion or moved by subsurface specializations into new zones. Finally, new surface macromolecules could be adsorbed onto or inserted directly into predefined membrane domains during the final differentiation of the spermatozoon. Once established, such surface domains may be stabilized by localized crosslinking, either to adjacent membrane components or to subsurface structural elements.

G. Gene Transcription during Spermatogenesis

Assembly of organelles and structural elements into the sperm cell occurs in a precise temporal sequence during spermiogenesis. These complicated morphological events predicate considerable need for protein synthesis at a time when the spermatid genome is condensing and becoming transcriptionally inactive. This demand for diverse proteins is met by the translation of gene products that are transcribed during meiotic prophase and early stages of spermiogenesis. Some mRNAs may be synthesized and translated during meiosis when the genome is active, and the proteins either incorporated into essential organelles or stored for subsequent biogenesis. Alternatively, specific meiotic mRNAs or their hnRNA precursors could be stored until required to encode for protein synthesis essential for assembling the sperm cell. Finally, certain genes activated during meiosis may continue to be expressed postmeiotically, while other unique genes may be transcribed exclusively from the haploid genome. There now is reasonable evidence to suggest that each of these possibilities may operate during spermatogenesis.

The relative transcriptional activities of the various mouse spermatogenic cells have been observed by autoradiography following the *in vivo* incorporation of [^{3}H]uridine (Monesi, 1964a, 1965a). High RNA synthetic rates occur in type A spermatogonia and then decline progressively in intermediate and type B spermatogonia to reach low levels in preleptotene spermatocytes. RNA synthesis is not detectable during early meiotic prophase. At zygonema, however, the rate increases rapidly to attain a peak in midpachytene spermatocytes before declining again through diplotene to undetectable levels during the two reduction divisions. Throughout meiosis, the condensed X and Y chromosomes do not appear to incorporate RNA precursors (Monesi, 1965b). While low levels of RNA synthesis are observed in early spermatids, no uridine incorporation is detectable after steps 8 to 9 of spermiogenesis. In Chinese and Syrian hamsters, the transcription profiles of spermatocytes and spermatids resemble those occuring in the mouse (Utakoji *et al.*, 1968). Later studies using high-resolution autoradiography confirm these early observations and also demonstrate ribosomal RNA (rRNA) synthesis in early meiotic prophase (Kierszenbaum and Tres, 1974a).

These studies do not allow for variations in membrane permeabilities and intracellular uridine pool sizes which could account for the observed differences in synthetic activity during meiosis and spermiogenesis. Nevertheless, *in vitro* studies on isolated pachytene spermatocytes and round spermatids suggest that the earlier data probably are valid. It should be noted that the two cell types synthesize RNA at comparable rates when both are expressed on a haploid genome basis (Loir, 1972).

1. Characterization of RNA Synthesized during Meiosis

The precise nuclear localization and identity of the nascent RNA molecules have been assessed by autoradiography, permitting tentative identification of rRNA and mRNA precursors that are synthesized in distinct regions of the spermatocyte nucleus. During the zygotene-to-midpachytene interval in both the mouse and the hamster, [³H]uridine is incorporated at low levels into the nucleolar masses adjacent to certain autosomal basal knobs (Kierszenbaum and Tres, 1974a). This synthesis presumably represents transcription of ribosomal DNA cistrons that are localized in nucleolar organizer regions (Hsu et al., 1975). Later, during midpachynema in mouse spermatocytes, these nucleolar bodies migrate toward the condensed sex chromosomes and coalesce to form the characteristic nucleolus (for review, see Kierszenbaum and Tres, 1978). By contrast, meiotic hnRNA synthesis in mouse spermatocytes is localized primarily to perichromosomal regions of the autosomes (Kierszenbaum and Tres, 1974a). In an *in vitro* study of human spermatocytes, Tres (1975) observed a peak of rRNA synthesis in late zygotene, followed by a prominent peak of hnRNA synthesis at midpachynema.

Biochemical analysis of RNA synthesis during spermatogenesis has been hampered by the cellular complexity of the mammalian testis. Despite these difficulties, diverse techniques have been used to characterize RNA transcribed during meiosis. Based on sedimentation analysis and base composition studies, hnRNA was shown to be the predominant species synthesized by decapsulated hamster testes (Muramatsu et al., 1968). Synthesis of hnRNA and low levels of rRNA have also been detected in cultured segments of seminiferous tubules containing midpachytene spermatocytes (Söderström and Parvinen, 1976). Despite problems of interpretation, both research groups tentatively attribute the major synthetic activity to pachytene spermatocytes. RNA synthesis has since been assessed directly in pachytene spermatocytes isolated from the rat (Grootegoed et al., 1977a) and the mouse (Geremia et al., 1978). These *in vitro* investigations demonstrate more convincingly that pachytene spermatocytes can synthesize rRNA and hnRNA, as identified by polyacrylamide gel electrophoresis (Grootegoed et al., 1977a) and sucrose gradient centrifugation (Geremia et al., 1978).

In somatic nuclei, intervening sequences (exons) in many large hnRNA molecules are deleted in the formation of cytoplasmic mRNAs (Miller, 1981; Perry, 1981). Therefore, the synthesis of hnRNA in spermatogenic cells is insufficient evidence for the formation of specific messenger sequences, particularly since much of the RNA synthesized remains in the nucleus until diplonema (Monesi, 1965a). Analysis by poly(U)-Sepharose chromatography indicates one-third of the *de novo* synthesized hnRNA in pachytene spermatocytes is polyadenylated (Söderström, 1976). By the same criterion, one-third of the polysomal RNA also is polyadenylated (Geremia *et al.*, 1978), suggesting that some hnRNA molecules are processed during meiotic prophase to yield cytoplasmic mRNAs (D'Agostino *et al.*, 1978).

RNA synthesis in isolated pachytene spermatocytes is not affected by additions of FSH and/or testosterone, thus supporting the concept that hormonal regulation of spermatogenesis is mediated by Sertoli cells (Grootegoed *et al.*, 1978). Although some investigators have reported androgen-binding activity in spermatogenic cells (Galena *et al.*, 1974; Sanborn *et al.*, 1975; Tsai *et al.*, 1977), both genetic (Lyon *et al.*, 1975) and biochemical (Grootegoed *et al.*, 1977b) evidence strongly suggest that these cells do not contain specific androgen receptors.

2. Transcription from Haploid Genes

The occurrence of RNA synthesis in haploid spermatids has been a point of contention for many years. Using high-resolution autoradiography, Kierszenbaum and Tres (1975) failed to find functional nucleoli and concluded that spermatids synthesize hnRNA. Recently, a cytochemical technique for selectively staining transcriptionally active nucleolar organizer regions (Goodpasture and Bloom, 1975; Bloom and Goodpasture, 1976) suggests that rRNA synthesis may occur during early spermiogenesis in a number of species, including the mouse (Schmid *et al.*, 1977).

Biochemical studies suggest that early spermatids synthesize both rRNA and mRNA. Following intratesticular injections of [^{3}H]uridine, Grootegoed *et al.* (1977a) recovered labeled 18 S, 28 S, and high M_r RNA species from isolated spermatids (steps 1–8). These cells, when labeled *in vitro*, exhibit similar RNA synthetic profiles as determined by sucrose gradient analysis (Geremia *et al.*, 1978; D'Agostino *et al.*, 1978). Analysis by poly(U)-Sepharose chromatography also suggests that approximately one-third of the cytoplasmic RNA synthesized in these cells is polyadenylated (Geremia *et al.*, 1978) and that some molecules, apparently active mRNAs, are bound to polysomes (Geremia *et al.*, 1978; D'Agostino *et al.*, 1978). It should be emphasized that these studies need to provide convincing evidence of cell purity and viability.

Similar results are obtained when oligo(dT)-cellulose chromatography is used to resolve 6 to 15 S poly[A$^+$]RNA (Erickson *et al.*, 1980a).

In seeking more definitive evidence, Erickson *et al.* (1980b) isolated total RNA from discrete populations of mouse spermatogenic cells and performed *in vitro* translation using the rabbit reticulolysate system. The translation products were screened for synthesis of protamines and phosphoglycerate kinase (PKG-2). Only minimal levels of [^{3}H]arginine were incorporated into the presumptive protamines, making it difficult to draw conclusions concerning the postmeiotic expression of these genes. The six-fold increase in the amount of PKG-2 translated following input of late spermatid RNA does not provide convincing evidence for the occurrence of haploid gene expression. Definitive evidence for the exclusive transcription of haploid genes will require specific use of cDNA probes prepared from testicular mRNA. While several research groups currently have such cDNA libraries, there are no reports on their use for analysis of postsegregational gene transcription.

3. Prolonged Stability of "Meiotic" RNA

RNA synthesized during meiotic prophase must have an unusually long half-life if it is to be used to direct translational events 10 to 15 days later during spermiogenesis. Autoradiographic evidence suggests that nuclear RNA in spermatocytes is released into the cytoplasm just prior to the first meiotic division where it remains throughout spermiogenesis (Monesi, 1964a), until the portion remaining is discarded within the residual body (Monesi, 1964a; Loir, 1972).

Estimates of the amount of stable RNA transcribed in spermatocytes vary considerably. RNA synthesized in isolated seminiferous tubule segments containing midpachytene spermatocytes apparently is stable for 36 hours (Söderström and Parvinen, 1976), even after a prolonged chase in the presence of actinomycin D (Söderström, 1976). By contrast, Grootegoed *et al.* (1977a) found RNA synthesized in isolated pachytene spermatocytes to be labile within 4 hours of incubation. This lability, however, may reflect degeneration of the cultured cells which can survive for only a few hours *in vitro*. The stability of RNA *in vivo* is probably much greater than this, since some fraction of the RNA synthesized in pachytene spermatocytes is preserved during spermiogenesis, some through advanced spermatid stages (Geremia *et al.*, 1977; Bellvé, 1982).

Attempts to characterize the stable RNA molecules in mammalian spermatids have not been definitive, although a major proportion is thought to be hnRNA (Söderström and Parvinen, 1976; Söderström, 1976). Support for the existence of stable mRNA is derived from the extensive characterization of trout protamine mRNAs (for reviews, see

Dixon *et al.*, 1977; Iatrou and Dixon, 1978). These mRNAs are first evident in the cytoplasm of primary spermatocytes and continue to accumulate during spermiogenesis (Iatrou *et al.*, 1978). The protamine mRNAs are processed and stored in the cytoplasm as distinct ribonucleoprotein particles prior to the synthesis of protamine in condensing spermatids. Thus, at least this one family of mRNAs is stored for 15 to 30 days during spermatogenesis.

Synthesis and processing of preribosomal RNA may be slow in mammalian primary spermatocytes (Galdieri and Monesi, 1974; Stefanini *et al.*, 1974; Söderström and Parvinen, 1976; Grootegoed *et al.*, 1977a). The 32 S ribosomal precursor accumulates in pachytene spermatocytes, suggesting the final step of the maturation sequence is rate limiting in these cells as it can be in somatic tissues. Those rRNA precursors synthesized during meiosis may be stored and used for translational events in spermatids.

H. Temporal Appearance and Synthesis of Spermatozoan Proteins

Protein synthesis is detectable by autoradiography at nearly all stages of spermatogenesis in the mouse (Monesi, 1964b, 1965a). The incorporation of ^{3}H-labeled amino acids occurs at increasing rates during the differentiation of type A spermatogonia and then declines substantially in type B spermatogonia. All meiotic cells synthesize protein. Maximal synthesis occurs at midpachynema and then continues at moderate levels through the meiotic reduction divisions to step 11 of spermiogenesis (Monesi, 1964b, 1965a). A peak in ^{3}H]arginine and ^{3}H]leucine incorporation is evident in elongating spermatids (Monesi, 1965a; Lee and Dixon, 1972). Generally, however, the incorporation of precursors into protein declines markedly during the maturation phase and is not detectable in step 16 spermatids (Monesi, 1964b, 1965a). This apparent decline in protein synthesis correlates with the regression of the highly structured endoplasmic reticulum in the rat (Clermont and Rambourg, 1978). Although valuable, these studies do not provide information either on the complexity of proteins being synthesized or on whether they have only a transient existence or are destined for assembly into the mature spermatozoon.

The temporal pattern of protein synthesis for the spermatozoon can be studied by utilization of the known kinetics of spermatogenesis. This differentiative process transforms undifferentiated spermatogonia into mature spermatozoa in a precise temporal sequence (Oakberg, 1956; Bellvé *et al.*, 1975; Meistrich *et al.*, 1975). Therefore, following an intratesticular injection of [³H]leucine, the sequence in which iso-topically labeled proteins appear in caudal spermatozoa reflects their ontogeny. Sperm components can also be processed into different fractions: the SDS-soluble proteins derived from the plasma membrane, acrosome, axoneme, and matrix and cristae of the mitochondria; the SDS-insoluble tail elements including structural proteins of the neck region, outer dense fibers, fibrous sheath, and outer membranes of the mitochondria; and the SDS-insoluble head comprising the perinuclear theca and nucleus (Bellvé *et al.*, 1975; O'Brien and Bellvé, 1980a; Bellvé, 1982). Assessment of the temporal appearance of [³H]leucine in these sperm fractions led to the observation that the SDS-soluble proteins were synthesized primarily during meiotic prophase and at declining levels during spermiogenesis (O'Brien and Bellvé, 1980b). In contrast, synthesis of the SDS-insoluble components of the sperm head and tail almost exclusively occurs during spermiogenesis, coincident with the assembly of these structures.

The complexity of proteins synthesized during meiotic prophase is substantial (> 250 species) but diminishes markedly as the cell progresses through spermiogenesis (Boitani *et al.*, 1980; Kramer and Erickson, 1982). Many proteins detected in autoradiographs of two-dimensional polyacrylamide gels are synthesized by both pachytene spermatocytes and spermatids, while the synthesis of others occurs in a stage-dependent manner. Presumably, some of the proteins incorporating [³⁵S]methionine exclusively during spermiogenesis are structural constituents of the nucleus and tail. These proteins could be translated from stored meiotic mRNA or they may represent products of haploid gene transcription.

1. Proteins Appearing during Meiosis

Meiotic prophase, a key transitional period in spermatogenesis, is characterized by the appearance of novel enzyme activities and structural proteins. In three mammalian species unique surface antigens appear in pachytene spermatocytes and are expressed by cells at all later stages of differentiation (O'Rand and Romrell, 1977; Millette and Bellvé, 1977; Tung and Fritz, 1978; Romrell *et al.*, 1982). H-2 and Ia histocompatibility antigens, although not testis-specific, also appear on the surface of mouse primary spermatocytes (Fellous *et al.*, 1976a, b). A variety of cell surface proteins have been identified on mouse primary spermatocytes (Millette and Moulding, 1981), but it is not known whether these also exist on cells prior to meiosis. Another surface constituent, the sulfatoxylgalactosyl glycerolipid, appears to be synthesized initially during meiotic prophase (Kornblatt, 1979). Mitochondrial enzymes change during meiotic prophase concomitant with the ultrastructural transformation of these organelles. Two testis isozymes, LDH-C_4 and cytochrome c_t, are first detectable in midpachytene spermatocytes (Hintz and Goldberg, 1977; Wheat et al., 1977). The activity of another mitochondrial enzyme, carnitine acetyltransferase, also is elevated in a mixture of spermatogenic cells predominantly containing pachytene spermatocytes (Vernon et al., 1971). During development of the rat the testis-specific cytoplasmic enzymes, cyclic nucleotide phosphodiesterase f (Monn et al., 1972) and sperm type hexokinase (Sosa et al., 1972), appear concomitantly with the inception of primary and secondary spermatocytes, respectively. The presence of these two isozymes in mature sperm suggests that their synthesis actually occurs in precursor germ cells. Yet only preliminary conclusions can be drawn from such developmental studies, since Sertoli cells mature concurrently with meiotic germ cells, as do a variety of other cell types present in the testis (Bellvé et al., 1977a).

The appearance of these protein constituents during meiosis coincides with the peak of protein synthesis at midpachynema. However, measurements of enzyme activity or detection of an antigen do not necessarily imply de novo synthesis of these macromolecules. In this regard LDH-C_4 is the only known enzyme whose biosynthetic profile has been monitored throughout spermatogenesis (Meistrich et al., 1977). Synthesis of LDH-C_4 first occurs in midpachytene spermatocytes and reaches maximal levels at late pachynema before declining during spermiogenesis to barely detectable levels in late spermatids.

Chromosomal proteins, both histones and non-histones (NHCP), undergo changes during meiosis. At least three atypical histones, two identified as testis-specific histone 1 species and another a histone 2 S, appear during early development of the mammalian testis (Branson et al., 1975; Shires et al., 1975, 1976; Levinger et al., 1978). The testis-specific designation may be premature, however, since relatively few somatic tissues have been examined in these comparative studies. Furthermore, Kistler and Geroch (1975) have observed small amounts of one atypical testis histone 1 in a variety of other tissues. This particular histone 1 species, perhaps present in low amounts in differentiating spermatogonia, increases relative to the somatic histone 1 when early primary spermatocytes appear in the testis. By contrast, the atypical histone 2S is detectable only after the appearance of primary spermatocytes (Grimes et al., 1975a; Kumaroo et al., 1975; Mills et al., 1977). Although both "testis-specific" histones are labeled by incubation of isolated pachytene spermatocytes with [³H]lysine (Brock et al., 1977, 1980), synthesis of these basic proteins has not been monitored at earlier stages of meiotic prophase or in spermatogonia. These histones persist in early spermatids (Brock *et al.*, 1977), and then along with somatic histones are eliminated from the nucleus by elongating spermatids (Grimes *et al.*, 1977).

Studies of the developing rat testis suggest the complement of NHCPs change when meiotic cells begin to appear (Kadohama and Turkington, 1974; Mills and Means, 1977). These two investigations, using different techniques, present conflicting data concerning the general trend of these changes. In mammals only one meiotic NHCP has been isolated and partially characterized. Designated R protein, this DNA-binding protein is detected only in zygotene and pachytene spermatocytes and therefore may be important in the synapsis of the homologous chromosomes (Mather and Hotta, 1977). Perhaps only a few "meiotic" nuclear proteins are assembled into the mature sperm nucleus (O'Brien and Bellvé, 1980b).

2. Proteins Appearing during Spermiogenesis

Both cytoplasmic and nuclear proteins apparently are synthesized by mammalian spermatids. In the guinea pig, where proacrosomal granules are formed in secondary spermatocytes, acrosomal antigens are detectable at, or just prior to, the initiation of spermiogenesis (Toullet *et al.*, 1973; Radu and Voisin, 1975). Sperm-specific antigens also appear in the acrosome during rabbit spermiogenesis (Johnson and Hunter, 1972a). Isozymes of the acrosomal enzymes hyaluronidase (Zaneveld *et al.*, 1973), N-acetyl-β-galactosidase and β-galactosidase (Majumder and Turkington, 1974) and the nonacrosomal testicular isozyme of phosphoglycerate kinase (Vandeberg *et al.*, 1976) first appear in the developing testis coincident with spermatids (for review, see Goldberg, 1977). Other metabolic enzymes, including α-glycerophosphate dehydrogenase (Schenkman *et al.*, 1965) and phosphamidase (Meyer and Weinmann, 1957), show increased activities at later stages of spermiogenesis. In addition, Romrell and O'Rand (1978) and Millette and Bellvé (1980) provide preliminary evidence for a dramatic increase in the number of surface antigenic sites during mammalian spermiogenesis, particularly in late spermatids. Unfortunately, except for LDH-X, the actual synthesis of spermatidal proteins has not been monitored.

As spermiogenesis proceeds, the complexity of nuclear proteins diminishes substantially as the histones and NHCPs are eliminated from the cell (Marushige and Marushige, 1974; Platz *et al.*, 1975). Studies in three mammals suggest that these proteins are transiently replaced by multiple basic proteins which are not detectable in epididymal sperm. These include the testis-specific protein (TP) identified by Kistler *et al.* (1973) which, according to its primary structure, is not a derivative of either histones or protamine (Kistler *et al.*, 1975b). Proteins with similar size and amino acid composition have also been isolated from human testis (Kistler *et al.*, 1975a). Subsequently, several other spermatidal basic proteins have been identified in the rat (Grimes *et al.*, 1975b, 1977; Platz *et al.*, 1976) and the ram (Loir and Lanneau, 1978). Since these proteins are synthesized in a defined temporal sequence during late spermiogenesis, they may facilitate the orderly condensation and elongation of the nucleus prior to the appearance of protamines (Grimes *et al.*, 1977; Loir and Lanneau, 1978; Mayer and Zirkin, 1979; Mayer *et al.*, 1981).

In mammalian sperm the principal nuclear proteins are the arginine- and cysteine-rich protamines whose temporal synthesis has been monitored in the mouse (Bellvé *et al.*, 1975) and rat (Calvin, 1976a). In autoradiographic studies, Monesi (1964b, 1965a) noted a prominent peak of [^{3}H]arginine incorporation into nuclei of steps 11 to 14 spermatids, an observation compatible with the recovery of isotopically labeled sperm from the distal excurrent ducts 11–13 days later (Kopečný and Pavlok, 1975; Goldberg *et al.*, 1977). The basic proteins being synthesized by late spermatids were identified conclusively as protamines by direct biochemical methods in the mouse (Bellvé *et al.*, 1975; Ecklund and Levine, 1975) and in the rat (Grimes *et al.*, 1977).

IV. MATURATION OF SPERMATOZOA IN THE EPIDIDYMIS

Eutherian sperm released from the seminiferous tubules are not capable of fertilization. Following transport through the rete testis and ductule efferentes, sperm enter the epididymis and undergo morphological and biochemical changes to acquire fertilizing capacity (for review, see Hamilton, 1977; Bedford, 1979). These maturational changes include structural alterations in both the sperm head and tail, changes in surface properties and constituents, and the acquisition of sustained forward motility. Thus far, no specific maturational change can be equated with the functional maturity of sperm although motility is an essential component. While earlier studies focused on resolving the question of whether intrinsic or extrinsic factors are responsible for these maturational changes (Orgebin-Crist, 1967; Bedford, 1967), recent efforts have clearly demonstrated that the epididymis actively promotes posttesticular differentiation of mammalian sperm (see Hamilton, 1977; Bedford, 1979). Moreover, many aspects of sperm maturation and viability now are known to be dependent on androgens, which mediate their effects by promoting and maintaining normal function of the epididymis (Orgebin-Crist et al., 1975; Hamilton, 1977).

The epididymis, a highly coiled duct, has three major regions: the caput, corpus, and cauda. Although the precise location of sperm maturation varies among species, the ability to fertilize usually is achieved by the time the sperm have entered the distal segment of the epididymis (Waites, 1980), where sperm are stored until ejaculation. Absorptive and secretory activity of the epithelium are considered responsible for the unique composition of epididymal plasma (Hamilton, 1977). During epididymal transit, sperm are concentrated 20-fold or more (Brooks, 1979) and are exposed to changes in their fluid environment including decreasing pH (Levine and Kelly, 1978; Howards et al., 1979), altered inorganic ion composition (Jones, 1978; Howards et al., 1979), and a marked accumulation of carnitine and glycerylphosphorylcholine (Brooks et al., 1974; Jones, 1978). Furthermore, specific proteins secreted by the epididymis appear to interact directly with sperm (Lea et al., 1978; Voglmayr et al., 1980; Moore, 1980).

A. Structural Changes in the Spermatozoon

Two ultrastructural features of sperm maturation—cytoplasmic droplet migration and acrosome remodeling—have been observed in mammalian species (Bedford, 1979). After spermiation a remnant of cytoplasm remains attached to the sperm in the neck region. During epididymal transit this cytoplasmic droplet migrates caudally along the midpiece and is eventually lost. At present the functional significance of this event remains obscure. Marked alterations in acrosomal shape have also been described in the guinea pig (Fawcett and Hollenberg, 1963), the chinchilla (Fawcett and Phillips, 1969a), and the pig-tailed macaque (Hoffer et al., 1981). Less prominent shape changes and reduction in acrosomal size occur in several other mammals (cf. Bedford, 1979). In addition, crystalline cores appear within the acrosomal contents of rabbit sperm during epididymal maturation (Fléchon, 1975). Once again, however, the physiological role of these ultrastructural changes has not been elucidated.

During epididymal passage in several species the plasma membrane appears to become loosened and marginally separated from the acrosome (Bedford, 1965; Fawcett and Phillips, 1969a). This change simply may be due to a fixation artifact (Jones, 1971) or may reflect changes in membrane permeability during sperm maturation (Hamilton, 1977). Alternatively, the apparent separation of plasma and acrosomal membranes could be related to the disappearance of flocculent material from the intervening space, at least in the rat (Suzuki and Nagano, 1980). The latter investigators also describe surface changes in the region overlying the acrosome during epididymal transit, including an apparent disorganization of hexagonal arrangements of membrane particles and alterations in surface glycocalyx material. Completion of these changes in the proximal cauda is correlated with the acquistion of fertilizing ability in this species and may reflect preparation of the cell surface for participation in capacitation and the acrosome reaction.

Although changes in nuclear and tail morphology generally do not occur as sperm traverse the epididymis, several sperm structures generally become more resistant to sonication (Henle *et al.*, 1938), detergents (Calvin and Bedford, 1971; Bedford and Calvin, 1974a), and trypsin (Meistrich *et al.*, 1976). These include the nucleus, perinuclear theca, basal plate, connecting piece, outer dense fibers, fibrous sheath, and outer mitochondrial membranes. Their increased structural stability has been attributed to a progressive increase in intra- and intermolecular disulfide cross-links among the constituent proteins during epididymal transit (Calvin and Bedford, 1971; Bedford and Calvin, 1974a).

B. Alterations in Cell-Surface Constituents

The surface of the mature sperm exhibits regions having distinct biochemical and functional properties. The acrosome reaction and gamete fusion are both restricted to discrete surface domains, suggesting that the membrane constituents in these regions may play crucial roles in fertilization. It is significant, therefore, that a number of surface properties, including charge density, adhesiveness, and resistance to cold shock, are altered during passage through the epididymis (Hamilton, 1977; Bedford, 1979). Furthermore, recent studies in several mammalian species have revealed striking posttesticular changes in plasma membrane constituents, particularly glycoproteins. These changes have received considerable attention because they may offer new molecular insights concerning the establishment and maintenance of sperm membrane domains and the development of contraceptive techniques that do not interfere with testicular function.

During epididymal transit sperm show marked losses in cholesterol and all classes of phospholipids, except choline plasmalogen (for review, see Voglmayr, 1975; Brooks, 1979). This is the major class of sperm phospholipid and may represent a metabolically inert membrane constituent while other phospholipids could be used as energy substrates (Selivonchick *et al.*, 1980). Also, the proportion of unsaturated fatty acids in the phospholipid fraction increases as sperm pass through the epididymis (Scott *et al.*, 1967; Poulos *et al.*, 1973). None of these lipid changes have yet been localized to the plasma membrane. However, observed changes in membrane permeability (Hamilton, 1977) and the greater susceptibility of cauda epididymal sperm to cold shock (Hammerstedt *et al.*, 1979) are consistent with expected physiochemical changes resulting from a loss of phospholipids and cholesterol and/or increases in unsaturated fatty acids.

Similar measurements of total protein content of bull spermatozoa indicate a concomitant loss of protein during epididymal maturation, with major quantitative and compositional changes occurring in the lipoprotein fraction (Lavon *et al.*, 1971). Although the plasma membrane has been implicated as the site of these biochemical changes (Lavon *et al.*, 1971), shedding of the cytoplasmic droplet also must account for some of the losses in protein and lipid as sperm traverse the epididymis (Voglmayr, 1975). More recently, investigators have used a variety of surface probes to document epididymal changes in sperm surface proteins, including both losses and additions of specific constituents.

Lectins with different sugar specificities define changes in the number and distribution of sugar residues on the sperm surface during epididymal transit. Concanavalin A (con A) binding sites may increase (Gordon *et al.*, 1975; Fournier-Delpech *et al.*, 1977), decrease (Fournier-Delpech and Courot, 1980), or remain unchanged (Nicolson and Yanagimachi, 1979), depending on species and experimental protocol. Similar changes have been observed with other lectins including *Ricinis communis* agglutinin and wheat germ agglutinin (Nicolson *et al.*, 1977). In addition, decreases in lectin-mediated agglutinability and changes in the pattern of lectin binding on the sperm surface have been observed following epididymal transit (for review, see Nicolson and Yanagimachi, 1979; also, Olson and Danzo, 1981). Recently, variations in lectin binding have been correlated with changes in specific surface glycoproteins on rat sperm (Olson and Danzo, 1981). These investigators detected an apparent loss (15–25%) of con A binding sites, reflecting a decrease in labeling of two high M_r components that is partly offset by increased binding to an M_r-37,000 glycoprotein.

Isotopic surface labeling also has revealed epididymal changes in sperm membrane proteins (Olson and Hamilton, 1978). For instance, a 37,000-M_r surface glycoprotein(s) of rat sperm is labeled when cauda, but not caput, cells are exposed to ^{3}H-labeled sodium borohydride. By contrast, lactoperoxidase-catalyzed iodination labels a comparable $37,000\text{-}M_r$ surface component in both caput and cauda sperm (Olson and Danzo, 1981). Although the identity of these labeled constituents has not been established, the results may reflect glycosylation of a surface protein during epididymal transit, since both the con A and ^{3}H-labeled sodium borohydride procedures label externally oriented sugar residues. Additional epididymal variations in sperm membrane proteins have been detected following ^{125}I surface labeling of tyrosine and histidine residues in the rat (Olson and Danzo, 1981), rabbit (Nicolson et al., 1979; Oliphant and Singhas, 1979), and ram (Voglmayr et al., 1980).

Recently, Feuchter et al. (1981) prepared monoclonal antibodies recognizing surface determinants that are detected only on sperm recovered from distal segments of the mouse epididymis. Other immunological probes depict a loss and/or modification of specific glycoprotein(s) on the surface of boar sperm during epididymal maturation (Bostwick et al., 1980; Hunter and Schellpfeffer, 1981). Although these surface components have not yet been isolated and characterized, the results provide additional evidence for the dynamic nature of the sperm surface during epididymal maturation.

Several explanations may account for the observed epididymal variations in sperm surface proteins (see Olson and Hamilton, 1978; Feuchter et al., 1981). First, new plasma membrane components could either be synthesized de novo or derived from some preexisting intracellular pool. Second, reactive sites could either be lost or unmasked on the sperm surface following the removal of peripheral membrane constituents or the limited hydrolysis of peptide or saccharide moieties. Third, posttranslational modifications such as phosphorylation or glycosylation also may alter sperm surface proteins. Such enzymatic alterations are possible, particularly in view of the protein kinase activity associated with the sperm surface (Majumder, 1978) and the galactosyltransferase activity in rat epididymal samples (Hamilton and Gould, 1980). The results of Olson and Hamilton (1978) and Olson and Danzo (1981) are consistent with glycosylation of sperm surface constituents in the epididymis. Finally, new proteins could bind to the sperm surface after being secreted by the epididymal epithelium. Coating antigens were proposed in earlier immunological studies (Hunter, 1969; Barker and Amann, 1971; Johnson and Hunter, 1972b; Killian and Amann, 1973). One such epididymal antigen is recognized by a monoclonal antibody (Vernon et al., 1982), which will greatly facilitate further studies on the physiological function of this mouse sperm-surface constituent.

Sperm-binding acidic glycoproteins secreted by the rat epididymis have been identified in several investigations of posttesticular sperm maturation (Lea *et al.*, 1978; Garberi *et al.*, 1979; Brooks and Higgins, 1980; Bayard *et al.*, 1981). One component characterized in each of these studies has an M_r of 30,000 to 40,000. Secretion of these glycoproteins, probably from the principal cells (Lea *et al.*, 1978; Bayard *et al.*, 1981), appears to be androgen-dependent and restricted to particular regions of the epididymis. Comparable epididymal glycoproteins also exist in the ram (Voglmayr *et al.*, 1980), rabbit, and hamster (Moore, 1980). Similar characteristics of these proteins include acidic isoelectric points, androgen-dependence, and localization in specific epididymal regions (Moore, 1980).

Other studies have examined in detail the synthetic and secretory capabilities of the epididymis both *in vivo* (Flickinger, 1979; Fain-Maurel *et al.*, 1981) and *in vitro* (Orgebin-Crist and Jahad, 1978; Jones *et al.*, 1980, 1981). High-resolution autoradiography of protein metabolism in the mouse epididymis generally confirms typical anabolic pathways for synthesis, Golgi processing, and secretion of protein(s) into the lumen, although secretory vesicles and exocytosis have not been observed (Flickinger, 1979; Fain-Maurel *et al.*, 1981). These investigations also suggest that smooth endoplasmic reticulum may participate in the synthesis and/or vectorial transport of proteins in the caput epithelial cells. Following *in vitro* incorporation of [^{35}S]methionine, rat and rabbit epididymal proteins show similar regional variations in synthetic profiles and dependence on circulating androgens and/or factors in testicular fluid (Jones *et al.*, 1980, 1981). Measurements of dolichol concentration and synthesis in the epididymis provide evidence for active glycoprotein synthesis in this organ (Wenström and Hamilton, 1980). These latter investigators found substantial concentrations of dolichols, which participate in the assembly of *N*-glycosylated glycoproteins, in both the testis and epididymis, with the highest concentrations in the corpus epididymis.

The binding of glycoproteins to sperm during epididymal transit could account for a number of observed changes in surface properties such as charge density and adhesiveness (for review, see Bedford, 1975). Visible markers, including colloidal iron and conjugated lectins, indicate that the distribution of negative charge and/or sugar residues on sperm is increased during epididymal maturation (Courtens and Fournier-Delpech, 1979; Nicolson and Yanagimachi, 1979). This increase in anionic charges at the sperm surface, both at the phospholipid–water interface and in the glycocalyx region (Bedford, 1963; Hammerstedt *et al.*, 1979), may be primarily due to the addition of sialic acid residues (Holt, 1980). Perhaps related to the variations in charge density and distribution is the increased tendency for mature sperm to agglutinate in many mammalian species (Bedford, 1975).

Several investigations have provided evidence that epididymal glycoproteins contribute to the development of sperm fertilizing capability. Substantial quantities of surface-bound epididymal proteins apparently are lost when rat sperm are incubated *in utero* or under *in vitro* conditions favoring capacitation (Kohane *et al.*, 1980). These investigators suggest that bound glycoproteins may play a protective role in preventing the acrosome reaction from occurring prematurely. In both rabbits and hamsters, antisera prepared against individual sperm-binding glycoproteins from the epididymis were effective in significantly reducing *in vivo* fertilization rates, thus suggesting that these proteins may participate in sperm-egg recognition or binding (Moore, 1981). Finally, the forward motility protein identified by Hoskins and associates (1979) is a glycoprotein, apparently of epididymal origin (see below).

C. Acquisition of Motility

During epididymal transit mammalian spermatozoa acquire the capacity for progressive motility. This capacity is observed as a transition from circular or whiplashlike movements of caput sperm to vigorous forward motion of sperm isolated from the cauda epididymis (for reviews, see Hamilton, 1977; Hoskins *et al.*, 1978). Although definitive evidence of *in situ* immotility is lacking (Brooks, 1979), spermatozoa apparently are quiescent in the epididymis and are activated during ejaculation or transfer to appropriate *in vitro* conditions (Jones, 1978). Thus, the acquisition of sperm motility involves both maturational changes and a triggering event at ejaculation.

Energy supply apparently is not a limiting factor in the initiation of motility. Spermatozoa can metabolize a large variety of exogenous substrates (Voglmayr, 1975; Brooks, 1979) and also can accumulate carnitine, a potential endogenous substrate for energy metabolism, during epididymal migration (Casillas, 1973; Brooks *et al.*, 1974; Casillas and Chaipayungpan, 1979). Furthermore, ATP concentrations are similar in testicular and ejaculated ram spermatozoa (Voglmayr, 1975). Observed epididymal variations in sperm metabolism, including altered rates of glycolysis and respiration, may be secondary consequences of the development of motility capacity (Harrison, 1977).

Cyclic AMP (cAMP) levels clearly play a role in the regulation of sperm motility (for reviews, see Hoskins and Casillas, 1975; Garbers and Kopf, 1980). Earlier studies of Garbers *et al.* (1971a) indicated that the motility of bovine cauda epididymal sperm is stimulated by a variety of cyclic nucleotide phosphodiesterase inhibitors. Subsequent studies have demonstrated similar stimulatory effects of both phosphodiesterase inhibitors and cAMP analogs on cauda epididymal or ejaculated sperm in a number of mammalian species (Garbers et al., 1971b, 1973a,b; Frenkel et al., 1973; for review, see Garbers and Kopf, 1980). Apparently, both intensity (evaluated by subjective criteria or more quantitative measures such as beat frequency) and percentage of motile sperm are enhanced by these treatments (Schoenfeld et al., 1973; Lindemann, 1978). Furthermore, observed stimulatory effects on motility are mediated by increases in intracellular cAMP concentrations which precede alterations in sperm metabolism (Garbers et al., 1973a,b).

Immature sperm do not show consistent responses to phosphodiesterase inhibitors or cAMP analogs, perhaps because differences exist among cells recovered from different species and different locations within the reproductive tract. Testicular sperm of at least two species are not stimulated by these agents (Cascieri et al., 1976; Wyker and Howards, 1977), while treated caput epididymal sperm generally exhibit limited flagellar activity without forward progression (Hoskins et al., 1975, 1978; Wyker and Howards, 1977). Thus, cAMP alone is not sufficient for the initiation of normal forward motility (Hoskins et al., 1978).

Certain sperm maturational changes that occur during epididymal transit may be related to the acquisition of motility. The cyclic AMP content of bovine sperm increases twofold in the epididymis (Hoskins et al., 1974). This increase does not appear to be due to sperm adenyl cyclase activity, which is several times greater in the caput compared to the cauda epididymis (Casillas et al., 1980). Instead, cAMP levels may be regulated primarily by the sperm cAMP phosphodiesterase activity that decreases significantly along the bovine epididymis (Stephens et al., 1979). Hoskins and associates (1978, 1979) have postulated that the development of progressive motility depends upon at least two factors—increased intracellular cAMP levels and the binding of a specific forward motility protein (FMP) to the sperm surface. Bovine FMP has been characterized as a heat-stable glycoprotein, M_r 37,500, originating in the epididymis and binding to sperm as they traverse this organ (Acott and Hoskins, 1978, 1981; Brandt et al., 1978). Similar activity has been identified in the seminal plasma from several mammals, and bovine FMP stimulates forward motility of other mammalian spermatozoa (Acott et al., 1979). The significance of these observations has not been fully determined, however, particularly in light of a recent report indicating that earlier estimates of FMP activity were at least 50% too high (Stephens *et al.*, 1981).

A number of recent investigations have begun to further define the relationship between elevated cAMP levels and enhanced sperm motility. Using detergent-extracted bull spermatozoa, Lindemann (1978) has presented evidence that cAMP may activate the flagellar system directly. Alternately, the effect of cAMP on sperm motility may be mediated via protein phosphorylation according to the classical model of cAMP action. Multiple sperm cAMP-dependent protein kinases have been characterized (Hoskins *et al.*, 1972; Garbers *et al.*, 1973c), and potential substrates for these enzymes are recovered in membrane and cytosolic fractions of sperm (Huacuja *et al.*, 1977; Brandt and Hoskins, 1980). Brandt and Hoskins (1980) have provided indirect evidence that the phosphorylation of a 55,000-M_r protein may be correlated with motility. Subsequently, Tash and Means (1982), using detergent-lysed dog sperm, demonstrated that cAMP stimulates motility and protein phosphorylation under identical experimental conditions, while calcium has inhibitory effects on both. Tubulin and perhaps a dynein subunit may be among the sperm proteins phosphorylated in association with cAMP-enhanced motility (Tash and Means, 1982). Both stimulatory and inhibitory effects of calcium on sperm motility have been reported, and the observed differences may be related to concentration dependence and species specificity (for review, see Garbers and Kopf, 1980). The precise relationship between cAMP and calcium as modulators of sperm motility have not been well defined, although interactive effects of ion transport (Peterson *et al.*, 1979) and adenyl cyclase activities (Hyne and Garbers, 1979) have been described.

Treatment of spermatozoa with typical mammalian hormones generally does not result in enhanced motility or elevated cAMP levels (Hoskins and Casillas, 1975; Garbers and Kopf, 1980). However, other factors, including acetylcholine (Nelson, 1978) and a low-molecular-weight sperm constituent that may be taurine (Bavister *et al.*, 1978; Mrsny *et al.*, 1979), have been identified as potential activators of sperm motility.

V. DISCUSSION

The biogenesis and molecular organization of the mammalian spermatozoon have been topics of intense research during the past decade. Progress stemming from these studies has been facilitated greatly by the recent endeavors to integrate morphological, immunological, and biochemical techniques. These approaches, coupled with new methods for cell separation and fractionation, have enabled investigators to identify and to localize many novel constituents of the sperm cell. Consequently, much more now is known concerning the cell's many structural and regulatory proteins, which generally exist in discrete cellular organelles and have distinct developmental origins during meiosis and spermiogenesis. Yet, still fewer than 100 sperm components have been characterized biochemically and assigned physiological functions, even though a complex array of proteins comprise certain structures and organelles. Presumably, many constituents are involved in protecting the genome, energy metabolism, motility, capacitation, acrosome reaction, ovum recognition, and fertilization. Other components may subserve less obvious but essential events after fertilization, during formation of the male pronucleus and subsequent embryogenesis. The complexity of these diverse processes affirms the necessity and the challenge of resolving the underlying molecular mechanisms.

The mature spermatozoon is the product of germ cell differentiation. Once committed to meiosis the germ cell acquires a variety of novel components. These include constituents associated with chromatin, cytoplasmic organelles and flagellum, and the plasma membrane, which, in most instances, are assembled into the polarized sperm cell during spermiogenesis. Other components are adsorbed to the cell surface during epididymal maturation. Preliminary evidence suggests that these processes occur in an integrated temporal sequence during spermatogenesis. However, this conclusion is based on limited evidence. Considerably more research is required to define the molecular events that initiate and regulate the differentiation of germ cells. Direct evidence to support the "sustentacular" role of the Sertoli cells is just becoming available and undoubtedly will be a main focus of research on mammalian spermatogenesis.

ACKNOWLEDGMENTS

The preparation of this chapter was funded, in part, by research grants HD 08270 and HD 12700 and Center grant HD 06916 from the National Institute of Child Health and Human Development. Dr. Deborah A. O'Brien is a Medical Foundation Research Fellow, sponsored by the Medical Foundation, Inc., Boston, Massachusetts. The authors extend their appreciation to Steven Borack of the photographic unit and to Mrs. Barbara Lewis for help in preparing the manuscript.

REFERENCES

Acott, T. S., and Hoskins, D. D. (1978). Bovine sperm forward motility protein: Partial purification and characterization. *J. Biol. Chem.* **253,** 6744–6750.

Acott, T. S., and Hoskins, D. D. (1981). Bovine sperm forward motility protein: Binding to epididymal spermatozoa. *Biol. Reprod.* **24,** 234–240.

Acott, T. S., Johnson, D. J., Brandt, H., and Hoskins, D. D. (1979). Sperm forward motility protein: Tissue distribution and species cross reactivity. *Biol. Reprod.* **20,** 247–252.

Adams, G. M. W., Huang, B., Piperno, G., and Luck, D. J. L. (1981). The central pair microtubular complex of *Chlamydomonas* flagella: Polypeptide composition as revealed by analysis of mutants. *J. Cell Biol.* **91,** 69–76.

Afzelius, B. (1959). Electron microscopy of the sperm tail: Results obtained with a new fixative. *J. Biophys. Biochem. Cytol.* **5,** 269–278.

Agutter, P. S., and Richardson, J. C. W. (1980). Nuclear non-chromatin proteinaceous structures: Their role in the organization and function of the interphase nucleus. *J. Cell Sci.* **44,** 395–435.

Allison, A. C., and Hartree, E. F. (1970). Lysosomal enzymes in the acrosome and their possible role in fertilization. *J. Reprod. Fertil.* **21,** 501–515.

Amos, L. A., Linck, R. W., and Klug, A. (1976). Molecular structure of flagellar microtubules. *Cold Spring Harbor Conf. Cell Proliferation* **3** (Book C), 847–867.

André, J. (1962). Contribution à la connaissance du chondriome. Etude de ses modifications ultrastructurales pendant la spermatogénèse. *J. Ultrastruct. Res., Suppl.* **3,** 1–85.

Artzt, K., Dubois, P., Bennett, D., Condamine, H. Babinet, C., and Jacob, F. (1973). Surface antigens common to mouse cleavage embryos and primitive teratocarcinoma cells in culture. *Proc. Natl. Acad. Sci. U.S.A.* **70,** 2988–2992.

Artzt, K., Bennett, D., and Jacob, F. (1974). Primitive teratocarcinoma cells express a differentiation antigen specified by a gene at the T-locus in the mouse. *Proc. Natl. Acad. Sci. U.S.A.* **71,** 811–814.

Austin, C. R., and Bishop, M. W. H. (1958a). Some features of the acrosome and perforatorium in mammalian spermatozoa. *Proc. R. Soc. London, Ser. B* **149,** 234–240.

Austin, C. R., and Bishop, M. W. H. (1958b). Role of the rodent acrosome and perforatorium in fertilization. *Proc. R. Soc. London, Ser. B* **149,** 241–248.

Baccetti, B., and Afzelius, B. A. (1976). The biology of the sperm cell. *Monogr. Dev. Biol.* **10,** 81–108.

Baccetti, B., Pallini, V., and Burrini, A. G. (1973). The accessory fibers of the sperm tail. I. Structure and chemical composition of the bull coarse fibers. *J. Submicrosc. Cytol.* **5,** 237–256.

Baccetti, B., Pallini, V., and Burrini, A. G. (1976a). The accessory fibers of the sperm tail. II. Their role in binding zinc in mammals and cephalopods. *J. Ultrastruct. Res.* **54,** 261–275.

Baccetti, B., Pallini, V., and Burrini, A. G. (1976b). The accessory fibers of the sperm tail. III. High-sulfur and low-sulfur components in mammals and cephalopods. *J. Ultrastruct. Res.* **57,** 289–308.

Baccetti, B., Bigliardi, E., and Burrini, A. G. (1980). The morphogenesis of vertebrate perforatorium. *J. Ultrastruct. Res.* **71,** 272–287.

Balhorn, R. (1982). A model for the structure of chromatin in mammalian sperm. *J. Cell Biol.* **93,** 298–305.

Balhorn, R., Gledhill, B. L., and Wyrobek, A. J. (1977). Mouse sperm chromatin proteins: Quantitative isolation and partial characterization. *Biochemistry* **16**, 4074–4080.

Barker, L. D. S., and Amann, R. P. (1971). Epididymal physiology. II. Immunofluorescent analyses of epithelial secretion and absorption, and of bovine sperm maturation. *J. Reprod. Fertil.* **26**, 319–332.

Bartoov, B., and Messer, G. Y. (1976). Isolation of mitochondria from ejaculated ram spermatozoa. *J. Ultrastruct. Res.* **57**, 68–76.

Bavister, B. D., Rogers, B. J., and Yanagimachi, R. (1978). The effects of cauda epididymal plasma on the motility and acrosome reaction of hamster and guinea pig spermatozoa in vitro. *Biol. Reprod.* **19**, 358–363.

Bayard, F., Duguet, L., Mazzuca, M., and Faye, J. C. (1981). Study of a glycoprotein produced by the rat epididymis. *In* "Reproductive Processes and Contraception" (K. W. McKerns, ed.), pp. 393–405. Plenum, New York.

Bearer, E. L., and Friend, D. S. (1982). Modifications of anionic-lipid domains preceding membrane fusion in guinea pig sperm. *J. Cell Biol.* **92**, 604–615.

Bechtol, K. B., Brown, S. C., and Kennett, R. H. (1979). Recognition of differentiation antigens of spermatogenesis in the mouse by using antibodies from spleen cell-myeloma hybrids after syngeneic immunization. *Proc. Natl. Acad. Sci. U.S.A.* **76**, 363–367.

Bedford, J. M. (1963). Morphological changes in rabbit spermatozoa during passage through the epididymis. *J. Reprod. Fertil.* **5**, 169–177.

Bedford, J. M. (1965). Changes in fine structure of the rabbit sperm head during passage through the epididymis. *J. Anat.* **99**, 891–906.

Bedford, J. M. (1967). Effect of duct ligation on the fertilizing ability of spermatozoa from different regions of the rabbit epididymis. *J. Exp. Zool.* **166**, 271–282.

Bedford, J. M. (1968). Ultrastructural changes in the sperm head during fertilization in the rabbit. *Am. J. Anat.* **123**, 329–358.

Bedford, J. M. (1972). An electron microscopic study of sperm penetration into the rabbit egg after natural mating. *Am. J. Anat.* **133**, 213–254.

Bedford, J. M. (1975). Maturation, transport, and fate of spermatozoa in the epididymis. *In* "Handbook of Physiology" (D. W. Hamilton and R. O. Greep, eds.), Sect. 7, Vol. V, pp. 303–317. Am. Physiol. Soc., Washington, D.C.

Bedford, J. M. (1979). Evolution of the sperm maturation and sperm storage functions of the epididymis. *In* "The Spermatozoon" (D. W. Fawcett and J. M. Bedford, eds.), pp. 7–21. Urban & Schwarzenberg, Baltimore, Maryland.

Bedford, J. M., and Calvin, H. I. (1974a). Changes in -S-S-linked structures in the sperm tail during epididymal maturation, with comparative observations in sub-mammalian species. *J. Exp. Zool.* **187**, 181–204.

Bedford, J. M., and Calvin, H. I. (1974b). The occurrence and possible functional significance of -S-S-crosslinks in sperm heads, with particular reference to eutherian mammals. *J. Exp. Zool.* **188**, 137–156.

Bedford, J. M., Bent, M. J., and Calvin, H. I. (1973). Variations in the structural character and stability of the nuclear chromatin in morphologically normal human spermatozoa. *J. Reprod. Fertil.* **33**, 19–29.

Bellvé, A. R. (1979). The molecular biology of mammalian spermatogenesis. *In* "Oxford Reviews of Reproductive Biology" (C. A. Finn, ed.), pp. 159–261. Oxford Univ. Press (Clarendon), London and New York.

Bellvé, A. R. (1982). Biogenesis of the mammalian spermatozoon. *In* "Prospects for Sexing Mammalian Sperm" (R. P. Amann and G. E. Seidel, Jr., eds.), pp. 69–102, Colorado Assoc. Univ. Press, Boulder.

Bellvé, A. R., and Carraway, R. (1978). Characterization of two basic chromosomal proteins isolated from mouse spermatozoa. *J. Cell Biol.* **79**, 177a.

Bellvé, A. R., Anderson, E., and Hanley-Bowdoin, L. (1975). Synthesis and amino acid composition of basic proteins in mammalian sperm nuclei. *Dev. Biol.* **47**, 349–365.

Bellvé, A. R., Cavicchia, J. C., Millette, C. F., O'Brien, D. A., Bhatnagar, Y. M., and Dym, M. (1977a). Spermatogenic cells of the prepuberal mouse. Isolation and morphological characterization. *J. Cell Biol.* **74**, 68–85.

Bellvé, A. R., Millette, C. F., Bhatnagar, Y. M., and O'Brien, D. A. (1977b). Dissociation of the mouse testis and characterization of isolated spermatogenic cells. *J. Histochem. Cytochem.* **25**, 480–494.

Bendet, I. J., and Bearden, J., Jr. (1972). Birefringence of bull sperm. II. Form birefringence of bull sperm. *J. Cell Biol.* **55**, 501–510.

Bennett, D., Goldberg, E., Dunn, L. C., and Boyse, E. A. (1972). Serological detections of a cell-surface antigen specified by the T (brachyury) mutant gene in the house mouse. *Proc. Natl. Acad. Sci. U.S.A.* **69**, 2076–2080.

Berezny, R. (1979). Dynamic properties of the nuclear matrix. *In* "The Cell Nucleus" (H. Busch, ed.), Vol. 7, Part 1, pp. 413–456. Academic Press, New York.

Bernstein, M. H., and Teichman, R. J. (1972). Regional differentiation in the heads of spermatozoa of rabbit, man and bull. *Am. J. Anat.* **133**, 165–178.

Bernstein, M. H., and Teichman, R. J. (1973). A chemical procedure for the extraction of the acrosomes of mammalian spermatozoa. *J. Reprod. Fertil.* **33**, 239–244.

Bloom, S. E., and Goodpasture, C. (1976). An improved technique for selective staining of nucleolar organizer regions in human chromosomes. *Hum. Genet.* **34**, 199–206.

Bloom, W., and Fawcett, D. W. (1975). "A Textbook of Histology," p. 821. Saunders, Philadelphia, Pennsylvania.

Bode, J., and Lesemann, D. (1977). The anatomy of cooperative binding between protamines and DNA. *Hoppe-Seyler's Z. Physiol. Chem.* **358**, 1505–1512.

Boitani, C., Geremia, R., Rossi, R., and Monesi, V. (1980). Electrophoretic pattern of polypeptide synthesis in spermatocytes and spermatids of the mouse. *Cell Differ.* **9**, 41–49.

Bostwick, E. F., Bentley, M. D., Hunter, A. G., and Hammer, R. (1980). Identification of a surface glycoprotein or porcine spermatozoa and its alteration during epididymal maturation. *Biol. Reprod.* **23**, 161–169.

Bradbury, E. M., Prince, W. C., and Wilkinson, G. R. (1962). Polarized infrared studies of nucleoproteins. I. Nucleoprotamines. *J. Mol. Biol.* **4**, 39–49.

Bradley, F. M., Meth, B. M., and Bellvé, A. R. (1981). Structural proteins of the mouse spermatozoan tail: An electrophoretic analysis. *Biol. Reprod.* **24**, 691–701.

Brandt, H., and Hoskins, D. D. (1980). A cAMP-dependent phosphorylated motility protein in bovine epididymal sperm. *J. Biol. Chem.* **255**, 982–987.

Brandt, H., Acott, T. S., Johnson, D. J., and Hoskins, D. D. (1978). Evidence for an epididymal origin of bovine sperm forward motility protein. *Biol. Reprod.* **19**, 830–835.

Branson, R. E., Grimes, S. R., Jr., Yonuschot, G., and Irvin, J. L. (1975). The histones of rat testis. *Arch. Biochem. Biophys.* **168**, 403–412.

Brock, W., Trostle, P., and Meistrich, M. (1977). Synthesis of testis-specific histones in pachytene spermatocytes. *J. Cell Biol.* **75**, 167a.

Brock, W. A., Trostle, P. K., and Meistrich, M. L. (1980). Meiotic synthesis of testis histones in the rat. *Proc. Natl. Acad. Sci. U.S.A.* **77**, 371–375.

Brokaw, C. J., Luck, D. J. L., and Huang, B. (1982). Analysis of the movement of *Chlamydomonas* flagella: The function of the radial spoke system is revealed by comparison of wild type and mutant flagella. *J. Cell Biol.* **92**, 722–732.

Brooks, D. E. (1979). Biochemical environment of sperm maturation. *In* "The Spermatozoon" (D. W. Fawcett and J. M. Bedford, eds.), pp. 43–53. Urban & Schwarzenberg, Baltimore, Maryland.

Brooks, D. E., and Higgins, S. J. (1980). Characterization and androgen-dependence of proteins associated with luminal fluid and spermatozoa in the rat epididymis. *J. Reprod. Fertil.* **59,** 363–375.

Brooks, D. E., Hamilton, D. W., and Mallek, A. H. (1974). Carnitine and glycerylphosphorylcholine in the reproductive tract of the male rat. *J. Reprod. Fertil.* **36,** 141–160.

Brown, C. R., and Harrison, R. A. P. (1978). The activation of proacrosin in spermatozoa from ram, bull and boar. *Biochim. Biophys. Acta* **526,** 202–217.

Brown, C. R., and Hartree, E. F. (1974). Distribution of a trypsin-like proteinase in the ram spermatozoon. *J. Reprod. Fertil.* **36,** 195–198.

Brown, C. R., and Hartree, E. F. (1975). An acrosin inhibitor in ram spermatozoa that does not originate from the seminal plasma. *Hoppe-Seyler's Z. Physiol. Chem.* **356,** 1909–1913.

Bryan, J., and Wilson, L. (1971). Are cytoplasmic microtubules heteropolymers? *Proc. Natl. Acad. Sci. U.S.A.* **8,** 1762–1766.

Bryan, J. H. D., and Unnithan, R. R. (1972). Non-specific esterase activity in bovine acrosomes. *Histochem. J.* **4,** 413–419.

Burgos, M. H., and Fawcett, D. W. (1955). Studies on the fine structure of the mammalian testis. I. Differentiation of the spermatids in the cat *(Felis domestica). J. Biophys. Biochem. Cytol.* **1,** 287–299.

Calvin, H. I. (1976a). Comparative analysis of the nuclear basic proteins in rat, human, guinea pig, mouse and rabbit spermatozoa. *Biochim. Biophys. Acta* **434,** 377–389.

Calvin, H. I. (1976b). Isolation and subfractionation of mammalian sperm heads and tails. *Methods Cell Biol.* **13,** 85–104.

Calvin, H. I. (1979). Electrophoretic evidence for the identity of the major zinc-binding polypeptides in the rat sperm tail. *Biol. Reprod.* **21,** 873–882.

Calvin, H. I., and Bedford, J. M. (1971). Formation of disulphide bonds in the nucleus and accessory structures of mammalian spermatozoa during maturation in the epididymis. *J. Reprod. Fertil., Suppl.* **13,** 65–75.

Calvin, H. I., Hwang, F. H.-F., and Wohlrab, H. (1975). Localization of zinc in a dense fiber-connecting piece fraction of rat sperm tails analogous chemically to hair keratin. *Biol. Reprod.* **13,** 228–239.

Campanella, G., Gabbiani, G., Baccetti, B., Burrini, A. G., and Pallini, V. (1979). Actin and myosin in the vertebrate acrosomal region. *J. Submicrosc. Cytol.* **11,** 53–71.

Cascieri, M., Amann, R. P., and Hammerstedt, R. H. (1976). Adenine nucleotide changes at initiation of bull sperm motility. *J. Biol. Chem.* **251,** 787–793.

Casillas, E. R. (1973). Accumulation of carnitine by bovine spermatozoa during maturation in the epididymis. *J. Biol. Chem.* **248,** 8227–8232.

Casillas, E. R., and Chaipayungpan, S. (1979). The distribution of carnitine and acetylcarnitine in the rabbit epididymis and the carnitine content of spermatozoa during maturation. *J. Reprod. Fertil.* **56,** 439–444.

Casillas, E. R., Elder, C. M., and Hoskins, D. D. (1980). Adenylate cyclase activity of bovine spermatozoa during maturation in the epididymis and the activation of sperm particulate adenylate cyclase by GTP and polyamines. *J. Reprod. Fertil.* **59,** 297–302.

Clarke, G. N., and Yanagimachi, R. (1978). Actin in mammalian sperm heads. *J. Exp. Zool.* **203,** 125–132.

Clermont, Y., and Rambourg, A. (1978). Evolution of the endoplasmic reticulum during rat spermiogenesis. *Am. J. Anat.* **151**, 191–212.

Clermont, Y., Einberg, E., Leblond, C. P., and Wagner, S. (1955). The perforatorium—An extension of the nuclear membrane of the rat spermatozoon. *Anat. Rec.* **121**, 1–12.

Clermont, Y., Lalli, M., and Rambourg, A. (1981). Ultrastructural localization of nicotinamide adenine dinucleotide phosphatase (NADPase), thiamine pyrophosphatase (TPPase), and cytidine monophosphate (CMPase) in the Golgi apparatus of early spermatids of the rat. *Anat. Rec.* **201**, 613–622.

Coelingh, J. P., Monfoort, C. H., Rozijn, T. H., Leuven, J. A. G., Schiphof, R., Steyn-Parve, E. P., Braunitzer, G., Schrank, B., and Ruhfus, A. (1972). The complete amino acid sequence of the basic nuclear protein of bull spermatozoa. *Biochim. Biophys. Acta* **285**, 1–14.

Courtens, J. L., and Fournier-Delpech, S. (1979). Modifications in the plasma membranes of epididymal ram spermatozoa during maturation and incubation *in utero*. *J. Ultrastruct. Res.* **68**, 136–148.

Courtens, J. L., Courot, M., and Fléchon, J. E. (1976). The perinuclear substance of boar, bull, ram and rabbit spermatozoa. *J. Ultrastruct. Res.* **57**, 54–64.

D'Agostino, A., Geremia, R., and Monesi, V. (1978). Post-meiotic gene activity in spermatogenesis of the mouse. *Cell Differ.* **7**, 175–183.

De Martino, C., Floridi, A., Marcante, M. L., Malorni, W., Barcellona, P. S., Bellocci, M., and Silvestrini, B. (1979). Morphological, histochemical and biochemical studies on germ cell mitochondria of normal rats. *Cell Tissue Res.* **196**, 1–22.

Dixon, G. H., Davies, P. L., Ferrier, L. N., Gedamu, L., and Iatrou, K. (1977). The expression of protamine genes in developing trout sperm cells. *In* "The Molecular Biology of the Mammalian Genetic Apparatus" (P. Ts'o, ed.), pp. 355–379. Elsevier/North-Holland Biomedical Press, New York.

Dooher, G. B., and Bennett, D. (1973). Fine structural observations on the development of the sperm head in the mouse. *Am. J. Anat.* **136**, 339–362.

Dooher, G. B., and Bennett, D. (1977). Spermiogenesis and spermatozoa in sterile mice carrying different lethal *T/t* locus haplotypes: A transmission and scanning electron microscopic study. *Biol. Reprod.* **17**, 269–288.

Ecklund, P. S., and Levine, L. (1975). Mouse sperm basic nuclear protein. Electrophoretic characterization and fate after fertilization. *J. Cell Biol.* **66**, 251–262.

Eddy, E. M., Clark, J. M., Gong, D., and Fenderson, B. A. (1981). Origin and migration of primordial germ cells in mammals. *Gamete Res.* **4**, 333–362.

Edelman, G. M., and Millette, C. F. (1971). Molecular probes of spermatozoon structures. *Proc. Natl. Acad. Sci. U.S.A.* **68**, 2436–2440.

Elias, P. M., Friend, D. S., and Goerke, J. (1979). Membrane sterol heterogeneity: Freeze fracture detection with saponins and filipin. *J. Histochem. Cytochem.* **27**, 1247–1260.

Erickson, R. P., and Martin, S. R. (1974). The relationship of mouse spermatozoal to mouse testicular cathepsins. *Arch. Biochem. Biophys.* **165**, 114–120.

Erickson, R. P., Gachelin, G., Fellous, M., and Jacob, F. (1977). Absorption analysis of H-2 D and K antigens on spermatozoa. *J. Immunogenet.* **4**, 47–51.

Erickson, R. P., Erickson, J. M., Betlach, C. J., and Meistrich, M. L. (1980a). Further evidence for haploid gene expression during spermatogenesis: Heterogeneous, poly[A]-containing RNA is synthesized postmeiotically. *J. Exp. Zool.* **214**, 13–19.

Erickson, R. P., Kramer, J. M., Rittenhouse, J., and Salkeld, A. (1980b). Quantitation of mRNAs during mouse spermatogenesis: Protamine-like histone and phosphoglycerate kinase-2 mRNAs increase after meiosis. *Proc. Natl. Acad. Sci. U.S.A.* **77**, 6086–6090.

Evans, R. W., and Setchell, B. P. (1978). The effect of rete testis fluid on the metabolism of testicular spermatozoa. *J. Reprod. Fertil.* **52**, 15–19.

Evenson, D. P., Witkin, S. S., deHarven, E., and Bendich, A. (1978). Ultrastructure of partially decondensed human spermatozoal chromatin. *J. Ultrastruct. Res.* **63**, 178–187.

Fain-Maurel, M. A., Dadoune, J. P., and Alfonsi, M. F. (1981). High-resolution autoradiography of newly formed proteins in the epididymis after incorporation of tritiated amino acids. *Arch. Androl.* **6**, 249–266.

Farquhar, M. D., and Palade, G. F. (1981). The Golgi apparatus (complex)—(1954–1982)—from artifact to center stage. *J. Cell Biol.* **91**, 77s–103s.

Favard, P., and André, J. (1970). The mitochondria of spermatozoa. *In* "Comparative Spermatology" (B. Baccetti, ed.), pp. 415–429. Academic Press, New York.

Fawcett, D. W. (1958). The structure of the mammalian spermatozoon. *Int. Rev. Cytol.* **7**, 195–234.

Fawcett, D. W. (1965). The anatomy of the mammalian spermatozoon with particular reference to the guinea pig. *Z. Zellforsch. Mikrosk. Anat.* **67**, 279–296.

Fawcett, D. W. (1970). A comparative view of sperm ultrastructure. *Biol. Reprod., Suppl.* **2**, 90–127.

Fawcett, D. W. (1972). Observations on cell differentiation and organelle continuity in spermatogenesis. *In* "International Symposium: The Genetics of the Spermatozoon" (R. A. Beatty and S. Gluecksohn-Waelsch, eds.), pp. 37–68. Bogtrykkeriet Forum, Copenhagen.

Fawcett, D. W. (1975a). The mammalian spermatozoon. *Dev. Biol.* **44**, 394–436.

Fawcett, D. W. (1975b). Morphogenesis of the mammalian sperm acrosome in new perspective. *In* "The Functional Anatomy of the Spermatozoon" (B. A. Afzelius, ed.), pp. 199–210. Pergamon, Oxford.

Fawcett, D. W., and Hollenberg, R. D. (1963). Changes in the acrosomes of guinea pig spermatozoa during passage through the epididymis. *Z. Zellforsch. Mikrosk. Anat.* **60**, 276–292.

Fawcett, D. W., and Phillips, D. M. (1969a). Observations on the release of spermatozoa and on changes in the head during passage through the epididymis. *J. Reprod. Fertil., Suppl.* **6**, 405–418.

Fawcett, D. W., and Phillips, D. M. (1969b). The fine structure of the neck region of the mammalian spermatozoon. *Anat. Rec.* **165**, 153–184.

Fawcett, D. W., and Phillips, D. M. (1970). Recent observations on the ultrastructure and development of the mammalian spermatozoon. *In* "Comparative Spermatology" (B. Baccetti, ed.), pp. 13–28. Academic Press, New York.

Fawcett, D. W., and Porter, K. R. (1954). A study of the fine structures of ciliated epithelia. *J. Morphol.* **94**, 221–281.

Fawcett, D. W., Eddy, E. M., and Phillips, D. M. (1970). Observations on the fine structure and relationships of the chromatoid body in mammalian spermatogenesis. *Biol. Reprod.* **2**, 129.

Fawcett, D. W., Anderson, W. A., and Phillips, D. M. (1971). Morphogenetic factors influencing the shape of the sperm head. *Dev. Biol.* **26**, 220–251.

Feit, H., Slusarek, L., and Shelanski, M. L. (1971). Heterogeneity of tubulin subunits. *Proc. Natl. Acad. Sci. U.S.A.* **68**, 2028–2031.

Fellous, M., Gachelin, G., Buc-Caron, M.-H., Dubois, P., and Jacob, F. (1974). Similar location of an early embryonic antigen on mouse and human spermatozoa. *Dev. Biol.* **41**, 331–337.

Fellous, M., Erickson, R. P., Gachelin, G., Dubois, P., and Jacob F. (1976a). The time of appearance of Ia antigens during spermatogenesis in the mouse. Relationship between Ia antigens and H-2, β-2 microglobulin and F9 antigens. *Folia Biol. (Prague)* **22**, 381–386.

Fellous, M., Erickson, R. P., Gachelin, G., and Jacob, F. (1976b). The time of appearance of Ia antigens during spermatogenesis in the mouse. *Transplantation* **22**, 440–444.

Feuchter, F. A., Vernon, R. B., and Eddy, E. M. (1981). Analysis of the sperm surface with monoclonal antibodies: Topographically restricted antigens appearing in the epididymis. *Biol. Reprod.* **24**, 1099–1110.

Feughelman, M., Langridge, R., Seeds, W. E., Stokes, A. R., Wilson, H. R., Hooper, C. W., Wilkins, M. H. F., Barclay, R. K., and Hamilton, L. D. (1955). Molecular structure of deoxyribose nucleic acid and nucleoprotein. *Nature (London)* **175**, 834–838.

Fine, R. E. (1971). Heterogeneity of tubulin. *Nature New Biol. (London)* **233**, 283–284.

Fink, E., Fritz, H., Jaumann, E., Schiebler, H., Förg-Brey, B., and Werle, E. (1973). Protein proteinase inhibitors in males sex glands and their secretions. *Protides Biol. Fluids* **20**, 425–431.

Fisher, J., Langsam, J., and Bartoov, B. (1977). Ram sperm mitochrondrial DNA. *Cell Biol. Int. Rep.* **1**, 535–540.

Fléchon, J.-E. (1974). Freeze-fracturing of rabbit spermatozoa. *J. Microsc. (Paris)* **19**, 59–64.

Fléchon, J.-E. (1975). Ultrastructural and cytochemical modification of rabbit spermatozoa during epididymal transport. *In* "The Biology of Spermatozoa" (E. S. E. Hafez and C. G. Thibault, eds.), pp. 36–45. Karger, Basel.

Flickinger, C. J. (1979). Synthesis, transport and secretion of proteins in the initial segment of the mouse epididymis as studied by electron microscope radioautography. *Biol. Reprod.* **20**, 1015–1030.

Fournier-Delpech, S., and Courot, M. (1980). Glycoproteins of ram sperm plasma membrane. Relationship of protein having affinity for Con A to epididymal maturation. *Biochem. Biophys. Res. Commun.* **96**, 756–761.

Fournier-Delpech, S., Danzo, B. J., and Orgebin-Crist, M.-C. (1977). Extraction of concanavalin A affinity material from rat testicular and epididymal spermatozoa. *Ann. Biol. Anim., Biochim., Biophys.* **17**, 207–213.

Franke, W. W., Grund, C., Fink, A., Weber, K., Jockusch, B. M., Zentgraf, H., and Osborn, M. (1978). Location of actin in the microfilament bundles associated with the junctional specializations between Sertoli cells and spermatids. *Biol. Cell.* **31**, 7–14.

Franke, W. W., Scheer, U., Krohne, G., and Jarasch, E.-D. (1981). The nuclear envelope and the architecture of the nuclear periphery. *J. Cell Biol.* **91**, 39s–50s.

Franklin, L. E., Barros, C., and Fussell, E. N. (1970). The acrosome region and the acrosome reaction in sperm of the golden hamster. *Biol. Reprod.* **3**, 180–200.

Frenkel, G., Peterson, R. N., and Freund, M. (1973). The role of adenine nucleotides and the effect of caffeine and dibutyryl cyclic AMP on the metabolism of guinea pig epididymal spermatozoa. *Proc. Soc. Exp. Biol. Med.* **144**, 420–425.

Friend, D. S. (1977). The organization of the spermatozoa membrane. *In* "Immunology of Gametes" (M. Edidin and M. H. Johnson, eds.), pp. 5–30. Cambridge Univ. Press, London and New York.

Friend, D. S. (1982). Plasma membrane diversity in a highly polarized cell. *J. Cell Biol.* **93**, 243–249.

Friend, D. S., and Fawcett, D. W. (1974). Membrane differentiations in freeze-fractured mammalian sperm. *J. Cell Biol.* **63**, 641–664.

Friend, D. S., and Heuser, J. E. (1981). Orderly particle arrays on the mitochondrial outer membrane in rapidly-frozen sperm. *Anat. Rec.* **199**, 159–169.

Fuster, C. D., Farrell, D., Stern, F. A., and Hecht, N. B. (1977). RNA polymerase activity in bovine spermatozoa. *J. Cell Biol.* **74**, 698–706.

Gaastra, W., Lukkes-Hofstra, J., and Kolk, A. H. J. (1978). Partial covalent structure of two basic chromosomal proteins from human spermatozoa. *Biochem. Genet.* **16**, 525–529.

Galdieri, M., and Monesi, V. (1974). Ribosomal RNA in mouse spermatocytes. *Exp. Cell Res.* **85**, 287–295.

Galena, H. J., Pillai, A. K., and Terner, C. (1974). Progesterone and androgen receptors in non-flagellate germ cells of the rat testis. *J. Endocrinol.* **63**, 223–237.

Garberi, J. C., Kohane, A. C., Cameo, M. S., and Blauzier, J. A. (1979). Isolation and characterization of specific rat epididymal proteins. *Mol. Cell. Endocrinol.* **13**, 73–82.

Garbers, D. L., and Kopf, G. S. (1980). The regulation of spermatozoa by calcium and cyclic nucleotides. *Adv. Cyclic Nucleotide Res.* **13**, 251–306.

Garbers, D. L., Lust, W. D., First, N. L., and Lardy, H. A. (1971a). Effects of phosphodiesterase inhibitors and cyclic nucleotides on sperm respiration and motility. *Biochemistry* **10**, 1825–1831.

Garbers, D. L., First, N. L., Sullivan, J. J., and Lardy, H. A. (1971b). Stimulation and maintenance of ejaculated bovine spermatozoan respiration and motility by caffeine. *Biol. Reprod.* **5**, 336–339.

Garbers, D. L., First, N. L., and Lardy, H. A. (1973a). The stimulation of bovine epididymal sperm metabolism by cyclic nucleotide phosphodiesterase inhibitors. *Biol. Reprod.* **8**, 589–598.

Garbers, D. L., First. N. L., Gorman, S. K., and Lardy, H. A. (1973b). The effects of cyclic nucleotide phosphodiesterase inhibitors on ejaculated porcine spermatozoan metabolism. *Biol. Reprod.* **8**, 599–606.

Garbers, D. L., First. N. L., and Lardy, H. A. (1973c). Properties of adenosine 3',5'-monophosphate-dependent protein kinases isolated from bovine epididymal spermatozoa. *J. Biol. Chem.* **248**, 875–879.

Gardner, P. J. (1966). Fine structure of the seminiferous tubule of the Swiss mouse. The spermatid. *Anat. Rec.* **155**, 235–250.

Garner, D. L., and Easton, M. P. (1977). Immunofluorescent localization of acrosin in mammalian spermatozoa. *J. Exp. Zool.* **200**, 157–162.

Gaunt, S. J. (1982). A 28K-dalton cell surface autoantigen of spermatogenesis: Characterization using a monoclonal antibody. *Dev. Biol.* **89**, 92–100.

Geremia, R., Boitani, C., Conti, M., and Monesi, V. (1977). RNA synthesis in spermatocytes and spermatids and preservation of meiotic RNA during spermiogenesis in the mouse. *Cell Differ.* **5**, 343–355.

Geremia, R., D'Agostino, A., and Monesi, V. (1978). Biochemical evidence of haploid gene activity in spermatogenesis of the mouse. *Exp. Cell Res.* **111**, 23–30.

Gibbons, I. R. (1966). Studies on the adenosine triphosphatase activity of 14S and 30S dynein from cilia of *Tetrahymena. J. Biol. Chem.* **241**, 5590–5596.

Gibbons, I. R. (1981). Cilia and flagella of eukaryotes. *J. Cell Biol.* **91**, 107s–124s.

Gibbons, I. R., and Rowe, A. J. (1965). Dynein: A protein with adenosine triphosphatase activity from cilia. *Science* **149**, 424–426.

Gibbons, I. R., Fronk, E., Gibbons, B. H., and Ogawa, K. (1976). Multiple forms of dynein in sea urchin sperm flagella. *Cold Spring Harbor Conf. Cell Proliferation* **3** (Book C), 915–932.

Goldberg, E. (1977). Isozymes in testes and spermatozoa. *Isozymes: Curr. Top. Biol. Med. Res.* **1**, 79–124.

Goldberg, E. H., Boyse, E. A., Bennett, D., Scheid, M., and Carlswell, E. A. (1971). Serological demonstration of H-Y (male) antigen on mouse sperm. *Nature (London)* **232**, 478–480.

Goldberg, R. B., Geremia, R., and Bruce, W. R. (1977). Histone synthesis and replacement during spermatogenesis in the mouse. *Differentiation* **7**, 167–180.

Gonzales, L. W., and Meizel, S. (1973). Acid phosphatases of rabbit spermatozoa. I. Electrophoretic characterization of the multiple forms of acid phosphatase in rabbit spermatozoa and other semen constituents. *Biochim. Biophys. Acta* **320**, 166–179.

Goodpasture, C., and Bloom, S. E. (1975). Visualization of nucleolar organizer regions in mammalian chromosomes using silver staining. *Chromosoma* **53**, 37–50.

Goodpasture, J. C., Polakoski, K. L., and Zaneveld, L. J. D. (1980). Acrosin, proacrosin, and acrosin inhibitor of human spermatozoa: Extraction, quantitation, and stability. *J. Androl.* **1**, 16–27.

Gordon, M., and Bensch, K. G. (1968). Cytochemical differentiation of the guinea pig sperm flagellum with phosphotungstic acid. *J. Ultrastruct. Res.* **24**, 33–50.

Gordon, M., Dandekar, P. V., and Bartoszewicz, W. (1974). Ultrastructural localization of surface receptors for concanavalin A on rabbit spermatozoa. *J. Reprod. Fertil.* **36**, 211–214.

Gordon, M., Dandekar, P. V., and Bartoszewicz, W. (1975). The surface coat of epididymal, ejaculated and capacitated sperm. *J. Ultrastruct. Res.* **50**, 199–207.

Gordon, M., Dandekar, P. V., and Eager, P. R. (1978). Identification of phosphastases on the membranes of guinea pig sperm. *Anat. Rec.* **191**, 123–133.

Gould, S. F., and Bernstein, M. H. (1975). The localization of bovine sperm hyaluronidase. *Differentiation* **3**, 123–132.

Grimes, S. R., Jr., Chae, C.-B., and Irvin, J. L. (1975a). Effect of age and hypophysectomy upon relative proportions of various histones in rat testis. *Biochem. Biophys. Res. Commun.* **64**, 911–917.

Grimes, S. R., Jr., Platz, R. D., Meistrich, M. L., and Hnilica, L. S. (1975b). Partial characterization of a new basic nuclear protein from rat testis elongated spermatids. *Biochem. Biophys. Res. Commun.* **67**, 182–189.

Grimes, S. R., Jr., Meistrich, M. L., Platz, R. D., and Hnilica, L. S. (1977). Nuclear protein transitions in rat testis spermatids. *Exp. Cell Res.* **110**, 31–39.

Grootegoed, J. A., Grollé-Hey, A. H., Rommerts, F. F. G., and van der Molen, H. J. (1977a). Ribonucleic acid synthesis *in vitro* in primary spermatocytes isolated from rat testis. *Biochem. J.* **168**, 23–31.

Grootegoed, J. A., Peters, M. J., Mulder, E., Rommerts, F. F. G., and van der Molen, H. J. (1977b). Absence of a nuclear androgen receptor in isolated germinal cells of rat testis. *Mol. Cell Endocrinol.* **9**, 159–167.

Grootegoed, J. A., Rommerts, F. F. G., and van der Molen, H. J. (1978). Hormonal regulation of spermatogenesis. Studies with isolated germinal cells and Sertoli cells. *Horm. Cell Regul.* **2**, 55–69.

Gusse, M., and Chevaillier, P. (1980). Electron microscopic evidence for the presence of globular structures in different sperm chromatins. *J. Cell Biol.* **87**, 280–284.

Hamilton, D. W. (1977). The epididymis. *In* "Frontiers in Reproduction and Fertility Control" (R. O. Greep and M. A. Koblinsky, eds.), pp. 411–426. MIT Press, Cambridge, Massachusetts.

Hamilton, D. W., and Gould, R. P. (1980). Galactosyl transferase activity associated with rat epididymal spermatozoon maturation. *Anat. Rec.* **196**, 71A.

Hammerstedt, R. H., Keith, A. D., Hay, S., Deluca, N., and Amann, R. P. (1979). Changes in ram sperm membranes during epididymal transit. *Arch. Biochem. Biophys.* **196**, 7–12.

Harrison, R. A. P. (1977). The metabolism of mammalian spermatozoa. *In* "Frontiers of Reproduction and Fertility Control" (R. O. Greep and M. A. Koblinsky, eds.), pp. 379–401. MIT Press, Cambridge, Massachusetts.

Hartree, E. F. (1977). Spermatozoa, eggs and proteinases. *Biochem. Soc. Trans.* **5**, 375–394.

Hecht, N. B. (1974). A DNA polymerase isolated from bovine spermatozoa. *J. Reprod. Fertil.* **41**, 345–354.

Henderson, S. A. (1970). The time and place of meiotic crossing-over. *Annu. Rev. Genet.* **4**, 295–324.

Henle, W., Henle, G., and Chambers, L. A. (1938). Studies on the antigenic structure of some mammalian spermatozoa. *J. Exp. Med.* **68**, 335–352.

Hermo, L., Clermont, Y., and Rambourg, A. (1979). Endoplasmic reticulum–Golgi apparatus relationships in the rat spermatid. *Anat. Rec.* **193**, 243–256.

Hermo, L., Rambourg, A., and Clermont, Y. (1980). Three-dimensional architecture of the cortical region of the Golgi apparatus in rat spermatids. *Am. J. Anat.* **157**, 357–373.

Herr, J. C., and Eddy, E. M. (1980). Detection of mouse sperm antigens by a surface labeling and immunoprecipitation approach. *Biol. Reprod.* **22**, 1263–1274.

Hintz, M., and Goldberg, E. (1977). Immunohistochemical localization of LDH-X during spermatogenesis in mouse testes. *Dev. Biol.* **57**, 375–384.

Hirtzer, P. G., and Bellvé, A. R. (1979). Displacement of protamines from mouse sperm heads with divalent cations. *J. Cell Biol.* **83**, 222a.

Hoffer, A. P., Shalev, M., and Frisch, D. H. (1981). Ultrastructure and maturational changes in spermatozoa in the epididymis of the pigtailed monkey, *Macaca nemestrina. J. Androl.* **3**, 140–146.

Holt, W. V. (1980). Surface-bound sialic acid on ram and bull spermatozoa: Deposition during epididymal transit and stability during washing. *Biol. Reprod.* **23**, 847–857.

Hoskins, D. D., and Casillas, E. R. (1975). Function of cyclic nucleotides in mammalian spermatozoa. *In* "Handbook of Physiology" (D. W. Hamilton and R. O. Greep, eds.), Sect. 7, Vol. V, pp. 453–460. Am. Physiol. Soc., Washington, D.C.

Hoskins, D. D., Casillas, E. R., and Stephens, D. T. (1972). Cyclic AMP dependent protein kinases of bovine epididymal spermatozoa. *Biochem. Biophys. Res. Commun.* **48**, 1331–1338.

Hoskins, D. D., Stephens, D. T., and Hall, M. L. (1974). Cyclic adenosine 3′,5′-monophosphate and protein kinase levels in developing bovine spermatozoa. *J. Reprod. Fertil.* **37**, 131–133.

Hoskins, D. D., Hall, M. L., and Munsterman, D. (1975). Induction of motility in immature bovine spermatozoa by cyclic AMP phosphodiesterase inhibitors and seminal plasma. *Biol. Reprod.* **13**, 168–176.

Hoskins, D. D., Brandt, H., and Acott, T. S. (1978). Initiation of sperm motility in the mammalian epididymis. *Fed. Proc. Fed. Am. Soc. Exp. Biol.* **37**, 2534–2542.

Hoskins, D. D., Johnson, D., Brandt, H., and Acott, T. S. (1979). Evidence for a role for a forward motility protein in the epididymal development of sperm motility. *In* "The Spermatozoon" (D. W. Fawcett and J. M. Bedford, eds.), pp. 43–53. Urban & Schwarzenberg, Baltimore, Maryland.

Howards, S., Lechene, C., and Vigersky, R. (1979). The fluid environment of the maturing spermatozoon. *In* "The Spermatozoon" (D. W. Fawcett and J. M. Bedford, eds.), pp. 35–41. Urban & Schwarzenberg, Baltimore, Maryland.

Hrudka, F. (1978). A morphological and cyctochemical study on isolated sperm mitochondria. *J. Ultrastruct. Res.* **63**, 1–19.

Hsu, T. C., Spirito, S. E., and Pardue, M. L. (1975). Distribution of 18 + 28S ribosomal genes in mammalian genomes. *Chromosoma* **53**, 25–36.

Huacuja, L., Delgado, N. M., Merchant, H., Pancardo, R. M., and Rosado, A. (1977). Cyclic AMP-induced incorporation of ^{33}Pi into human spermatozoa membrane components. *Biol. Reprod.* **17**, 89–96.

Huang, B., Ramanis, Z., and Luck, D. J. K. (1982). Suppressor mutations in *Chlamydomonas* reveal a regulatory mechanism for flagella function. *Cell* **28**, 115–124.

Hunter, A. G. (1969). Differentiation of rabbit sperm antigens from those of seminal plasma. *J. Reprod. Fertil.* **20**, 413–418.

Hunter, A. G., and Schellpfeffer, D. A. (1981). Concentrations of sperm, protein and a sperm membrane glycoprotein within boar epididymal luminal fluids. *J. Anim. Sci.* **52**, 575–579.

Hutson, S. M., Van Dop, C., and Lardy, H. A. (1977). Mitochondrial metabolism of pyruvate in bovine spermatozoa. *J. Biol. Chem.* **252**, 1309–1315.

Hyne, R. V., and Garbers, D. L. (1979). Regulation of guinea pig sperm adenylate cyclase by calcium. *Biol. Reprod.* **21**, 1135–1142.

Iatrou, K., and Dixon, G. H. (1978). Protamine messenger RNA: Its life history during spermatogenesis in rainbow trout. *Fed. Proc., Fed. Am. Soc. Exp. Biol.* **37**, 2526–2533.

Iatrou, K., Spira, A. W., and Dixon, G. H. (1978). Protamine messenger RNA: Evidence for early synthesis and accumulation during spermatogenesis in rainbow trout. *Dev. Biol.* **64**, 82–98.

Illisson, L. (1966). The fine structure of the mature spermatozoan head and neck of the mouse. *J. Anat.* **100**, 949–950.

Inoué, S., and Sato, H. (1962). Arrangement of DNA in living sperm: A biophysical analysis. *Science* **136**, 1122–1124.

Irons, M. J., and Clermont, Y. (1982). Formation of outer dense fibers during spermiogenesis in the rat. *Anat. Rec.* **202**, 463–471.

Johnson, W. L., and Hunter, A. G. (1972a). Immunofluorescent evaluation of the male rabbit reproductive tract for sites of secretion and absorption of seminal antigens. *Biol. Reprod.* **6**, 13–22.

Johnson, W. L., and Hunter, A. G. (1972b). Seminal antigens: Their alteration in the genital tract of female rabbits and during partial *in vitro* capacitation with beta amylase and beta glucuronidase. *Biol. Reprod.* **7**, 332–340.

Jones, R. (1978). Comparative biochemistry of mammalian epididymal plasma. *Comp. Biochem. Physiol. B* **61B**, 365–370.

Jones, R., Brown, C. R., von Glos, K. I., and Parker, M. G. (1980). Hormonal regulation of protein synthesis in the rat epididymis. Characterization of androgen-dependent and testicular fluid-dependent proteins. *Biochem. J.* **188**, 667–676.

Jones, R., von Glos, K. I., and Brown, C. R. (1981). Characterization of hormonally regulated secretory proteins from the caput epididymis of the rabbit. *Biochem. J.* **196**, 105–114.

Jones, R. C. (1971). Studies of the structure of the head of boar spermatozoa from the epididymis. *J. Reprod. Fertil., Suppl.* **13**, 51–64.

Jutte, N. H. P. M., Grootegoed, J. A., Rommerts, F. F. G., and van der Molen, H. J.

(1981). Exogenous lactate is essential to metabolic activities in isolated rat spermatocytes and spermatids. *J. Reprod. Fertil.* **62**, 399–405.

Kadohama, N., and Turkington, R. W. (1974). Changes in acidic chromatin proteins during the hormone-dependent development of rat testis and epididymis. *J. Biol. Chem.* **249**, 6225–6233.

Kaya, M., and Harrison, R. G. (1976). The ultrastructural relationships between Sertoli cells and spermatogenic cells in the rat. *J. Anat.* **121**, 279–290.

Keyhani, E., and Storey, B. T. (1973). Energy conservation capacity and morphological integrity of mitochondria in hypotonically treated rabbit spermatozoa. *Biochim. Biophys. Acta* **305**, 557–569.

Khorlin, A. Y., Vikka, I. V., and Milishnikov, A. N. (1973). Subunit structure of testicular hyaluronidase. *FEBS Lett.* **31**, 107–110.

Kierszenbaum, A. L., and Tres, L. L. (1974a). Nucleolar and perichromosomal RNA synthesis during meiotic prophase in the mouse testis. *J. Cell Biol.* **60**, 39–53.

Kierszenbaum, A. L., and Tres, L. L. (1974b). Transcription sites in spread meiotic prophase chromosomes from mouse spermatocytes. *J. Cell Biol.* **63**, 923–935.

Kierszenbaum, A. L., and Tres, L. L. (1975). Structural and transcriptional features of the mouse spermatid genome. *J. Cell Biol.* **65**, 258–270.

Kierszenbaum, A. L., and Tres, L. L. (1978). RNA transcription and chromatin structure during meiotic and postmeiotic stages of spermatogenesis. *Fed. Proc., Fed. Am. Soc. Exp. Biol.* **37**, 2512–2516.

Killian, G. J., and Amann, R. P. (1973). Immunoelectrophoretic characterization of fluid and sperm entering and leaving the bovine epididymis. *Biol. Reprod.* **9**, 489–499.

Kistler, W. S., and Geroch, M. E. (1975). An unusual pattern of lysine-rich histone components is associated with spermatogenesis in rat testis. *Biochem. Biophys. Res. Commun.* **63**, 378–384.

Kistler, W. S., Geroch, M. E., and Williams-Ashman, H. G. (1973). Specific basic proteins from mammalian testes. Isolation and properties of small basic proteins from rat testes and epididymal spermatozoa. *J. Biol. Chem.* **248**, 4532–4543.

Kistler, W. S., Geroch, M. E., and Williams-Ashman, H. G. (1975a). A highly basic small protein associated with spermatogenesis in the human testis. *Invest. Urol.* **12**, 346–350.

Kistler, W. S., Noyes, C., Hsu, R., and Heinrikson, R. L. (1975b). The amino acid sequence of a testis-specific basic protein that is associated with spermatogenesis. *J. Biol. Chem.* **250**, 1847–1853.

Kistler, W. S., Keim, P. S., and Heinrikson, R. L. (1976). Partial structural analysis of the basic chromosomal protein of rat spermatozoa. *Biochim. Biophys. Acta* **427**, 752–757.

Klugerman, A., and Kornblatt, M. J. (1980). The subcellular localization of testicular sulfogalactoglycerolipid. *Can. J. Biochem.* **58**, 225–229.

Koehler, J. K. (1966). Fine structure observations in frozen-etched bovine spermatozoa. *J. Ultrastruct. Res.* **16**, 359–375.

Koehler, J. K. (1970). A freeze-etching study of rabbit spermatozoa with particular reference to head structures. *J. Ultrastruct. Res.* **33**, 598–614.

Koehler, J. K. (1972). Human sperm head ultrastructure: A freeze-etching study. *J. Ultrastruct. Res.* **39**, 520–539.

Koehler, J. K. (1973). Studies on the structure of the water buffalo spermatozoa. *J. Ultrastruct. Res.* **44**, 355–368.

Koehler, J. K. (1975). Studies on the distribution of antigenic sites on the surface of rabbit spermatozoa. *J. Cell Biol.* **67**, 647–659.

Koehler, J. K. (1978). The mammalian sperm surface: Studies with specific labeling techniques. *Int. Rev. Cytol.* **54,** 73–108.

Koehler, J. K. (1981). Lectins as probes of the spermatozoon surface. *Arch. Androl.* **6,** 197–217.

Koehler, J. K., and Perkins, W. D. (1974). Fine structure observations on the distribution of antigenic sites on guinea pig spermatozoa. *J. Cell Biol.* **60,** 789–795.

Kohane, A. C., González Echeverría, F. M. C., Piñeiro, L., and Blaquier, J. A. (1980). Interaction of proteins of epididymal origin with spermatozoa. *Biol. Reprod.* **23,** 737–742.

Kolk, A. H. J., and Samuel, T. (1975). Isolation, chemical and immunological characterization of two strongly basic nuclear proteins from human spermatozoa. *Biochim. Biophys. Acta* **393,** 307–319.

Koo, G. C., Stackpole, C. W., Boyse, E. A., Hammerling, U., and Lardis, M. P. (1973). Topographical localization of H-Y antigen on mouse spermatozoa by immunoelectronmicroscopy. *Proc. Natl. Acad. Sci. U.S.A.* **70,** 1502–1505.

Kopečný, V., and Pavlok, A. (1975). Autoradiographic study of mouse spermatozoan arginine-rich nuclear protein in fertilization. *J. Exp. Zool.* **191,** 85–96.

Koren, E., and Milkovíc, S. (1973). 'Collagenase-like' peptidase in human, rat and bull spermatozoa. *J. Reprod. Fertil.* **32,** 349–356.

Kornblatt, M. J. (1979). Synthesis and turnover of sulfogalactoglycerolipid, a membrane lipid, during spermatogenesis. *Can. J. Biochem.* **57,** 255–258.

Kossel, A. (1928). "The Protamines and Histones." Longmans, Green, New York.

Kramer, J. M., and Erickson, R. P. (1982). Analysis of stage-specific protein synthesis during spermatogenesis of the mouse by two-dimensional gel electrophoresis. *J. Reprod. Fertil.* **64,** 139–144.

Krimer, D. B., and Esponda, P. (1978). Preferential staining of the post-acrosomal lamina of mouse spermatids. *Mikroskopie* **34,** 55–59.

Kumaroo, K. K., Jahnke, G., and Irvin, J. L. (1975). Changes in basic chromosomal proteins during spermatogenesis in the mature rat. *Arch. Biochem. Biophys.* **168,** 413–424.

Lalli, M., and Clermont, Y. (1981). Structural changes in the head component of the rat spermatid during late spermiogenesis. *Am. J. Anat.* **160,** 419–434.

Lavon, U., Volcani, R., and Danon, D. (1971). The proteins of bovine spermatozoa from the caput and cauda epididymis. *J. Reprod. Fertil.* **24,** 219–232.

Lea, O. A., Petrusz, P., and French, F. S. (1978). Purification and localization of acidic epididymal glycoprotein (AEG): A sperm coating protein secreted by the rat epididymis. *Int. J. Androl., Suppl.* **2,** 592–607.

Leblond, C. P., and Clermont, Y. (1952). Spermiogenesis of rat, mouse, hamster and guinea pig as revealed by the "periodic acid–fuschin sulfurous acid" technique. *Am. J. Anat.* **90,** 167–216.

Le Bouteiller, P. P., Toullet, F., Righenzi, S., and Voisin, G. A. (1979). Ultrastructural localization of guinea pig spermatozoal autoantigens on germinal cells by immunoperoxidase techniques. *J. Histochem. Cytochem.* **27,** 857–866.

Lee, I. P., and Dixon, R. L. (1972). Antineoplastic drug effects on spermatogenesis studied by velocity sedimentation cell separation. *Toxicol. Appl. Pharmacol.* **23,** 20–41.

Leeuwenhoek, A. (1680). *In* "The Collected Letters," Vol. III, Lett. No. 57, p. 205. Amsterdam, 1948.

Levine, N., and Kelly, H. (1978). Measurement of pH in the rat epididymis in vivo. *J. Reprod. Fertil.* **52,** 333–335.

Levinger, L. F., Carter, C. W., Jr., Kumaroo, K. K., and Irvin, J. L. (1978). Cross-referencing testis-specific nuclear proteins by two-dimensional gel electrophoresis. *J. Biol. Chem.* **253**, 5232–5234.

Linck, R. W. (1973). Chemical and structural differences between cilia and flagella from the lamellibranch *Aequipecten irradians. J. Cell Sci.* **12**, 951–981.

Linck, R. W., and Langevin, G. L. (1981). Reassembly of flagellar B (αβ) tubulin into singlet microtubules: Consequences for cytoplasmic microtubule structure and assembly. *J. Cell Biol.* **89**, 323–337.

Linck, R. W., Olson, G. E., and Langevin, G. L. (1981). Arrangement of tubulin subunits and microtubule-associated proteins in the central-pair microtubule apparatus of squid (*Loligo pealii*) sperm flagella. *J. Cell Biol.* **89**, 309–322.

Lindemann, C. B. (1978). A cAMP-induced increase in the motility of demembranated bull sperm models. *Cell* **13**, 9–18.

Lindemann, C. B., and Gibbons, I. R. (1975). Adenosine triphosphate-induced motility and sliding of filaments in mammalian sperm extracted with Triton X-100. *J. Cell Biol.* **65**, 147–162.

Lingwood, C., and Schachter, H. (1981). Localization of sulfatoxygalactosylacylalkylglycerol at the surface of rat testicular germinal cells by immunocytochemical techniques: pH dependence of a nonimmunological reaction between immunogobulin and germinal cells. *J. Cell Biol.* **89**, 621–630.

Loir, M. (1972). Protein and ribonucleic acid metabolism in spermatocytes and spermatids of the ram (*Ovis aries*). I. Incorporation and fate of ³H-uridine. *Ann. Biol. Anim., Biochim., Biophys.* **12**, 203–219.

Loir, M., and Courtens, J.-L. (1979). Nuclear organization in ram spermatids. *J. Ultrastruct. Res.* **67**, 309–324.

Loir, M., and Lanneau, M. (1978). Partial characterization of ram spermatidal basic nuclear proteins. *Biochem. Biophys. Res. Commun.* **80**, 975–982.

Luduena, R. F., and Woodward, D. O. (1973). Isolation and partial characterization of α- and β-tubulin from outer doublets of sea-urchin sperm and microtubules of chick-embryo brain. *Proc. Natl. Acad. Sci. U.S.A.* **70**, 3594–3598.

Lung, B. (1968). Whole-mount electron microscopy of chromatin and membranes in bull and human sperm heads. *J. Ultrastruct. Res.* **22**, 485–493.

Lung, B. (1972). Ultrastructure and chromatin disaggregation of human sperm head with thioglycolate treatment. *J. Cell Biol.* **52**, 179–186.

Lyon, M. F., Glenister, P. H., and Lamoreux, M. L. (1975). Normal spermatozoa from androgen-resistant germ cells of chimaeric mice and the role of androgen in spermatogenesis. *Nature (London)* **258**, 620–622.

McIntosh, J. R., and Porter, K. R. (1967). Microtubules in the spermatids of domestic fowl. *J. Cell Biol.* **35**, 153–173.

McRorie, R. A., and Williams, W. L. (1974). Biochemistry of mammalian fertilization. *Annu. Rev. Biochem.* **43**, 777–803.

McRorie, R. A., Turner, R. B., Bradford, M. M., and Williams, W. L. (1976). Acrolysin, the aminoproteinase catalyzing the initial conversion of proacrosin to acrosin in mammalian fertilization. *Biochem. Biophys. Res. Commun.* **71**, 492–498.

Majumder, G. C. (1978). Occurrence of cyclic AMP-dependent protein kinase on the outer surface of rat epididymal spermatozoa. *Biochem. Biophys. Res. Commun.* **83**, 829–836.

Majumder, G. C., and Turkington, R. W. (1974). Acrosomal and lysosomal isoenzymes of β-galactosidase and N-acetyl-β-glucosaminidase in rat testis. *Biochemistry* **13**, 2857–2864.

Mann, T. (1964). "The Biochemistry of Semen and of the Male Reproductive Tract." Wiley, New York.

Mann, T., and Lutwak-Mann, C. (1981). "Male Reproductive Function and Semen." Springer-Verlag, Berlin and New York.

Mansy, S., Engström, S. K., and Peticolas, W. L. (1976). Laser Raman identification of an interaction site on DNA for arginine containing histones in chromatin. *Biochem. Biophys. Res. Commun.* **68**, 1242–1247.

Marushige, Y., and Marushige, K. (1974). Properties of chromatin isolated from bull spermatozoa. *Biochim. Biophys. Acta* **340**, 498–508.

Marushige, Y., and Marushige, K. (1975). Enzymatic unpacking of bull sperm chromatin. *Biochim. Biophys. Acta* **403**, 180–191.

Mather, J., and Hotta, Y. (1977). A phosphorylatable DNA-binding protein associated with a lipoprotein fraction from rat spermatocyte nuclei. *Exp. Cell Res.* **109**, 181–189.

Mayer, J. F., and Zirkin, B. R. (1979). Spermatogenesis in the mouse. 1. Autoradiographic studies of nuclear incorporation and loss of ^{3}H-amino acids. *J. Cell Biol.* **81**, 403–410.

Mayer, J. F., Chang, T. S. K., and Zirkin, B. R. (1981). Spermatogenesis in the mouse. 2. Amino acid incorporation into basic nucleoproteins of mouse spermatids and spermatozoa. *Biol. Reprod.* **25**, 1041–1051.

Meistrich, M. L., Hughes, T. J., and Bruce, W. R. (1975). Alteration of epididymal sperm transport and maturation in mice by oestrogen and testosterone. *Nature (London)* **258**, 145–147.

Meistrich, M. L., Reid, B. O., and Barcellona, W. J. (1976). Changes in sperm nuclei during spermiogenesis and epididymal maturation. *Exp. Cell Res.* **99**, 72–78.

Meistrich, M. L., Trostle, P. K., Frapart, M., and Erickson, R. P. (1977). Biosynthesis and localization of lactate dehydrogenase X in pachytene spermatocytes and spermatids of mouse testes. *Dev. Biol.* **60**, 428–441.

Meizel, S. (1972). Biochemical detection and activation of an inactive form of a trypsin-like enzyme in rabbit testes. *J. Reprod. Fertil.* **31**, 459–462.

Meizel, S. (1978). The mammalian sperm acrosome reaction, a biochemical approach. *Dev. Mamm.* **3**, 1–61.

Meizel, S., and Cotham, J. (1972). Partial characterization of a new bull sperm arylaminidase. *J. Reprod. Fertil.* **28**, 303–307.

Mello, M. L. S., and Vidal, B. de C. (1973). Linear dichroism and anomalous dispersion of the birefringence on sperm heads. *Acta Histochem.* **45**, 109–114.

Meyer, J., and Weinmann, J. P. (1957). Phosphamidase activity during spermatogenesis in the rat. *Am. J. Anat.* **101**, 461–475.

Meischer, F. (1878). Die Spermatozoen einiger Wirbeltiere; ein Beitrag zur Histochemie. *Verh. Naturforsch. Ges. Basel* **6**, 138.

Miller, O. L. (1981). The nucleolus, chromosomes, and visualization of genetic activity. *J. Cell Biol.* **91**, 15s–27s.

Millette, C. F. (1977). Distribution and mobility of lectin binding sites on mammalian spermatozoa. *In* "Immunobiology of Gametes" (M. Edidin and M. H. Johnson, eds.), pp. 51–71. Cambridge Univ. Press, London and New York.

Millette, C. F., and Bellvé, A. R. (1977). Temporal expression of membrane antigens during mouse spermatogenesis. *J. Cell Biol.* **74**, 86–97.

Millette, C. F., and Bellvé, A. R. (1980). Selective partitioning of plasma membrane antigens during mouse spermatogenesis. *Dev. Biol.* **79**, 309–324.

Millette, C. F., and Moulding, C. T. (1981). Cell surface marker proteins during mouse spermatogenesis: Two-dimensional gel electrophoretic analysis. *J. Cell Sci.* **48**, 367–382.

Millette, C. F., O'Brien, D. A., and Moulding, C. T. (1980). Isolation of plasma membranes from purified mouse spermatogenic cells. *J. Cell Sci.* **43**, 279–299.

Mills, N. C., and Means, A. R. (1977). Nonhistone chromosomal proteins of the developing rat testis. *Biol. Reprod.* **17**, 769–779.

Mills, N. C., Van, N. T., and Means, A. R. (1977). Histones of rat testis chromatin during early postnatal development and their interactions with DNA. *Biol. Reprod.* **17**, 760–768.

Mirzabekov, A. D., San'ko, D. F., Kolchinsky, A. M., and Melnikova, A. F. (1977). Protein arrangement in the DNA grooves in chromatin and nucleoprotamine *in vitro* and *in vivo* revealed by methylation. *Eur. J. Biochem.* **75**, 379–389.

Mita, M., and Hall, P. F. (1982). Metabolism of round spermatids from rats: Lactate as the preferred substrate. *Biol. Reprod.* **26**, 445–455.

Mohri, H., Mohri, T., and Ernster, L. (1965). Isolation and enzymic properties of the midpiece of bull spermatozoa. *Exp. Cell Res.* **38**, 217–246.

Mollenhauer, H. H., and Morré, D. J. (1978). Polyribosomes associated with forming acrosome membranes in guinea pig spermatids. *Science* **200**, 85–86.

Monesi, V. (1964a). Ribonucleic acid synthesis during mitosis and meiosis in the mouse testis. *J. Cell Biol.* **22**, 521–532.

Monesi, V. (1964b). Autoradiographic evidence of a nuclear histone synthesis during mouse spermiogenesis in the absence of detectable quantities of nuclear ribonucleic acid. *Exp. Cell Res.* **36**, 683–688.

Monesi, V. (1965a). Synthetic activities during spermatogenesis in the mouse. RNA and protein. *Exp. Cell Res.* **39**, 197–224.

Monesi, V. (1965b). Differential rate of ribonucleic acid synthesis in the autosomes and sex chromosomes during male meiosis in the mouse. *Chromsoma* **17**, 11–21.

Monfoort, C. H., Schiphof, R., Rozijn, T. H., and Steyn-Parvé, E. P. (1973). Amino acid composition and carboxyl-terminal structure of some basic chromosomal proteins of mammalian spermatozoa. *Biochim. Biophys. Acta* **322**, 173–177.

Monn, E., Desautel, M., and Christiansen, R. O. (1972). Highly specific testicular adenosine $3'$–$5'$-monophosphate phosphodiesterase associated with sexual maturation. *Endocrinology* **91**, 716–720.

Montamat, E. E., and Blanco, A. (1976). Subcellular distribution of the lactate dehydrogenase isozyme specific for testis and sperm. *Exp. Cell Res.* **103**, 241–245.

Moore, H. D. M. (1980). Localization of specific glycoproteins secreted by the rabbit and hamster epididymis. *Biol. Reprod.* **22**, 705–718.

Moore, H. D. M. (1981). Glycoprotein secretions of the epididymis in the rabbit and hamster: Localization on epididymal spermatozoa and the effect of specific antibodies on fertilization *in vivo*. *J. Exp. Zool.* **215**, 77–85.

Mortimer, D., and Thompson, T. E. (1976). Nuclear pores in the spermatozoon of the rat. *Experientia* **32**, 104–105.

Morton, D. B. (1975). Acrosomal enzymes: Immunochemical localization of acrosin and hyaluronidase in ram spermatozoa. *J. Reprod. Fertil.* **45**, 375–378.

Mrsny, R. J., and Meizel, S. (1981). Potassium ion influx and Na^+,K^+-ATPase activity are required for the hamster sperm acrosome reaction. *J. Cell Biol.* **91**, 77–82.

Mrsny, R. J., Waxman, L., and Meizel, S. (1979). Taurine maintains and stimulates motility of hamster sperm during capacitation *in vitro*. *J. Exp. Zool.* **210**, 123–128.

Mukerji, S. K., and Meizel, S. (1975). The molecular transformation of rabbit testis proacrosin into acrosin. *Arch. Biochem. Biophys.* **168**, 720–721.

Mukerji, S. K., and Meizel, S. (1979). Rabbit testis proacrosin. Purification, molecular weight estimation, and amino acid and carbohydrate composition of the molecule. *J. Biol. Chem.* **254**, 11721–11728.

Muramatsu, M., Utakoji, T., and Sugano, H. (1968). Rapidly-labeled nuclear RNA in Chinese hamster testis. *Exp. Cell Res.* **53**, 278–283.

Musick, W. D. L., and Rossmann, M. G. (1979). The structure of mouse lactate dehydrogenase isoenzyme C_4 at 2.9 Å resolution. *J. Biol. Chem.* **254**, 7611–7620.

Myles, D. G., Primakoff, P., and Bellvé, A. R. (1980). Topographical organization of the mammalian sperm cell surface. *J. Cell Biol.* **87**, 98a.

Myles, D. G., Primakoff, P., and Bellvé, A. R. (1981). Surface domains of the guinea pig sperm defined with monoclonal antibodies. *Cell* **23**, 433–439.

Nakamura, M., Hino, A., Yasumasu, I., and Kato, J. (1981). Stimulation of protein synthesis in round spermatids from rat testes by lactate. *J. Biochem. (Tokyo)* **89**, 1309–1315.

Nelson, L. (1978). Chemistry and neurochemistry of sperm motility control. *Fed. Proc., Fed. Am. Soc. Exp. Biol.* **37**, 2543–2549.

Nicander, L., and Bane, A. (1962). Fine structure of boar spermatozoa. *Z. Zellforsch. Mikrosk. Anat.* **57**, 390–405.

Nicander, L., and Bane, A. (1966). Fine structure of the sperm head in some mammals with particular reference to the acrosome and the subacrosomal substance. *Z. Zellforsch. Mikrosk, Anat.* **72**, 496–515.

Nicolson, G. L. (1982). Mammalian sperm plasma membrane. *In* "Prospects for Sexing Mammalian Sperm" (R. P. Amann and G. E. Seidel, eds.), pp. 5–16. Colorado Assoc. Univ. Press, Boulder.

Nicolson, G. L., and Yanagimachi, R. (1972). Terminal saccharides on sperm plasma membranes: Identification by specific agglutinins. *Science* **177**, 276–279.

Nicolson, G. L., and Yanagimachi, R. (1974). Mobility and restriction of mobility of plasma membrane lectin-binding components. *Science* **184**, 1294–1296.

Nicolson, G. L., and Yanagimachi, R. (1979). Cell surface changes associated with the epididymal maturation of mammalian spermatozoa. *In* "The Spermatozoon" (D. W. Fawcett and J. M. Bedford, eds.), pp. 187–194. Urban & Schwarzenberg, Baltimore, Maryland.

Nicolson, G. L., Usui, N., Yanagimachi, R., Yanagimachi, H., and Smith, J. R. (1977). Lectin-binding sites on the plasma membranes of rabbit spermatozoa. Changes in surface receptors during epididymal maturation and after ejaculation. *J. Cell Biol.* **74**, 950–962.

Nicolson, G. L., Brodginski, A. B., Beattie, G., and Yanagimachi, R. (1979). Cell surface changes in the proteins of rabbit spermatozoa during epididymal passage. *Gamete Res.* **2**, 153–162.

Oakberg, E. F. (1956). Duration of spermatogenesis in the mouse and timing of stages of the cycle of the seminiferous epithelium. *Am. J. Anat.* **99**, 507–516.

O'Brien, D. A., and Bellvé, A. R. (1980a). Protein constituents of the mouse spermatozoon. I. An electrophoretic characterization. *Dev. Biol.* **75**, 386–404.

O'Brien, D. A., and Bellvé, A. R. (1980b). Protein constituents of the mouse spermatozoon. II. Temporal synthesis during spermatogenesis. *Dev. Biol.* **75**, 405–418.

Ogawa, K., and Mohri, H. (1972). Studies on flagellar ATPase from sea urchin spermatozoa. I. Purification and some properties of the enzyme. *Biochim. Biophys. Acta* **256**, 142–155.

Ogawa, K., Mohri, T., and Mohri, H. (1977). Identification of dynein as the outer arms of sea urchin sperm axonemes. *Proc. Natl. Acad. Sci. U.S.A.* **74**, 5006–5010.

Ogawa, K., Negishi, S., and Obika, M. (1982). Immunological dissimilarity in protein component (dynein 1) between outer and inner arms within sea urchin sperm axonemes. *J. Cell Biol.* **92**, 706–713.

Oliphant, G., and Singhas, C. A. (1979). Iodination of rabbit sperm plasma membrane: Relationship of specific surface proteins to epididymal function and sperm capacitation. *Biol. Reprod.* **21**, 937–944.

Olson, G. E. (1979). Isolation of the fibrous sheath and perforatorium of rat spermatozoa. *In* "The Spermatozoon" (D. W. Fawcett and J. M. Bedford, eds.), pp. 395–400. Urban & Schwarzenberg, Baltimore, Maryland.

Olson, G. E., and Danzo, B. J. (1981). Surface changes in rat spermatozoa during epididymal transit. *Biol. Reprod.* **24**, 431–443.

Olson, G. E., and Hamilton, D. W. (1978). Characterization of the surface glycoproteins of rat spermatozoa. *Biol. Reprod.* **19**, 26–35.

Olson, G. E., and Linck, R. W. (1977). Observations of the structural components of flagellar axonemes and central pair microtubules from rat sperm. *J. Ultrastruct. Res.* **62**, 21–43.

Olson, G. E., and Sammons, D. W. (1980). Structural chemistry of outer dense fibers of rat sperm. *Biol. Reprod.* **22**, 319–332.

Olson, G. E., Hamilton, D. W., and Fawcett, D. W. (1976a). Isolation and characterization of the fibrous sheath of rat epididymal spermatozoa. *Biol. Reprod.* **14**, 517–530.

Olson, G. E., Hamilton, D. W., and Fawcett, D. W. (1976b). Isolation and characterization of the perforatorium of rat spermatozoa. *J. Reprod. Fertil.* **47**, 293–297.

Olson, G. E., Lifsics, M., Fawcett, D. W., and Hamilton, D. W. (1977). Structural specializations in the flagellar plasma membrane of opossum spermatozoa. *J. Ultrastruct. Res.* **59**, 207–221.

O'Rand, M. G. (1977). Restriction of a sperm surface antigen's mobility during capacitation. *Dev. Biol.* **55**, 260–270.

O'Rand, M. G., and Porter, J. P. (1979). Isolation of a sperm membrane sialoglycoprotein autoantigen from rabbit testes. *J. Immunol.* **122**, 1248–1254.

O'Rand, M. G., and Romrell, L. J. (1977). Appearance of cell surface auto- and isoantigens during spermatogenesis in the rabbit. *Dev. Biol.* **55**, 347–358.

O'Rand, M. G., and Romrell, L. J. (1980a). Appearance of regional surface autoantigens during spermatogenesis: Comparison of anti-testis and anti-sperm autoantisera. *Dev. Biol.* **75**, 431–441.

O'Rand, M. G., and Romrell, L. J. (1980b). Identification of rabbit sperm autoantigen as a ricinus communis I receptor. *Gamete Res.* **3**, 317–322.

Orgebin-Crist, M.-C. (1967). Maturation of spermatozoa in rabbit epididymis: Fertilizing ability and embryonic mortality in does inseminated with epididymal spermatozoa. *Ann. Biol. Anim., Biochim., Biophys.* **7**, 373–389.

Orgebin-Crist, M.-C., and Jahad, N. (1978). The maturation of rabbit epididymal spermatozoa in organ culture: Inihibition by antiandrogens and inhibitors of ribonucleic acid and protein synthesis. *Endocrinology* **103**, 46–53.

Orgebin-Crist, M.-C., Danzo, B. J., and Davies, J. (1975). Endocrine control of the development and maintenance of sperm fertilizing ability in the epididymis. *In* "Handbook of Physiology" (D. W. Hamilton and R. O. Greep, eds.), Sect. 7, Vol. V, pp. 319–338. Am. Physiol. Soc., Washington, D.C.

Pallini, V. (1979). Isolation of mitochondria from bull epididymal spermatozoa. *In* "The Spermatozoon" (D. W. Fawcett and J. M. Bedford, eds.), pp. 401–410. Urban & Schwarzenberg, Baltimore, Maryland.

Pallini, V., and Bacci, E. (1979). Bull sperm selenium is bound to a structural protein of mitochondria. *J. Submicrosc. Cytol.* **11**, 165–170.

Pallini, V., Baccetti, B., and Burrini, A. G. (1979). A peculiar cysteine-rich polypeptide related to some unusual properties of mammalian sperm mitochondria. *In* "The Spermatozoon" (D. W. Fawcett and J. M. Bedford, eds.), pp. 141–151. Urban & Schwarzenberg, Baltimore, Maryland.

Parrish, R. F., and Polakoski, K. L. (1979). Mammalian sperm proacrosin–acrosin system. *Int. J. Biochem.* **10**, 391–395.

Pedersen, H. (1972a). The postacrosomal region of the spermatozoa of man and *Macaca arctoides. J. Ultrastruct. Res.* **40**, 366–377.

Pedersen, H. (1972b). Further observations on the fine structure of the human spermatozoa. *Z. Zellforsch. Mikrosk, Anat.* **123**, 305–315.

Perry, R. P. (1981). RNA processing comes of age. *J. Cell Biol.* **91**, 28s–38s.

Peterson, R. N., Seyler, D., Bundman, D., and Fruend, M. (1979). The effect of theophylline and dibutyryl cyclic AMP on the uptake of radioactive calcium and phosphate ions by boar and human spermatozoa. *J. Reprod. Fertil.* **55**, 385–390.

Philippe, M., and Chevaillier, P. (1976). Further characterization of a DNA polymerase activity in mouse sperm nuclei. *Biochim. Biophys. Acta* **447**, 188–202.

Phillips, D. M. (1972a). Substructure of the mammalian acrosome. *J. Ultrastruct. Res.* **38**, 591–604.

Phillips, D. M. (1972b). Comparative analysis of mammalian sperm motility. *J. Cell Biol.* **53**, 561–573.

Phillips, D. M. (1975a). Cell surface structure of rodent sperm heads. *J. Exp. Zool.* **191**, 1–8.

Phillips, D. M. (1975b). Mammalian sperm structure. *In* "Handbook of Physiology" (D. W. Hamilton and R. O. Greep, eds.), Sect. 7, Vol. V, pp. 405–419. Am. Physiol. Soc., Washington, D.C.

Phillips, D. M. (1977a). Surface of the equatorial segment of the mammalian acrosome. *Biol. Reprod.* **16**, 128–137.

Phillips, D. M. (1977b). Mitochondrial disposition in mammalian spermatozoa. *J. Ultrastruct. Res.* **58**, 144–154.

Phillips, D. W. (1980). Observations on mammalian spermiogenesis using surface replicas. *J. Ultrastruct. Res.* **72**, 103–111.

Pikó, L. (1969). Gamete structure and sperm entry in mammals. *In* "Fertilization. Comparative Morphology, Biochemistry, and Immunology" (C. B. Metz and A. Monroy, eds.), Vol. 2, pp. 325–403. Academic Press, New York.

Piperno, G., Huang, B., and Luck, D. J. L. (1977). Two-dimensional analysis of flagellar proteins from wild-type and paralyzed mutants of *Chlamydomonas reinhardtii. Proc. Natl. Acad. Sci. U.S.A.* **74**, 1600–1604.

Plattner, H. (1971). Bull spermatozoa: A re-investigation by freeze-etching using widely different cryofixation procedures. *J. Submicrosc. Cytol.* **3**, 19–32.

Platz, R. D., Grimes, S. R., Jr., Meistrich, M. L., and Hnilica, L. S. (1975). Changes in nuclear proteins of rat testis cells separated by velocity sedimentation. *J. Biol. Chem.* **250**, 5791–5800.

Platz, R. D., Grimes, S. R., Jr., Meistrich, M. L., and Hnilica, L. S. (1976). Synthesis and phosphorylation of nuclear proteins in rat testis spermatids. *J. Cell Biol.* **70**, 106a.

Polakoski, K. L., and Parrish, R. F. (1977). Boar proacrosin. Purification and preliminary activation studies of proacrosin isolated from ejaculated boar sperm. *J. Biol. Chem.* **252**, 1888–1894.

Polakoski, K. L., Williams, W. L., and McRorie, R. A. (1972). Purification and properties of acrosin, an arginyl proteinase, from sperm acrosomes. *Fed. Proc., Fed. Am. Soc. Exp. Biol.* **31**, 278.

Pongsawasdi, P., and Svasti, J. (1976). The heterogeneity of the protamines from human spermatozoa. *Biochim. Biophys. Acta* **434**, 462–473.

Poulos, A., Voglmayr, J. D., and White, I. G. (1973). Phospholipid changes in spermatozoa during passage through the genital tract of the bull. *Biochim. Biophys. Acta* **306**, 194–202.

Premkumar, E., and Bhargava, P. M. (1972). Transcription and translation in bovine spermatozoa. *Nature (London) New Biol.* **240**, 139–143.

Premkumar, E., and Bhargava, P. M. (1973). Isolation and characterization of newly synthesized RNA and protein in mature bovine spermatozoa and effects of inhibitors on these syntheses. *Indian J. Biochem. Biophys.* **10**, 239–253.

Price, J. M. (1973). Biochemical and morphological studies of outer dense fibers of rat spermatozoa. *J. Cell Biol.* **59**, 272a.

Primakoff, P., Myles, D. G., and Bellvé, A. R. (1980a). Biochemical analysis of the released products of the mammalian acrosome reaction. *Dev. Biol.* **80**, 324–331.

Primakoff, P., Myles, D. G., and Bellvé, A. R. (1980b). Topographical organization of the mammalian sperm cell surface. *J. Cell Biol.* **87**, 98a.

Puwaravutipanich, T., and Panyim, S. (1975). The nuclear basic proteins of human testes and ejaculated spermatozoa. *Exp. Cell Res.* **90**, 153–158.

Radu, I., and Voisin, G. A. (1975). Ontogenesis of spermatozoa auto-antigens in guinea pig. *Differentiation* **3**, 107–114.

Rattner, J. B., and Brinkley, B. R. (1972). Ultrastructure of mammalian spermiogenesis. III. The organization and morphogenesis of the manchette during rodent spermiogenesis. *J. Ultrastruct. Res.* **41**, 209–218.

Robinson, R., and Fritz, I. B. (1981). Metabolism of glucose by Sertoli cells in culture. *Biol. Reprod.* **24**, 1032–1041.

Romrell, L. J., and O'Rand, M. G. (1978). Capping and ultrastructural localization of sperm surface isoantigens during spermatogenesis. *Dev. Biol.* **63**, 76–93.

Romrell, L. J., Bellvé, A. R., and Fawcett, D. W. (1976). Separation of mouse spermatogenic cells by sedimentation velocity. A morphological characterization. *Dev. Biol.* **49**, 119–131.

Romrell, L. J., O'Rand, M. G., Sandow, P. R., and Porter, J. P. (1982). Identification of surface antigens which appear during spermatogenesis. *Gamete Res.* **5**, 35–48.

Russell, L., and Frank, B. (1978). Characterization of rat spermatocytes after plastic embedding. *Arch. Androl.* **1**, 5–18.

Sanborn, B. M., Steinberger, A., Meistrich, M. L., and Steinberger, E. (1975). Androgen binding sites in testis cell fractions as measured by nuclear exchange assay. *J. Steroid Biochem.* **6**, 1459–1465.

Sandoz, D. (1970). Evolution des ultrastructures au cours de la formation de l'acrosome du spermatozoide chez la souris. *J. Microsc. (Paris)* **9**, 535–558.

Satir, P. (1965). Studies on cilia. II. Examination of the distal region of the ciliary shaft and the role of the filaments in motility. *J. Cell Biol.* **26**, 805–834.

Satir, P. (1968). Studies on cilia. III. Further studies on the cilium tip and a "sliding filament" model of ciliary motion. *J. Cell Biol.* **39**, 77–94.

Schachner, M., Wortham, K. A., Carter, L. D., and Chaffee, J. K. (1975). NS-4 (Nervous system antigen-4), a cell surface antigen of developing and adult mouse brain and sperm. *Dev. Biol.* **44**, 313–325.

Schenkman, J. B., Richert, D. A., and Westerfeld, W. W. (1965). α-Glycerophosphate dehydrogenase activity in rat spermatozoa. *Endocrinology* **76**, 1055–1061.

Schmid, M., Hofgartner, F. J., Zenzes, M. T., and Engel, W. (1977). Evidence for postmeiotic expression of ribosomal RNA genes during male gametogenesis. *Hum. Genet.* **38**, 279–284.

Schoenfeld, C., Amelar, R. D., and Dubin, L. (1973). Stimulation of ejaculated human spermatozoa by caffeine. A preliminary report. *Fertil. Steril.* **24**, 772–775.

Schrader, F., and Leuchtenberger, C. (1951). The cytology and chemical nature of some constituents of the developing sperm. *Chromosoma* **4**, 404–428.

Schwartz, M. A., and Koehler, J. K. (1979). Alterations in lectin binding to guinea pig spermatozoa accompanying *in vitro* capacitation and the acrosome reaction. *Biol. Reprod.* **21**, 1295–1307.

Scott, T. W., Voglmayr, J. E., and Setchell, B. P. (1967). Lipid composition and metabolism in testicular and ejaculated ram spermatozoa. *Biochem. J.* **102**, 456–461.

Seeds, N. W. (1975). Cerebellar cell surface antigens of mouse brain. *Proc. Natl. Acad. Sci. U.S.A.* **72**, 4110–4114.

Seiguer, A. C., and Castro, A. E. (1972). Electron microscopic demonstration of arylsulfatase activity during acrosome formation in the rat. *Biol. Reprod.* **7**, 31–42.

Selivonchick, D. P., Schmid, P. E., Natarajan, V., and Schmid, H. H. O. (1980). Structure and metabolism of phospholipids in bovine epididymal spermatozoa. *Biochim. Biophys. Acta* **618**, 242–254.

Shams-Borhan, G., Huneau, D., and Fléchon, J.-E. (1979). Acrosin does not appear to be bound to the inner acrosomal membrane of bull spermatozoa. *J. Exp. Zool.* **209**, 143–149.

Shaper, J. H., Pardoll, D. M., Kaufmann, S. H., Barrack, E. R., Vogelstein, B., and Coffery, D. S. (1979). The relationship of the nuclear matrix to cellular structure and function. *Adv. Enzyme Regul.* **17**, 213–248.

Shires, A., Carpenter, M. P., and Chalkley, R. (1975). New histones found in mature mammalian testes. *Proc. Natl. Acad. Sci. U.S.A.* **72**, 2714–2718.

Shires, A., Carpenter, M. P., and Chalkley, R. (1976). A cysteine-containing H2B-like histone found in mature mammalian testis. *J. Biol. Chem.* **251**, 4155–4158.

Sipski, M. L., and Wagner, T. E. (1977). The total structure and organization of chromosomal fibers in eutherian sperm nuclei. *Biol. Reprod.* **16**, 428–440.

Smith, B. V., and Lacy, D. (1959). Residual bodies of seminiferous tubules of the rat. *Nature (London)* **184**, 249–251.

Söderström, K.-O. (1976). Characterization of RNA synthesis in mid-pachytene spermatocytes of the rat. *Exp. Cell Res.* **102**, 237–245.

Söderström, K.-O., and Parvinen, M. (1976). RNA synthesis in different stages of rat seminiferous epithelial cycle. *Mol. Cell. Endocrinol.* **5**, 181–199.

Solari, A. J. (1974). The behavior of the XY pair in mammals. *Int. Rev. Cytol.* **38**, 273–317.

Sosa, A., Altamirano, E., Hernández, P., and Rosado, A. (1972). Developmental pattern of rat testis hexokinase. *Life Sci.* **11** (Part II), 493–498.

Srivastava, P. N., and Abou-Issa, H. (1977). Purification and properties of rabbit spermatozoal acrosomal neuraminidase. *Biochem. J.* **161**, 193–200.

Srivastava, P. N., Adams, C. E., and Hartree, E. F. (1965). Enzymic action of acrosomal preparations on the rabbit ovum *in vitro*. *J. Reprod. Fertil.* **10**, 61–67.

Srivastava, P. N., Zaneveld, L. J. D., and Williams, W. L. (1970). Mammalian sperm acrosomal neuraminidases. *Biochem. Biophys. Res. Commun.* **39**, 575–582.

Srivastava, P. N., Munnell, J. F., Yang, C. H., and Foley, C. W. (1974). Sequential release of acrosomal membranes and acrosomal enzymes of ram spermatozoa. *J. Reprod. Fertil.* **36**, 363–372.

Stackpole, C. W., and Devorkin, D. (1974). Membrane organization in mouse spermatozoa revealed by freeze-etching. *J. Ultrastruct. Res.* **49**, 167–187.

Stambaugh, R. (1978). Enzymatic and morphological events in mammalian fertilization. *Gamete Res.* **1**, 65–85.

Stambaugh, R., and Buckley, J. (1969). Identification and subcellular localization of the enzymes effecting penetration of the zona pellucida by rabbit spermatozoa. *J. Reprod. Fertil.* **19**, 423–432.

Stambaugh, R., and Buckley, J. (1970). Comparative studies of the acrosomal enzymes of rabbit, rhesus monkey and human spermatozoa. *Biol. Reprod.* **3**, 275–282.

Stedman, E., and Stedman, E. (1947). The chemical nature and functions of the components of cell nuclei. *Cold Spring Harbor Symp. Quant. Biol.* **12**, 224–236.

Stefanini, M., Oura, C., and Zamboni, L. (1969). Ultrastructure of fertilization in the mouse. 2. Penetration of sperm into the ovum. *J. Submicrosc. Cytol.* **1**, 1–23.

Stefanini, M., DeMartino, C., D'Agostino, A., Agrestini, A., and Monesi, V. (1974). Nucleolar activity of rat primary spermatocytes. *Exp. Cell Res.* **86**, 166–170.

Stephens, D. T., Wang, J., and Hoskins, D. D. (1979). The cyclic AMP phosphodiesterase of bovine spermatozoa: Multiple forms, kinetic properties and changes during development. *Biol. Reprod.* **20**, 483–491.

Stephens, D. T., Acott, T. S., and Hoskins, D. D. (1981). A cautionary note on the determination of forward motility protein activity with bovine epididymal spermatozoa. *Biol. Reprod.* **25**, 945–949.

Stephens, R. E. (1970a). Thermal fractionation of outer fiber doublet microtubules into A- and B- subfiber components. *J. Mol. Biol.* **47**, 353–363.

Stephens, R. E. (1970b). Isolation of nexin—the linkage protein responsible for maintenance of the nine-fold configuration of flagellar axonemes. *Biol. Bull. (Woods Hole, Mass.)* **139**, 438.

Stephens, R. E. (1974). Enzymatic and structural proteins of the axoneme. *In* "Cilia and Flagella" (M. A. Sleigh, ed.), pp. 39–76. Academic Press, New York.

Storey, B. T., and Kayne, F. J. (1977). Energy metabolism of spermatozoa. VI. Direct intramitochondrial lactate oxidation by rabbit sperm mitochondria. *Biol. Reprod.* **16**, 549–556.

Storey, B. T., and Kayne, F. J. (1978). Energy metabolism of spermatozoa. VII. Interactions between lactate, pyruvate and malate as oxidative substrates for rabbit sperm mitochondria. *Biol. Reprod.* **18**, 527–536.

Strauch, A. R., Luna, E. J., and LaFountain, J. (1980). Biochemical analysis of actin in crane-fly gonial cells: Evidence for actin in spermatocytes and spermatids—but not in sperm. *J. Cell Biol.* **86**, 315–325.

Suau, P., and Subirana, J. A. (1977). X-ray diffraction studies of nucleoprotamine structure. *J. Mol. Biol.* **117**, 909–926.

Summers, K. (1974). ATP-induced sliding of microtubules in bull sperm flagella. *J. Cell Biol.* **60**, 321–324.

Summers, K. E., and Gibbons, I. R. (1971). Adenosine triphosphate-induced sliding of tubules in trypsin treated flagella of sea urchin sperm. *Proc. Natl. Acad. Sci. U.S.A.* **68**, 3092–3096.

Susi, F. R., and Clermont, Y. (1970). Fine structural modifications of the rat chromatoid body during spermatogenesis. *Am. J. Anat.* **129**, 177–192.

Susi, F. R., Leblond, C. P., and Clermont, Y. (1971). Changes in the Golgi apparatus during spermiogenesis in the rat. *Am. J. Anat.* **130**, 251–268.

Suzuki, F. (1981). Changes in intramembrane particle distribution in epidiymal spermatozoa of the boar. *Anat. Rec.* **199**, 361–376.

Suzuki, F., and Nagano, T. (1980). Epididymal maturation of rat spermatozoa studied by thin sectioning and freeze-fracture. *Biol. Reprod.* **22**, 1219–1231.

Swyer, G. I. M. (1947). The release of hyaluronidase from spermatozoa. *Biochem. J.* **41**, 413–417.

Tamblyn, T. M. (1980). Identification of actin in boar epididymal spermatozoa. *Biol. Reprod.* **22**, 727–734.

Tang, X.-M., Lalli, M. F., and Clermont, Y. (1982). A cytochemical study of the Golgi apparatus of the spermatid during spermiogenesis in the rat. *Am. J. Anat.* **163**, 283–294.

Tash, J. S., and Means, A. R. (1982). Regulation of protein phosphorylation and motility of sperm by cyclic adenosine monophosphate and calcium. *Biol. Reprod.* **26**, 745–763.

Teichman, R. J., and Bernstein, M. H. (1971). Fine structure localizations of acid phosphatase in rabbit and bull sperm heads. *J. Reprod. Fertil.* **27**, 243–248.

Teichman, R. J., Fujimoto, M., and Yanagimachi, R. (1972). A previously unrecognized material in mammalian spermatozoa as revealed by malachite green and pyronine. *Biol. Reprod.* **7**, 73–81.

Teichman, R. J., Cummins, J. M., and Takei, G. M. (1974). The characterization of a malachite green stainable, glutaraldehyde extractable phospholipid in rabbit spermatozoa. *Biol. Reprod.* **10**, 565–577.

Telkka, A., Fawcett, D. W., and Christensen, A. K. (1961). Further observations on the structure of the mammalian sperm tail. *Anat. Rec.* **141**, 231–245.

Teuscher, C., Wild, G. C., and Tung, K. S. K. (1982). Immunochemical analysis of guinea pig sperm autoantigens. *Biol. Reprod.* **26**, 218–229.

Tobias, P. S., and Schumacher, G. F. B. (1977). Observation of two proacrosins in extracts of human spermatozoa. *Biochem. Biophys. Res. Commun.* **74**, 434–439.

Toullet, F., Voisin, G. A., and Neminrovsky, M. (1973). Histoimmunochemical localization of three guinea-pig spermatozoal antigens. *Immunology* **24**, 635–653.

Tres, L. L. (1975). Nucleolar RNA synthesis of meiotic prophase spermatocytes in the human testis. *Chromosoma* **53**, 141–151.

Tsai, Y.-H., Sanborn, B. M., Steinberger, A., and Steinberger, E. (1977). The interaction of testicular androgen-receptor complex with rat germ cell and Sertoli cell chromatin. *Biochem. Biophys. Res. Commun.* **75**, 366–372.

Tsanev, R., and Avramova, Z. (1981). Nonprotamine nucleoprotein ultrastructures in mature ram sperm nuclei. *Eur. J. Cell Biol.* **24**, 139–145.

Tung, K. S. K., Han, L.-P. B., and Evan, A. P. (1979). Differentiation autoantigen of testicular cells and spermatozoa in the guinea pig. *Dev. Biol.* **68**, 224–238.

Tung, K. S. K., Okada, A., and Yanagimachi, R. (1980). Sperm autoantigens and fertilization. I. Effects of antisperm autoantibodies on rouleaux formation, viability, and acrosome reaction of guinea pig spermatozoa. *Biol. Reprod.* **23**, 877–886.

Tung, K. S. K., Yanagimachi, H., and Yanagimachi, R. (1982). Sperm autoantigens and fertilization. III. Ultrastructural localization of guinea pig autoantigens. *Anat. Rec.* **22**, 241–253.

Tung, P. S., and Fritz, I. B. (1978). Specific surface antigens on rat pachytene spermatocytes and successive classes of germinal cells. *Dev. Biol.* **64**, 297–315.

Utakoji, T., Muramatsu, M., and Sugano, H. (1968). Isolation of pachytene nuclei from the Syrian hamster testis. *Exp. Cell Res.* **53**, 447–458.

Vandeberg, J. L., Cooper, D. W., and Close, P. J. (1976). Testis specific phosphoglycerate kinase B in mouse. *J. Exp. Zool.* **198**, 231–240.

Van Dop, C., Hutson, S. M., and Lardy, H. A. (1977). Pyruvate metabolism in bovine epididymal spermatozoa. *J. Biol. Chem.* **252**, 1303–1308.

Vernon, R. B., Muller, C. H., Herr, J. C., Feuchter, F. A., and Eddy, E. M. (1982). Epididymal secretion of a mouse sperm surface component recognized by a monoclonal antibody. *Biol. Reprod.* **26**, 523–535.

Vernon, R. G., Go, V. L. W., and Fritz, I. B. (1971). Studies on spermatogenesis in rats. II. Evidence that carnitine acetyltransferase is a marker enzyme for the investigation of germ cell differentiation. *Can. J. Biochem.* **49**, 761–767.

Voglmayr, J. K. (1975). Metabolic changes in spermatozoa during epididymal transit. *In* "Handbook of Physiology" (D. W. Hamilton and R. O. Greep, eds.), Sect. 7, Vol. V, pp. 437–451. Am. Physiol. Soc., Washington, D.C.

Voglmayr, J. K., Fairbanks, G., Jackowitz, M. A., and Colella, J. R. (1980). Post-testicular developmental changes in the ram sperm cell surface and their relationship to luminal fluid proteins of the reproductive tract. *Biol. Reprod.* **22**, 655–667.

Waites, G. M. H. (1980). Functional relationships of the mammalian testes and epididymis. *Aust. J. Biol. Sci.* **33**, 355–370.

Walker, M. H. (1971). Studies on the arrangement of nucleoprotein in elongate sperm heads. *Chromosoma* **34**, 340–354.

Warner, F. D. (1976). Cross-bridge mechanisms in ciliary motility: The sliding-bending conversion. *Cold Spring Harbor Conf. Cell Proliferation* **3** (Book C), 891–914.

Warrant, R. W., and Kim, S.-H. (1978). α-Helix–double helix interaction shown in the structure of a protamine-transfer RNA complex and a nucleoprotamine model. *Nature (London)* **271**, 130–135.

Weintraub, H. (1975). Release of discrete subunits after nuclease and trypsin digestion of chromatin. *Proc. Natl. Acad. Sci. U.S.A.* **72**, 1212–1216.

Wenström, J. C., and Hamilton, D. W. (1980). Dolichol concentration and biosynthesis in rat testis and epididymis. *Biol. Reprod.* **23**, 1054–1059.

Westergaard, M., and von Wettstein, D. (1972). The synaptonemal complex. *Annu. Rev. Genet.* **6**, 71–110.

Wheat, T. E., Hintz, M., Goldberg, E., and Margoliash, E. (1977). Analyses of stage-specific multiple forms of lactate dehydrogenase and of cytochrome c during spermatogenesis in the mouse. *Differentiation* **9**, 37–41.

Witkin, S. S., Evenson, D. P., and Bendich, A. (1977). Chromatin organization and the existence of a chromatin-associated DNA-generating system in human sperm. *In* "The Molecular Biology of the Mammalian Genetic Apparatus" (P. Ts'o, ed.), pp. 345–354. Elsevier/North-Holland Biomedical Press, New York.

Witman, G. B., Carlson, K., and Rosenbaum, J. L. (1972). *Chlamydomonas* flagella. II. The distribution of tubulins 1 and 2 in the outer doublet microtubules. *J. Cell Biol.* **54**, 540–555.

Wooding, F. B. P. (1973). The effect of Triton X-100 on the ultrastructure of ejaculated bovine sperm. *J. Ultrastruct. Res.* **42**, 502–516.

Wooding, F. B. P., and O'Donnell, J. M. (1971). A detailed ultrastructural study of the head membranes of ejaculated bovine sperm. *J. Ultrastruct. Res.* **35**, 71–85.

Woolley, D. M. (1970). The midpiece of the mouse spermatozoon: Its form and development as seen by surface replication. *J. Cell Sci.* **6**, 865–879.

Woolley, D. M., and Fawcett, D. W. (1973). The degeneration and disappearance of the centrioles during the development of the rat spermatozoon. *Anat. Rec.* **177,** 289–302.

Working, P K., and Meizel, S. (1981). Evidence that an ATPase functions in the maintenance of the acidic pH of the hamster sperm acrosome reaction. *J. Biol. Chem.* **256,** 4708–4711.

Working, P. K., and Meizel, S. (1982). Preliminary characterization of a Mg^{2+} ATPase in hamster sperm head membranes. *Biochem. Biophys. Res. Commun.* **104,** 1060–1065.

Wyker, R., and Howards, S. S. (1977). Micropuncture studies of the motility of rete testis and epididymal spermatozoa. *Fertil. Steril.* **28,** 108–112.

Yanagimachi, R., and Noda, Y. D. (1970a). Ultrastructural changes in the hamster sperm head during fertilization. *J. Ultrastruct. Res.* **31,** 465–485.

Yanagimachi, R., and Noda, Y. D. (1970b). Electron microscope studies of sperm incorporation into the golden hamster egg. *Am. J. Anat.* **128,** 429–437.

Yanagimachi, R., and Teichman, R. J. (1972). Cytochemical demonstration of acrosomal proteinase in mammalian and avian spermatozoa by a silver proteinate method. *Biol. Reprod.* **6,** 87–97.

Yanagisawa, K., Bennett, D., Boyse, E. A., Dunn, L. C., and Dimeo, A. (1974). Serological identification of sperm antigens specified by lethal *t*-alleles in the mouse. *Immunogenetics* **1,** 57–67.

Yang, C. H., and Srivastava, P. M. (1974). Separation and properties of hyaluronidase from ram sperm acrosomes. *J. Reprod. Fertil.* **37,** 17–25.

Zamboni, L., and Stefanini, M. (1971). The fine structure of the neck of mammalian spermatozoa. *Anat. Rec.* **169,** 155–172.

Zamboni, L., Zemjanis, R., and Stefanini, M. (1971). The fine structure of monkey and human spermatozoa. *Anat. Rec.* **169,** 129–154.

Zaneveld, L. J. D., Robertson, R. T., Kessler, M., and Williams, W. L. (1971). Inhibition of fertilization *in vivo* by pancreatic and seminal plasma trypsin inhibitors. *J. Reprod. Fertil.* **25,** 387–392.

Zaneveld, L. J. D., Dragoje, B. M., and Schumacher, G. F. B. (1972a). Acrosomal proteinase and proteinase inhibitor of human spermatozoa. *Science* **177,** 702–703.

Zaneveld, L. J. D., Polakoski, K. L., and Williams, W. L. (1972b). Properties of a proteolytic enzyme from rabbit sperm acrosomes. *Biol. Reprod.* **6,** 30–39.

Zaneveld, L. J. D., Polakoski, K. L., and Schumacher, G. F. B. (1973). Properties of acrosomal hyaluronidase from bull spermatozoa. Evidence for its similarity to testicular hyaluronidase. *J. Biol. Chem.* **248,** 564–570.

Zirkin, B. R., Chang, T. S. K., and Heaps, J. (1980). Involvement of an acrosinlike proteinase in the sulfhydryl-induced degradation of rabbit sperm nuclear protamine. *J. Cell Biol.* **85,** 116–121.

3

Morphological, Biochemical, and Immunochemical Characterization of the Mammalian Zona Pellucida

BONNIE S. DUNBAR

139

Mechanism and Control of Animal Fertilization
Copyright © 1983 by Academic Press, Inc.
All rights of reproduction in any form reserved.
ISBN 0-12-328520-8

I. INTRODUCTION

Of the many aspects of the fertilization process, the encounter between the sperm and the zona pellucida is one of the most significant.
Oocytes of many species are surrounded by egg envelopes which include the zona pellucida of mammals (Austin, 1961; Pikó, 1969) and
fish (Nakano, 1969) and the vitelline envelopes of invertebrates
(Heller and Raftery, 1976; Glabe and Vacquier, 1977) and amphibians
(Wolf *et al.*, 1976). The mammalian zona pellucida is the extracellular
glycoprotein structure surrounding the mammalian oocyte. It is
formed during the development of the oocyte, surrounds the embryo
after fertilization, and remains in this locale until implantation. The
zona is important in the initial stages of fertilization since the sperm
must bind to and penetrate this structure before fusing with the oocyte
plasma membrane (Austin and Braden, 1965; Austin, 1975; Stambaugh, 1978).

Initial studies using some rodent species suggested that sperm attachment to the zona was species-specific (Austin and Braden, 1956;
Yanagimachi, 1977). These studies prompted the search for specific
"sperm receptors" on the surface of the zona. Such receptors have been
described for invertebrate species such as those associated with sea
urchin vitelline envelopes (Aketa, 1973; Kinsey and Lennarz, 1981).
Although limited evidence has been presented for such receptors in
mammals (Gwatkin and Williams, 1977; Peterson *et al.*, 1981), the
universality of this phenomenon is yet to be proved. For instance, the
species-specificity of sperm–zona interaction has been described for
some species of mammals, including mouse, hamster, guinea pig, and
rat (Austin and Braden, 1956; Yanagimachi, 1977; Schmell and
Gulyas, 1980), but less specificity is exhibited by other mammalian
species, such as the rabbit (Bedford, 1977; Swenson and Dunbar, 1982).
Other factors affecting sperm–zona interaction also vary among species. These factors include sperm capacitation (the changes that occur
in the sperm which make it capable of fertilizing the ova), which is a
requirement in sperm binding *in vitro* to zonae of mice (Saling *et al.*,
1978) and in physiologically significant binding in hamsters
(Hartmann and Hutchison, 1974, 1977), but not in pig or rabbit (Peterson *et al.*, 1980; Swenson and Dunbar, 1982). The requirement for
calcium in sperm–zona interaction also varies according to species,
since this divalent ion is essential for sperm binding to zonae of mice
(Saling *et al.*, 1978) but is not essential for rabbit sperm–zona interaction *in vitro* (Swenson and Dunbar, 1982). Until there is a better understanding of the macromolecular composition of zonae and of sperm

membranes, the exact nature of these interactions will not be clearly understood.

The zona also plays a role in the "block to polyspermy." This process, which will be discussed in more detail elsewhere in this volume, prevents abnormal fertilization and embryo cleavage which result from entry of more than one male pronuclei (Austin and Braden, 1956). The block is presumably due to changes in the zona that are thought to be due to the ova cortical granule contents which are released following sperm–egg plasma membrane fusion (Barros and Yanagimachi, 1977; Gwatkin et al., 1973) and varies among species (Yanagimachi, 1977). To date, however, there is limited information available on the precise chemical nature of the zona reaction of mammalian oocytes, because it has not been possible to obtain sufficient numbers of ova or embryos for detailed chemical characterization.

II. ISOLATION OF MAMMALIAN ZONAE PELLUCIDAE

Since few mammalian oocytes were available, early studies on the physical and chemical properties of zonae pellucidae have been restricted to microscopic methods or to methods that could be adapted to the analysis of small amounts of material (Soupart and Noyes, 1964; Pikó, 1969; Gould et al., 1971; Bleil and Wassarman, 1980a,b,c; Stegner and Wartenberg, 1961). More recently, methods have been developed that allow the large-scale isolation of porcine (Dunbar et al., 1980; Dunbar and Raynor, 1980; Wood et al., 1981; Oikawa, 1978; Sacco, 1981), cow (Gwatkin et al., 1980), and rabbit zonae pellucidae (Wood et al., 1981). Recently an apparatus was designed to rupture ovarian follicles en masse, leaving the ovary intact (Wood et al., 1981). This apparatus has been found to be more efficient in the time required for preparation as well as in the numbers of oocytes which can be isolated from ovaries. This system makes it possible to isolate up to 400,000 pig oocytes and zonae or 30,000 rabbit oocytes and zonae in 4–5 hours.

Many attempts have been made to isolate zonae from mouse, hamster, and rat ovaries with these en masse zonae isolation methods, since these animals are the models that have been used in the majority of mammalian fertilization studies. To date all such attempts have failed. A primary reason for these failures is because the oocyte diameter as well as the zonae width of these rodent species is smaller than those of the pig or rabbit (Table I). A second reason is that the popula-

TABLE I

Summary of the Relative Sizes of Zonae Pellucidae of a Variety of Mammalian Species[a]

Species	Zona width (μm)	References
Opossum	1–2	J. M. Bedford, personal communication
Mouse	5	Lowenstein and Cohen, 1964
Hamster	8	Austin, 1961[b]
Human	13	Austin, 1961[b]
Sheep (mature)	14.5	Wright et al., 1977
Sheep (immature)	14.5	Wright et al., 1977
Rabbit	15	Austin, 1965[b]
Pig	16	J. M. Dunbar, unpublished
Cow	27	Wright et al., 1977

[a] Values taken from mature ova except where indicated.
[b] Values extrapolated from diagrams.

tions of oocytes obtained from rodent ovaries are not homogenous in size as are those isolated from pig and rabbit ovaries. Finally, rodent zonae are far more fragile and cannot be mechanically manipulated as can those from species having larger zonae (B. S. Dunbar, unpublished observations).

III. MORPHOLOGICAL PROPERTIES OF ZONAE PELLUCIDAE

The morphological properties of zonae have been studied by light as well as by scanning and transmission electron microscopy. These studies have suggested that the zonae of some species such as the human (Stegner and Wartenberg, 1961), pig (Dickmann and Dziuk, 1964; Hedrick and Fry, 1980), and rabbit (Sacco, 1981) are composed of more than one layer as compared to other species such as the mouse (Cholewa-Stewart and Massaro, 1972) or the rat (Sacco, 1981).

Scanning electron microscopy of the zonae of all species examined to date has demonstrated that the outer surface of the zonae has a fenestrated lattice-like appearance (Phillips and Shalgi, 1980; Jackowski and Dumont 1979; Dudkiewicz et al., 1976; Russel et al., 1980). The outer surface of the rabbit zona is illustrated in Fig. 1a. This fenestrated structure may be formed during oocyte maturation as the result of cytoplasmic processes of follicular cells, which are formed during development, being extended through the zona to make contact with

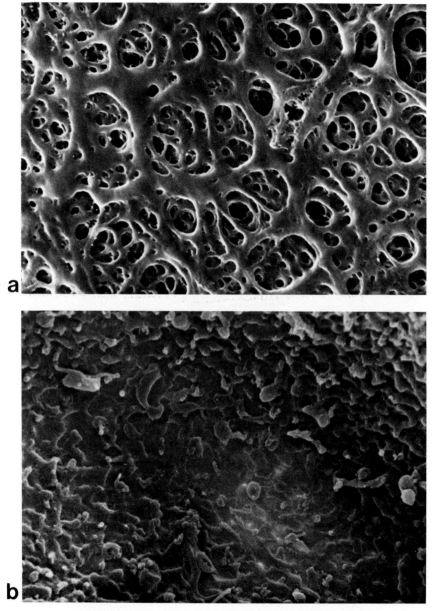

Fig. 1.   Scanning electron micrograph of rabbit zona pellucida. (a) Outer surface. (b) Inner surface. (Courtesy of David M. Phillips, The Population Council.)

the oocyte (Anderson and Albertini, 1976; Van Blerkom and Motta, 1979; Dekel and Phillips, 1979). Such processes of the inner layer of follicular cells which extend through the zona are illustrated in Fig. 2. The inner portion of the zona of the hamster has been found to contain a surface that is morphologically distinct from the outer surface (Phillips and Shalgi, 1980). This morphological distinction has also been observed in the rabbit zona of an ovulated ova (D. M. Phillips and B. S. Dunbar, unpublished, see Fig. 1b). These morphological observations are consistent with the lectin-binding properties of zona which also demonstrate the variability of the properties of outer and inner surfaces of zonae. (Nicolson *et al.*, 1975; Dunbar *et al.*, 1980; Dunbar, 1980).

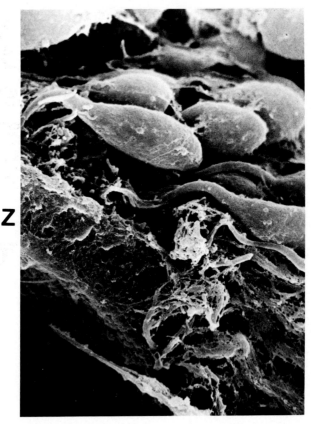

Fig. 2. Scanning electron micrograph of rabbit follicular cells with processes extending through the zona pellucida (z). (Courtesy of David M. Phillips, The Population Council.)

IV. PHYSICAL AND CHEMICAL PROPERTIES OF ZONAE PELLUCIDAE

A. Solubility Properties

1. Physicochemical Parameters

Studies have been carried out to examine the efficacy of a variety of parameters to cause dissolution of zonae pellucidae. Solubilization has been evaluated by light microscopy. Visual criteria of zona dissolution are limited by their subjective nature and do not necessarily correlate with biochemical methods (Dunbar et al., 1980). However, such information is useful as a means of comparing zonae pellucidae of different species. A summary of conditions which affect the dissolution of the zonae assessed by microscopic criteria are listed in Table II. This summary indicates that species variation in zonae exists since a variety of conditions affect dissolution differentially. As an example, the zonae of rodents appear to be more sensitive to pH than those of other species.

More detailed chemical studies in which protein analysis of pig zonae are used have now been reported (Dunbar et al., 1980). Pig zonae can be solubilized by conditions which do not break covalent bonds (heat at basic pH). These conditions result in supramacromolecular complexes of zona macromolecules. Dissociation into individual macromolecules can be carried out by the reduction of disulfide bonds in the presence of detergent (Dunbar et al., 1980, 1981).

2. Effect of Enzymes on Zonae

Proteolytic enzymes have been shown to cause dissolution of zonae pellucidae (see Table III). Again there appears to be considerable variation among species with respect to the susceptibility of zonae to enzymatic digestion. Earlier studies gave conflicting results which could be due to impurities or to the variation of specific activities of enzyme preparations which were available. These studies do demonstrate, however, that there is species variation in the enzymatic dissolution of zonae.

A variety of enzymes, including proteolytic enzymes, have been detected in mammalian sperm, although there are considerable quantitative and qualitative species differences (Stambaugh, 1978; McRorie and Williams, 1974). Some of these enzymes, including acrosin (the well-characterized trypsinlike proteolytic enzyme in the sperm acrosome), are thought to be critical in sperm penetration of the zona pellucida (McRorie and Williams, 1974; Fritz et al., 1975; Hartree, 1977), but their specific role(s) have yet to be directly characterized.

TABLE II

Summary of Conditions Known to Effect Dissolution of Zonae Pellucidae[a]

Species	Temperature (°C)	pH	Solubilization reagents	Reference
Mouse	68–70			Cholewa-Stewart and Massaro, 1972
		4.1		Gwatkin, 1964
	37	4.51	(10 minutes)	Inoue and Wolf, 1974[b,c]
			0.75 M Mercaptoethanol (15 minutes)	Inoue and Wolf, 1974[c]
			0.375 M Dithiothreitol (31 minutes)	
			0.75 M Thioglycolate (130 minutes)	
Rat			0.25 M Mercaptoethanol (22 minutes)	Inoue and Wolf, 1975[c]
		3		Austin, 1961
		5		Hall, 1935
		13		Braden, 1952
Rabbit		<3		Braden, 1952
		13		Braden, 1952

Species		Time (min)	Solubilization method	Reference
	60		1.5 M Mercaptoethanol 1% Sodium dodecyl sulfate (SDS) 0.01 M Mercaptoethanol (heated at 60°C for 60 minutes)	Gould et al., 1971 B. S. Dunbar, unpublished[d]
Pig	<3.8	60	1% SDS + 0.01 Mercaptoethanol > 6 M urea > Triton X-100 + 0.01 M mercaptoethanol (heated at 60°C for 120 minutes)	Dunbar et al., 1980[d]
Hamster			0.01 M Mercaptoethanol (25°C, 5 minutes) 0.001 M Mercaptoethanol (5 minutes)	Oikawa et al., 1973 Inoue and Wolf, 1975

[a] Zona dissolution determined by light microscopy except where indicated.
[b] Rate of dissolution in low pH found to be temperature dependent.
[c] Dissolution time is mean time for 50% of all zonae to dissolve.
[d] Solubilization of zonae estimated by determination of the amount of solubilized protein as compared to the insoluble pellet after centrifugation.

148

TABLE III

Summary of Enzymes Shown to Effect the Dissolution of Zonae Pellucidae of Unfertilized Ova[a]

Species	% Zona/time needed for dissolution (enzyme concentration)			Reference
	Pronase	Trypsin	Chymotrypsin	
Mouse	100%/34 minutes (0.5%)	No effect/60 minutes	No effect/60 minutes	Wright et al., 1977
CBA genotype			90%/180 minutes (0.003%)	Gwatkin, 1964
				Kaleta and Majewska, 1979
KE genotype			22%/180 minutes (0.003%)	Kaleta and Majewska, 1979
F (CBAXKE)			65%/180 minutes (0.003%)	Kaleta and Majewska, 1979
	50%/60 minutes (0.005%)	49%/60 minutes (0.005%)	52%/60 minutes (0.005%)	Aonuma et al., 1978
	ng[b]/3 minutes (0.5%)			Mintz, 1962

Species				Reference
Hamster	ng/2–10 minutes (0.01%)	ng/2–10 minutes (0.01%)	ng/2–10 minutes) (.01%)	Chang and Hunt, 1956[d]
Rabbit		ng/30–100 minutes (0.1%)	No effect (0.1%)	Chang and Hunt, 1956
		ng/20 minutes (0.1%)		Bedford and Cross, 1978
	100%/15 minutes[c] (0.01%)	100%/20 minutes (0.5%)		D. Drell and B. S. Dunbar, unpublished observations
Rat		ng/20–120 minutes (0.1%)	ng/10 minutes + (0.1%)	Chang and Hunt, 1956
Cow	100%/263 minutes (0.5%)			Wright et al., 1977
Sheep	100%/144 minutes (0.5%)			Wright et al., 1977
Pig	100%/30 minutes[c] (0.5%)	No effect/180 minutes (2%)		D. Drell and B. S. Dunbar, unpublished

[a] Dissolution determined by light microscopic criteria.

[b] ng = not given.

[c] Proteinase K.

[d] Hyaluronidase and papain had no visible effect on rabbit, rat, or hamster eggs.

Microscopic evidence for the involvement of proteolytic digestion of zonae by sperm enzymes has been obtained. Linear arrays of sites of proteolytic activity detected by silver proteinate have been observed during sperm penetration of the rabbit zona pellucida (Stambaugh and Smith, 1976). Acrosin has been shown to remove the zona pellucida from rabbit ova *in vitro* although zona lysis *in vitro* does not correlate with acrosin content of sequential acrosomal extracts (Srivastava, 1973). The use of sperm extracts rather than isolated enzymes results in more rapid lysis of the zona *in vitro;* therefore, the requirement of more than one enzyme in zona digestion has been considered (McRorie and Williams, 1974).

Other evidence has been presented which suggests that the penetration of spermatozoa through the rabbit zona may not require the activity of a trypsinlike enzyme (Bedford and Cross, 1978). These studies show that the addition of wheat germ agglutinin to the rabbit zonae will reduce the susceptibility of digestion by trypsin or acrosin, but that sperm can still penetrate the zona and complete fertilization. Additional studies have shown that protease activity is involved in sperm binding to the hamster and mouse zonae (Hartmann and Hutchison, 1974; Saling, 1981) but is not necessary for sperm penetration (Saling, 1981).

A preliminary report by Hedrick and Wardrip (1980) has shown that proteins of the pig zona pellucida, characterized by two-dimensional gel electrophoresis, are modified by trypsin. These reports have been confirmed by studies which show that pig zonae remain intact (as determined microscopically) after trypsin treatment, but that zonae proteins are chemically altered since a change in protein patterns was visualized by two-dimensional gel electrophoresis (B. S. Dunbar, unpublished; Dunbar and Roberts, 1982). Since it is now possible to isolate large quantities of zonae, detailed studies can be carried out directly to examine the effects of sperm enzymes on zona proteins.

B. Characterization of Zona Pellucida Proteins by Gel Electrophoresis

1. One-Dimensional Gel Electrophoresis

The analyses of zonae pellucidae proteins by one-dimensional gel electrophoresis are summarized in Table IV. The protein-staining patterns of pig zonae obtained from studies using one-dimensional gel electrophoresis have shown that zona proteins exhibit considerable heterogeneity. These proteins have, therefore, not been resolved read-

TABLE IV

Analysis of Zona Proteins by One-Dimensional Polyacrylamide Gel Electrophoresis

Species	sample preparation and solubilization	Page method (% acrylamide)	Number zonae used/gel	Protein identification	Major proteins identified (molecular weight) $\times 10^{-3}$	References
Mouse	[125I]iodosulfanilic acid labeling; frozen four times, (−70°C), then thawed (60°C) in 2% SDS, pH 6.8	Laemmli (1970) (7%)		Radioautography		Bleil and Wassarman, 1980b
	(a) Unreduced				3 (200;120;83)	
	(b) Reduced (50 mM dithiothreitol)				1 (85)	
	Not given	Laemmli (1970) (7%)	750	Coomassie blue (Bleil and Wassarman, 1980b)	3 (200;120;83)	
Rat	2% SDS, pH 6.8; 2% β-mercaptoethanol; heat 2 minutes, 95°C	Laemmli (1970) (10%)	109	Silver stain (Merril et al., 1981)	1 (105–200)	Wolgemuth and Garvin, 1981
Rabbit	2% SDS, 2% mercaptoethanol; heat 5 minutes, 95°C, pH 6.8	Laemmli (1970) (7.5%)	6000	Coomassie blue	1 (70–110)	Dunbar et al., 1981
Pig	2% SDS, 2% mercaptoethanol heat 5 minutes, 95°C, pH 6.8	Laemmli (1970) (7.5%)	6000	Coomassie blue	1 (50–80)	Dunbar et al., 1981
	100°C, 3 minutes, 10% β-mercaptoethanol	Laemmli (1970)	4000	Coomassie blue	1 (60)	Gwatkin et al., 1980
Cow	100°C, 3 minutes; 10% β-mercaptoethanol	Laemmli (1970)	4000	Coomassie blue	3 (100;50;25)	Gwatkin et al., 1980

ily using conventional electrophoresis methods (Dunbar *et al.*, 1980, 1981; Dunbar, 1980; Sacco, 1981; Gwatkin *et al.*, 1980). The major pig zonae proteins revealed by sodium dodecyl sulfate polyacrylamide gel electrophoresis followed by protein staining with Coomassie blue were found to have molecular weights ranging from 40,000 to 70,000 (Dunbar *et al.*, 1980) as compared to the major proteins of rabbit zonae which have molecular weights ranging from 70,000 to 100,000. Gwatkin *et al.* (1980) reported a similar molecular weight range (50,000–80,000) for the proteins of pig zona and also reported molecular weight ranges for proteins associated with the cow zona of 25,000, 50,000, and 100,000.

One-dimensional polyacrylamide gel electroporesis of mouse zona proteins resolved three proteins (Bleil and Wassarman, 1980a,b). It is interesting that three predominant proteins could be detected by Coomassie blue staining when only 750 mouse zonae were applied to the gel. Since these authors have reported the mouse zona to contain 4.8 ng of protein, a total of 3.6 μg total protein was applied to this gel. This quantity of protein was further found to be widely spread among Coomassie blue staining, this amount of protein would be less than is generally detectable by Coomassie blue staining (Fairbanks *et al.*, 1971). It has further been shown by conventional Coomassie blue staining of polyacrylamide gels that several thousand pig zonae or rabbit zonae, each of which contains approximately seven times more protein than those reported for mouse zonae, are necessary for detection of the major zona proteins (Dunbar *et al.*, 1980; Gwatkin *et al.*, 1980). Recent studies have also shown that 150 rat or Rhesus monkey zonae could be detected by the protein–silver stain methods in one-dimensional gels (D. J. Wolgemuth, personal communication). Since this method has been reported to be a 100-fold more sensitive than the Coomassie blue methods (Merril, *et al.*, 1981), this quantity would be equivalent to 15,000 mouse zonae needed for detection by Coomassie blue staining. The future use of the silver stains and two-dimensional polyacrylamide gel electrophoresis methods may resolve these discrepancies.

2. Characterization of Zona Proteins by Two-Dimensional Gel Electrophoresis

Since zona proteins exhibit extreme heterogeneity when resolved with one-dimensional gel electrophoresis, improved resolution of these proteins has been obtained with high-resolution two-dimensional gel electrophoresis. These studies are summarized in Table V. Bleil and Wassarman (1980b) have employed two separate methods of two-di-

TABLE V

Analysis of Zonae Proteins by Two-Dimensional Polyacrylamide Gel Electrophoresis Methods

Species	Sample preparation	PAGE method (% acrylamide) 2nd dimension	No. zonae/gel	Protein detection method	Major proteins identified [MW × 10⁻³ (*pI*)]		References
Mouse	(1) pH 2.5 → [¹²⁵I]iodosulfanilic acid labeling; ¹²⁵I-labeled total zonae combined with ¹²⁵I-labeled zona protein 1 → frozen two times, (−70°C), thawed → 60°C	O'Farrell, 1975 (9%)		Radioautography	ZP1 red ZP2 ZP3	−(5.9)ᵃ −(4.3) −(3.7)	Bleil and Wassarman, 1980
	(2) Same as (1) above or ³H-labeled dansyl chloride labeling instead of ¹²⁵I	Reduction electrophoresis (a) SDS PAGE 1st dimension (b) 50 m*M* dithiothreitol → SDS PAGE 2nd dimension		Radioautography	ZP1 ZP2 ZP3	120–140 100–150ᵇ 60–100ᵇ	Bleil and Wassarman, 1980
	(3) "Lysis buffer" (O'Farrell, 1975)	Garrels, 1979 (5–15% gradient)		Radioautography	1 2	116–122ᶜ 90–92ᶜ	Sacco et al., 1981
	(4) 2% SDS; 2% β-mercaptoethanol, pH 9.4, 95°C, 10 minutes	Anderson et al., 1979 (10–20% gradient)	1000	Silver stain (Upjohn) Sammons et al., 1981	1 2	130–200ᶜ 85–140ᶜ	Dunbar and Wolgemuth, unpublished, Fig. 3
Pig	(5) Same as (4)	6000		Coomassie blue	1 2 3	49–119ᶜ 70–101ᶜ 95–118ᶜ	Dunbar et al., 1981 Fig. 4
	(6) Same as (3)	Same as (3)		Radioautography	1	82–118ᶜ	Sacco et al., 1981

(Continued)

TABLE V—*Continued*

Species	Sample preparation	PAGE method (% acrylamide) 2nd dimension	No. zonae/gel	Protein detection method	Major proteins identified [MW × 10^{-3} (pI)]		References
Rabbit	(7) Same as (4)	Same as (4)	6000	Coomassie blue	2	58–96[c]	Dunbar et al., 1981
					3	40–74[c]	
					1	68–125[c]	
					2	81–100[c]	
					3	100–132[c]	
	(8) Same as (3)	Same as (3)		Radioautography	1	100–118[c]	Sacco et al., 1982
					2	83–110[c]	
					3	80–92[c]	
Squirrel monkey	(9) Same as (3)	Same as (3)		Radioautography	1	63–78[c]	
					2	63–70[c]	
					3	47–51[c]	
					4	43–47[c]	
Human	(10) Same as (3)	Same as (3)		Radioautography	1	80–120[c]	
					2	73	
					3	59–65[c]	

[a] pIs correspond to the iodosulfanililic acid-modified zona pellucida proteins and may not be the same as the pIs of the unmodified protein (Bleil and Wassarman, 1980).

[b] Estimated from Fig. 7 (Bleil and Wassarman, 1980).

[c] Proteins give wide range of relative pIs (due to posttranslational modification of proteins).

mensional electrophoresis using mouse zonae which have been radiolabeled with either [^{125}I]iodosulfanilic acid or ^{3}H-labeled dansyl chloride. The first employed separation of zona proteins in the first dimension using nonreducing conditions, followed by separation in SDS-PAGE after reduction of the proteins with dithiothreitol. Three proteins were apparent in radioautographs of these gels. The second method employed isoelectric focusing of reduced [^{125}I]iodosulfanilic acid-labeled zonae in the first dimension followed by separation of these proteins in SDS-PAGE. Three proteins that migrated as single spots having basic relative pI's were detected. The authors admit that the iodosulfanilic acid-modified proteins might not have isolectric points identical to the pI's of unmodified proteins; therefore, the protein patterns obtained from these studies might differ from unmodified proteins. This chemical modification might also affect the charge heterogeneity frequently observed in glycosylated proteins (Anderson and Anderson, 1977) as well as the binding of SDS to the proteins which could alter the apparent molecular weights. These may result in the variations in the two-dimensional PAGE pattern obtained by Bleil and Wassarman as compared to those obtained by Sacco (1981) who used ^{125}I-labeled chloramine-T or by B. S. Dunbar and D. J. Wolgemuth (unpublished) who did not chemically modify mouse zonae prior to electrophoresis (Fig. 3).

Two-dimensional gel electrophoresis patterns of the zona proteins of other species (pig, rabbit, human, squirrel monkey) appear to be more complex than those of the mouse (Dunbar *et al.*, 1981; Sacco *et al.*, 1982). Direct protein staining of pig or rabbit zona proteins by Coomassie blue shows that there are three major protein families, each demonstrating both size and charge heterogeneity (Fig. 4; Dunbar *et al.*, 1981). The more sensitive silver stain, which stains different proteins different colors (Adams and Sammons, 1981; Sammons *et al.* 1981), has now been used to show the presence of an additional low-molecular-weight glycoprotein family (<15,000) (B. S. Dunbar, unpublished). These studies have further shown that the major protein family of the pig zona has two components which stain two separate colors when this silver stain method is used. The additional observation that there are two distinct zona antigens which originate at the acidic end of the isoelectric focusing gel (Dunbar *et al.*, 1980) gives further evidence that the major protein of pig zona actually contains two proteins. A preliminary report by Hedrick and Wardrip (1981) has provided evidence that differences in carbohydrate content can also account for part of this heterogeneity observed in two-dimensional PAGE patterns. Sacco *et al.* (1982) have analyzed ^{125}I-labeled (chloramine-T method) zonae of pig, human, squirrel monkey, rabbit, and mouse. The

acidic   basic

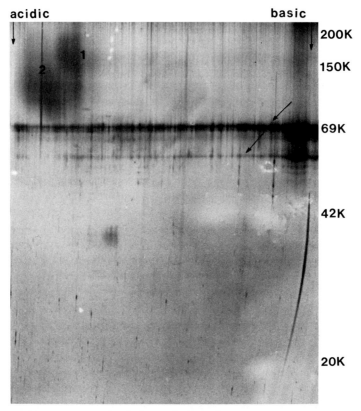

Fig. 3. Two-dimensional gel electrophoresis of mouse zonae pelucidae (1000 mechanically isolated zonae from ovulated mouse ova). Samples solubilized and isoelectric focused in 2% SDS, 2% β mercaptoethanol (pH9.5, 95°C, 10 min). pI range: acidic end, pH 3.8 (arrow indicates position of SDS bulb at acidic end of gel); basic end, pH 8.5. Second dimension is a 10–20% logarithmic gradient gel. Silver stain method (Gelcode, Upjohn; Sammons *et al.*, 1981) used to stain proteins. Two major proteins stained orange-brown. Arrows indicate silver stain artifacts always present at 69,000 and 50,000 molecular weight range. Molecular weights determined with rat heart used as standard (Giometti *et al.*, 1980).

pig, human, and rabbit zonae were found to contain three major protein families, all exhibiting considerable microheterogeneity, while four protein families were associated with the squirrel monkey, and only two were observed with mouse zonae. The patterns obtained for the radiolabeled pig and rabbit zonae in these studies were similar to those obtained by direct staining of these proteins (Dunbar *et al.*, 1981). These investigations collectively demonstrate the dramatic variation in proteins among different species as well as the complexity of the chemical composition of zona proteins. They further demonstrate

acidic   basic

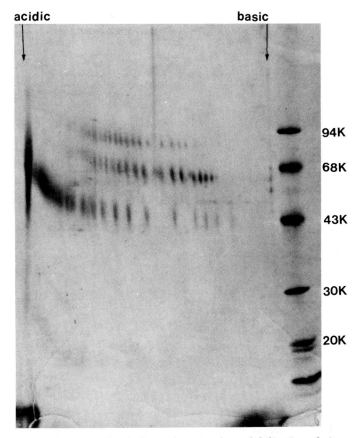

Fig. 4. Two-dimensional gel electrophoresis after solubilization of pig zonae pellucidae (approximately 6000). Samples solubilized and isoelectric focused as for mouse zonae (see Fig. 3). Second dimension is SDS-PAGE using a 10–20% linear gradient gel. Coomassie blue protein staining was used and molecular weight markers include: phosphorylase B, 94,000; bovine serum albumin, 68,000; ovalbumin, 43,000; carbonic anhydrase, 30,000; soybean trypsin inhibitor, 20,000.

the importance of the use of high-resolution two-dimensional electrophoresis for optimal resolution of zona proteins, particularly in the comparison of those of different species.

V. CHARACTERIZATION OF ZONA PELLUCIDA ANTIGENS AND OF ANTIBODIES DIRECTED TOWARD THEM

Studies on zonae pellucidae have been of increasing interest since immunization with zonae pellucidae has been shown to reduce fertility. Of the proposed immunological contraceptive methods, immunization with zonae pellucidae antigens has distinct advantages. (1) These methods are not abortive but would inhibit fertilization. (2) Low titers of antibodies would be adequate to block fertilization since there are limited numbers of oocytes with zonae and since these oocytes would be exposed to antibodies in the follicular fluid for long periods of time. (3) The zona antigens studied to date are tissue specific. (4) The zonae of a variety of animal species are immunologically cross-reactive; therefore, sources of antigenic material are readily available for purification and characterization (Shivers, 1974, 1975, 1977; Dunbar and Shivers, 1976; Sacco and Shivers, 1978).

The studies of antibodies to zonae pellucidae antigens have been of further interest since early studies suggested that some infertile women have antibodies to zonae antigens. These antibodies were implicated, therefore, in infertility (Shivers and Dunbar, 1977; Mori *et al.,* 1978, 1979). Before it will be possible to evaluate critically the use of such a method of immunological contraception or to determine the clinical implications of antibodies to zonae antigens in infertility, it is imperative that zona antigens and antibodies directed toward them be better characterized.

A. Methods Used to Detect Antibodies to Zona Pellucida Antigens

To date, most investigators have used microscopic methods to study antibodies to zonae pellucidae antigens since limited numbers of isolated zonae have been available. More recently, methods to isolate large numbers of oocytes from the pig, cow, and rabbit have allowed detailed studies of antibodies to the zonae of these species (Dunbar *et al.,* 1980; Dunbar, 1980; Gwatkin *et al.,* 1980). Because these large-scale isolation methods have not proved as successful in rodent species (Dunbar, 1980), microscopic methods continue to be the acceptable methods for detection of antibodies to zonae in these species.

1. Indirect Immunofluorescence

Indirect immunofluorescence has been the most popular method used to detect antibodies to zonae antigens in the sera of animals that have been immunized with ovarian antigens as well as in the sera of infertile women. These methods generally involve incubation of isolated oocytes or isolated zonae in the primary antisera, followed by incubation in a fluorescein-conjugated second antibody. Although this has been the primary method for detection of antibodies to zonae in infertile women, there have now been reports of positive binding reactions in sera of men as well as in fertile and infertile women (Sacco and Moghissi, 1979; Mori *et al.*, 1978, 1979; Dakhno *et al.*, 1980). These studies have shown that extensive absorption with tissue homogenates or with red blood cells is required before specific antibodies to zona can be detected. More recently it has been shown that a variety of hyperimmune sera (complete Freund's adjuvant plus protein antigen-induced antibody) do not demonstrate any immunological cross-reactivity with zona antigens when immunoelectrophoresis or radio-immunoassay methods are used, although these antisera frequently give positive fluorescence (Gerrity *et al.*, 1981). The immunofluorescence observed with sera of hyperimmunized animals was evenly distributed throughout the zonae as compared with the "rim" fluorescence characteristic of antisera prepared against intact or heat-solubilized pig zonae. Positive fluorescence may result, therefore, from the nonspecific trapping of immunoglobulins (possibly immune complexes). This is a possibility, since immunization with serum proteins in complete Freund's adjuvant can induce serum sickness caused by increased serum immune complexes (Haakenstad and Mannik, 1978). Further studies have shown that rabbits with induced serum sickness have immune complexes localized specifically in the zona pellucida (Albini *et al.*, 1979). The studies by Mori *et al.* (1978, 1979) have revealed that extensive absorption of sera with red blood cells will remove binding activity observed by immunofluorescence. Since blood group substances are present in sera (Kabat, 1956) and can be absorbed from circulating fluids onto cell surfaces (Race and Sanger, 1968), these factors may also affect immunofluorescence results. Reviews of immunofluorescence methods have further emphasized that it is important to purify fluorescein-conjugated immunoglobulins by DEAE affinity chromatography to reduce nonspecific charge binding (Kawamura, 1977). Detailed studies that use purified Fab fragments, as well as purified fluorescein-conjugated immunogloblins, in conjunction with other specific antibody-detection methods may resolve some of the conflicting reports of the presence of antibodies to zonae antigens when immunofluorescence techniques are used.

2. Zonae Precipitation Reaction (ZPR)

The zona precipitation reaction is the change in light-scattering properties detected by light- or dark-field microscopy. The ZPR has been attributed to the binding of antibodies to the outer region of the zona pellucida (Ownby and Shivers, 1972; Garavagno *et al.*, 1974; Dudkiewicz *et al.*, 1976; Sacco, 1977; Dunbar and Shivers, 1976). Scanning microscopy has also demonstrated surface changes of pig zonae after they were treated with antibodies to pig ovary (Dudkiewicz *et al.*, 1976). Garavagno *et al.* (1974) demonstrated with light microscopy that the ZPR was observed only on the outer surface of the hamster zona, while Fléchon and Gwatkin (1980) have shown with transmission electron microscopy that antibody to cow zonae localizes at the exterior as well as the interior surfaces of zonae. This discrepancy in the appearance of the ZPR may be due either to a variation in the species used or to the differences in methods of preparation used for light or electron microscopy. The immunochemical phenomenon responsible for the surface precipitation reaction is not clearly understood. A recent report by Ahuja and Tzartos (1981) has shown, however, that if Fab fragments from rabbit antihamster ovary homogenate are used instead of intact immunoglobulins, the zona precipitation reaction is absent. Furthermore, these antibodies did not inhibit fertilization as did the nondigested antisera. More detailed studies will have to be carried out to quantitate the specific titers of Fab fragments prepared against specific zonae antigens. Quantitative studies on Fab fragments as compared with the immunoglobulins from which they were prepared must also be completed before it will be possible to understand the differences in the biological activity of the bivalent and monovalent antibodies.

3. Passive Hemagglutination Assay

Tsunoda and Chang (1976a) have used a passive hemagglutination assay to detect ovarian antigens. The methods used were those described by Herbert (1977). Serum dilutions of antisera to ovary homogenate of up to 2^{12} were reported to react with ovarian antigens, although exact details of the experimental methods were not given.

4. Immunodiffusion and Immunoelectrophoresis Methods

Many early studies used antibodies to whole ovarian tissue as the source for antibodies in immunoprecipitation studies (Ownby and Shivers, 1972; Sacco and Shivers, 1973; Tsunoda and Chang, 1976b,c). Because of the complexity of ovarian tissue and because of the limited sensitivity and resolution of immunodiffusion methods (Ouchterlony and Nillson, 1978), it is difficult to determine which ovarian antigens were recognized in these studies.

It is now possible to prepare antisera with titers sufficient to obtain precipitating antibodies to isolated pig and rabbit zonae (Dunbar *et al.*, 1980; Dunbar and Raynor, 1980) as well as to cow zonae (Gwatkin *et al.*, 1980). Tsunoda *et al.* (1981) have used immunoelectrophoresis studies to show that one antigen in ovarian homogenate could be detected when goat antisera to isolated bovine zonae were used. This antigen was not found in other tissues examined. Recently, antibodies to purified zona proteins, isolated from both one-dimensional (Dunbar and Raynor, 1980) and two-dimensional electrophoresis polyacrylamide gels, have been raised (Wood and Dunbar, 1981). Rocket and crossed immunolectrophoresis methods, as compared with immunodiffusion methods, have resulted in better resolution as well as in the detection of greater numbers of zona antigens (Dunbar and Raynor, 1980; Wood and Dunbar, 1981). Thses studies have demonstrated clearly that there are multiple zona-specific antigens associated with both the pig and rabbit zonae pellucidae when optimal antigen-antibody ratios were determined for immunoelectrophoresis methods.

5. Radioimmunoassay Methods (RIA)

Radioimmunoassay methods to detect and to quantitate antibodies to zona antigens have now been described by Palm *et al.* (1979) and Gerrity *et al.* (1981). Palm *et al.* (1979) used the second antibody reagent and Gerrity *et al.* (1981) used *Staphylococcus aureus* (protein A-coated) cells as the immunoabsorbent in the RIA. These assays have been shown to be more sensitive than microscopic methods, since antibodies can be detected in serum dilutions of up to 5×10^5. Both RIA assays were used to detect antibodies specific against zona antigens.

B. Immunochemical Characterization of Ovarian and Zona Pellucida Antigens

Many investigators have used ovarian tissue as a source of immunogenic material to characterize zona pellucida antigens (Porter, 1965; Shahini *et al.*, 1972; Ownby and Shivers, 1972; Tsunoda and Chang, 1976b,c,d; Sacco and Shivers, 1973). It has been shown that serum proteins in pig follicular fluid (Dunbar *et al.*, 1981) are predominant proteins and are potential antigens. Hundreds of polypeptides in ovarian tissue can further be resolved in two-dimensional polyacrylamide gels after staining with Gelcode silver stain (Upjohn Co.) (B. S. Dunbar, unpublished results). Since serum albumin alone has been shown to contain a minimum of six nonrepeating antigenic determinants (Benjamin and Teale, 1978), it would be expected that vast numbers of antibodies of different specificities would be generated when an animal is exposed to ovarian tissue. Although many of the complexities of this system can be simplified by absorption of immune sera with a variety of tissues (Ownby and Shivers, 1972; Sacco and Shivers, 1973; Sacco, 1977; Tsunoda and Chang, 1976a,b,c), the operational immunogenicity of one antigen might be quite different when injected with hundreds of other antigens. It is difficult, therefore, to compare directly the immunological response obtained when ovarian tissue is used as the immunogen as opposed to isolated zona antigens.

More detailed studies have been carried out that examine the immunogenicity of isolated pig zonae in rabbits as well as rabbit zonae in both rabbits and guinea pigs. Studies by Dunbar and Raynor (1980) have demonstrated that the immunogenicity of the pig zona is complex, since the immunological response is dependent on the amount of zona protein as well as on the solubilization conditions used to prepare zonae prior to immunization. These studies demonstrated that as many as four pig zona-specific antigens can be detected with cross-immunoelectrophoresis methods that use rabbit antisera prepared against intact or heat-solubilized zonae (Dunbar et al., 1980). These studies also suggest that when intact zonae are used as the immunogen, antibodies are induced which recognize a unique structural antigenic determinant. This type of antigenic determinant appears to be similar to that described for the recognition of structural antigens of the H3-H4 complex of calf thymus histones as well as for other protein conformations (Habeeb, 1977; Cinader, 1977). Further studies have shown that binding of antibodies (prepared against intact pig zonae) in the RIA is dependent on the temperature used to solubilize zonae prior to radiolabeling (Gerrity et al., 1981) as well as on the method of iodination used (D. M. Wood and B. S. Dunbar, unpublished results).

In more recent studies, crossed immunoelectrophoresis patterns were obtained with antisera to rabbit zonae (after electrophoresis of rabbit zonae) which were remarkably similar to those patterns observed when antisera to pig zonae (after electrophoresis of pig zonae) were used (Wood and Dunbar, 1981). Purified zona proteins have now been obtained from two-dimensional polyacrylamide electrophoresis gels. Antibodies have been prepared against these isolated components which give precipitation reactions in immunoelectrophoretic studies (Wood and Dunbar, 1981). The antisera to two purified rabbit zona proteins have now been used in RIA as well as in immunoelectrophoresis studies to demonstrate directly that there are at least two immunologically cross-reactive antigens between pig and rabbit zonae pellucidae. These studies have further shown that two of these antigens are immunochemically identical since crossed-line immunoelectrophoresis methods demonstrate immunoprecipitate fusion. Other investigators have used similar immunoelectrophoresis methods to study zonae antigens. Gwatkin and Williams (1978) using rocket immunoelectrophoresis methods, observed one diffuse immunoprecipitin arc when rabbit antiserum to bovine zonae was used. Tsunoda *et al.* (1981) used goat antisera prepared against cow zonae. In their studies one immunoprecipitation line was obtained when immunoelectrophoresis was carried out against ovarian homogenate. No immunoprecipitin lines were observed against other tissues in these studies. The variation in the numbers of antigens detected could be accounted for by the methods of immunization or by the methods of immunoelectrophoresis, particularly the antigen:antibody ratios.

VI. THE EFFECTS OF ANTIBODIES TO OVARIAN AND ZONA PELLUCIDA ANTIGENS ON FERTILITY

Since the early observations of Porter (1965), Porter *et al.* (1970), Shivers *et al.* (1972), and Shahini *et al.* (1972) that antibodies to ovarian antigens can reduce fertility, there have been numerous studies to determine the causes of this fertility reduction. Most of these studies have concentrated on the antigens associated with the zona pellucida, since antibodies to these antigens could readily be detected by immunofluorescence and/or the zona precipitation reaction. Many of these earlier studies have been reviewed by Dunbar and Shivers (1976), Shivers (1977), Shivers *et al.* (1978), Tsunoda and Sugie (1979), Aitken and Richardson (1980), Sacco (1981), and Dunbar (1982). As the review by Dunbar (1982) provides a detailed tabulated summary of the effects of antibodies to ovarian and zona antigens on fertility, only an overview of earlier studies will be given here.

A. The Effect of Antibodies to Zonae Pellucidae on Sperm–Egg Interaction

Many investigators have used ovarian tissue as the immunogen for preparation of antisera in fertility studies because it was difficult to isolate sufficient numbers of zonae for immunization. Hetero- or alloimmunization with ovarian tissue was found dramatically to reduce or inhibit fertility *in vitro* by preventing sperm from binding to the surface of the zona (Jilek and Pavlok, 1975; Shivers *et al.*, 1982; Garavagno *et al.*, 1974; Oikawa and Yanagimachi, 1975; Tsunoda and Chang, 1976b,c,d; Mahi and Yanagimachi, 1979; Aitken *et al.*, 1981; Ahuja and Tzartos, 1981). In these studies, antibodies to zona antigens were detected with microscopic methods. These antibodies were presumed to be responsible for the reduction in fertilization rates since absorption of antisera with other tissues did not affect the inhibition of sperm binding or fertilization. More recently, studies to examine the inhibition of sperm binding to zonae *in vitro* have been extended to antibodies prepared against isolated eggs (with or without cumulus cells) or to isolated zonae pellucidae (Gwatkin *et al.*, 1977; Tsunoda, 1977; Tsunoda and Sugie, 1977).

The results of these studies show that heteroantisera prepared against eggs or zonae inhibit sperm binding to zonae or reduce fertilization *in vitro*. This reduction of fertilization *in vitro*, however, was found to depend on the species of oocytes used in the sperm binding studies relative to the species against which the antibodies to zonae were formed. Studies using mouse and hamster ova showed little effect on the fertilization rate *in vitro* if isologous antizona antisera were used instead of heterologous antisera (Gwatkin *et al.*, 1977).

B. The Effects of Passive Immunization with Antibodies to Ovarian Antigens on Fertility

Passive immunization with heteroantisera to ovarian tissue has been shown to reduce or inhibit fertility (Shahini *et al.*, 1972; Oikawa and Yanagimachi, 1975; Yanagimachi *et al.*, 1976; Tsunoda and Chang, 1976b,c,d, 1977). The effects were found to depend on the time of immunization before mating as well as on the quantities of sera or immunoglobulins administered. Reductions in fertility were generally concluded to be due to antibodies to zonae pellucidae, since microscopic methods could detect antibodies and since absorption of antisera with nonovarian tissues did not change the inhibitory effects. As with the fertilization studies carried out *in vitro*, the reduction of fertility was found to be less pronounced when animals (mice or rats) were passively immunized with rabbit antisera to a heterologous ovarian tissue (hamster) (Tsunoda and Chang, 1977).

C. The Effects of Active Immunization with Ovarian Tissue or with Isolated Zonae Pellucidae on Fertility

There have been fewer studies performed in which active immunization rather than passive immunization was used, again, because of the limitations on the numbers of available zonae. Investigations carried out by immunization of animals with ovarian homogenates have demonstrated a reduction in fertility, although it is difficult to conclude from such studies which immunogens are responsible (Tsunoda and Chang, 1976d, Aitken and Richardson, 1980; Gwatkin *et al.*, 1977;

Gwatkin and Williams, 1978; Dunbar *et al.*, 1981). The observations by Dunbar *et al.* (1981) in the rabbit, however, revealed that not only is the antifertility effect more pronounced when zonae from a heterologous species are used (e.g., pig versus rabbit zonae), but that the methods used to solubilize the zonae are also important in the inhibition of fertility. Even more dramatic was the observation that, of the rabbits heteroimmunized with pig zonae, none ovulated normally in response to hCG injections or cervical stimulation (during artificial insemination). This effect appears to be dependent on antibodies to a structural zona antigenic determinant, since the zonae which had been solubilized with detergents prior to immunization did not exhibit this effect. Shivers *et al.* (1982) have reported reduction in fertility in dogs immunized with intact pig zonae. Of the three dogs tested, one had normal pups even though antizona antibody titers detected by immunofluorescence methods were similar to one dog that did not conceive. Normal ovarian structure was found in the immunized animals except for the appearance of amorphous, granular zonae. Since both the numbers of zonae used to immunize animals as well as the antibody detection methods were different, it is not yet possible to compare the effects of active immunization of rabbits with pig zonae (Wood *et al.*, 1981) with the immunization of dogs with pig zonae.

Recent studies by Sacco *et al.* (1982) have shown that female mice heteroimmunized with pig zonae pellucidae developed significant antibody titers, although these antibodies had no significant effect on their fertility. Similar studies by Drell *et al.* (1982) showed that rats immunized with pig zonae had no reduction in fertility even though significantly high titers of antibodies to zonae were present. No cross-reactivity between mouse and pig zona proteins was detected with sensitive RIA methods, although cross-reactivity was observed among porcine, human, rabbit, and squirrel monkey (Sacco *et al.*, 1982). It has been concluded, therefore, that the human, squirrel monkey, and rabbit zonae are antigenically more similar to pig zonae than are either rat or mouse. Wood and Dunbar (1981) demonstrated directly that at least two pig and rabbit zonae antigens are immunochemically cross-reactive and exhibit immunological identity, since immunoprecipitin arcs fuse in crossed-immunoelectrophoresis studies and antisera to two isolated rabbit zona proteins bind pig zona proteins.

Other RIA studies have shown that the Rhesus monkey zona is immunochemically similar to the pig zona (D. M. Wood, B. S. Dunbar, and D. J. Wolgemuth, unpublished observations). To date, all attempts in which sensitive specific assays other than immunofluorescence were used have failed to demonstrate immunological cross-reactivity between mouse or rat with either pig or rabbit zonae (B. S. Dunbar, unpublished observations). These recent studies collectively suggest that rodent (rat and mouse) zonae have different major antigenic determinants than those of other species which have morphologically larger zonae (pig, human, rabbit, squirrel monkey, and Rhesus monkey).

Earlier studies demonstrated the immunochemical similarity between zonae of different species (Gwatkin et al., 1977; Shivers et al., 1978). Many of these studies used antibodies to ovarian tissue and the primary method of antibody detection was immunofluorescence. In view of some of the more recent discussions concerning the specificity of immunofluorescence for the detection of antibodies to zonae antigens (Sacco and Moghiss, 1979; Gerrity et al., 1981), including the need for extensive tissue absorptions to obtain specificity (Mori et al., 1979; Dakhno et al., 1980), more direct methods are now available (e.g. RIA and immunoelectrophoresis) which will have to be used to demonstrate the immunological cross-reactivity of the zonae antigens of different species. The studies which have used specific methods to detect and quantitate zona proteins suggest that rodent (rat and mice) species are not adequate models for the study of the effects of antizona antibodies on human fertility (Sacco et al., 1982; Drell et al., 1982).

D. The Role of Antibodies to Zonae Pellucidae in Infertile Women and Aging Animals

Several early studies in which immunofluorescence methods were used have demonstrated that antibodies that react with zonae pellucidae are found in the sera of some infertile women (Shivers and Dunbar, 1977; Mori et al., 1978). Immunofluorescence methods and tests for the inhibition of sperm binding to zona indicated that there were autoantibodies to zona in the sera of aging women as well as aging animals (Trounson et al., 1980; Tsunoda and Chang, 1979). These studies led to the conclusion that such an autoimmune phenomenon might occur naturally in aging animals, although specific antibodies to zonae antigens have yet to be characterized. Recently, Nishimoto et al. (1980), using immunofluorescence techniques, reported low incidences (4%) of antizona binding activity in the sera of aging women the sera had been absorbed by red blood cells.

Zona-binding activity has also been observed in the sera of fertile males, as well as of fertile females, when immunofluorescence methods were used (Sacco and Moghissi, 1979; Dakhno et al., 1980). The studies by Dakhno et al. (1980) found that all the antizona activity of the human sera tested could not be eliminated with red blood cells. Mori *et al.* (1979), however, reported that after absorption with red blood cells to remove hemagglutinins, some human sera still gave positive immunofluorescence reactions. Since neither Palm *et al.(1979) nor Gerrity et al.* (1981) have observed any cross-reactivity with pig red blood cells or other pig tissues, it is not clear why such cross-reactivity is seen in human sera. The significance of these observations is uncertain at this time.

Since immunofluorescence methods have been the only techniques to date which have detected the presence of antibodies to zonae antigens in human sera, it is essential to confirm these observations with alternative methods such as radioimmunoassays. Preliminary studies in which radioimmunoassay was used to screen for antibodies to zonae serum of over 150 infertile women failed to detect significant quantities of antibodies that recognize pig zonae. Some patients with ovarian cancers, however, demonstrated significant antibody levels (B. S. Dunbar, unpublished results). Now that RIA methods are available, it will be possible to screen sera from large numbers of patients to determine whether antibodies to zonae are a factor in infertility.

VII. CONCLUDING REMARKS

Until recently studies on all aspects of the zona pellucida have been limited. Recent improved methodologies for isolating large numbers of oocytes, as well as sensitive methods for protein analysis, are allowing a more rapid characterization of the macromolecular composition of zona proteins. The information obtained to date has demonstrated striking differences in the zonae of different species. Future studies on the biological roles and the chemical and immunological properties of zonae must take these species variations into consideration.

REFERENCES

Adams, L. D., and Sammons, D. W. (1981). A unique silver staining procedure for color characterization of polypeptides. *In* "Electrophoresis 81" (R. C. Allen and P. Arnaud, ed.), pp. 155–167. de Gruyter, New York.

Ahuja, K. K., and Tzartos, S. J. (1981). Investigation of sperm receptors in the hamster zona pellucida by using univalent (Fab) antibodies to hamster ovary. *J. Reprod. Fertil.* **61,** 257–264.

Aitken, R. J., and Richardson, D. W. (1980). Immunization against zona pellucida antigens. *In* "Immunological Aspects of Reproduction and Fertility Control" (J. P. Heap, ed.), pp. 173–201. MTP Press Ltd., Lancaster, England.

Aitken, R. J., and Richardson, D. W. (1981). Mechanism of sperm binding inhibition by anti-zona antisera. *Gamete Res.* **4,** 41–47.

Aitken, R. J., Rudak, E. A. Richardson, D. W., Dor, J., Djahanbakkch, O., and Templeton, A. A. (1981). The influence of anti-zona and antisperm antibodies on sperm-egg interactions. *J. Reprod. Fertil.* **62,** 597–606.

Aketa, K. (1973). Physiological studies on the egg surfaces component responsible for sperm-egg binding in sea urchin fertilization. I. Effect of sperm-binding protein on the fertilizing capacity of sperm. *Exp. Cell Res.* **70,** 439–441.

Albini, B., Ossi, E., Newland, C., Noble, B., and Andres, G. (1979). Deposition of immune complexes in the ovarian follicle of rabbits with experimental chronic serum sickness I. Immunopathology. *Lab. Invest.* **41,** 446–454.

Anderson, E., and Albertini, D. F. (1976). Gap junctions between the oocyte and companion follicle cells in the mammalian ovary. *J. Cell Biol.* **71,** 680–686.

Anderson, L., and Anderson N. G. (1977). High resolution two-dimensional electrophoresis of human plasma proteins. *Proc. Natl. Acad. Sci. U.S.A.* **74,** 5421–5425.

Anderson, N. G., Anderson, N. L., and Tollaksen, S. L. (1979). "Operation of the ISO-Dalt System", Aubl. ANL–BIM–79–2. Argonne Natl. Lab., Argonne, Illinois.

Aonuma, S. M., Okabe, Y., Kawai, D. D., and Kawaguchi, M. (1978). The change of solubility properties of zona pellucida to proteases related to fertilizability of mouse ova in vitro. *Chem. Pharm. Bull.* **26,** 405–410.

Austin, C. R. (1961). "The Mammalian Egg." Thomas, Springfield, Illinois.

Austin, C. R. (1965). "Fertilization," Found. Dev. Biol. Ser. Prentice-Hall, Englewood Cilffs, New Jersey.

Austin, C. R. (1975). Membrane fusion events in fertilization. *J. Reprod. Fertil.* **44,** 155–166.

Austin, C. R., and Braden, A. W. H. (1956). Early reactions of the rodent egg to spermatozoan penetration. *J. Exp. Biol.* **33,** 358–365.

Barros, C., and Yanagimachi, R. (1971). Induction of zona reaction in golden hamster eggs by cortical granule material. *Nature (London)* **233,** 268–269.

Bedford, J. M. (1977). Sperm/egg interaction: The specificity of human spermatozoa. *Anat. Rec.* **188,** 477–488.

Bedford, J. M., and Cross, N. L. (1978). Normal penetration of rabbit spermatozoa through a trypsin-and acrosin-resistant zona pellucida. *J. Reprod. Fertil.* **54,** 385–392.

Benjamin, D. C., and Teale, J. M. (1978). The antigenic structure of bovine serum albumin. *J. Biol. Chem.* **253,** 8087–8092.

Bleil, J. D., and Wassarman, P. M. (1980a). Mammalian sperm-egg interaction: Identification of a glycoprotein in mouse egg zonae pellucidae possessing receptor activity for sperm. *Cell* **20,** 873–882.

Bleil, J. D., and Wassarman, P. M. (1980b). Structure and function of the zona pellucida: Identification and characterization of the proteins of the mouse oocytes zona pellucida. *Dev. Biol.* **76,** 185–202.

Bleil, J. D., and Wassarman, P. M. (1980c). Synthesis of zona pellucida proteins by denuded and follicle-enclosed mouse oocytes during culture *in vitro*. *Proc. Natl. Acad. Sci. U.S.A.* **77,** 1029–1033.

Braden, A. W. H. (1952). Properties of the membranes of rat and rabbit eggs. *Aust. J. Sci. Res.* **5,** 460–471.

Chang, M. C., and Hunt, D. M. (1956). Effects of proteolytic enzymes on the zona pellucida of fertilized and unfertilized mammalian eggs. *Exp. Cell. Res.* **11**, 497–499.

Cholewa-Stewart, J., and Massaro, E. J. (1972). Thermally induced dissolution of the murine zona pellucida. *Biol. Reprod.* **7**, 166–169.

Cinader, B. (1977). Enzyme-antibody interactions. *Methods Immunol. Immunochem.* **4**, 313–335.

Dakhno, F. V., Hjort, T., and Grischenko, V. I. (1980). Evaluation of immunofluorescence on pig zona pellucida for detection of anti-zona antibodies in human sera. *J. Reprod. Immunol.* **20**, 281–291.

Dekel, N., and Phillips, D. M. (1979). Maturation of the rat cumulus oophorus: A scanning electron microscopic study. *Biol. Reprod.* **21**, 9–18.

Dekel, N., Kraicer, P. F., Phillips, D. M., Sanchez, R. S., and Segal, S. J. (1978). Cellular associations in the rat oocyte-cumulus cell complex: Morphology and ovulatory changes. *Gamete Res.* **1**, 47–57.

Dickmann, Z., and Dziuk, P. J., (1964). Sperm penetration of the zonae pellucida of the pig egg. *J. Exp. Biol.* **41**, 603–608.

Drell, D., Wood, D., and Dunbar, B. (1982). Heteroimmunization with porcine zonae pellucidae in rats: Absence of correlation of antibody to zonae with infertility. *Biol. Reprod.* (submitted for publication).

Dudkiewicz, A. B., Shivers, C. A., and Williams, W. L. (1976). Ultrastructure of hamster zona pellucida treated with zona-precipitating antibody. *Biol. Reprod.* **14**, 175–185.

Dunbar, B. S. (1980). Model systems to study the relationship between antibodies to zonae and infertility. Comparison of rabbit and porcine zonae pellucidae. *Int. Congr. Anim. Reprod. Artif. Insemin. [Proc.],* 9th, 1980 Vol. II, pp. 191–199.

Dunbar, B. S., (1982). Characterization of antibodies to zonae pellucidae antigens and their role in fertility. *In* "International Congress on Reproductive Immunology" (T. Wegmann and T. Gill, eds.). Oxford Univ. Press, London and New York (in press).

Dunbar, B. S., and Raynor, B. D. (1980). Characterization of porcine zona pellucida antigens. *Biol. Reprod.* **22**, 941–954.

Dunbar, B. S., and Roberts, S. (1982). The major glyco-protein family of the porcine zona pellucida contains two protein species. *Fed. Proc., Fed. Am. Soc. Exp. Biol.* (in press).

Dunbar, B. S., and Shivers, C. A. (1976). Immunological aspects of sperm receptors on the zona pellucida of mammalian eggs. *In* "Immunology of Receptors" (B. Cinader, ed.), pp. 509–519. Dekker, New York.

Dunbar, B. S., Wardrip, N. J., and Hedrick, J. L. (1980). Isolation, physiochemical properties and the macromolecular composition of the zona pellucida from porcine oocytes. *Biochemistry* **19**, 356–365.

Dunbar, B. S., Liu, C., and Sammons, D. W. (1981). Identification of the three major proteins of porcine and rabbit zonae pellucidae by high resolution two-dimensional gel electrophoresis: Comparison with follicular fluid, sera, and ovarian cell proteins. *Biol. Reprod.* **24**, 1111–1124.

Fairbanks, G., Steck, T. G., and Wallach, D. F. H. (1971). Electrophoretic analysis of the major polypeptides of the human erythrocyte membrane. *Biochemistry* **10**, 2606–2616.

Fléchon, J. E., and Gwatkin, R. B. L. (1980). Immunochemical studies on the zona pellucida of cow blastocytes. *Gamete Res.* **3**, 141–148.

Fritz, H., Schleuning, W.-D., Schiessler, H., Wendt, V., and Winkler, G. (1975). Boar, bull and human sperm acrosin-isolation, properties and biological aspects. *Cold Spring Harbor Conf. Cell Proliferation* **2**, 715–735.

Garavagno, A., Posada, J., Barros, C., and Shivers, C. A. (1974). Some characteristics of the zona pellucida antigen in the hamster. *J. Exp. Zool.* **189**, 37–50.

Garrels, J. I. (1979). Two dimensional gel electrophoresis and computer analysis of proteins synthesized by clonal cell lines. *J. Biol. Chem.* **254**, 7961–7977.

Gerrity, M., Niu, E., and Dunbar, B. S. (1981). A specific radioimmunoassay for evaluation of serum antibodies to zona pellucida antigens. *J. Reprod. Immunol.* **3**, 59–70.

Giometti, C. S., Anderson, N. G., Tollaksen, S. L., Edwards, J. J., and Anderson, N. L. (1980). Analytical techniques for cell fractions. XXVII. Use of heart proteins as reference standards in two-dimensional electrophoresis. *Anal. Biochem.* **102**, 47–58.

Glabe, C. G., and Vacquier, V. D. (1977). Isolation and characterization of the vitelline layer of sea urchin eggs. *J. Cell Biol.* **75**, 410–421.

Gould, K., Zaneveld, L. J. D., Srivastava, P. N., and Williams, W. L. (1971). Biochemical changes in the zona pellucida of rabbit ova induced by fertilization and sperm enzymes. *Proc. Soc. Exp. Biol. Med.* **136**, 6–10.

Gwatkin, R. B. L. (1964). Effect of enzymes and acidity on the zona pellucida of the mouse egg before and after fertilization. *J. Reprod. Fertil.* **7**, 99–105.

Gwatkin, R. B. L., and Williams, D. T. (1977). Receptor activity of the hamster and mouse solubilized zona pellucida before and after the zona reaction. *J. Reprod. Fertil.* **49**, 55–59.

Gwatkin, R. B. L., and Williams, D. T. (1978). Immunization of female rabbits with heat-solubilized bovine zonae: Production of anti-zona antibody and inhibition of fertility. *Gamete Res.* **1**, 19–26.

Gwatkin, R. B. L., Williams, D. T., and Anderson, O. F. (1973). Zona reaction of mammalian eggs: Properties of the cortical granule protease (cortin) and its receptor substrate in hamster eggs. *J. Cell Biol.* **59**, 128a.

Gwatkin, R. B. L., Williams, D. T., and Carlo, D. J. (1977). Immunization of mice with heat-solubilized hamster zonae: Production of anti-zona antibody and inhibition of fertility. *Fertil. Steril.* **28**, 871–877.

Gwatkin, R. B. L., Anderson, O. F., and Williams, D. T. (1980). Large scale isolation of bovine, and pig zonae pellucidae: Chemical, immunological, and receptor properties. *Gamete Res.* **3**, 217–231.

Haakenstad, A. O., and Mannik, M. (1978). The biology of the immune complexes. *In* "Autoimmunity" (N. Talal, ed.), pp. 277–360. Academic Press, New York.

Habeeb, A. F. S. A. (1977). Influence of conformation on immunochemical properties of proteins. *In* "Immunochemistry of Proteins" (M. Z. Atassi, ed.), Vol. 1, pp. 163–230. Plenum, New York.

Hall, B. (1935). The reactions of rat and mouse eggs to the hydrogen ion. *Proc. Soc. Exp. Biol. Med.* **32**, 747–478.

Hartmann, J. F., and Hutchison, C. F. (1974). Nature of the pre-penetration contact interaction between hamster gametes in vitro. *J. Reprod. Fertil.* **36**, 49–57.

Hartmann, J. F., and Hutchison, C. F. (1977). Involvement of two carbohydrate-containing components in the binding of uncapacitated spermatozoa to eggs of the golden hamster in vitro. *J. Exp. Zool.* **201**, 383–390.

Hartree, E. F. (1977). Spermatozoa, eggs and proteinases. *Biochem. Soc. Trans.* **5**, 375–394.

Hedrick, J. L., and Frye, G. N. (1980). Immunocytochemical studies on the porcine zona pellucida. *J. Cell Biol.* **87**, 136a.

Hedrick, J. L., and Wardrip, N. (1980). The macromolecular composition of the porcine zona pellucida. *Fed. Proc., Fed. Am. Soc. Exp. Biol.* **39,** Abstr. 2516.

Hedrick, J. L., and Wardrip, N. (1981). Microheterogeneity in the glycoproteins of the zona pellucida is due to the carbohydrate moiety. *J. Cell Biol.* **91,** 177a.

Heller, E., and Raftery, M. A. (1976). The vitelline envelope of eggs from the giant keyhole limpet. *Megathura crenulata.* II. Product formed by lysis with sperm enzyme and dithiothreitol. *Biochemistry* **15,** 1199–1203.

Herbert, W. J. (1977). Passive haemagglutination. *In* "Handbook of Experimental Immunology" (D. M. Weir, ed.), pp. 720–747. Blackwell, Oxford.

Inoue, M., and Wolf, D. P. (1974). Comparative solubility properties of the zona pellucida of unfertilized mouse ova. *Biol. Reprod.* **11,** 558–565.

Inoue, M., and Wolf, D. P. (1975). Comparative solubility properties of rat and hamster zona pellucida. *Biol. Reprod.* **12,** 535–540.

Jackowski, S., and Dumont, J. N. (1979). Surface alterations of the mouse zona pellucida and ovum following in vitro fertilization: Correlation with cell cycle. *Biol. Reprod.* **20,** 150–161.

Jilek, F., and Pavlok, A. (1975). Antibodies against mouse ovaries and their effect on fertilization *in vitro* and *in vivo* in the mouse. *J. Reprod. Fertil.* **42,** 377–380.

Kabat, E. A. (1956), "Blood Group Substances: Their Chemistry and Immunochemistry," pp. 100–105. Academic Press, New York.

Kaleta, E., and Majewsha, I. (1979). Inheritance of solubility properties of the zona pellucida of mouse oocytes. *Genet. Pol.* **20,** 258–264.

Kawamura, A. (1977). "Fluorescent Antibody Techniques and Their Applications," 2nd ed. Univ. Park Press, Baltimore, Maryland.

Kinsey, W. H., and Lennarz, W. J. (1981). Isolation of a glycopeptide fraction from the surface of the sea urchin egg that inhibits sperm-egg binding and fertilization. *J. Cell Biol.* **91,** 325–331.

Laemmli, U. K. (1970). Cleavage of structural proteins during the assembly of the head of bacteriophage T4. *Nature (London)* **227,** 680–685.

Lowenstein, J. E., and Cohen, A. I. (1964). Dry mass, lipid content and protein content of the intact and zona-free mouse zona. *J. Embryol. Exp. Morphol.* **12,** 113–121.

McRorie, R. A., and Williams, W. L. (1974). Biochemistry of mammalian fertilization. *Annu. Rev. Biochem.* **43,** 777–803.

Mahi, C. A., and Yanagimachi, R. (1979). Prevention of *in vitro* fertilization of canine oocytes by anti-ovary antisera: A potential approach to fertility control in the bitch. *J. Exp. Zool* **210,** 129–135.

Merril, C. R., Goldman, D., Sedman, S. A., and Ebert, M. H. (1981). Ultrasensitive stain for proteins in polyacrylamide gels shows regional variation in cerebrospinal fluid proteins. *Science* **211,** 1437–1438.

Mintz, B. (1962). Experimental study of the developing mammalian egg: Removal of the zona pellucida. *Science* **138,** 594–597.

Mori, T., Nishimoto, T., Kitagawa, M., Noda, Y., Nishimura, T., and Oikawa, T. (1978). Possible presence of autoantibodies to zona pellucida in infertile women. *Experientia* **34,** 797–799.

Mori, T., Nishimoto, T., Kohda, H., Takai, I., Nishimura, T., and Oikawa, T. (1979). A method for specific detection of autoantibodies to the zona pellucida in infertile women. *Fertil. Steril.* **32,** 67–72.

Nicolson, G. L., Yanagimachi, R., and Yanagimachi, H. (1975). Ultrastructural localization of lectin-binding sites on the zona pellucida and plasma membrane of mammalian eggs. *J. Cell Biol.* **66,** 263–274.

Nishimoto, T., Mori, T., Yamada, I., and Nishimura, T. (1980). Autoantibodies to zona pellucida in infertile and aged women. *Fertil. Steril.* **34,** 552–556.

O'Farrell, P. H. (1975). High resolution two dimensional electrophoresis of proteins. *J. Biol. Chem.* **250,** 4007–4021.

Oikawa, T. (1978). A simple method for the isolation of a large number of ova from pig ovaries. *Gamete Res.* **1,** 265–267.

Oikawa, T., and Yanagimachi, R. (1975). Block of hamster fertilization by anti-ovary antibody. *J. Reprod. Fertil.* **45,** 487–494.

Oikawa, T., Yanagimachi, R., and Nicolson, G. L. (1973). Wheat germ agglutinin blocks mammalian fertilization. *Nature (London)* **241,** 256–259.

Ouchterlony, O., and Nillson, L. A. (1978). Immunodiffusion and immunoelectrophoresis. *In* "Handbook of Experimental Immunology" (D. M. Weir, ed.), pp. 19.1–19.44. Blackwell, Oxford.

Ownby, C. L., and Shivers, C. A. (1972). Antigens of the hamster ovary and effects of anti-ovary serum on eggs. *Biol. Reprod.* **6,** 310–318.

Palm, V. S., Sacco, A. G., Syner, F. N., and Subramanian, M. G. (1979). Tissue specificity of porcine zona pellucidae antigen(s) tested by radioimmunoassay. *Biol. Reprod.* **21,** 709–713.

Peterson, R. N., Russell, L. D., Bundman, D., and Freund, M. (1980). Sperm-egg interaction: Evidence for boar sperm plasma membrane receptors for porcine zona pellucidae. *Science* **207,** 73–74.

Peterson, R. N., Russell, L. D., Bundman, D., Conway, M., and Freund, M. (1981). The interaction of living boar sperm and sperm plasma membrane vesicles with the porcine zona pellucida. *Dev. Biol.* **84,** 144–156.

Phillips, D. M., and Shalgi, R. M. (1980). Surface properties of the zona pellucida. *J. Exp. Zool.* **213,** 1–8.

Pikó, L. (1969). Gamete structure and sperm entry in mammals. In "Fertilization" (C. B. Metz and A. Monrey, eds.), Vol. 2, pp. 325–403. Academic Press, New York.

Porter, C. W. (1965). Ovarian antibodies in female guinea pigs. *Int. J. Fertil.* **10,** 257–260.

Porter, C. W., Highfill, D., and Winovich, R. (1970). Guinea pig ovary and testis: Demonstration of common gonad specific antigens in the ovary and testis. *Int. J. Fertil.* **15,** 171–176.

Race, R. R., and Sanger, R. (1968). "Blood Groups in Man," 5th ed. Davis, Philadelphia, Pennsylvania.

Russel, L. D., Peterson, R. N., Blumershine, R., Freund, M. (1980). Morphological observations on the binding of boar sperm to porcine zona pellucida. *Scan. Electron Micros.* **3,** 407–412.

Sacco, A. G. (1977). Antigenic cross-reactivity between human and pig zona pellucida. *Biol. Reprod.* **16,** 164–173.

Sacco, A. G. (1981). Immunocontraception: Consideration of the zona pellucida as a target antigen. *Obstet. Gynecol. Annu.* **10,** 1–26.

Sacco, A. G., and Moghissi, K. S. (1979). Anti-zona pellucida activity in human sera. *Fertil. Steril.* **31,** 503–506.

Sacco, A. G., and Shivers, C. A. (1973). Comparison of antigens in the ovary, oviduct and uterus of the rabbit and other mammalian species. *J. Reprod. Fertil.* **32,** 421–427.

Sacco, A. G., and Shivers, C. A. (1978). Immunologic inhibition of development. *In* "Methods in Mammalian Reproduction" (J. C. Daniel, Jr., ed.), pp. 203–227. Academic Press, New York.

Sacco, A. G., Subramanian, M. G., and Yurewicz, E. C. (1981). Active immunization of mice with porcine zonae pellucidae: Immune response and effect on fertility. *J. Exp. Zool.* (in press).

Sacco, A. G., Yurewicz, E. C., Subramanian, M. G., and Demayo, F. J. (1982). Zona pellucida composition: Species cross-reactivity and contraceptive potential of antiserum to a partially purified pig zona antigen. *Biol. Reprod.* (in press).

Saling, P. M. (1981). Involvement of trypsin-like activity in binding of mouse spermatozoa to zona pellucidae. *Proc. Natl. Acad. Sci. U.S.A.* **78,** 6231–6235.

Saling, P. M., Storey, B. T., and Wolf, D. P. (1978). Calcium-dependent binding of mouse epididymal spermatozoa to the zona pellucida. *Dev. Biol.* **65,** 515–525.

Sammons, D. W., Adams, L. D., and Nishizawa, E. E. (1981). Ultrasensitive silver-based color staining of polypeptides in polyacrylamide gels *Electrophoresis (Weinheim, Fed. Repub. Ger.)* **2,** 135–141.

Schmell, E. D., and Gulyas, B. J. (1980). Mammalian sperm-egg recognition and binding *in vitro*. Specificity of sperm interactions with live and fixed eggs in homologous and heterologous inseminations of hamster, mouse and guinea pig oocytes. *Biol. Reprod.* **23,** 1075–1085.

Shahini, S. K., Padbidri, J. R., and Rao, S. S. (1972). Immunological studies with the reproductive organs, adrenals, and spleen of the female mouse. *Int. J. Fertil.* **17,** 161–165.

Shivers, C. A. (1974). Immunological interference with fertilization. *In* "Immunological Approaches to Fertility Control" (E. Diczfalusy, ed.), pp. 223–242. Karolinska Inst., Stockholm.

Shivers, C. A. (1975). Antigens of ovum as a potential basis for the development of contraceptive vaccine. *Int. Symp. Immunol. Reprod., 3rd, 1975,* pp. 881–891.

Shivers, C. A. (1977). The zona pellucida as a possible target in immunocontraception. *In* "Immunological Influence on Human Fertility" (B. Boettcher, ed.), pp. 13–24. Academic Press, New York.

Shivers, C. A., and Dunbar, B. S. (1977). Autoantibodies to zona pellucida: A possible cause for infertility in women. *Science* **197,** 1187–1190.

Shivers, C. A., Dudkiewicz, A. B., Franklin, L. E., and Russell, E. N. (1972). Inhibition of sperm-egg interaction by specific antibody. *Science* **178,** 1211–1213.

Shivers, C. A., Gengozian, N., Franklin, S., and McLaughlin, C. L. (1978). Antigenic cross-reactivity between human and marmoset zonae pellucidae, a potential target for immunocontraception. *J. Med. Primatol.* **7,** 242–248.

Shivers, C. A., Sieg, P. M., and Kitchen, H. (1982). Pregnancy prevention in the dog: Potential for an immunological approach. *J. Am. Anim. Hosp. Assoc.* (in press).

Soupart, P., and Noyes, R. W. (1964). Sialic acid as a component of the zona pellucida of the mammalian ovum. *J. Reprod. Fertil.* **8,** 251–253.

Srivastava, P. N. (1973). Location of the zona lysin. *Biol. Reprod.* **9,** 84 (abstract).

Stambaugh, R. (1978). Enzymatic and morphological events in mammalian fertilization. *Gamete Res.* **1,** 65–85.

Stambaugh, R., and Smith, M. (1976). Sperm proteinase release during fertilization of rabbit ova. *J. Exp. Zool.* **197,** 121–125.

Stegner, H. E., and Wartenberg. H. (1961). Elektronenmikroskopische und histochemische untersuchen uber struktur und bildung der zona pellucida menshlicher lin zellen. *Z. Zellforsch. Mikrosk. Anat.* **53,** 702–713.

Swenson, C. E., and Dunbar, B. S. (1982). Specificity of sperm-zona interaction. *J. Exp. Zool.* **219,** 97–104.

Trounson, A. D., Shivers, C. A., McMaster, R., and Lopata, A. (1980). Inhibition of sperm binding and fertilization of human ova by antibody to porcine zona pellucida and human sera. *Arch. Androl.* **4**, 29–36.

Tsunoda, Y. (1977). Inhibitory effect of anti-mouse egg serum on fertilization in vitro and in vivo in the mouse. *J. Reprod. Fertil.* **50**, 353–355.

Tsunoda, Y., and Chang, M. C. (1976a). *In vivo* and *in vitro* fertilization of hamster, rat and mouse eggs after treatment with anti-hamster ovary antiserum. *J. Exp. Zool.* **195**, 409–416.

Tsunoda, Y., and Chang, M. C. (1976b). Reproduction in rats and mice isoimmunized with homogenate of ovary or testis with epididymis, or sperm suspensions. *J. Reprod. Fertil.* **46**, 379–382.

Tsunoda, Y., and Chang, M. C. (1976c). Effect of anti-rat ovary antiserum on the fertilization of the mouse and hamster eggs in vivo and in vitro. *Biol. Reprod.* **14**, 354–361.

Tsunoda, Y., and Chang, M. C. (1976d). The effect of passive immunization with hetero and isoimmune anti-ovary antiserum on the fertilization of mouse, rat, and hamster eggs. *Biol. Reprod.* **15**, 361–365.

Tsunoda, Y., and Chang, M. C. (1977). Further studies of antisera on the fertilization of mouse, rat, and hamster eggs in vivo and in vitro. *Int. J. Fertil.* **22**, 129–139.

Tsunoda, Y., and Chang, M. C. (1979). The suppressive effect of sera from old female mice on *in vitro* fertilization and blastocyst development. *Biol. Reprod.* **20**, 355–361.

Tsunoda, Y., and Sugie, T. (1977). Inhibition of fertilization in mice by anti-zona pellucida antiserum. *Jpn. J. Zootech. Sci.* **48**, 784–786.

Tsunoda, Y., and Sugie, T. (1979). Inhibitory effect on fertilization *in vitro* and *in vivo* by zona pellucida antibody and the titration of this antibody. *In* "Recent Advances in Reproduction and Regulation of Fertility" (G. P. Dalway, ed.), pp. 123–133. Elsevier/North-Holland Biomedical Press, Amsterdam.

Tsunoda, Y., Soma, T., and Sugie, T. (1981). Inhibition of fertilization in cattle by passive immunization with anti-zona pellucida serum. *Gamete Res.* **4**, 133–138.

Van Blerkom, J., and Motta, P. (1979). "The Cellular Basis of Mammaliam Reproduction." Urban & Schwarzenberg, Baltimore, Maryland.

Wolf, D. P., Nishihara, T., West, D. M., Wyrick, R. E., and Hedrich, J. L. (1976). Isolation, physicochemical properties and the macromolecular composition of the vitelline and fertilization envelopes from *Xenopus laevis* eggs. *Biochemistry* **15**, 3671–3678.

Wolgemuth, D. J., and Garvin, D. D. (1981). Ultrastructure and biochemical characterization of gene expression in follicular oocytes in neonatal and prepubertal rats. *In* "Proceedings of the Fifth Workshop on Developmental and Function of Reproductive Organs" (A. G. Beyskov, ed), pp. 289–298. Excerpta Medica, Amsterdam.

Wood, D. M., and Dunbar, B. S. (1981). Direct-detection of two cross-reactive antigens between porcine and rabbit zonae pellucidae by radioimmunoassay and immunoelectrophoresis. *J. Exp. Zool.* **217**, 423–433.

Wood, D. M., Liu, C., and Dunbar, B. S. (1981). The effect of alloimmunization and heteroimmunization with zonae pellucidae on fertility in rabbits. *Biol. Reprod.* **25**, 439–450.

Wright, R. W., Jr., Cupps, P. T., Goskins, C. T., and Hillers, J. K. (1977). Comparative solubility properties of the zona pellucida of unfertilized murine, ovine and bovine ova. *J. Anim. Sci.* **44**, 850–853.

Yanagimachi, R. (1977). Specificity of sperm-egg interaction. *In* "Immunobiology of Gametes" (M. Edidin and M. H. Johnson, eds.), pp. 187–207. Cambridge Univ. Press, London and New York.
Yanagimachi, R., Winkelhake, J. L., and Nicholson, G. L. (1976). Immunological block to mammalian fertilization: Survival and organ distribution of immunoglobulin which inhibits fertilization in vivo. *Proc. Natl. Acad. Sci. U.S.A.* **73**, 2405–2408.

4

Mechanisms of Mammalian Sperm Capacitation

ERIC D. CLEGG

Mechanism and Control of Animal Fertilization
Copyright © 1983 by Academic Press, Inc.
All rights of reproduction in any form reserved.
ISBN 0-12-328520-8

I. INTRODUCTION

A. Previous Reviews

The topics of capacitation and the acrosome reaction in mammalian sperm have been reviewed comprehensively several times over the last several years. Early observations were covered by Bedford (1970). Subsequent reviews by McRorie and Williams (1974), Austin (1975), Gwatkin (1977), Bedford and Cooper (1978), Meizel (1978), Rogers (1978), Green (1978a), and Yanagimachi (1981) have been valuable in summarizing the literature and presenting working hypotheses on the subjects.

With the availability of those reviews, particularly that by Yanagimachi (1981), it is not necessary to embark upon another comprehensive review that would be largely repetitive. Instead, emphasis will be placed here on evaluation of the current status of the field, and an attempt will be made to indicate where research in the area is (and/or should be) headed. This treatment will build on the material covered in those reviews. In so doing, some concepts will be introduced or reintroduced that do not seem to be receiving much consideration presently. The primary purpose is to stimulate new thinking in the hope that it will contribute to further productive research.

B. Distinction between Capacitation and the Acrosome Reaction

Capacitation has been a functional term used to indicate the changes in mammalian sperm that must occur in the female or in *in vitro* incubations as preparation for the induction of the acrosome reaction. The scope of the term capacitation has been expanded by some investigators to include other events (not yet identified) that might be required prior to fertilization.

In this chapter, emphasis is placed on those aspects of capacitation that seem to relate directly to preparation for the acrosome reaction. The mechanism for the induction of the acrosome reaction is also discussed. The current state of knowledge does not allow a clear distinction in all cases to be made between events that are strictly capacitation or the acrosome reaction. Capacitation and the acrosome reaction are often combined in discussion of topics where assignment of an event to one or the other does not seem at present to be prudent.

C. *In Vivo* versus *in Vitro* Experiments

Initially, studies of capacitation were limited to *in vivo* experiments in which females were either mated naturally or artificially inseminated. This approach allowed investigation of many parameters related to the site and timing of capacitation (judged by ability to fertilize). Morphological characteristics could also be studied. However, such approaches have severe limitations, not the least of which is the small number of sperm that can be retrieved under normal conditions from the female, particularly from the oviduct. Consequently, experiments requiring measurement of alterations in sperm components during capacitation *in vivo* are difficult. Other problems include the surgical or postmortem manipulations necessary to recover the sperm and an inability to manipulate satisfactorily the environment to which the sperm are exposed. Sperm are always exposed to the secretions of the female reproductive tract in *in vivo* experiments. Thus, it is not possible to use well-defined conditions or to change those conditions sufficiently to meet the demands of many experiments.

Alternative approaches became possible with the development of techniques for capacitation and fertilization *in vitro* (see Chapter 7). Although completely defined conditions have still not been achieved, much better control of experimental conditions is possible. For example, sperm can be exposed sequentially to different components, as in the experiments of Yanagimachi and Usui (1974) in which calcium was shown to allow the acrosome reaction after completion of capacitation in a calcium-free medium.

However, as with most good things, there is also a cost. In the study of the mechanisms by which capacitation can be induced *in vitro*, it has been necessary substantially to simplify media. Conditions have been developed that appear to result in the same end point as that reached in the *in vivo* process, but it is not assured that the end point is attained in the same way. Ultimately, observations made with *in vitro* techniques must be tested under more physiologic conditions to determine if mechanisms discovered with *in vitro* experiments acually operate under physiologic conditions. A related requirement is that events that are observed during capacitation must be distinguished from those that are obligatory components of capacitation. This point applies, of course, when interest is in the mechanisms of capacitation as they occur *in vivo*. However, successful *in vitro* capacitation and fertilization have provided important clinical benefits without regard to how they are accomplished (e.g., Steptoe and Edwards, 1978).

II. PROPERTIES OF SPERM PLASMA MEMBRANE

In this section, the pertinent properties of the plasma membrane of mature sperm, either ejaculated or from the cauda epididymis, will be identified. A similar discussion of the properties of the outer acrosomal membrane is not included because of the paucity of information about that membrane.

A. Lipids

There is no compelling evidence to indicate that the plasma membrane of mammalian sperm differs markedly from the general properties predicted by the fluid mosaic model (Singer and Nicolson, 1972). With one exception, there are no quantitative reports on the phospholipid and sterol contents of sperm plasma membrane, although the various lipid classes have been measured extensively in whole sperm.

It appears valid to assume that lipids extracted from whole sperm are obtained almost entirely (> 90%) from the cell membranes. However, there may be substantial differences in the lipid compositions of the four membrane types (plasma, acrosomal, nuclear, and mitochondrial membranes). Further, if the regional differences in the plasma membrane (demonstrated) and possible differences between the inner and outer acrosomal membranes (not yet addressed) are considered, it is not possible to assume from such studies that the lipids are similar, even between different areas of the same membrane.

Nevertheless, there is little doubt that the plasma membrane contains both phospholipids and sterols, although additional work must be done to quantify them in a variety of species. The phospholipids of whole sperm have been measured by numerous laboratories (see Mann and Lutwak-Mann, 1981). Quantitatively, phospholipids are the predominant lipid class. Although studied much less extensively, sperm also contain substantial amounts of cholesterol plus a smaller amount of desmosterol. In addition to the free cholesterol, cholesteryl sulfate and cholesteryl fatty acyl esters have been found in whole sperm. In our laboratory, plasma membrane (PM) preparations of >70% purity from ejaculated pig sperm contained 57.8% of the total lipid as phospholipid, 12.7% as cholesterol, and a trace amount of cholesteryl acyl ester (D. D. Lunstra and E. D. Clegg, unpublished results). The protein-to-lipid ratio was 59:41 for six replicates. More recently, Davis *et al.* (1980) measured total phopholipid, cholesterol, and cholesteryl ester in a PM fraction from epididymal rat sperm. Even though the purity of these PM preparations was less than ideal, these compounds were definitely components of the membrane in ratios that were similar to PM from other cells.

B. Intramembrane Proteins

Another feature of the fluid mosaic model (Singer and Nicolson, 1972) is the presence of proteins in the hydrophobic region of the membrane. Freeze-etching techniques (Friend *et al.*, 1977; Kinsey and Koehler, 1976) have demonstrated in the sperm of several species the characteristic particles within the plasma membrane that probably are intramembrane proteins. More direct evidence has revealed ATPases and adenylate cyclase which are considered to be inserted into the sperm plasma membrane (see Garbers and Kopf, 1980).

C. Surface Components

Most attention (although still quite limited in scope) has focused on the external surface of the plasma membrane, but the properties of the internal surface may also be important. It is clear that the properties of the external surface undergo almost continuous change from spermatogenesis through capacitation. One can assume that the plasma membrane contains hydrophobic regions of molecules that have hydrophilic portions exposed at the membrane surface. These hydrophilic portions could include carbohydrate and sialic acid from glycoproteins, glycolipids, and gangliosides. Some of the galactose units may be sulfated. The presence of sialic acid (see Bedford and Cooper, 1978, for discussion) and sulfated carbohydrate probably accounts for most of the negative surface charge displayed by sperm. These polar components, which are anchored to the membrane, could easily interact with other proteins and ions (possibly also with lipids) to which the cells are exposed sequentially during spermiogenesis, while passing through the excurrent ducts of the male, after mixing with the secretions of the accessory sex glands, and finally during capacitation. One can visualize a gradual change in the surface components caused by addition, modification, and removal of either entire molecules or portions thereof.

There is ample evidence that the surface of mammalian sperm is indeed in a state of continuous change. Bypassing changes that occur in the testis and epididymis, sperm from the cauda epididymis of swine undergo marked changes in surface properties when exposed to fluid produced by the seminal vesicles. Moore and Hibbitt (1975) showed with isoelectric focusing that ejaculated sperm from vesiculectomized boars focused at pH 4.5, whereas sperm from intact boars focused at pH 6.5. When sperm from vesiculectomized boars were exposed to seminal plasma from intact boars, the focusing point was increased to pH 5.8. These experiments were supplemented by studies in which basic proteins in seminal plasma, labeled with ^{131}I, were shown to be adsorbed to intact sperm (Moore and Hibbitt, 1976).

The nature of the negative surface charge of sperm is still open to question. This subject has been reviewed by Bedford and Cooper (1978). In general, sperm seem to emerge from the epididymis with a net negative surface charge (Fléchon, 1979). It is important to emphasize the term "net" since positively charged groups must also be present at approximately neutral pH (Fléchon and Morstin, 1975). Sources of positive charges could be basic amino acids in membrane proteins and phospholipids. Negative groups may be contributed by sialic acid on glycoproteins and gangliosides, by sulfated sugars or sterols, or by phospholipids. The assumption is made (but not proved) that the phosphoproteins of sperm are internal.

Hamster sperm show a substantial increase in sterol sulfate content during passage through the epididymis. Since the sperm are exposed to epididymal fluid thought to contain sterol sulfate and are able to accumulate the sterol during *in vitro* incubations, the assumption has been made that at least some of the sterol sulfate becomes associated with the plasma membrane (see Langlais *et al.*, 1981, for review). Recently, this same group (Langlais *et al.*, 1981) found that radiolabeled cholesteryl sulfate was bound selectively to the plasma membrane, with the majority localized in the acrosomal region.

Another potential source of negative surface charge is seminolipid (see Mann and Lutwak-Mann, 1981). This sulfated glycerogalactolipid contains galactose-sulfate, a fatty acid, and an alkyl ether, all linked to glycerol. No evidence exists yet as to the localization of this lipid in sperm once it has been incorporated, but it is the major glycolipid in the species studied thus far.

Sialic acid has long been thought to be the primary source of negative surface charge, but more recent work has cast some doubts on the concept (see Bedford and Cooper, 1978). In recent experiments with pig sperm (G. S. Svoboda and E. D. Clegg, unpublished results), we were unable to demonstrate the presence of sialic acid on the surface of either cauda epididymal or ejaculated sperm using sialic acid-specific lectin or selective hydrolyses, with or without mild treatment with trypsin or chymotrypsin.

Finally, sialic acid could be contributed by either sperm gangliosides (Bushway *et al.*, 1977) or surface glycoproteins. Numerous reports using electron microscopy with labeled lectins or staining with phosphotungstic acid have indicated that there are several types of carbohydrates exposed at the sperm surface. However, these have not specifically indicated that sialic acid is included.

That certain reactive groups are exposed at the sperm surface is recognized, but the only things known about specific membrane proteins are estimated molecular weight (usually of a denatured form) and whether or not they contain carbohydrate. Nothing is known about how the different surface components are attached to the plasma membrane or how they interact with each other.

Very little information is available about the nature of the internal surface of the plasma membrane. Since the plasma membrane and outer acrosomal membrane must closely approach each other in order to undergo the acrosome reaction, it is important to know what, if anything, exists as a barrier to that approach. Also, it is possible that a network of protein could exist at the inner surface of the plasma membrane to serve as an anchor for other membrane proteins. However, no evidence exists that microtubules or microfilaments play a role in capacitation or the acrosome reaction, although elements of both exist in mammalian sperm.

Both Stambaugh and Smith (1978) and Peterson et al. (1978) have observed microtubular structures in sperm that have undergone membrane vesiculations resembling the acrosome reaction, indicating that nonpolymerized tubulin is probably present in the acrosomal region of noncapacitated sperm. In addition, Peterson et al. (1978) showed formation of microfilamentlike structures associated with the plasma membrane in the equatorial segment and postacrosomal region, as well as in the membrane vesicles formed in the acrosomal region. The possibility that the microfilaments were actin polymers is strengthed by immunofluorescence evidence of actin (unpolymerized) in at least the postnuclear region of sperm and probably in the entire postacrosomal and midpiece regions (Talbot and Kleve, 1978; Clarke and Yanagimachi, 1978; Campanella et al., 1979; Tamblyn, 1980; Clarke et al., 1982). Actin has not yet been demonstrated conclusively in the acrosomal region. However, the possibility should not be ruled out in view of the observations of Peterson et al. (1978). It is possible that the immunofluorescence techniques are not sufficiently sensitive. Additional work is needed to clarify this point.

Tamblyn (1981) has now demonstrated that a myosinlike ATPase is present in bovine sperm. Myosin would be necessary for function of actin microfilaments. The location of the myosin is unknown.

Although no evidence exists for support, it is possible that a protein such as actin could exist at the inner surface of the plasma membrane and have a substantial influence on the distribution and mobility of intramembrane proteins. It could also serve as a barrier preventing close approach of the plasma and outer acrosomal membranes.

III. MECHANISMS OF CAPACITATION

The review by Yanagimachi (1981) summarized five hypotheses dealing with the mechanisms of capacitation and the acrosome reaction. These were based on papers by Gordon (1973), Gordon et al. (1978), Green (1978a), Meizel (1978), and Davis (1978). In addition, Yanagimachi proposed his own hypothesis in that review. Readers are referred to that review for summaries of those hypotheses. In this section, the key elements of those hypotheses will be discussed, along with other concepts proposed more recently. The discussion is intended to be provocative.

At the present time, the major steps occurring during capacitation and induction of the acrosome reaction appear to be the following:

1. Acquisition by the sperm of increased permeability to calcium.
2. Modification of membrane structure.
3. Activation of sperm adenylate cyclase.
4. Conversion of proacrosin to active acrosin.

While not all of these processes are proven to be obligatory for the acrosome reaction and successful fertilization, they are so intricately implicated that they must be treated as essential until proved otherwise. One of the challenges facing workers in this area is to devise methods for separating the different events from each other so they can be studied without confounding effects.

A. Availability of Calcium

The discussion of calcium must be quite complex. It will consider calcium availability in the fluids to which sperm are exposed, the possibility that entry of calcium into sperm is inhibited by seminal plasma, the mechanisms by which calcium might be accumulated by sperm, and the potential effects of intracellular calcium accumulation.

All available evidence indicates that elevated intracellular calcium is absolutely required for induction of the acrosome reaction. Elevated intracellular levels may also be involved in activation of acrosin, in membrane modifications prior to vesiculation, and in control of adenylate cyclase activity. Therefore, the factors influencing calcium availability and uptake are of utmost importance.

The secretions of the accessory sex glands of the male and the female reproductive tract contain calcium at levels exceeding 1 mM. This should be adequate for induction of the acrosome reaction, although the minimum required level has not been determined for most species. Therefore, under conditions of *in vivo* capacitation and fertilization, sperm are thought to be continuously exposed to calcium in sufficient amount. This is a dangerous assumption for several reasons. First, accessory sex gland secretions of many species contain substantial amounts of low-molecular-weight chelators, as well as proteins, which can bind calcium. As a result, not all of the calcium in seminal plasma is likely to be available to the sperm. Very little has been done to assess this factor. Also, it is entirely possible that availability of free calcium (or other ions and molecules) could vary substantially in fluids in different segments of the female reproductive tract, including different segments of the oviduct. Availability could also vary with the endocrine status of the female. Overstreet and co-workers (see Chapter 11) have demonstrated marked differences in sperm motility within particular parts of the rabbit oviduct as ovulation is approached, indicating that changes in the fluid environment of the sperm have indeed occurred with changing endocrine status of the female.

Second, even if sufficient free calcium is present in the extracellular fluid, sperm may not be able to take it up if they have been exposed to seminal plasma. Babcock *et al.* (1979) found that bovine sperm from the cauda epididymis rapidly accumulated exogenous calcium when it was supplied, whereas ejaculated sperm did not. They presented evidence that a component of the seminal plasma prevented calcium uptake. Although not documented, this may be a role of the decapacitation factor present in the seminal plasma (see McRorie and Williams, 1974). If this is a general occurrence with ejaculated sperm, then capacitation must include a mechanism to remove the inhibition by seminal plasma of calcium uptake.

Both the binding of calcium by components in male accessory sex gland secretions and inhibition of uptake of free calcium (as seen with bovine sperm) are factors which would only be present when ejaculated sperm are used for experimentation. Since the large majority of studies on capacitation *in vitro* have been done with sperm from the cauda epididymis, an important component of the capacitation mechanisms may have been missed.

The third consideration relative to calcium availability concerns the mechanisms for regulation of internal calcium level. Of particular interest is the calcium level in the cytoplasmic compartment between the plasma membrane and the outer acrosomal membrane. Work with other cell types (see Carafoli and Crompton, 1978) would indicate that it is safe to assume that calcium entry into sperm across the plasma membrane is not an active transport process. The active transport, via a Ca^{2+}-ATPase, should function in the opposite direction to keep cytoplasmic calcium concentration low. In that situation, which should pertain to sperm prior to capacitation, calcium diffusing into the sperm head would be pumped right back out at a cost of high-energy phosphate bonds. The work of Singh *et al.* (1980) may support that concept. In their experiments with guinea pig sperm, the calcium transport antagonist methoxyverapamil accelerated onset of the acrosome reaction when extracellular calcium was present. Compatibility of these results with the concepts advanced here would require that the methoxyverapamil antagonism be directed against the calcium pump, but not against the mechanism for large-scale influx at the time of the acrosome reaction. Gordon (1973) and Gordon *et al.* (1978) have presented cytochemical evidence that a Ca^{2+}-ATPase exists in the acrosomal region of rabbit and guinea pig sperm. They showed reaction products associated with both the plasma membrane and the outer acrosomal membrane. More recently, Bradley and Forrester (1980) have studied a Ca^{2+}, Mg^{2+}-ATPase in membrane preparations from ram sperm. The membrane vesicles actively accumulated calcium. Although the membrane vesicles used in this study were called plasma membrane, it is likely that a substantial amount of outer acrosomal membrane was also present. Evidence was not presented to refute that possibility. Nevertheless, the value of these observations is in the biochemical demonstration of the enzyme in one or both of the membranes in capacitation. If Ca^{2+}-dependent ATPases exist in both membranes, then the most likely situation for calcium transport is the pumping of calcium out of the cytoplasmic compartment to either the extracellular fluid or into the acrosome. Under conditions of restricted calcium permeability predicted by the work of Babcock *et al.* (1979), the very low cytoplasmic $[Ca^{2+}]$ probably precludes any significant accumulation of calcium inside the acrosome. The situation could change dramatically when the barrier to calcium influx through the plasma membrane is removed.

I hypothesize that an important component of capacitation or induction of the acrosome reaction is removal of such a barrier, rather than activation of a Ca^{2+}-dependent ATPase. Other potential roles of calcium include regulation, in part, of motility (Tash and Means, 1982), activation of adenylate cyclase, activation of acrosin and possibly phospholipase, and involvement in membrane fusion. These latter three roles will be discussed subsequently in this chapter.

Although direct involvement of calmodulin in capacitation has not been reported, it is likely that actions of calcium in the cytoplasm of sperm are mediated via that calcium-binding protein. Tash and Means (1982) found that the anticalmodulin drug W13 could markedly interfere with motility. Calmodulin has been demonstrated to be present in the head of sperm as well as in the flagellar region (Jones *et al.*, 1978, 1980; Feinberg *et al.*, 1981; Tash and Means, 1982).

B. Modification of Membrane Structure

Initial morphological studies of the alterations of sperm membranes during capacitation using standard techniques of transmission electron microscopy failed to demonstrate any changes that could be correlated with capacitation. However, with the availability of lectins and procedures for using antisperm (or antiseminal plasma) antibodies, it became apparent that the carbohydrate-containing extrinsic proteins (or possibly glycolipids) were altered under conditions promoting capacitation both *in vitro* and *in vivo* (see review by Koehler, 1978). In general, when cauda epididymal or ejaculated sperm from several species were labeled with either FITC- or ferritin-conjugated concanavalin A or *Ricinis communis* agglutinin, relatively uniform labeling of the plasma membrane was observed over the acrosomal region (if the sperm were prefixed). Temperature-induced movement (clustering) of lectin-binding components of the membrane was not observed in the acrosomal region of rabbit (Nicolson and Yanagimachi, 1974), hamster (Koehler, 1978), or guinea pig sperm (Schwarz and Koehler, 1979), but was seen in the postacrosomal region of rabbit sperm. In contrast, O'Rand (1977) observed redistribution of a surface antigen in cauda or ejaculated rabbit sperm when the sperm were labeled with fluorescent Fab antibody fragments against a single sperm antigen at low temperature and then allowed to warm. Exposure of the sperm to capacitation *in vivo* caused restriction of the mobility of the surface antigen. Ability to form temperature-induced patches (Nicolson and Yanagimachi, 1974) is usually taken as a sign that intrinsic membrane proteins are mobile within a fluid-phase membrane. However, as Koehler (1978) has indicated, failure to patch does not prove that the surface components are not mobile prior to capacitation.

When lectin-labeled sperm are incubated in the reproductive tract of females in estrus or under conditions conducive to capacitation *in vitro,* they show reduced binding of lectin in the acrosomal region when compared to noncapacitated sperm. In addition to the papers cited by Koehler (1978), similar results have been obtained for rat (Lewin *et al.*, 1979) and ram sperm (Courtens and Fournier-Delpech, 1979). Eventually, large patches cleared of bound lectin were formed.

Use of labeled antibodies reacting with antigens on the sperm surface has yielded similar results (see review by Koehler, 1978). Exposure of sperm to "capacitating" conditions *in vivo* or *in vitro* resulted in formation of areas that were incapable of binding antibody. Although such findings could result from selective masking of surface antigens, the favored interpretation is that at least some of the surface components of the sperm are removed from the acrosomal region of the plasma membrane during capacitation. That concept is supported by the observations of Oliphant (1976) in which it was demonstrated that removal of sperm-bound seminal plasma components facilitated induction of the acrosome reaction in rabbit sperm. More recently, Talbot and Franklin (1978) and Talbot and Chacon (1981) have shown that selected lectins caused head-to-head agglutination of noncapacitated guinea pig sperm, but the agglutination pattern shifted to one of primarily tail-to-tail agglutination during capacitation. In the experiments of Talbot and Chacon (1981), treatment of sperm with trypsin caused a shift in agglutination pattern similar to that seen during capacitation.

In a similar study using antibody against fibronectin, Koehler *et al.* (1980) found that ejaculated, but not cauda, epididymal rabbit sperm bound the antibody. *In vivo* capacitation caused a reduction in anti-fibronectin fluorescence.

Other approaches to the study of membrane-related events during capacitation have utilized surface replica and freeze-etch procedures. Friend *et al.* (1977) and Kinsey and Koehler (1978) demonstrated that areas cleared of intramembrane particles (presumed to be proteins) form in the plasma membrane in the acrosomal region during *in vitro* capacitation of guinea pig and hamster sperm. Extending this technique further, Friend (1980) showed by binding of filipin that areas cleared of sterol were produced in acrosomal region plasma membrane during *in vitro* capacitation of guinea pig sperm. The production of

Fig. 1. Thin section of the acrosomal cap portion of a guinea pig sperm head. In thin section, differences between noncapacitated and capacitated sperm are indistinguishable. A, acrosome. (Provided by Dr. D. S. Friend.)

Fig. 2. Freeze-fracture preparation of the acrosomal cap portion of the plasma membrane from noncapacitated guinea pig sperm. Patches of quilt-patterned membrane characterize this area of the cell. A, acrosome. (Reproduced from Friend and Fawcett, 1974.)

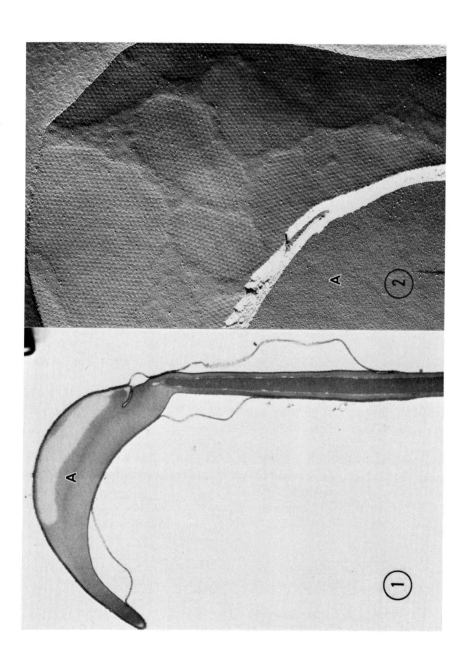

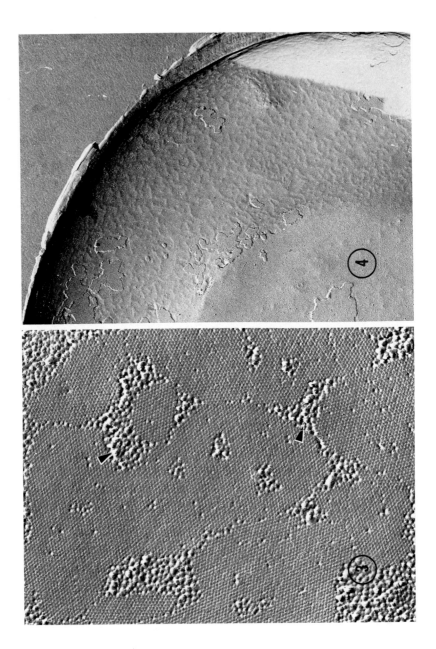

sterol-depleted patches was followed by depletion of intramembrane protein particles from the patches. Finally, Bearer and Friend (1982) used hemocyanin-conjugated polymyxin B as a probe to detect surface areas with exposed anionic lipids in guinea pig sperm. Cauda epididymal sperm bound polymyxin B in the distal acrosomal region. After incubation under conditions resulting in capacitation, the more proximal region of the plasma membrane over the acrosome also bound the antibiotic. Only a band of membrane over the tip of the nucleus was not affected. The equatorial segment and postacrosomal plasma membrane did not show affinity for polymyxin B before or after capacitation. These changes in intramembrane protein, sterol, and exposed anionic lipid distribution in guinea pig sperm are illustrated in Fig. 1–8.

Taken together, all of these morphological studies indicate that capacitation, in part, causes formation of specialized areas within the plasma membrane in the acrosomal region that are devoid of intramembrane proteins and of sterols and that have increased concentration of anionic phospholipid that is thought to be cardiolipin (Bearer and Friend, 1982). In support, D. D. Lunstra and E. D. Clegg (unpublished results) have detected cardiolipin in plasma membrane isolated from pig sperm. These specialized areas are thought to be fusigenic when the proper conditions for the acrosome reaction are provided. Although the exposed areas of anionic lipid seem to be on the outer surface of the plasma membrane, the membrane fusion of the acrosome reaction must occur between the outer surface of the outer acrosomal membrane and the inner surface of the plasma membrane. Thus, areas of anionic phospholipid should be present on the inner surface of the plasma membrane, but have not been clearly demonstrated. Although less well studied, cleared areas also appear in the outer acrosomal membrane (Friend, 1980).

The mechanisms by which these intramembrane alterations occur are unknown. Presumably, they are caused by one or more of the following:

1. Removal of components at the outer and/or inner surface that restrict mobility of intramembrane proteins.

Fig. 3. Freeze-fracture of a filipin-treated, noncapacitated guinea pig sperm. Filipin/sterol complexes (arrows), 200 to 250 Å in diameter, occupy the aisles between the quilted patches. (Provided by Dr. D. S. Friend.)

Fig. 4. Freeze-fracture of polymyxin B-treated, noncapacitated guinea pig sperm. The anterior acrosomal cap region of the plasma membrane wrinkles. Polymyxin B perturbs membranes rich in external leaflet anionic phospholipids. (Provided by Dr. E. L. Bearer.)

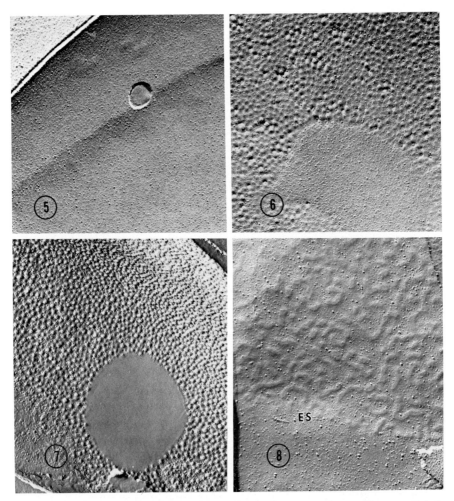

Fig. 5. Freeze-fracture of the acrosomal cap plasma membrane of a capacitated guinea pig sperm. The quilt pattern is gone, and intramembranous particles randomly adorn the membrane. (Provided by Dr. D. S. Friend.)

Fig. 6. Filipin/sterol complexes fill the membrane, except for circular microdomains which form a band across the head of capacitated guinea pig sperm. (Provided by Dr. D. S. Friend.)

Fig. 7. The filipin/sterol-free microdomains often contain few intramembranous particles in capacitated guinea pig sperm. (Reproduced from Friend, 1980.)

Fig. 8. In capacitated guinea pig sperm (and trypsinized sperm) the polymyxin B-induced wrinkles extend to the equatorial segment (ES) instead of being limited to the anterior acrosomal cap region. (Reproduced from Bearer and Friend, 1982.)

2. Shifts in affinities between membrane components caused by changing ionic balance or changing membrane composition.
3. Changes in membrane properties caused by activation and/or inactivation of membrane-bound proteins.

C. Alteration or Removal of Surface Proteins

Results using lectins and antibodies against sperm surface antigens indicate strongly that material on the outer surface of the plasma membrane is removed or altered during capacitation under both *in vivo* and *in vitro* conditions. Work using analytical methods has also led to that conclusion.

The facts that capacitation can be reversed by exposure of capacitated sperm to seminal plasma and that sperm in the same population can be recapacitated led to the strong suspicion that an interaction of seminal plasma proteins with the sperm surface was involved. The decapacitation factor or acrosome-stabilizing factor (Eng and Oliphant, 1978; ASF) has not yet been identified in most species.

A technique for facilitating capacitation in mouse, rabbit, and bovine sperm utilized a high-ionic-strength (HIS) medium having an osmolarity around 390 mOsm (see Oliphant and Eng, 1981). It was shown that protein was solubilized from sperm populations that became capable of fertilizing ova. Although it appears unlikely that the removal of surface proteins by HIS medium is the only requirement to complete capacitation in those species, the demonstration that removal of surface proteins was important to capacitation was a valuable contribution.

Several studies have appeared which evaluated the surface proteins of sperm before and after exposure to fluids of the female reproductive tract or under *in vitro* capacitation conditions. Oliphant and Singhas (1979; rabbit) and Esbenshade and Clegg (1980; pig) utilized lactoperoxidase-catalyzed iodination with intact sperm to demonstrate substantial alteration of surface proteins. The findings of Oliphant and Singhas (1979) included apparent removal of ASF from the rabbit sperm by HIS medium. The latter study included demonstration of removal of substantial quantities of specific proteins from pig sperm by fluids from the uterus and oviducts of gilts in estrus. Sperm from those incubations were capable of undergoing the acrosome reaction at the surface of ova. Davis and Gergely (1979) detected extensive hydrolysis of plasma membrane polypeptides when rat sperm were incubated *in vitro* in a Krebs-Ringer bicarbonate medium. The extent of hydrolysis was increased when bovine serum albumin was included in the medium.

D. Involvement of Membrane Lipids

Two of the more prominent theories concerning the physiologic mechanism(s) for membrane fusion involve the phospholipids of the membranes. One invokes the concept that activation of a phospholipase causes sufficient localized accumulation of lysophospholipids to result in the destruction of membrane integrity. The other postulates that divalent cations, particularly calcium, can interact with anionic phospholipids that are exposed at the membrane surface, bringing the two membranes into close proximity so that they can fuse. Consequently, increasing attention is being directed toward the membrane phospholipids.

Initial efforts to study the effect of capacitation on the phospholipids of sperm were done by Snider and Clegg (1975). In that study, phospholipids of whole pig sperm were analyzed quantitatively before and after incubation of semen (seminal plasma included) in the uterus or oviduct of gilts in estrus for up to 2 hours. A biphasic response was seen in both total phospholipid and phosphatidylcholine (PC) level. Both of these declined significantly on a "per sperm" basis, reaching their lowest values at 90 minutes. By 2 hours, which is considered to be the minimum capacitation time *in vivo* for the pig, both had returned to near the initial level. Phosphatidylinositol (PI), which was absent in control samples, appeared in all samples after 2 hours of incubation. Subsequently, this same group (Evans *et al.*, 1980) did a similar study in which washed sperm were introduced into ligated uterine segments of gilts in estrus containing oviductal flushings as well as the indigenous uterine secretions. In that experiment, the phospholipids were analyzed only at 0 and 2 hours by a more refined procedure that used selective hydrolyses and column chromatography. A striking finding was that 64% of the total pig-sperm phospholipid was either an alkyl ether (41%) or alkenyl ether phospholipid (23%). Scott *et al.* (1967) observed a similar combined level of ether phospholipids in ram sperm, but the alkenyl ether form predominated. Selivonchick *et al.* (1980) detected substantial amounts of ether phospholipids in bovine epididymal sperm. Evans *et al.* (1980) observed a significant increase in PC during *in utero* incubation, all of which was in the diacyl fraction. There were nonsignificant (statistically) increases in total phospholipid, PI, and cardiolipin. The role of the ether phospholipids in sperm function is unknown, but the possibility should be considered that they may be more resistant to enzymatic attack compared to the diacyl phospholipids.

Davis *et al.* (1979) incubated rat sperm in medium containing bovine serum albumin (BSA) and analyzed the cholesterol and phospholipid contents of both the albumin and the sperm. Cholesterol content decreased in sperm while phospholipid content increased. The opposite occurred in the extracellular albumin. Interestingly, the decline in sperm cholesterol was in the free cholesterol fraction, while the BSA showed an increase in cholesteryl ester. Unfortunately, no evidence was presented demonstrating that the sperm were capacitated during this treatment.

It must be recognized that the isolated plasma membrane was not analyzed in any of the preceding studies. Therefore, although evidence of changes in sperm phospholipids was obtained, the site(s) of the changes cannot be assigned. Additional experiments are needed to determine if the changes are localized in the plasma membrane or outer acrosomal membrane, and if the shifts in individual phospholipids are related to capacitation.

Recently, Fleming and Yanagimachi (1981) reported that incubation of guinea pig sperm in media containing a monoglyceride, diacyl phospholipids, or lysophospholipids, in addition to BSA, could reduce the time required to achieve the acrosome reaction. Specifically, lysophosphatidylcholine, lysophosphatidylethanolamine, and lysophosphatidylinositol all markedly reduced the time necessary to obtain the acrosome reaction, while the corresponding diacyl phospholipids or sphingomyelin were not particularly effective. Phosphatidylserine appeared to inhibit the acrosome reaction. A very interesting observation was that glyceryl monooleate caused the acrosome reaction within 10 minutes if calcium was present. Cholesterol was not effective. Thus, exposure of the sperm to agents (lysophospholipids) that have membrane-disrupting properties effectively facilitated the acrosome reaction *in vitro*. Although it is generally assumed that such added lipids can be incorporated within the lipid matrix of the plasma membrane of the sperm, proof that such is the case is lacking (see Evans and Setchell, 1978).

If accumulation of lysophospholipids within the membranes of sperm is a component of capacitation, then a mechanism must also exist for activation of a phospholipase that can act selectively on the membranes in the acrosomal region. Snider and Clegg (1975) did not detect lysophospholipids in pig sperm that had been incubated in the uterus.

Because whole sperm were analyzed, a small quantity of lysophospholipids present in membranes in the acrosomal region may have gone undetected.

Some evidence exists for the presence of a phospholipase in sperm. Lui and Meizel (1979), working with two phospholipase A inhibitors, were able to block acrosome reactions in hamster sperm. Mepacrine and *p*-bromophenacyl bromide inhibited induction of the acrosome reaction in both an *in vitro* capacitation system and in incubations with the divalent cation ionophore A23187. Llanos *et al.* (1982) have subsequently demonstrated that a phospholipase A is released from hamster sperm after the acrosome reaction. This does not indicate whether the enzyme was active before the acrosome reaction or where it might be acting in the sperm. The BSA used in those experiments did not contain phospholipase activity.

The phospholipase A released in the preceding experiments was activated by calcium, a general characteristic of such enzymes from other cells. It was active at pH 7.4 to 7.8, but not at pH 4.5. This is important, since the enzyme in sperm might be of acrosomal origin. If so, the pH of the intact acrosome of noncapacitated sperm is probably sufficiently low (Meizel and Deamer, 1978) that the enzyme would be inactive. An elevation of acrosomal pH during capacitation (to be discussed later), along with calcium influx, could activate the enzyme so that it could act on the membrane(s) in the acrosomal region. In studies involving effects of inhibitors on intact cells, uncertainties exist about the site and specificity of inhibitor action.

Another potential mechanism by which sperm membranes may be prepared for the acrosome reaction has been proposed by Davis *et al.* (1980) and Davis (1981). In that scheme, cholesterol is donated to sperm by "decapacitation" proteins or vesicles in seminal plasma to raise the cholesterol:phospholipid ratio of the sperm. Conversely, the serum proteins present in fluids of the female reproductive tract are proposed to sequester cholesterol from the sperm and/or donate additional phospholipid to the sperm. In either case, the key is suggested to be a lowering of the cholesterol:phospholipid ratio of the sperm during capacitation.

Sterol sulfates may play a role in capacitation, although this possibility has not received wide attention (see Langlais *et al.,* 1981, for summary of observations). A potentially important early finding was that very low concentrations of desmosteryl sulfate (desmosterol is a close relative of cholesterol) could inhibit *in vitro* fertilization by hamster sperm. Present evidence indicates that sperm accumulate sterol sulfate during transit through the epididymis, but then are exposed to sterol sulfatase activity in the female reproductive tract. According to the theory proposed by those investigators, sterol sulfates at the surface of sperm would be hydrolyzed, leaving free sterol in the membrane. Cleavage of membrane phospholipid by a phospholipase A or a lecithin:cholesterol acyltransferase could allow a free fatty acid from the phospholipid to be esterified to cholesterol, with the products being lysophospholipid and cholesteryl acyl ester. The mechanism could result in both lysophospholipid accumulation and an alteration in the cholesterol:phospholipid balance. The cholesteryl esters could be sequestered by albumin in the medium. It is also possible that acyltransferases responsible for esterification of cholesterol are activated by albumin. However, caution must be exercised until more is known about the existence, properties, and sites of action of such enzymes in sperm and in environments that are conducive to capacitation.

It should be noted that the hypothesis proposed by Langlais *et al.* (1981) provides a link between the concepts of lysophospholipid accumulation in the sperm membranes and alteration of the phospholipid and/or cholesterol contents of the membranes as factors in preparation of the membranes for the acrosome reaction.

E. Role of Cyclic Nucleotides

The roles of cyclic nucleotides and their related enzymes in capacitation remain unclear. The subject was reviewed comprehensively by Garbers and Kopf (1980), and a more general review on adenylate cyclase was presented by Ross and Gilman (1980).

Initially, observations were made in two laboratories that adenylate cyclase activity was increased under conditions that could produce capacitated or acrosome-reacted sperm. Morton and Albagli (1973) worked with *in vitro* incubation of hamster sperm, while Berger and Clegg (1983) incubated pig sperm *in utero*. In what is probably the most definitive work available on that subject, Hyne and Garbers (1979a) measured cAMP levels in guinea pig sperm incubated *in vitro* under varying conditions. Substantial elevation of intracellular cAMP (up to 30-fold) occurred very rapidly when sperm were added to media containing calcium, but only increased slightly (threefold) and in a transient manner when added to media without calcium. The calcium transport antagonist methoxyverapamil blocked the calcium-induced elevation of cAMP. After the sperm were capacitated in calcium-free medium, addition of calcium caused cAMP levels to increase within 1 minute and the acrosome reaction was maximized within 10 minutes. A key observation may be that 8-bromo-cAMP or 1-methyl-3-iso-

butylxanthine (a phosphodiesterase inhibitor) decreased the time necessary to attain the acrosome reaction when calcium was present. Also,
Peterson *et al.* (1978) found that dibutyryl cAMP, in the presence of
calcium, increased the proportion of pig sperm undergoing the A23187-
induced acrosome reaction. These experiments represent the strongest
evidence (albeit tenuous) that adenylate cyclase and cAMP are actually involved in capacitation. The strong possibility remains that elevated cAMP levels may be limited to involvement in activation of
motility and respiration.

Most of the recent work on this subject supports the concept that
elevation of intracellular cAMP in some way facilitates capacitation or
induction of the acrosome reaction. Several investigators have examined the effects of cAMP analogs or phosphodiesterase inhibitors on
induction of the acrosome reaction or the time required for penetration
of ova. Toyoda and Chang (1974; rat), Rosado *et al.* (1974; rabbit),
Reyes *et al.* (1978; rabbit), Hyne and Garbers (1979a; guinea pig),
Mrsny and Meizel (1980; hamster), and Fraser (1981; mouse) found
that added dibutyryl cAMP or 8-bromo-cAMP had a beneficial effect on
the above parameters. Dibutyryl cAMP and theophylline also facilitated onset of the A23187-induced acrosome reaction in pig and human
sperm (Peterson *et al.*, 1979). The single exception is the report by
Rogers and Garcia (1979; guinea pig) that dibutyryl cAMP and phosphodiesterase inhibitors could reduce the incidence of acrosome reactions and fertilization rate. The discrepancy may be due to the relatively high levels of cAMP analog and phosphodiesterase inhibitors
used. The cAMP level was much higher than physiologic levels. Also,
butyrate released from the dibutyryl cAMP may have had an inhibiting effect (Fraser, 1981). The use by Hyne and Garbers (1979a) of 8-
bromo-cyclic AMP at much lower concentration may explain their success in inducing the acrosome reaction in guinea pig sperm.

Inclusion of phosphodiesterase inhibitors in *in vitro* incubations has
yielded essentially the same result as cAMP analogs (Fraser, 1979;
Hyne and Garbers, 1979a; Mrsny and Meizel, 1980).

Two reports have appeared in which 8-bromo-cGMP induced very
rapid onset of acrosome reactions in guinea pig (Santos-Sacchi *et al.*,
1980; Santos-Sacchi and Gordon, 1980). They proposed that an elevated cGMP:cAMP ratio was important for induction of the acrosome
reaction. Again, caution must be exercised in the interpretation of
these results since very high levels (10 mM) of the cGMP analog were
used. Garbers and Kopf (1980) cite unpublished work from their laboratory in which oviductal fluid caused up to 50-fold increase in cGMP
in pig sperm without affecting cAMP level.

Calcium may be involved in regulation of sperm adenylate cyclase. Hyne and Garbers (1979b; guinea pig) showed that micromolar amounts of free calcium in the presence of Mg^{2+} produced a fourfold increase in activity compared to that with Mg^{2+} alone. They suggested that a component of the adenylate cyclase system in sperm (probably the catalytic protein) may be regulated by calcium via calmodulin.

It is important to consider the possibility that there may be more than one adenylate cyclase system present in sperm. Evidence for such a possibility is extremely scanty. Rosado *et al.* (1975) and Delgado *et al.* (1981) measured binding of cAMP to human sperm. They observed that the majority of the labeled cAMP (after cell disruption and fractionation) was associated with the midpiece-tail fraction. Also, Tash and Means (1982) found that cAMP acted on lysed dog sperm to stimulate both phosphorylation of proteins and motility. Under those conditions, calcium interfered with motility and inhibited cAMP-stimulated phosphorylation of some, but not all, of the proteins. A protein that may be tubulin was prominent among those not phosphorylated when calcium was added. If these results are combined with the demonstrated regional differences in surface properties of the sperm plasma membrane and with the possible separation of cytoplasmic compartments between the head and midpiece-tail regions, it does seem possible that cAMP produced by adenylate cyclases in different regions could have different functions. Further, adenylate cyclases in different regions could be regulated by differing mechanisms.

The mechanism for control of sperm adenylate cyclase is poorly understood. In so-called "normal" cells (see Ross and Gilman, 1980, for review), at least three types of membrane-bound proteins are required for hormonally activated adenylate cyclase activity. These are a catalytic protein, a regulatory protein, and receptor protein(s). The catalytic protein (C) is stimulated by Mn^{2+}. Catalytic activity of C can be stimulated by binding of guanine nucleotide (variable effects) or fluoride to the G/F regulatory protein. A regulatory GTPase cycle has been proposed to explain control of the enzyme via the GTP:GDP ratio. The role of the receptor protein(s) complexed with hormone is thought to be one of altering the affinity of the regulatory protein for guanine nucleotide.

In sperm, the enzyme is quite unique in that it is Mn^{2+}-stimulated but is not responsive to hormones, guanine nucleotides, fluoride, or cholera toxin (see Stengel and Hanoune, 1981). Apparent exceptions are the reports by Casillas *et al.* (1978) and Cheng and Boettcher (1979) of stimulation of sperm adenylate cyclase activity by the GTP analog Gpp(NH)p. A variant of an S49 lymphoma cell line (cyc$^-$) has similar properties and has been found to lack the G/F regulatory protein. Stengel and Hanoune (1981) have taken advantage of those experiments to show that apparent transfer of the regulatory protein to ram sperm from human erythrocytes conferred hormone sensitivity as well as activation by guanine nucleotide and fluoride to the sperm adenylate cyclase. The most obvious interpretation is that sperm adenylate cyclase appears to lack the regulatory protein and that the observed effects in cauda epididymal or ejaculated sperm are due to divalent cation or guanine nucleotide effects, either directly on the catalytic protein or on the surrounding lipid milieu.

F. Role of Catecholamines

Adrenal extracts have been found to influence the ability of hamster sperm to achieve the acrosome reaction *in vitro* (see Meizel, 1978, for initial observations). Two different factors have been elucidated as necessary for that *in vitro* system. Taurine or hypotaurine seems to allow hamster sperm to remain motile for a sufficient period of time to achieve capacitation (Meizel *et al.*, 1980; Leibfried and Bavister, 1981). In addition, catecholamines or other α- and β-adrenergic agonists are required, apparently for both optimal motility and for attainment of the acrosome reaction in that system (Bavister *et al.*, 1979; Cornett *et al.*, 1979; Meizel and Working, 1980; Meizel, 1981).

It is tempting to speculate that the catecholamines should serve to activate the adenylate cyclase in the sperm plasma membrane. However, sperm adenylate cyclase is thought to be unresponsive to exogenous catecholamines for reasons discussed previously. There has been no demonstration that catecholamines can activate sperm adenylate cyclase. Thus, it seems likely that the catecholamines are acting by another as yet unidentified mechanism.

Support for the existence of an alternate mode of action of catecholamines is provided by Cornett and Meizel (1980) who were unable to demonstrate binding of the β-adrenergic antagonist 9-aminoacrydylpropanolol to β-adrenergic receptors of hamster sperm. However, a recent abstract from that laboratory (Meizel and Turner, 1982) indicates that induction of the acrosome reaction in hamster sperm by biogenic amines, including serotonin, 5-methoxytryptamine, dopamine, and epinephrine, was inhibited by serotonin or dopamine receptor antagonists. Thus, the mode of action of catecholamines is very much open to question and deserves substantial attention, particularly since sperm may be exposed to catecholamines in the female reproductive tract. Caution should be exercised since all of the above work was done with one species. Earlier studies were done with very high levels of catecholamines, but Meizel (1981) has now indicated that similar results were obtained with levels closer to the physiologic range.

G. Activation and Role of Acrosin in Capacitation and the Acrosome Reaction

In addition to the long-standing proposed role of acrosin in penetration of the zona pellucida, evidence suggests a role of acrosin, or at least an acrosomal enzyme, possibly phospholipase, in the acrosome reaction (see Meizel, 1978). Both low-molecular-weight trypsin inhibitors and phospholipase inhibitors prevented the acrosome reaction when added to capacitated hamster sperm (Lui and Meizel, 1979). The A23187-induced acrosome reaction was also inhibited. However, Perreault et al. (1982) found that permeable trypsin inhibitors allowed the membrane vesiculation of the acrosome reaction but interfered with dispersion of the acrosomal matrix in in vitro capacitated guinea pig sperm. Green (1978b) obtained a similar result in the guinea pig with A23187-induced acrosome reactions. The different results could be dismissed as a difference between species, but there are other possible explanations, including potential differences in cytoplasmic or acrosomal pH and availability of calcium to the acrosomal matrix.

Recent studies by Working and Meizel (1981, 1982) have dealt with the possibility that an increase in acrosomal pH during capacitation could assist in conversion of proacrosin to active acrosin. Proacrosin is stable at low pH, but is converted to acrosin if the pH is elevated to 6 or higher (see review by Parrish and Polakoski, 1979). Acrosomal pH in hamster sperm appears to be less than 5 prior to capacitation (Meizel and Deamer, 1978). If this is the case in general, an increase in acrosomal pH would at least facilitate activation of the enzyme. Working and Meizel (1981) presented evidence for a proton pump that could serve to maintain an acidic acrosomal pH. The proton ionophore FCCP, in combination with the potassium ionophore valinomycin, was able to dissipate the proton gradient between the acrosome and the cytoplasm of hamster sperm. In that situation, an influx of potassium into the acrosome due to the influence of valinomycin was used to maintain electrochemical equilibrium. The same workers (Working and Meizel, 1982) also found a Mg^{2+}-ATPase in the membrane vesicles released from hamster sperm by the acrosome reaction. It was interesting that the enzyme was inhibited by calcium. Since such vesicles are composed of mixed plasma and outer acrosomal membrane, localization of the enzyme in the outer acrosomal membrane was precluded. If the enzyme was present in the outer acrosomal membrane, it could provide a mechanism for translocating protons into or out of the acrosome. No evidence is available on the direction of transport in the membrane vesicles.

The role of calcium in conversion of proacrosin to acrosin is uncertain. Autoactivation of rabbit and hamster proacrosin to acrosin (measuring esterase activity) was reported to be accelerated by Ca^{2+} and inhibited by Zn^{2+} (see Meizel and Mukerji, 1976). The activation was optimal at pH 8. In contrast, Polakoski and Parrish (1977) found that calcium inhibits conversion of purified pig proacrosin to acrosin. However, once an active form of acrosin was obtained, the proteolytic activity of the purified enzyme was activated at calcium concentrations of 2–50 mM (Parrish and Polakoski, 1981). Other divalent cations, with the exception of Zn^{2+}, which was not tested, were also able to stimulate activity. The optimal pH range was 7–8.

Parrish et al. (1979) also found that conversion of purified proacrosin from pig sperm to m_α-acrosin, the first active form, was accelerated by glycosaminoglycans in vitro. The ability of glycosaminoglycans to stimulate proacrosin to acrosin conversion in intact sperm has not been demonstrated.

Substantial uncertainty still exists over the role of acrosin in capacitation. Whether or not this proteolytic and esterolytic enzyme does have a role in the acrosome reaction, conversion of proacrosin to an active form of acrosin probably occurs during capacitation. In pig sperm, such activation occurs during incubation of the sperm in utero (Polakoski et al., 1979). If, as proposed in this chapter, cytoplasmic calcium is kept at a low concentration in vivo until induction of the acrosome reaction, then perhaps only an increase in acrosomal pH is sufficient for conversion of proacrosin to acrosin. To have a role in the acrosome reaction, active acrosin then would need to pass through the outer acrosomal membrane (probably after attacking that membrane) to act on components in the intermembrane space and/or on the inner surface of the plasma membrane. Such activity could remove a barrier between the membranes, allowing them to approach each other sufficiently closely to permit membrane fusion. Obviously, much work remains to be done before the role of acrosin prior to fertilization is understood.

H. Potential Role of Complement

A possible role of the complement system in capacitation or induction of the acrosome reaction has been mostly ignored. Cabot and Oliphant (1978) demonstrated that the acrosome reaction induced in rabbit sperm by bovine follicular fluid was prevented by antibody against the bovine C component of complement. Other evidence in that paper suggested that the alternate complement pathway was involved. More recently, Suarez *et al.* (1981) detected immunoglobulin (probably IgG) bound to the surface of sperm from the epididymis. This surface immunoglobulin could bind C_{1q} with subsequent breakdown of the sperm acrosome (Suarez and Oliphant, 1982). Seminal plasma interfered with the fixation of complement. Whether or not this was a true acrosome reaction remains to be determined. Nevertheless, the possibility that at least some portion of the complement system may be involved in induction of the acrosome reaction should be examined closely. Complement is virtually absent in fluids from the rabbit uterus and oviduct (Cabot and Oliphant, 1978). However, follicular fluid contains substantial amounts of complement. Since the acrosome reaction is induced selectively *in vivo* when sperm are in contact with the cumulus cells or the zona pellucida, this may be the component triggering the acrosome reaction under physiologic conditions. This possibility will be considered in more detail in the next section.

I. Proposed Events in Capacitation and Induction of the Acrosome Reaction *in Vivo*

Much less is known about the events occurring in sperm in the female reproductive tract than those occurring during *in vitro* capacitation. At the same time, some of the more drastic treatments (such as high ionic strength medium and high pH) that can be at least partially effective *in vitro* can be eliminated as possibilities for the *in vivo* system. It is important to consider that the changes in sperm *in vivo* that are components of capacitation are probably mimicked with some *in vitro* systems by treatments quite unlike those functioning *in vivo*. It is also important to state, since little is known with certainty about the mechanisms *in vivo*, that proof for the preceding statement is tenuous at best.

As viewed by this investigator, the following events are suggested for capacitation and induction of the acrosome reaction *in vivo*. A basic assumption is made that elevation of calcium in the cytoplasm between the plasma and outer acrosomal membranes is the key event just prior to initiation of the acrosome reaction. Much of the emphasis is placed on preparation of sperm for that entry of calcium and on the consequences of that entry.

1. Removal and/or alteration of surface components. This could include removal of the decapacitation or acrosome-stabilizing factor(s), removal of surface-bound enzyme inhibitors (such as a protease inhibi-

tor), removal of barrier(s) to transport mechanisms, exposure or preparation of surface receptor sites for interaction with an acrosome reaction-inducing factor and for sperm–ovum recognition, and removal of surface cross-linking structures that restrict mobility of intramembrane components.

2. Preparation of the plasma membrane and probably the outer acrosomal membrane for fusion when a sufficient level of calcium is present in the cytoplasm between the plasma membrane and outer acrosomal membrane. This would involve localized alteration of the membrane lipid composition and possibly removal of a barrier preventing close approach of the two membranes. A mechanism resembling those proposed by Langlais *et al.* (1981) and Davis (1981) seems most probable to me at this time (see Section III,D). Such a mechanism could explain the apparent necessity for albumin in even the simplest *in vitro* systems. The alteration of membrane lipids, combined with removal of surface cross-linking components, would cause increased susceptibility to membrane fusion and altered permeability/transport properties.

3. Activation of sperm adenylate cyclase. The most obvious possibility is that phosphorylation of proteins are required for activation of motility which, in turn, facilitates ovum penetration. Since motility activation is accompanied by stimulation of sperm respiration, an increase in cAMP probably causes an increase in metabolic rate (perhaps indirectly) and/or a shift in substrate utilization. The metabolic changes could affect cytoplasmic pH. A more direct role of cAMP in regulation of membrane properties should not be ruled out. The possibility of differential activation of adenylate cyclase and different modes of action of cAMP in different regions of sperm (flagellar versus acrosomal regions, for instance) should be considered.

4. Activation of acrosin. The conflicting reports, involving only two species, make it impossible at this time to assign a direct role to acrosin in the alteration of membrane properties prior to the acrosome reaction. However, conversion of proacrosin to acrosin within the acrosome is probably an important component of capacitation. Part of that conversion process should include elevation of acrosomal pH. The *in vivo* experiments of Polakoski *et al.* (1979) indicate that proacrosin-to-acrosin conversion is accomplished during capacitation when cytoplasmic calcium is proposed to be low. The concept that acrosomal enzyme(s) activated by calcium may act on membrane and intermembrane components just prior to the acrosome reaction should be considered.

5. Influx of calcium. An important component of this proposed se-

quence is the concept that calcium, although present in the extracellular fluid, would not be available in substantial amounts to intracellular compartments of the sperm head until just before the acrosome reaction, even though it may be available earlier in the mitochondrial region. Low levels of cytoplasmic calcium in the acrosomal region after ejaculation may be sufficient to stimulate adenylate cyclase activation but be insufficient to induce membrane fusion. The basic assumption is made that elevation of calcium in the cytoplasm between the plasma membrane and outer acrosomal membrane is the key event just prior to initiation of the acrosome reaction. If that is true, then the factor inducing the acrosome reaction under physiologic conditions should act by causing a substantial increase in calcium influx. This could be accomplished in several ways, including insertion of ionophore-type molecules into the membrane, sufficient destruction of membrane integrity such that the barrier to massive calcium influx is removed, and/or inhibition of the calcium pump(s) responsible for maintenance of low cytoplasmic calcium level. This concept may well be an important point where some *in vitro* capacitation methods differ substantially from the physiologic process.

If complement is involved in induction of the acrosome reaction, its action could be explained as causing sufficient perturbation of membrane integrity such that the barrier to influx of calcium is destroyed. Regardless of the mechanism for the increased calcium influx, the final component in the induction of the acrosome reaction is proposed to be interaction of calcium with membrane lipids (both within and between the membranes) in such a way that areas of membrane susceptible to fusion are drawn into sufficient proximity for fusion and vesiculation to occur.

In contrast to many methods for capacitation *in vitro,* the vast majority of acrosome reactions *in vivo* occur only when sperm are in the close vicinity of either cumulus cells or the zona pellucida. (See Chapter 7 and Chapter 10.) Therefore, the factor inducing the calcium influx probably exists in the matrix between cumulus cells and in the zona matrix. It is not clear if the factor is in solution so that it can diffuse away from these sources or if it is bound. The entire ovum plus cumulus cells is bathed in follicular fluid prior to ovulation and would have ample opportunity to soak up the fluid, much as a sponge would trap a solution. The possibility also exists that the inducing factor could originate from the vitellus itself. In either case, it is a function of the female reproductive tract, via secretions of the various segments, to remove the barrier to action by that factor. This should involve a stepwise process with the cervix and/or uterus serving initially to remove seminal plasma and to begin acting on adsorbed surface components. Once sperm are in the oviduct, this process of surface alteration can be completed. An area of research that requires much further attention is the extent (and manner) to which secretions (and their ability to induce the required alterations in sperm) of the uterus, isthmus, and ampulla change relative to the time of ovulation. The work of Overstreet and co-workers with the rabbit (see Chapter 11) indicates quite clearly that properties of those oviductal segments can change substantially as ovulation is approached.

IV. CONCLUDING COMMENTS

The primary impetus for research on capacitation has been the need for acceptable contraceptive methods. That need still remains. However, there are other related needs that should also receive increased attention. Despite the importance of population control, infertility is tragic in human populations and very costly in farm animal populations. Research is needed on infertility due to both noninfectious and infectious causes in a wide variety of animals.

In the last 10 years, progress has been impressive in identifying processes that occur in sperm during capacitation. However, that progress also has demonstrated that capacitation is complex and still inadequately understood. There is virtually no area of investigation within the subject of capacitation in which work can be considered to be completed. Many of these areas have been identified in this chapter. Work on the subject must continue at levels of increasing depth, with the most advanced techniques available for morphological and biochemical evaluation being used. It is important that capacitation be understood as it occurs in the intact animal. The number of species used as models should be increased so that a broader spectrum of animal types is represented.

REFERENCES

Austin, C. R. (1975). Membrane fusion events in fertilization. *J. Reprod. Fertil.* **44,** 155–166.
Babcock, D. F., Singh, J. P., and Lardy, H. A. (1979). Alteration of membrane permeability to calcium ions during maturation of bovine spermatozoa. *Dev. Biol.* **69,** 85–93.

Bavister, B. D., Chen, A. F., and Fu, P. C. (1979). Catecholamine requirement for hamster sperm motility in vitro. *J. Reprod. Fertil.* **56**, 507–513.

Bearer, E. L., and Friend, D. S. (1982). Modifications of anionic-lipid domains preceding membrane fusion in guinea pig sperm. *J. Cell Biol.* **92**, 604–615.

Bedford, J. M. (1970). Sperm capacitation and fertilization in mammals. *Biol. Reprod., Suppl.* **2**, 128–158.

Bedford, J. M., and Cooper, G. W. (1978). Membrane fusion events in the fertilization of vertebrate eggs. *In* "Membrane Fusion" (G. Poste and G. L. Nicolson, eds.), pp. 65–125. Elsevier/North-Holland Biomedical Press, Amsterdam.

Berger, T., and Clegg, E. D. (1983). Adenylate cyclase activity in porcine sperm in response to female reproductive tract secretions. *Gamete Res.* **7** (in press).

Bradley, M. P., and Forrester, I. T. (1980). A [Ca^{2+} + Mg^{2+}]-ATPase and active Ca^{2+} transport in the plasma membranes isolated from ram sperm flagella. *Cell Calcium* **1**, 381–390.

Bushway, A. A., Clegg, E. D., and Keenan, T. W. (1977). Composition and synthesis of gangliosides in bovine testis, sperm and seminal plasma. *Biol. Reprod.* **17**, 432–442.

Cabot, C. L., and Oliphant, G. (1978). The possible role of immunological complement in induction of rabbit sperm acrosome reaction. *Biol. Reprod.* **19**, 666–672.

Campanella, C., Gabbiani, G., Baccetti, B., Burrini, A. G., and Pollini, V. (1979). Actin and myosin in the vertebrate acrosomal region. *J. Submicrosc. Cytol.* **11**, 53–71.

Carafoli, E., and Crompton, M. (1978). The regulation of intracellular calcium. *Curr. Top. Membr. Transp.* **10**, 151–216.

Casillas, E. R., Elder, C. M., and Hoskins, D. D. (1978). Adenylate cyclase activity in maturing bovine spermatozoa: Activation by GTP and polyamines. *Fed. Proc., Fed. Am. Soc. Exp. Biol.* **37**, 1688 (abstr.).

Cheng, C. Y., and Boettcher, B. (1979). Effects of cholera toxin and 5'-guanylylimidodiphosphate on human spermatozoal adenylate cyclase activity. *Biochem. Biophys. Res. Commun.* **91**, 1–9.

Clarke, G. N., and Yanagimachi, R. (1978). Actin in mammalian sperm heads. *J. Exp. Zool.* **205**, 125–132.

Clarke, G. N., Clarke, F. M., and Wilson, S. (1982). Actin in human spermatozoa. *Biol. Reprod.* **26**, 319–327.

Cornett, L. E., and Meizel, S. (1980). 9-AAP, a fluorescent β-adrenergic antagonist, enters the hamster sperm acrosome in a manner inconsistent with binding to β-adrenergic receptors. *J. Histochem. Cytochem.* **28**, 462–464.

Cornett, L. E., Bavister, B. D., and Meizel, S. (1979). Adrenergic stimulation of fertilizing ability in hamster spermatozoa. *Biol. Reprod.* **20**, 925–929.

Courtens, J. L., and Fournier-Delpech, S. (1979). Modifications in the plasma membranes of epididymal ram spermatozoa during maturation and incubation in utero. *J. Ultrastruct. Res.* **68**, 136–148.

Davis, B. K. (1978). Inhibition of fertilizing capacity in mammalian spermatozoa by natural and synthetic vesicles. *Symp. Pharmacol. Eff. Lipids [Pap.]* AOCS Monogr. No. 5, pp. 145–158.

Davis, B. K. (1981). Timing of fertilization in mammals: Sperm cholesterol/phospholipid ratio as a determinant of the capacitation interval. *Proc. Natl. Acad. Sci. U.S.A.* **78**, 7560–7564.

Davis, B. K., and Gergely, A. F. (1979). Studies on the mechanism of capacitation: Changes in plasma membrane proteins of rat spermatozoa during incubation in vitro. *Biochem. Biophys. Res. Commun.* **88**, 613–618.

Davis, B. K., Byrne, R., and Hungund, B. (1979). Studies on the mechanism of capacitation. II. Evidence for lipid transfer between plasma membrane of rat sperm and serum albumin during capacitation in vitro. *Biochim. Biophys. Acta* **558**, 257–266.

Davis, B. K., Byrne, R., and Bedigian, K. (1980). Studies on the mechanism of capacitation: Albumin-mediated changes in plasma membrane lipids during in vitro incubation of rat sperm cells. *Proc. Natl. Acad. Sci. U.S.A.* **77**, 1546–1550.

Delgado, N. M., Huacuja, L., Merchant, H., and Rosado, A. (1981). Differential distribution of cyclic-AMP receptors in human spermatozoa. *Arch. Androl.* **7**, 45–49.

Eng. L. A., and Oliphant, G. (1978). Rabbit sperm reversible decapacitation by membrane stabilization with a highly purified glycoprotein from seminal plasma. *Biol. Reprod.* **19**, 1083–1094.

Esbenshade, K. L., and Clegg, E. D. (1980). Surface proteins of ejaculated porcine sperm and sperm incubated in the uterus. *Biol. Reprod.* **23**, 530–537.

Evans, R. W., and Setchell, B. P. (1978). Association of endogenous phospholipids with spermatozoa. *J. Reprod. Fertil.* **53**, 357–362.

Evans, R. W., Weaver, D. E., and Clegg, E. D. (1980). Diacyl, alkenyl, and alkyl ether phospholipids in ejaculated, in utero-, and in vitro-incubated porcine spermatozoa. *J. Lipid Res.* **21**, 223–228.

Feinberg, J., Weinmann, J., Weinmann, S., Walsh, M. P., Harricane, M. C., Gabrion, J., and Demaille, J. G. (1981). Immunocytochemical and biochemical evidence for the presence of calmodulin in bull sperm flagellum. *Biochim. Biophys. Acta* **673**, 303–311.

Fléchon, J. E. (1979). Sperm glycoproteins of the boar, bull, rabbit and ram. II. Surface glycoproteins and free acidic groups. *Gamete Res.* **2**, 53–64.

Fléchon, J. E., and Morstin, J. (1975). Localisation des glycoprotéines et des charges négatives et positives dans le révètement de surface des spermatozoides éjacules de Lapin et de Taureau. *Ann. Histochem.* **20**, 291–300.

Fleming, A. D., and Yanagimachi, R. (1981). Effects of various lipids on the acrosome reaction and fertilizing capacity of guinea pig spermatozoa with special reference to the possible involvement of lysophospholipids in the acrosome reaction. *Gamete Res.* **4**, 253–273.

Fraser, L. R. (1979). Accelerated mouse sperm penetration in vitro in the presence of caffeine. *J. Reprod. Fertil.* **57**, 377–384.

Fraser, L. R. (1981). Dibutyryl cyclic AMP decreases capacitation time in vitro in mouse spermatozoa. *J. Reprod. Fertil.* **62**, 63–72.

Friend, D. S. (1980). Freeze-fracture alterations in guinea pig sperm membranes preceding gamete fusion. *In* "Membrane–Membrane Interactions" (N. B. Gilula, ed.), pp. 153–166. Raven Press, New York.

Friend, D. S., and Fawcett, D. W. (1974). Membrane differentiations in freeze-fractured mammalian sperm. *J. Cell Biol.* **63**, 641–664.

Friend, D. S., Orci, L., Perrelet, A., and Yanagimachi, R. (1977). Membrane particle changes attending the acrosome reaction in guinea pig spermatozoa. *J. Cell Biol.* **74**, 561–577.

Garbers, D. L., and Kopf, G. S. (1980). The regulation of spermatozoa by calcium and cyclic nucleotides. *Adv. Cyclic Nucleotide Res.* **13**, 251–306.

Gordon, M. (1973). Localization of phosphatase activity on the membrane of the mammalian sperm head. *J. Exp. Zool.* **185**, 111–120.

Gordon, M., Dandekar, P. V., and Eager, P. R. (1978). Identification of phosphatases on the membranes of guinea pig sperm. *Anat. Rec.* **191**, 123–134.

Green, D. P. L. (1978a). The mechanism of the acrosome reaction. *Dev. Mamm.* **3**, 65–81.

Green, D. P. L. (1978b). The activation of proteolysis in the acrosome reaction of guinea pig sperm. *J. Cell Sci.* **32**, 153–164.

Gwatkin, R. B. L. (1977). "Fertilization Mechanisms in Man and Animals." Plenum, New York.

Hyne, R. V., and Garbers, D. L. (1979a). Calcium-dependent increase in adenosine 3′,5′-monophosphate and induction of the acrosome reaction in guinea pig spermatozoa. *Proc. Natl. Acad. Sci. U.S.A.* **76**, 5699–5703.

Hyne, R. V., and Garbers, D. L. (1979b). Regulation of guinea pig sperm adenylate cyclase by calcium. *Biol. Reprod.* **21**, 1135–1142.

Jones, H. P., Bradford, M. M. McRorie, R. A., and Cormier, M. J. (1978). High levels of a calcium-dependent modulator protein in spermatozoa and its similarity to brain modulator protein. *Biochem. Biophys. Res. Commun.* **82**, 1264–1272.

Jones, H. P., Lenz, R. W., Palevitz, B. A., and Cormier, M. J. (1980). Calmodulin localization in mammalian spermatozoa. *Proc. Natl. Acad. Sci. U.S.A.* **77**, 2772–2776.

Kinsey, W. H., and Koehler, J. K. (1976). Fine structural localization of concanavalin A binding sites on hamster spermatozoa. *J. Supramol. Biol.* **5**, 185–198.

Kinsey, W. H., and Koehler, J. K. (1978). Cell surface changes associated with in vitro capacitation of hamster sperm. *J. Ultrastruct. Res.* **64**, 1–13.

Koehler, J. K. (1978). The mammalian sperm surface: Studies with specific labeling techniques. *Int. Rev. Cytol.* **54**, 73–108.

Koehler, J. K., Nudelman, E. D., and Hakomori, S. (1980). A collagen-binding protein on the surface of ejaculated rabbit spermatozoa. *J. Cell Biol.* **86**, 529–536.

Langlais, J., Zoolinger, M., Plante, L., Chapdelaine, A., Bleau, G., and Roberts, K. D. (1981). Localization of cholesteryl sulfate in human spermatozoa in support of a hypothesis for the mechanism of capacitation. *Proc. Natl. Acad. Sci. U.S.A.* **78**, 7266–7270.

Leibfried, M. L., and Bavister, B. D. (1981). The effects of taurine and hypotaurine on in vitro fertilization in the golden hamster. *Gamete Res.* **4**, 57–63.

Lewin, L. M., Weissenberg, R., Sobel, J. S., Marcus, Z., and Nebel, L. (1979). Differences in concanavalin A–FITC binding to rat spermatozoa during epididymal maturation and capacitation. *Arch. Androl.* **2**, 279–281.

Llanos, M. N., Lui, C. W., and Meizel, S. (1982). Studies of phospholipase A_2 related to the hamster sperm acrosome reaction. *J. Exp. Zool.* **221**, 107–117.

Lui, C. W., and Meizel, S. (1979). Further evidence in support of a role for hamster sperm hydrolytic enzymes in the acrosome reaction. *J. Exp. Zool.* **207**, 173–186.

McRorie, R. A., and Williams, W. L. (1974). Biochemistry of mammalian fertilization. *Annu. Rev. Biochem.* **43**, 777–803.

Mann, T., and Lutwak-Mann, C. (1981). "Male Reproductive Function and Semen." Springer-Verlag, Berlin and New York.

Meizel, S. (1978). The mammalian sperm acrosome reaction: A biochemical approach. *Dev. Mamm.* **3**, 1–64.

Meizel, S. (1981). Stimulation of sperm fertility in vitro by exogenous molecules. *Reproduccion* **5**, 169–176.

Meizel, S., and Deamer, D. W. (1978). The pH of the hamster sperm acrosome. *J. Histochem. Cytochem.* **26**, 98–105.

Meizel, S., and Mukerji, S. K. (1976). Biochemical studies of proacrosin and acrosin from hamster cauda epididymal spermatozoa. *Biol. Reprod.* **14**, 444–450.

Meizel, S., and Turner, K. O. (1982). Stimulation of the hamster sperm acrosome reaction by biogenic amines. *Biol. Reprod.* (Suppl. 1), **93** (abstr).

Meizel, S., and Working, P. K. (1980). Further evidence suggesting the hormonal stimulation of hamster sperm acrosome reactions by catecholamines in vitro. *Biol. Reprod.* **22**, 211–216.

Meizel, S., Lui, C. W., Working, P. K., and Mrsny, R. J. (1980). Taurine and hypotaurine: Their effects on motility, capacitation and the acrosome reaction of hamster sperm in vitro and their presence in sperm and reproductive tract fluids of several mammals. *Dev. Growth Differ.* **22**, 483–494.

Moore, H. D. M., and Hibbitt, K. G. (1975). Isoelectric focusing of boar spermatozoa. *J. Reprod. Fertil.* **44**, 329–332.

Moore, H. D. M., and Hibbitt, K. G. (1976). The binding of labelled basic proteins by boar spermatozoa. *J. Reprod. Fertil.* **46**, 71–76.

Morton, B., and Albagli, L. (1973). Modification of hamster sperm adenyl cyclase by capacitation in vitro. *Biochem. Biophys. Res. Commun.* **50**, 697–703.

Mrsny, R. J., and Meizel, S. (1980). Evidence suggesting a role for cyclic nucleotides in acrosome reactions of hamster sperm in vitro. *J. Exp. Zool.* **211**, 153–157.

Nicolson, G. L., and Yanagimachi, R. (1974). Mobility and restriction of mobility of plasma membrane lectin-binding components. *Science* **184**, 1294–1296.

Oliphant, G. (1976). Removal of sperm-bound seminal plasma components as a prerequisite to induction of the rabbit acrosome reaction. *Fertil. Steril.* **27**, 28–38.

Oliphant, G., and Eng. L. A. (1981). Collection of gametes in laboratory animals and preparation of sperm for in vitro fertilization. *In* "Fertilization and Embryonic Development in Vitro" (L. Mastroianni, Jr. and J. D. Biggers, eds.), pp. 11–26. Plenum, New York.

Oliphant, G., and Singhas, C. A. (1979). Iodination of rabbit sperm plasma membrane: Relationship of specific surface proteins to epididymal function and sperm capacitation. *Biol. Reprod.* **21**, 937–944.

O'Rand, M. G. (1977). Restriction of a sperm surface antigen's mobility during capacitation. *Dev. Biol.* **55**, 260–270.

Parrish, R. F., and Polakoski, K. L. (1979). Mammalian sperm proacrosin-acrosin system. *Int. J. Biochem.* **10**, 391–395.

Parrish, R. F., and Polakoski, K. L. (1981). Stimulation of proteolytic activity of boar sperm acrosin by divalent metal ions. *J. Reprod. Fertil.* **62**, 417–422.

Parrish, R. F., Wincek, T. J., and Polakoski, K. L. (1979). Glycosaminoglycan stimulation of the in vitro conversion of boar proacrosin into acrosin. *J. Androl.* **1**, 85–95.

Perreault, S. D., Zirkin, B. R., and Rogers, B. J. (1982). Effect of trypsin inhibitors on acrosome reaction of guinea pig spermatozoa. *Biol. Reprod.* **26**, 343–351.

Peterson, R. N., Russell, L., Bundman, D., and Freund, M. (1978). Presence of microfilaments and tubular structures in boar spermatozoa after chemically inducing the acrosome reaction. *Biol. Reprod.* **19**, 459–466.

Peterson, R. N., Seyler, D., Bundman, D., and Freund, M. (1979). The effect of theophylline and dibutyryl cyclic AMP on the uptake of radioactive calcium and phosphate ions by boar and human spermatozoa. *J. Reprod. Fertil.* **55**, 385–390.

Polakoski, K. L., and Parrish, R. F. (1977). Purification and preliminary activation studies of proacrosin isolated from ejaculated boar sperm. *J. Biol. Chem.* **252**, 1888–1894.

Polakoski, K. L., Clegg, E. D., and Parrish, R. F. (1979). Identification of the in vivo sperm proacrosin into acrosin conversion sequence. *Int. J. Biochem.* **10**, 483–488.

Reyes, A., Goicoechea, B., and Rosado, A. (1978). Calcium ion requirement for rabbit spermatozoal capacitation and enhancement of fertilizing ability by ionophore A23187 and cyclic adenosine 3':5'-monophosphate. *Fertil. Steril.* **29**, 451–455.

Rogers, B. J. (1978). Mammalian sperm capacitation and fertilization in vitro. A critique of methodology. *Gamete Res.* **1**, 165–223.

Rogers, B. J., and Garcia, L. (1979). Effect of cAMP on acrosome reaction and fertilization. *Biol. Reprod.* **21,** 365–372.

Rosado, A., Hicks, J. J., Reyes, A., and Blanco, I. (1974). Capacitation in vitro of rabbit spermatozoa with cyclic adenosine monophosphate and human follicular fluid. *Fertil. Steril.* **25,** 821–824.

Rosado, A., Huacuja, L., Delgado, N. M., Hicks, J. J., and Pancardo, R. M. (1975). Cyclic-AMP receptors in the human spermatozoa membrane. *Life Sci.* **17,** 1707–1714.

Ross, E. M., and Gilman, A. G. (1980). Biochemical properties of hormone-sensitive adenylate cyclase. *Annu. Rev. Biochem.* **49,** 533–564.

Santos-Sacchi, J., and Gordon M. (1980). Induction of the acrosome reaction in guinea pig spermatozoa by cGMP analogues. *J. Cell Biol.* **85,** 798–803.

Santos-Sacchi, J., Gordon, M., and Williams, W. L. (1980). Potentiation of the cGMP-induced guinea pig acrosome reaction by zinc. *J. Exp. Zool.* **213,** 289–291.

Schwarz, M. A., and Koehler, J. K. (1979). Alterations in lectin binding to guinea pig spermatozoa accompanying in vitro capacitation and the acrosome reaction. *Biol. Reprod.* **21,** 1295–1307.

Scott, T. W., Voglmayr, J. K., and Setchell, B. P. (1967). Lipid composition and metabolism in testicular and ejaculated ram spermatozoa. *Biochem. J.* **102,** 456–461.

Selivonchick, D. P., Schmid, P. C., Natarajan, V., and Schmid, H. H. O. (1980). Structure and metabolism of phospholipids in bovine epididymal spermatozoa. *Biochim. Biophys. Acta* **618,** 242–254.

Singer, S. J., and Nicolson, G. L. (1972). The fluid mosiac model of the structure of cell membranes. *Science* **175,** 720–731.

Singh, J. P., Babcock, D. F., and Lardy, H. A. (1980). Induction of accelerated acrosome reaction in guinea pig sperm. *Biol. Reprod.* **22,** 566–570.

Snider, D. R., and Clegg, E. D. (1975). Alteration of phospholipids in porcine spermatozoa during in vivo uterus and oviduct incubation. *J. Anim. Sci.* **40,** 269–274.

Stambaugh, R., and Smith, M. (1978). Tubulin and microtubule-like structures in mammalian acrosomes. *J. Exp. Zool.* **203,** 135–141.

Stengel, D., and Hanoune, J. (1981). The catalytic unit of ram sperm adenylate cyclase can be activated through guanine nucleotide regulatory component and prostaglandin receptors of human erythrocyte. *J. Biol. Chem.* **256,** 5394–5398.

Steptoe, P. C., and Edwards, R. G. (1978). Birth after reimplantation of a human embryo. *Lancet* **2,** 366.

Suarez, S. S., and Oliphant, G. (1982). I. Interaction of rabbit spermatozoa and serum complement components. *Biol. Reprod.* **27,** 473–483.

Suarez, S. S., Hinton, B. T., and Oliphant, G. (1981). Binding of a marker for immunoglobulins to the surface of rabbit testicular, epididymal, and ejaculated spermatozoa. *Biol. Reprod.* **25,** 1091–1097.

Talbot, P., and Chacon, R. (1981). Detection of modifications in the tail of capacitated guinea pig sperm using lectins. *J. Exp. Zool.* **216,** 435–444.

Talbot, P., and Franklin, L. E. (1978). Surface modification of guinea pig sperm during in vitro capacitation: An assessment using lectin-induced agglutination of living sperm. *J. Exp. Zool.* **203,** 1–14.

Talbot, P., and Kleve, M. G. (1978). Hamster sperm cross-react with antiactin. *J. Exp. Zool.* **204,** 131–136.

Tamblyn, T. M. (1980). Identification of actin in boar epididymal spermatozoa. *Biol. Reprod.* **22,** 727–734.

Tamblyn, T. M. (1981). Evidence for nonmuscle myosin in bovine ejaculated spermatozoa. *Gamete Res.* **4,** 499–506.

Tash, J. S., and Means, A. R. (1982). Regulation of protein phosphorylation and motility of sperm by cyclic adenosine monophosphate and calcium. *Biol. Reprod.* **26,** 745–763.

Toyoda, Y., and Chang, M. C. (1974). Capacitation of epididymal spermatozoa in a medium with high K/Na ratio and cyclic AMP for the fertilization of rat eggs in vitro. *J. Reprod. Fertil.* **36,** 125–134.

Working, P. K., and Meizel, S. (1981). Evidence that an ATPase functions in the maintenance of the acidic pH of the hamster sperm acrosome. *J. Biol. Chem.* **256,** 4708–4711.

Working, P. K., and Meizel, S. (1982). Preliminary characterization of an Mg^{2+}-ATPase in hamster sperm head membranes. *Biochem. Biophys. Res. Commun.* **104,** 1060–1065.

Yanagimachi, R. (1981). Mechanisms of fertilization in mammals. *In* "Fertilization and Embryonic Development In Vitro" (L. Mastroianni, Jr. and J. D. Biggers, eds.), pp. 81–188. Plenum, New York.

Yanagimachi, R., and Usui, N. (1974). Calcium dependence of the acrosome reaction and activation of guinea pig spermatozoa. *Exp. Cell Res.* **89,** 161–174.

5

Membrane Properties and Intracellular Ion Activities of Marine Invertebrate Eggs and Their Changes during Activation

SHELDON S. SHEN

I. INTRODUCTION

Nothing would more clearly demonstrate the sovereign role that electrolytes play in the phenomena of life than by causing, if possible, with their help, unfertilized eggs to develop into larvae. (Loeb, 1913)

This chapter is concerned primarily with the expanding body of knowledge on changes in membrane ionic permeabilities and intra-

Mechanism and Control of Animal Fertilization
Copyright © 1983 by Academic Press, Inc.
All rights of reproduction in any form reserved.
ISBN 0-12-328520-8

cellular ionic activities, which occur upon activation of eggs of marine invertebrates. This subject had its beginning at the turn of the century when the focus was on the parthenogenetic capabilities in different ionic compositions of seawater. However, due to the great numbers and diversity of treatments discovered, and the technical difficulties of demonstrating ionic changes during normal development, interest in the significance of ions during egg activation waned. A revival of interest has occurred in the past decade, due not only to the development of techniques to answer the questions left by earlier investigators but also to new findings that demonstrate the role of ions in the causal chain of events that occurs during activation of the egg. In this chapter, I shall focus primarily on the sea urchin egg, in which many of the ionic changes are best characterized. However, the role of ions during activation of eggs of other marine invertebrates is important to any unifying theory on the role of ions in early development. (For a discussion of ionic movements during activation of the male gamete, see Chapter 6.)

II. RESTING POTENTIAL

Like other living cells, sea urchin eggs have an unequal distribution of ions across the cell membrane (Rothschild and Barnes, 1953). Depending on the permeability characteristics of the egg membrane, a membrane potential or resting potential can be expected. Since sea urchin eggs are large (ranging from 70 to 140 μm) in comparison to somatic cells, impalement with intracellular microelectrodes should be facilitated and the resting potential, as well as its ionic basis, easily determined. However, this has not been the case and several problems are worth mentioning. Sea urchin eggs are protected by a jelly coat. Aside from impeding microelectrode penetration, the extracellular coat may act as a diffusion barrier, thus acting itself as a membrane. The jelly coat is usually removed by a variety of means prior to measurement of the resting potential; the effect of removal on the resting potential has not been studied. Since the resting potential is dependent on the selective permeability of the membrane, the leak current associated with microelectrode impalement may also present as an artifact. This problem is especially significant in determination of the resting potential of unfertilized sea urchin eggs, which have high membrane input resistance (Hagiwara and Jaffe, 1979). The age of the egg affects its morphology, respiration, and development (Harvey, 1956), and may also affect the resting potential of an unfertilized egg (Jaffe and Robinson, 1978; Dale and De Santis, 1981b). While the biological significance of the resting potential is uncertain, knowledge of the resting potential in intact eggs is important for deciphering the regulation of intracellular ion activities that are associated with metabolic activation of the egg. This point is discussed in later sections.

Early attempts to measure the resting potential generally reported no potential difference across the membrane of unfertilized echinoderm eggs (Gelfan, 1931; Rothschild, 1938a; Kamada and Kinosita, 1940; Scheer et al., 1954; Furshpan, 1955; Lundberg, 1955; Hori, 1958). The failure of reseachers to find any significant resting potential was due to several factors, including blunt electrodes, extensibility of the egg membrane, and vesiculation at the electrode tip (Chambers, 1922; Tyler and Monroy, 1955; Rothschild, 1956). The first definitive report of an inside negative resting potential was by Tyler et al. (1956) in eggs of the starfish Asterias forbesi. Hiramoto (1959a,b) later reported negative resting potentials in a variety of echinoderm eggs, including the sea urchins Hemicentrotus pulcherrimus and Clypeaster japonicus.

The resting potential of unfertilized sea urchin eggs has now been examined by a number of investigators. Reported resting potentials have ranged from −5 to −80 mV and have fallen into two general ranges of −5 to −20 mV (Hiramoto, 1959a; Higashi and Kaneko, 1971; Steinhardt et al., 1971, 1972; Ito and Yoshioka, 1972, 1973; Tupper, 1973; Higashi, 1974; Dale et al., 1978b; Taglietti, 1979; DeFelice and Dale, 1979; Dale and De Santis, 1981a,b) and −60 to −80 mV (Chambers et al., 1974a; Jaffe, 1976; MacKenzie and Chambers, 1977; Chambers and de Armendi, 1977a,b, 1979; Okamoto et al., 1977; Jaffe and Robinson, 1978). Several studies on the ionic bases of the more positive resting potential have concluded that the unfertilized egg membrane is anion-permeable and cation-impermeable (Steinhardt et al., 1971; Higashi and Kaneko, 1971; Ito and Yoshioka, 1973). The selectivity is, however, very poor, because the membrane potential changed less than 10 mV per 10-fold change in external Cl^- concentration. The ionic basis of the more negative resting potential is K^+-dependent (Chambers and de Armendi, 1977a,b, 1979; Jaffe and Robinson, 1978), a 55-mV change in membrane potential per 10-fold change in external K^+ concentration.

A number of observations suggests that low resting potentials of unfertilized eggs are a consequence of leakage current associated with microelectrode penetration. Even in the reports of hyperpolarized membrane, the resting potential immediately after electrode impalement was −8 to −12 mV. Within a few minutes, the amplitude of the negative resting potential increased to stable values of −60 to −80 mV

(Ito and Yoshioka, 1972; Jaffe and Robinson, 1978; Chambers and de Armendi, 1979). The increase in resting potential was accompanied by an increase in membrane resistance (Jaffe and Robinson, 1978). Eggs with large negative resting potentials are generally characterized by nonlinear current-voltage (I-V) relation, while eggs with depolarized membrane have a linear I-V relation (Jaffe and Robinson, 1978; Chambers and de Armendi, 1979; Fig. 1). As seen in Fig. 1, eggs with low resting potential may also have a nonlinear I-V relation. In these eggs, the injection of small hyperpolarizing current (-0.1---0.2 nA) is sufficient to lower the membrane potential to below -60 mV. Application of hyperpolarizing current can result in unfertilized eggs' spontaneously maintaining large negative resting potentials after the current has been switched off entirely (Chambers and de Armendi, 1979). The application of hyperpolarizing current may aid membrane sealing around the microelectrode (Brown and Flaming, 1977). Higher external Ca^{2+} concentrations may also speed recovery from penetration damage. Okamoto et al. (1977) reported resting potentials of -70 mV for sea urchin eggs in 30 mM Ca^{2+} seawater.

The resting potential of unfertilized sea urchin eggs has also been determined by tracer flux measurements (Chambers and de Armendi, 1977a,b; Jaffe and Robinson, 1978). By measuring ion fluxes, a resting potential of -70 mV was calculated by means of the constant-field equations. As a further check, the effect of external K^+ concentration on Na^+ influx was determined (Jaffe and Robinson, 1978). The results fitted closely with the theoretical expectations, assuming that the resting potential of the unfertilized egg is a K^+ diffusion potential. Therefore, the resting potential of unfertilized sea urchin eggs is K^+-dependent and in the range of -60 to -80 mV. Since the I-V relation is characterized by a negative slope conductance region (Fig. 1), a slight outward current would result in a large shift of the membrane potential. Thus, presence of leak current due to microelectrode penetration could shift the resting potential measured to a depolarized level (Hagiwara and Jaffe, 1979).

Two stable resting potential states have also been reported for the starfish oocyte (Miyazaki et al., 1975a; Shen and Steinhardt, 1976). Starfish oocytes with resting potentials ranging from -10 to -25 mV generally have a linear I-V relation and lower membrane input resistance, while oocytes with resting potentials ranging from -60 to -90 mV had a nonlinear I-V relation and higher membrane input resistance. Certain oocytes with depolarized membranes and nonlinear I-V relation were observed to stabilize at resting potentials more negative than -65 mV after hyperpolarizing current pulses (Miyazaki et

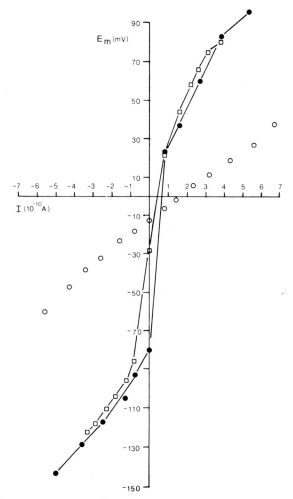

Fig. 1. The current-voltage (I-V) relation of unfertilized eggs of the sea urchin *Lytechinus pictus*. These relations were recorded from eggs of the same female within 2 hours of shedding and are representative of the results obtained with batches of eggs from other females. In the majority of eggs, resting potentials were either low, with a linear I-V relation (○) or more negative, with a nonlinear I-V relation (●). Occasionally, an egg would have a low resting potential with a nonlinear I-V relation (□). An action potential could be induced as an "off-response" to hyperpolarizing current pulses. Perturbation of the microelectrode impaled in eggs with a nonlinear I-V relation often shifted the I-V relation to a linear one and the resting potential to a more positive one, which suggested that the low resting potential and linear I-V relation of an unfertilized egg may be due to an increased leak current.

al., 1975a). The more negative resting potential is K^+-dependent (Hagiwara and Takahashi, 1974; Miyazaki *et al.,* 1975b; Shen and Steinhardt, 1976). The depolarized resting potential of oocytes with nonlinear I-V relation could be shifted to -70 mV by the replacement of external Na^+ ions with a nonpermeant cation (Miyazaki *et al.,* 1975a). Since the nonlinear I-V relation is characterized by a negative slope conductance region, a depolarized resting potential will be maintained by a slight outward current or a slight leak current. Therefore, it was concluded that differences in the resting potential state and I-V relation of starfish oocytes may be the result of differences in the amount of leak current caused by microelectrode penetration (Miyazaki *et al.,* 1975a).

Changes of membrane potentials and membrane resistances have been reported with starfish oocyte maturation induced by 1-methyladenine (Kanatani *et al.,* 1969; Miyazaki *et al.,* 1975a,b; Shen and Steinhardt, 1976; Moreau and Cheval, 1976; Dale *et al.,* 1979). In all cases reported to date, the specific membrane resistance of oocytes increased five- to seven-fold shortly after 1-methyladenine exposure. In most starfish species, membrane depolarization occurs with maturation (Miyazaki *et al.,* 1975b; Moreau and Cheval, 1976; Dale *et al.,* 1979) due to a loss of K^+ permeability and an increase in Na^+ permeability (Miyazaki *et al.,* 1975b; Doree, 1981). However, oocytes of *Patiria miniata* hyperpolarize after 1-methyladenine addition, due to a decrease in Na^+ permeability (Shen and Steinhardt, 1976). In view of the different changes of membrane potential with maturation of different starfish species and the lack of explanation for the biological significance of an increase in specific membrane resistance, the interpretation of electrophysiological changes induced by 1-methyladenine is still largely speculative (Masui and Clarke, 1979).

Since there is no known maturation-promoting factor for sea urchin oocytes, the electrophysiological changes accompanying maturation of sea urchin oocytes have not been studied. The resting potential of sea urchin oocytes has been reported to range from -50 to -90 mV (Jaffe and Robinson, 1978; Taglietti, 1979; DeFelice and Dale, 1979; Dale and De Santis, 1981b). Dale and De Santis (1981b) reported a depolarization of the sea urchin oocyte membrane with maturation. This polarization was induced by tetraethylammonium, which is a blocker of K channels (Tasaki and Hagiwara, 1957; Armstrong, 1971). The authors suggested that, following maturation, the unfertilized sea urchin egg would be characterized by a high resistance, low resting potential, indicating a predominance of a sparse population of linear and nonspecific ionic channels. Several difficulties exist with the interpretation of the data. If tetraethylammonium blocks K channels, one would expect a resting potential more dependent upon the leakage introduced by microelectrode impalement. Depolarization was observed in eight separate recordings, while in two oocytes, the germinal vesicle remained intact. Exposure to tetraethylammonium induced maturation in only approximately 15% of the sea urchin oocytes (Dale and De Santis, 1981b). These results suggest that depolarization may be a consequence of tetraethylammonium and electrode impalement, rather than maturation induced by tetraethylammonium.

Several reports have suggested that the resting potential of unfertilized eggs may be age-dependent. The frequency of eggs with large negative resting potentials may increase with time after being shed (Taglietti, 1979; DeFelice and Dale, 1979; Dale and De Santis, 1981b) or may vary with the condition of the female (Jaffe and Robinson, 1978; Dale and De Santis, 1981b). *In vitro* aging paralleled by an increase in K^+ conductance has been reported for starfish oocyte maturation induced by the addition of 1-methyladenine (Miyazaki, 1979; Miyazaki and Hirai, 1979). However, the optimal time for fertilization in the starfish is near germinal vesicle breakdown, while sea urchin oocytes complete meiosis prior to ovulation and fertilization. A systematic study of the effect of aging on the resting potential of sea urchin eggs is necessary.

Resting potentials have been measured in a variety of other marine invertebrate eggs, including echiuroid, annelid, tunicate, and mollusk. In the echiuroid *Urechis caupo,* a resting potential of -33 mV has been reported (Jaffe *et al.,* 1979). Since the potential shifted 20 mV per 10-fold change of external K^+ concentration and 10 mV per 10-fold change of external Na^+ concentration, the authors concluded that the resting potential is due largely to K^+ permeability with some Na^+ component. The resting potential of the *Urechis* oocyte is more negative than that of eggs, averaging -57 mV in seawater (Holland and Gould-Somero, 1981). Since a 10-fold increase in external K^+ concentration caused a membrane potential shift of 49 mV, the more negative resting potential of oocytes is due in part to a greater K^+ selectivity of the oocyte membrane. In the coelenterate *Renilla koellikeri,* the resting potential of the immature egg is about -70 mV and is K^+-dependent (Hagiwara *et al.,* 1981). Similar K^+-dependent resting potential has been reported for the immature and mature eggs of the annelid *Chaetopterus pergamentaceus* (Hagiwara and Miyazaki, 1977). Low resting potentials have been reported for the eggs of tunicates in seawater, ranging from 0 to -20 mV (Miyazaki *et al.,* 1974; Dale *et al.,* 1978a). Replacement of external Na^+ ions with Tris increased the membrane potential to more than -70 mV, which was K^+-dependent (Miyazaki et al., 1974). Finally, the resting potential of several species of mollusks has been reported. The resting potential of the unfertilized oocyte of Spisula solidissima is about -20 mV (Finkel and Wolf, 1980), similar to the K^+-dependent resting potential of the unfertilized egg of Ilyanassa obsoleta (Conrad et al., 1977; Moreau and Guerrier, 1981), while the resting potential of unfertilized Dentalium dentale eggs is about -70 mV (Jaffe and Guerrier, 1981). Thus, the resting potentials reported for other marine invertebrate eggs have ranged from those with small potentials and relatively nonspecific membranes to those with more negative potentials and K^+-selective membranes. Further investigations are necessary in some eggs with low resting potentials to eliminate the possibility of leakage artifact.

III. ACTION POTENTIAL

A property that appears common to many unfertilized marine invertebrate egg membranes studied to date is electrical excitability. Generation of an action potential in response to currents applied across the egg membrane was initially reported in eggs of the tunicate (Miyazaki et al., 1972, 1974) and subsequently in those of starfish (Hagiwara and Takahashi, 1974; Miyazaki et al., 1975a; Shen and Steinhardt, 1976), sea urchin (Jaffe, 1976; Okamoto et al., 1977; Chambers and de Armendi, 1977a,b, 1979; Jaffe and Robinson, 1978), annelid (Hagiwara and Miyazaki, 1977; Fox and Krasne, 1981), coelenterate (Hagiwara et al., 1981), echiuroid (Jaffe et al., 1979, Holland and Gould-Somero, 1981), and mollusk (Moreau and Guerrier, 1981). Several recent reviews discuss the electrical excitability of eggs and the changes during developmental differentiation (Hagiwara and Jaffe, 1979; Spitzer, 1979; Takahashi, 1979). Since the action potential of unfertilized eggs may be important during the fertilization response, the ionic bases of the action potential are briefly considered.

A depolarizing current pulse can elicit a regenerative response in unfertilized sea urchin eggs with resting potentials more negative than -60 mV (Jaffe, 1976; Okamoto et al., 1977; Jaffe and Robinson, 1978; Chambers and de Armendi, 1979). A typical action potential of Lytechinus pictus is seen in Fig. 2. In this example, the resting potential was -80 mV and the threshold potential was -57 mV. The action potential had a peak of $+21$ mV, a duration of 12.2 sec, and an inflection during the rising phase at -11 mV. These values are similar to

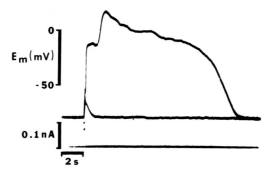

Fig. 2. Oscillograph record of an action potential of an unfertilized egg of the sea urchin *Lytechinus pictus*. An action potential was induced by a depolarizing 0.1 nA current pulse of 100 msec duration. A depolarizing 0.08 nA current pulse of 100 msec duration was subthreshold.

those described by Chambers and de Armendi (1979) for *Lytechinus variegatus*. In unfertilized eggs, with more positive resting potentials but with nonlinear I-V relation, an action potential is generated as an "off response" upon cessation of a hyperpolarizing current. Although a 100-fold reduction of external Na^+ concentration shortens the duration of the action potential, the amplitude is relatively unaffected (Chambers and de Armendi, 1979). Reduction of external Ca^{2+} concentration, however, decreases the peak amplitude of the action potential at 26 mV per ten-fold decrease (Chambers and de Armendi, 1979). These results indicate that the action potential of unfertilized sea urchin eggs is Ca^{2+}-dependent.

Since electrical excitability consists of changes in membrane permeability due to the opening or closing of ion channels, techniques such as that of voltage clamp, developed in the study of differentiated excitable membranes, have been applied for analysis of the ionic currents during action potential in the egg. The identification of the membrane currents in the unfertilized sea urchin egg has been performed under the voltage-clamp condition (Okamoto *et al.*, 1977). An inward current appeared when the egg membrane was depolarized above −50 mV, with a maximum current near −25 mV. The current shows both activation and inactivation, with membrane potential-dependent time courses. Since the inward current is increased markedly with enhancement of external Ca^{2+} concentration, is insensitive to external Na^+ concentration, and is greatly reduced with Mn^{2+}, Okamoto *et al.* (1977) suggested that the inward current is through calcium channels in the egg membrane. Furthermore, Sr^{2+} and Ba^{2+} ions could substitute for Ca^{2+} ions, similar to that observed for the voltage-dependent calcium channels of crustacean muscle fiber (Hagiwara et al., 1974).

The ionic currents during the action potential of other marine invertebrate eggs have been studied by the voltage-clamp technique. The properties of the egg membrane channels of tunicate and starfish differ from those of the sea urchin. Since the resting potential of tunicate eggs is small, the regenerative response is observed as an "off response" during the recovery phase of the membrane potential upon cessation of a hyperpolarizing current (Miyazaki et al., 1972, 1974). The "off response" of the tunicate egg has two components. The major component has a threshold value of -45 to -40 mV and has been identified as a Na^+-dependent action potential. The properties of the sodium channels are similar in many aspects to those of the Na^+ channel in adult tissues (Okamoto et al., 1976a,b; Ohmori and Yoshii, 1977). So far, voltage-dependent sodium channels in egg membrane have been identified only in the tunicate. The minor component has a threshold value near 0 mV. It is evident when all the Na^+ ions in the artificial seawater are replaced with Tris or choline (Miyazaki et al., 1974) or when the major component is inactivated by a conditioning depolarization pulse (Okamoto et al., 1976b). Because the minor component of the inward current is external Ca^{2+}-dependent, the channel is blocked by Mn^{2+}, Co^{2+}, and La^{3+}, and the channel is permeable to Sr^{2+} and Ba^{2+}; the minor component has been identified as a Ca^{2+}-dependent action potential (Okamoto et al., 1976a,b; Ohmori and Yoshii, 1977).

A Ca^{2+}-dependent action potential has been described in the starfishes Mediaster aequalis (Hagiwara et al., 1975), Asterina pectinifera (Miyazaki et al., 1975a), and Patiria miniata (Shen and Steinhardt, 1976), but was absent in Marthasterias glacialis (Moreau and Cheval, 1976). Detailed voltage clamp analysis of the eggs of Mediaster shows two types of inward current channels (Hagiwara et al., 1975). The inward current of both channels is carried by Ca^{2+} ions, but the two channels are separated by the following criteria. (1) Activation and inactivation of the two channels have different membrane potential dependencies. Channel I is activated at -55 to -50 mV and channel II is activated at -7 to -6 mV. (2) The time course of the two currents is different with the inactivation of channel II being substantially slower than that of channel I. (3) The two inward currents have different ion concentration dependence. Channel II is more easily saturated. (4) The two channels have different sensitivities to blocking cations, such as

Mg^{2+} and Co^{2+}. Channel II is substantially more sensitive than channel I. (5) Although the inward current is not carried by Na^+ ions, the Ca^{2+}-dependent current through channel I is sensitive to external Na^+, while that of channel II is Na^+ insensitive (Hagiwara et al., 1975).

A Ca^{2+}-dependent action potential is also present in the unfertilized eggs of annelids (Hagiwara and Miyazaki, 1977; Fox and Krasne, 1981), a coelenterate (Hagiwara et al., 1981), an echiuroid (Jaffe et al., 1979), and a mollusk (Moreau and Guerrier, 1981). Identification of the action potential as Ca^{2+}-dependent in these cases is supported by some or all of the following data. Replacement of external Na^+ concentration has no significant effect on the action potential. The peak amplitude and rise time of the action potential is dependent on the external Ca^{2+} concentration. Known blockers of Ca^{2+} currents through membranes suppress the action potential. Ba^{2+} and Sr^{2+} ions can replace Ca^{2+} ions as the permeant divalent. Presently, the data demonstrate the presence of electrical excitability in a wide range of marine invertebrate eggs. The biological significance of the voltage-sensitive ion channels, however, is unclear. The action potential may participate in the electrical changes at fertilization.

IV. FERTILIZATION POTENTIAL

The earliest perceivable electrophysiological response to fertilization in marine invertebrate eggs is a transient depolarization. Initially, this response was termed an activation potential, although the term was coined in reference to artificial activation (Maeno, 1959). Subsequently, for identification of the bioelectric response to fertilization, the term fertilization action potential was used (Steinhardt et al., 1971). Since regenerative responses are elicited by current pulses, the terms fertilization potential and activation potential are used when referring to the bioelectric response of eggs to sperm and parthenogenetic agents, respectively (Hagiwara and Jaffe, 1979).

Early in the 1900s, McClendon (1910a,b), Harvey (1910), Lyon and Shackell (1910), and Loeb (1910) presented evidence for a marked increase in sea urchin egg membrane permeability shortly after fertilization, including an increase in the electrical conductivity of a suspension of eggs (McClendon, 1910c). Lillie (1911) predicted a transient "action-current" due to alterations in the ionic permeabilities of the egg membrane with fertilization. However, evidence that the membrane potentials of animal eggs change during fertilization was not available until microelectrodes could be successfully implanted in an unfertilized egg.

Fertilization potential was initially described in a starfish, *Asterias forbesi* (Tyler *et al.*, 1956), as a positive-going shift of 5 to 10 mV of the membrane potential which lasted less than 1 minute, with a gradual return to a new stable resting potential even more negative than that of the unfertilized egg. The occurrence of a transient depolarization of the membrane upon insemination is common to marine invertebrates. Fertilization potentials have been observed in a wide variety of echinoids (Hiramoto, 1959a,b; Steinhardt *et al.*, 1971; Higashi and Kaneko, 1971; Ito and Yoshioka, 1972; Chambers *et al.*, 1974a; Miyazaki *et al.*, 1975b; Jaffe, 1976; Dale *et al.*, 1978b; Chambers and de Armendi, 1979; DeFelice and Dale, 1979; Miyazaki, 1979; Miyazaki and Hirai, 1979; Taglietti, 1979; Dale and De Santis, 1981a,b), an echiuroid (Jaffe *et al.*, 1979; Gould-Somero *et al.*, 1979; Holland and Gould-Somero, 1981), mollusks (Finkel and Wolf, 1978, 1980; Jaffe and Guerrier, 1981), an annelid (Hagiwara and Jaffe, 1979), and a tunicate (Dale *et al.*, 1978a).

The ionic bases of the fertilization potential have been extensively analyzed in echinoids and echiuroids. The initial event in the fertilization response of these eggs is the activation of the voltage-dependent calcium channels, which depolarize the membrane from -31 to $+12$ mV in *Asterina pectinifera* (Miyazaki and Hirai, 1979), -75 to $+20$ mV in *Lytechinus variegatus* (Chambers and de Armendi, 1979), and -37 to $+51$ mV in *Urechis caupo* (Jaffe *et al.*, 1979). However, the duration of depolarization during a fertilization potential exceeds that of an action potential, elicited by a depolarizing current pulse. Both the activation of voltage-dependent calcium channels and the maintained depolarization during the fertilization potential result from a slow transient increase in Na^+ permeability of the egg membrane (Jaffe *et al.*, 1979; Chambers and de Armendi, 1979). In sea urchin and starfish fertilization, inactivation of the calcium channels may precede the complete opening of Na^+ channels, such that the fertilization potential is characteristically biphasic (Chambers and de Armendi, 1979; Miyazaki and Hirai, 1979). In unfertilized echinoid eggs with more positive resting potentials, only the transient increase in Na^+ permeability is observed with fertilization (Steinhardt *et al.*, 1971, 1972; Ito and Yoshioka, 1973; Higashi, 1974; Dale *et al.*, 1978b; Taglietti, 1979; Miyazaki and Hirai, 1979; DeFelice and Dale, 1979; Dale and De Santis, 1981a,b), since the ionic mechanisms of the action potential are inactivated by the leak current. After about 45 to 60 seconds in sea urchin eggs and several minutes in *Asterina* and *Urechis* eggs, the membrane repolarizes. The falling phase of the fertilization potential results from an inactivation of the sodium channels and a large increase in K^+ permeability (Steinhardt et al., 1972; Higashi, 1974; Jaffe and Robinson, 1978; Jaffe et al., 1979; Chambers and de Armendi, 1979), except in Asterina (Miyazaki et al., 1975b; Miyazaki, 1979), where no increase in K^+ permeability has been detected.

Evidence consistent with the fertilization potential occurring as a result of membrane permeability changes to Ca^{2+}, Na^+, and K^+ comes from ion replacement, inhibitor, and radioactive tracer flux studies. Replacement of external Na^+ or Ca^{2+} dramatically shifts the peak amplitudes of the fertilization potential. A 100-fold reduction of external Na^+ concentration has little effect on the peak amplitude of the initial spike of the fertilization potential of sea urchin, but significantly suppresses the peak amplitude of the second positive shift. A 100-fold reduction of external Ca^{2+} concentration greatly decreases the initial peak amplitude of the fertilization potential of the sea urchin but not the amplitude of the second response phase (Chambers and de Armendi, 1979). These results suggest that the initial rapid depolarization of the sea urchin egg membrane upon insemination is similar to the Ca^{2+}-dependent action potential (Okamoto et al., 1977), while the second positive shift results from a slower developing increase in Na^+ permeability. Similar results are observed with the fertilization potential of Urechis (Jaffe et al., 1979). A 10-fold reduction of external Ca^{2+} concentration decreases the initial spike amplitude without having any significant effect on the later events of the fertilization response. On the other hand, a 10-fold reduction of external Na^+ concentration reduces the amplitude of the fertilization potential, after the first 15 seconds by 51 mV. The initial spike amplitude of the fertilization potential is also reduced when Na^+ concentration is lowered, since the fertilization potential amplitude is too small in 50 mM Na^+ seawater to initiate the Ca^{2+}-dependent action potential (Jaffe et al., 1979). Further evidence for an initial Ca^{2+}-dependent action potential during the fertilization response of Urechis is seen with the drug D-600, which blocks Ca^{2+} uptake into squid axon (Baker et al., 1973) and mammalian cardiac and smooth muscle (Kohlhardt et al., 1972) and inhibits the Ca^{2+}-dependent action potential of starfish eggs (Shen and Steinhardt, 1976). In the presence of D-600, the initial spike amplitude of the fertilization potential is reduced, while the average amplitude during the first minute after insemination is unchanged (Gould-Somero et al., 1979).

Radioactive tracer flux studies support the electrophysiological data. Increases in Ca^{2+} fluxes of sea urchin eggs (Azarnia and Chambers,

1969; Chambers *et al.*, 1970; Nakazawa *et al.*, 1970; Steinhardt and Epel, 1974; Paul and Johnston, 1978) and *Urechis* eggs (Johnston and Paul, 1977; Jaffe *et al.*, 1979; Gould-Somero *et al.*, 1979) have been observed at fertilization. In sea urchins, the rate of Ca^{2+} uptake increases nearly 200-fold during the first 3 seconds after insemination (Paul and Johnston, 1978). In *Urechis*, the Ca^{2+} influx is greatest during the first 15 seconds after insemination (Johnston and Paul, 1977). Similarly, Na^+ flux increases at fertilization of sea urchin eggs (Chambers and Chambers, 1949; Chambers, 1968, 1972; Johnson *et al.*, 1976; Payan *et al.*, 1981) and of *Urechis* eggs (Jaffe *et al.*, 1979). Corresponding to the time of termination of the fertilization potential, the Na^+ and Ca^{2+} permeabilities of the *Urechis* egg decrease (Jaffe *et al.*, 1979). In the sea urchin egg, Na^+ influx decreases by 1 minute after insemination (Payan *et al.*, 1981); however, a decrease in Ca^{2+} influx is less evident (Nakazawa *et al.*, 1970; Paul and Johnston, 1978). The continued uptake of Ca^{2+} in the sea urchin egg may be attributed to Ca^{2+} binding by surface coat materials (Paul and Johnston, 1978).

Further evidence for independent Na^+ and Ca^{2+} permeability changes during fertilization has been presented. Under polyspermic conditions, the Ca^{2+} influx of *Urechis* eggs is independent of the number of sperm incorporations in normal seawater; however, Na^+ influx increases with the number of sperm incorporated (Jaffe *et al.*, 1979). This observation supports the idea that Ca^{2+} influx is by way of the voltage-gated calcium channels, while Na^+ influx is by way of sperm-gated sodium channels. Further evidence for localized gating of egg sodium channels by sperm has been reported (Gould-Somero, 1981). With utilization of a perforated nickel screen, such that the *Urechis* egg is exposed to two chambers with different Na^+ content, the average fertilization potential amplitude corresponds to the Na^+ content of the chamber to which sperm were added. The observation of multiple depolarization steps during polyspermic fertilization of the sea urchin egg (Jaffe, 1976; Dale *et al.*, 1978b; Taglietti, 1979; DeFelice and Dale, 1979; Dale and De Santis, 1981a,b) suggests a similar localized sperm activation of sea urchin egg sodium channels. The mechanism of sperm-gating of egg sodium channels remains to be determined. Direct involvement of the inward Ca^{2+} current is unlikely, since a fertilization potential is not observed after generation of action potentials with current pulses, and step depolarizations are observed in eggs with more positive resting potentials, which lack the initial Ca^{2+}-dependent action potential. Furthermore, when Ca^{2+} influx is reduced by either low external Ca^{2+} seawater (Chambers and de Armendi, 1979) or D-600 (Gould-Somero *et al.*, 1979), the sperm-gated sodium channels are not blocked.

Although permeability changes to Na^+ and Ca^{2+} ions are significant during the fertilization potential, permeability to other ions may also be involved. If the internal Na^+ concentration of sea urchin eggs is near 27 mM and the amplitude of the fertilization potential is Na^+-dependent, the expected Nernst potential is +69 mV, which is far greater than the measured peak amplitude mean of +20 mV (Chambers and de Armendi, 1979). Miyazaki (1979) has analyzed the I-V relations before and during the fertilization potential of the starfish egg. The equilibrium potential for the channels opened at fertilization is +15 mV, which is less positive than the expected Na^+ or Ca^{2+} equilibrium potential. These results suggest that during the fertilization potential, the egg membrane permeabilities are not strictly limited to Na^+ or Ca^{2+} ions. Following fertilization, in sea urchins and *Urechis,* an increase in K^+ permeability becomes significant during the falling phase of the fertilization potential (Steinhardt et al., 1971, 1972; Tupper, 1973; Higashi, 1974; Jaffe et al., 1979).

The repolarization of the membrane of the sea urchin egg is associated with the large increase in K^+ permeability shortly after insemination. The increase in K^+ permeability was initially demonstrated with radioactive tracer flux studies (Chambers, 1949; Chambers and Chambers, 1949; Monroy and Tyler, 1958; Tyler and Monroy, 1956, 1959; Tyler, 1958; Tupper, 1973) and subsequently by electrophysiological measurements (Steinhardt et al., 1971, 1972; Tupper, 1973; Ito and Yoshioka, 1973; Higashi, 1974). By 10 minutes after insemination, the increased K^+ permeability is reflected in the five- to eight-fold decrease in the membrane input resistance of unfertilized sea urchin eggs (Jaffe and Robinson, 1978). With the decreased input resistance, the leak current due to impalement has much less effect on the membrane potential. Thus, the reported resting potential of fertilized sea urchin eggs has generally been close to −70 mV and K^+-dependent (Hiramoto, 1959a,b; Steinhardt et al., 1971, 1972; Higashi and Kaneko, 1971; Ito and Yoshioka, 1972, 1973; Tupper, 1973; Higashi, 1974; Jaffe and Robinson, 1978; Dale and De Santis, 1981b). One apparent result of the increased K^+ conductance of fertilized sea urchin eggs is a loss of electrical excitability by 10 minutes after insemination (S. S. Shen, unpublished observations). The possibility of a loss of the voltage-dependent calcium channels with fertilization has not been excluded.

A number of morphological changes occur during the fertilization potential of sea urchin and other marine invertebrate eggs (Epel, 1978a; Schuel, 1978; Vacquier, 1981). Two events, sperm–egg interaction and cortical granule dehiscence, may evoke the fertilization potential. The ionic mechanisms underlying the fertilization potential preexist in the egg membrane, since similar potential shifts are elicited by parthenogenetic agents, such as pronase, trypsin, or ionophores (Steinhardt *et al.*, 1971; Steinhardt and Epel, 1974; Chambers *et al.*, 1974a,b). However, which step in the process of sperm–egg interaction initiates the opening of the channels is unclear. The general sequence of sperm–egg interaction can be subdivided into sperm–egg binding, sperm–egg fusion, and sperm entry. The latter event is apparently unnecessary for generation of the fertilization potential. Pretreatment of marine invertebrate eggs with cytochalasin B or D will prevent sperm pronuclear incorporation (Gould-Somero *et al.*, 1977; Longo, 1978; Byrd and Perry, 1980; Schatten and Schatten, 1980). Although cytochalasin B or D altered some of the electrical parameters, the fertilization potential was not blocked (Dale and De Santis, 1981a). Another inhibitor that acts during sperm–egg interaction is erythrosin B, which may block gamete fusion but not binding (Carroll and Levitan, 1978a,b). Elevation of the fertilization membrane and activation of the sea urchin egg are blocked by erythrosin B (Carroll and Levitan, 1978a). In addition, erythrosin B reversibly increases the K^+ permeability of the unfertilized sea urchin egg and blocks the fertilization potential (Levitan and Carroll, 1977), suggesting that sperm–egg fusion, rather than sperm–egg binding, is necessary for initiating the fertilization potential. When unfertilized eggs are depolarized, more positive than $+5$ mV with current, sperm binding occurs but without a fertilization potential (Jaffe, 1976). Under polyspermic conditions, there is a high degree of correlation between the number of 1- to 2-mV step depolarizations seen electrophysiologically and the number of sperm pronuclei located within the egg (DeFelice and Dale, 1979).

The exocytosis of the cortical granules, the cortical reaction, more than doubles the plasma membrane area of the sea urchin egg (Eddy and Shapiro, 1976). The change in plasma membrane area is reflected by a 1.7-fold increase in membrane capacitance (Jaffe *et al.*, 1978). A latent period of 30 to 45 seconds between the rise of the activation potential and the increase in membrane capacitance is observed, which correlates with the latent period between insemination and cortical vesicle disappearance determined by light or electron microscopy (Allen and Griffin, 1958; Pasteels, 1965; Paul and Epel, 1971; Chandler and Heuser, 1979). This latency suggests that the rising phase of the fertilization potential is not a consequence of the cortical reaction. However, Dale and De Santis (1981b) have suggested that, at least in the sea urchins *Paracenterotus lividus* and *Sphaerechinus granularis,* the fertilization potential is a result of the cortical reaction. Evidence favoring this viewpoint is the absence of fertilization potential in oocytes (Taglietti, 1979; Hagiwara and Jaffe, 1979; DeFelice and Dale,

1979; Dale and De Santis, 1981b), which may be incapable of the cortical reaction (Hagstrom and Lonning, 1961). However, the absence of a fertilization potential may be due to a 5- to 30-fold greater K^+ conductance of the oocyte (Jaffe and Robinson, 1978). In *Urechis,* where most of the cortical granules remain intact through the first cleavage (Gould-Somero and Holland, 1975; Paul, 1975), the fertilization potential is independent of the cortical reaction.

The repolarization of the membrane during the falling phase of the fertilization potential is not a consequence of the cortical reaction. An increase in K^+ conductance can be initiated by treatment of unfertilized sea urchin eggs with ammonia, which does not trigger the cortical reaction (Steinhardt and Mazia, 1973). In the starfish oocyte, the K^+ permeability is dependent on the internal Na^+ concentration (Hagiwara and Yoshii, 1979). However, in the sea urchin egg, increased K^+ permeability is probably not a consequence of increased intracellular Na^+ concentration, since the exposure of unfertilized eggs to ammonia does not stimulate Na^+ entry (Payan et al., 1981). Instead, the increased K^+ permeability is a consequence of an increase in the intracellular pH with fertilization (Shen and Steinhardt, 1980).

Several hypotheses have been proposed for the role of the fertilization potential during fertilization. Evidence for its function as a rapid block to polyspermy has been described for several marine invertebrates (L. A. Jaffe, 1976, 1980; Gould-Somero et al., 1979; Miyazaki, 1979; Miyazaki and Hirai, 1979). However, other investigators claim an absence of a rapid electrical, precortical block to polyspermy (Byrd and Collins, 1975; DeFelice and Dale, 1979; Dale and De Santis, 1981b). This subject is considered more closely elsewhere in this volume (see Chapter 8). Another possible function of the fertilization potential is the initiation of development. Since in most marine invertebrate eggs, the resting potentials of the unfertilized and fertilized eggs are about -70 mV, the possible role of the fertilization potential in egg activation can be examined by restriction of the transient potential changes during the fertilization potential. Voltage clamping the sea urchin egg at -70 mV does not prevent development (MacKenzie and Chambers, 1977), nor does activation of the sea urchin egg occur when the unfertilized egg is depolarized with current or high K^+ seawater (Hagiwara and Jaffe, 1979). Thus, at least in the sea urchin, the potential changes at fertilization may not be of importance for initiation of development. However, the ionic currents associated with the fertilization potential and changes of intracellular ion activities are important for triggering development not only of sea urchin eggs but of the eggs of other marine invertebrates as well.

V. INTRACELLULAR ION ACTIVITIES

Although changes of the membrane potential at fertilization in the sea urchin may not be directly associated with initiation of development, changes of intracellular ion activities and associated ionic currents do trigger some of the events of early development (discussed in Section VI). Observations of changes in intracellular ion activities and associated developmental effects have, for the most part, been limited to sea urchins. However, a number of observations on other marine invertebrate eggs suggests that changes of ionic activities are important and widespread in early development.

A. Potassium

Fertilization of the sea urchin egg results in a five- to eight-fold increase in K^+ conductance during the first 10 minutes. Measurement of internal K^+ concentration with a K^+-selective microelectrode during this interval gives a constant value of 200 to 240 mM (Steinhardt et $al.$, 1971). These values are consistent with estimates by spectrophotometric techniques of 200 to 210 mM (Rothschild and Barnes, 1953; Tupper, 1973; Chambers, 1975a; Robinson, 1976). Estimation of internal K^+ concentration in other marine invertebrate eggs, including starfish (Tyler et $al.$, 1956; Miyazaki et $al.$, 1975a; Hagiwara and Yoshii, 1979), tunicate (Miyazaki et $al.$, 1974), echiuroid (Jaffe et $al.$, 1979), and coelenterate (Hagiwara et $al.$, 1981) is in a similar range of 185 to 240 mM, except for the starfish $Patiria$ $miniata$. K^+-selective microelectrode measurement of internal K^+ level was 350 mM in the immature oocyte, which increased to near 480 mM with maturation (Shen and Steinhardt, 1976).

On the basis of isotope exchange experiments, a nonhomogeneity of K^+ distribution in the unfertilized sea urchin egg was suggested (Chambers et $al.$, 1948; Tyler and Monroy, 1959; Tupper, 1973, 1974; Chambers, 1975a). According to this viewpoint, only 30% of the internal K^+ ions of the unfertilized egg is exchangeable with external K^+ ions. Fertilization initiates a gradual process of decompartmentalization of K^+ ions, such that by the cleavage stage, embryos exhibit 70–80% exchangeability of the total internal K^+ content (Tupper, 1973). The two-compartment hypothesis was reinvestigated by Robinson (1976), using both K^+ influx and efflux experiments. He concluded that at least 80–90% of the internal K^+ content of unfertilized sea urchin eggs is exchangeable. A single K^+ compartment is compatible with the observation that the internal K^+ concentration is nearly constant during fertilization. Otherwise, with the two-compartment hypothesis, the inexchangeable K^+ ions would have to be sequestered in impermeable organelles, which occupy 70% of the unfertilized egg volume. This would be in sharp conflict with the 30% estimation of organelle volume (Robinson, 1976).

Exposure of unfertilized sea urchin eggs to 500 mM K^+ for up to 2 hours does not cause egg activation or the loss of fertilizability after return to normal seawater (Hagiwara and Jaffe, 1979). After fertilization, exposure of the zygote to artificial seawater containing 100 mM K^+ does not affect the normal pattern of protein and DNA syntheses (Tupper, 1973, 1974). However, the developing sea urchin embryo is susceptible to isotonic KCl. Immersion of fertilized eggs in isotonic KCl at pH 6, 0.5 to 1.5 minutes after insemination will immediately arrest further development (Chambers and Chambers, 1949). However, the inhibition of development is attributable to the removal of external Na^+ ions, which are required in millimolar amounts for development (Chambers, 1975b, 1976). Unlike sea urchin eggs, high K^+ seawater is effective in activating other marine invertebrate eggs: the annelid *Chaetopterus* (Lillie, 1902, 1906; Brachet, 1938; Zampetti-Bosseler *et al.*, 1973; Ikegami *et al.*, 1976; Hagiwara and Miyazaki, 1977), other annelids (Treadwell, 1902; Scott, 1903, 1906), the mollusk *Spisula* (Allen, 1953; Ii and Rebhun, 1979), and the echiuroid *Urechis* (Jaffe *et al.*, 1979). Interestingly, the absence of external K^+ ions is equally effective in activating *Spisula* eggs (Allen, 1953). Furthermore, high K^+ seawater is ineffectual in activating *Chaetopterus* eggs if Ca^{2+} ions are absent (Ikegami *et al.*, 1976) or *Spisula* eggs if Ca^{2+} or Na^+ ions are removed (Ii and Rebhun, 1979). These results suggest that K^+-stimulated activation is not mediated directly through its effects on the membrane potential.

B. Sodium

Estimation of intracellular Na^+ concentration of unfertilized sea urchin eggs has been reported from 22 to 52 mM (Rothschild and Barnes, 1953; Chambers, 1972, 1975b; Payan *et al.*, 1981). In the first 5 minutes following fertilization, the Na^+ content is increased 20–30% (Chambers, 1972; Payan *et al.*, 1981). By 10 minutes after fertilization, the Na^+ content is restored to levels present in unfertilized eggs (Chambers, 1972, 1975b). Chambers (1975b) reported that the Na^+ content then remains essentially constant, while Payan *et al.* (1981) reported a continued slow drop of internal Na^+ level to a new stable value of 13.8 mEq. Estimation of the internal Na^+ concentration has been reported for very few other marine invertebrate eggs: the echi-uroid *Urechis* of 13 mM (Jaffe *et al.*, 1979) and the starfish *Mediaster* of 10–15 mM (Hagiwara and Yoshii, 1979).

Measurements of Na$^+$ fluxes are consistent with the changes of internal Na$^+$ content after fertilization of the sea urchin egg. Chambers and Chambers (1949) were the first to report a low Na$^+$ uptake by unfertilized eggs, which is increased dramatically following insemina-tion. In the first 5 minutes after insemination, both Na$^+$ influx and efflux are increased (Chambers, 1972; Johnson *et al.*, 1976; Payan *et al.*, 1981). The net Na$^+$ uptake is increased nearly 660-fold (Chambers, 1972). From 15 to 60 minutes after fertilization, Na$^+$ influx balanced Na$^+$ efflux (Chambers, 1972). However, another laboratory has reported a net Na$^+$ efflux by 6 minutes after insemination (Payan *et al.*, 1981). In the presence of 2 mM ouabain, Na$^+$ efflux is reduced by 80% (Chambers, 1975b). These data suggest that an increased Na$^+$ permeability after fertilization is followed by activation of Na$^+$, K$^+$ ATPase. A similar increase in Na$^+$ uptake has been reported to occur during the first 10 minutes following insemination of *Urechis* eggs (Jaffe *et al.*, 1979) or oocytes (Holland and Gould-Somero, 1981) and during ionophore activation of oocytes of the starfish *Asterias rubens* (Peaucellier and Doree, 1981). The initial increase of Na$^+$ influx most likely corresponds to the increased Na$^+$ permeability during the fertil-ization potential (Hagiwara and Jaffe, 1979), although some fraction of the increased Na$^+$ fluxes may be due to the activation of Na$^+$/H$^+$ and Na$^+$/Na$^+$ exchanges.

Sodium has emerged as the one cation in the external medium essen-tial for the activation of the sea urchin egg, both by sperm and iono-phore (Chambers, 1975b, 1976; Johnson *et al.*, 1976). K$^+$, Mg^{2+}, and Ca^{2+} ions are not required (Chambers *et al.*, 1974a; Steinhardt and Epel, 1974; Chambers, 1980), although divalent cations may be neces-sary for sperm–egg fusion (Sano and Kanatani, 1980; Sano *et al.*, 1980). Sea urchin eggs inseminated in choline substituted for Na$^+$ seawater do not undergo either cytoplasmic or nuclear activation un-less at least 2–3 mM Na$^+$ ions are present (Chambers, 1975b, 1976). The Na$^+$ requirement diminishes with time, such that by 10 minutes after insemination, eggs transferred to Na$^+$-free seawater develop through the blastula stage (Chambers, 1975b, 1976). Li$^+$ and NH$_4^+$ can substitute for Na$^+$ (Chambers, 1975b, 1976; Johnson *et al.*, 1976; Nishioka and Cross, 1978). This Na$^+$ requirement for activation be-tween 0.5 and 10 minutes postinsemination has been linked to the increased intracellular pH, which is discussed in the next section. The

Na^+ requirement for K^+-stimulated activation of *Spisula* eggs may also be linked to changes of internal pH (Ii and Rebhun, 1979).

C. Hydrogen

Interest in intracellular pH changes with fertilization can be traced back to the turn of the century. Jacques Loeb (1913) reported the activation of sea urchin and other marine invertebrate eggs by exposure to both acids and bases. After a brief exposure of unfertilized eggs of the sea urchin *Strongylocentrotus purpuratus* to acids, elevation of the fertilization membrane is observed upon return to normal seawater. Weak acids, such as butyric acid, are effective at 1 mM after a 2-minute exposure, while strong acids, such as HCl, require a 10-minute exposure at 2 mM. Loeb concluded that the physiological action of the acids is not determined by the diffusion of hydrogen ions into the egg but by the diffusion of undissociated acid. Activation of acid-treated eggs requires the return of the eggs to normal seawater. Loeb observed fertilization membrane formation when the eggs are transferred from the butyric acid solution into an alkaline mixture of NaCl, KCl, and $CaCl_2$, but a proper membrane is not formed when the eggs are transferred into a neutral mixture. Interestingly, eggs returned to a neutral mixture could be fertilized and develop. Butyric acid-treated eggs could develop to larvae by a further treatment with neutral hypertonic seawater for 20–50 minutes. Treatment with the 1.5- to 1.6-fold concentrated seawater induces cytasters, necessary for cell division (Loeb, 1913; Brandriff *et al.,* 1975).

Parthenogenetic activation of sea urchin eggs can be induced by both strong and weak bases (Loeb, 1913). Similar to the efficiencies of strong and weak acids, weak bases are more effective than strong ones. Larvae development could be induced by following the exposure to the weak base solution with the hypertonic seawater treatment. In some respects, however, the action of weak bases differs from that of weak acids. (1) While only a short exposure to acid will induce membrane formation (longer treatments are lethal), the action of bases requires a longer time of exposure. (2) The action of acids is not prevented by the presence of KCN, but the action of bases is sensitive to KCN or anoxia. (3) Elevation of fertilization membrane does not occur during the treatment with bases, but only afterward, during the hypertonic seawater treatment. (4) Low concentrations (1–2 mM) of NH_4OH are as effective as higher concentrations for inducing egg activation.

Activation of other marine invertebrate eggs by exposure to weak acids or bases have been reported for the starfishes *Asterias* and *Asterina* (Loeb, 1913), the annelids *Polynoe* (Loeb, 1913) and *Thalassema* (Lefevre, 1907), the mollusks *Spisula* (Allen, 1953; Finkel and Wolf, 1980; Guerrier *et al.*, 1981) and *Barnea* (Dube and Guerrier, 1982), and the echiuroid *Urechis* (Hiraiwa and Kawamura, 1936; Tyler and Bauer, 1937).

The possibility of the parthenogenetic activity of weak acids and weak bases being exerted through alteration of intracellular pH was initially studied with colorimetric indicators. With neutral red, the presence of CO_2 or NH_3 is found readily to change the intracellular pH of eggs (Warburg, 1910; Chambers, 1928). Furthermore, consistent with the observations of Loeb, living cells are much less permeable to strong acid or base than to weak acid or base (Jacobs, 1920). However, Needhan and Needhan (1926) and Chambers and Pollack (1927), using a variety of indicators, failed to find a difference in intracellular pH in unfertilized and fertilized eggs of several marine invertebrates. Alkalinization of the cytoplasm at fertilization was first detected by cell homogenate studies (Johnson *et al.*, 1976; Lopo and Vacquier, 1977). The pH of unfertilized egg homogenates of the sea urchin *Strongylocentrotus purpuratus* is about 6.48 and rises to near 6.76 by 4 minutes after fertilization, with an initial small transient decrease between 30 and 60 seconds after insemination (Johnson *et al.*, 1976). In another homogenate study, the pH was observed to reach a peak alkaline value by 10 minutes after insemination and then to decline steadily, reaching the unfertilized level by 70 minutes after insemination (Lopo and Vacquier, 1977). However, numerous artifacts are possible with intracellular pH estimates when homogenates are used. Apart from the obvious difficulties created by the necessary time gaps between homogenization and measurement of pH, it is well established that injury to cell contents releases acid and gives lowered pH values (Chambers and Chambers, 1961).

The development of the recessed-tip, H^+-sensitive microelectrode (Thomas, 1974, 1976) made possible the direct measurement of the intact egg cytoplasmic pH. Unfertilized eggs of the sea urchin *Lytechinus pictus* maintain a steady intracellular pH near 6.9; and 60–90 seconds after insemination, the cytoplasm rapidly alkalinizes to a new steady value near 7.3, reached in 6–8 minutes (Shen and Steinhardt, 1978). The intracellular pH of fertilized eggs continues to remain alkaline for at least 60 minutes after fertilization, although some fluctuations are observed (Steinhardt *et al.*, 1978). A possible artifact currently exists with intracellular ion activity measurements of unfertilized sea urchin eggs made with ion-sensitive microelectrodes.

Due to the high input resistance of the egg membrane and the additional impalement with an ion-sensitive microelectrode, the measured resting potential of the unfertilized egg is near -10 mV, rather than -70 mV. Thus, microelectrode determination of intracellular ion activity may not reflect true values in the intact egg. Several lines of evidence suggest that the measured internal pH of unfertilized eggs is close to the pH of intact eggs, despite the small resting potential. Estimated values of the internal pH in unfertilized *S. purpuratus* and *L. pictus* eggs, by the distribution of 5,5-dimethyl-2, 4-oxazolidine-dione (DMO), are 7.08 and 6.86, respectively (Johnson and Epel, 1981), and by [^{31}P]NMR are 7.12 and 7.02, respectively (Winkler *et al.*, 1982). Preliminary experiments also indicate that the internal pH of unfertilized eggs is insensitive to the membrane potential. Clamping the membrane potential more negative than -70 mV or more positive than $+15$ mV in excess of 15 minutes has little or no effect on the internal pH (S. S. Shen and R. A. Steinhardt, unpublished observations).

The increase in intracellular pH at fertilization of sea urchin eggs has also been substantiated by the DMO, [^{31}P]NMR, and fluorimetric techniques (Gillies and Deamer, 1979; Johnson and Epel, 1981; Whitaker and Steinhardt, 1981; Winkler *et al.*, 1982). Fig. 3 shows the chemical shift of the intracellular P_i with fertilization of *S. purpuratus* eggs, corresponding to an increase in internal pH from 7.12 to 7.55. An absence of an increase in the internal pH, determined by [^{31}P]NMR technique, after fertilization of three other species of sea urchins has been reported (Inoue and Yoshioka, 1980). The reason for the discrepancy between the [^{31}P]NMR measurements of Winkler *et al.* (1982) and Inoue and Yoshioka (1980) is not clear. However, a significant possibility may be the failure of Inoue and Yoshioka (1980) to bubble air through the egg suspensions, which could result in anoxia. Anoxia will depress the intracellular pH change normally seen during fertilization (S. S. Shen and R. A. Steinhardt, unpublished observations). Furthermore, the maintenance of the alkaline internal pH of fertilized eggs appears to be dependent on metabolic energy (Shen and Steinhardt, 1980; Winkler *et al.*, 1982, Fig. 3). It may also be possible that changes in intracellular pH during fertilization are not universal among marine invertebrates, even among sea urchin species. The intracellular pH of the starfish *Pisaster ochraceus,* as measured by the DMO method (Johnson and Epel, 1980, 1982) and the starfish *Asterias rubens,* as measured with the homogenate method (Peaucellier and Doree, 1981), does not change significantly after activation.

Exposure of unfertilized sea urchin eggs to weak acids and weak

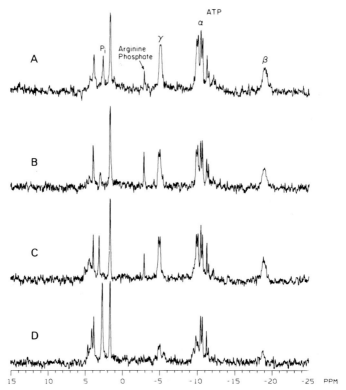

Fig. 3. [^{31}P]NMR spectra of unfertilized and fertilized eggs of the sea urchin *Strongylocentrotus purpuratus*. (A) The spectrum of unfertilized eggs showed the P_i peak at 2.53 ppm, which corresponds to an intracellular pH of 7.12. (B) The spectrum of fertilized eggs showed a shift of the P_i peak to 2.90 ppm, which corresponds to an intracellular pH of 7.55. (C) The spectrum of unfertilized eggs 20 minutes after treatment with 10 mM NH$_4$Cl, showed that the intracellular pH has shifted to 7.76. (D) The spectrum of fertilized eggs 30 minutes after treatment with 0.5 mM dinitrophenol, an uncoupler of oxidative phosphorylation, which showed that the intracellular pH has dropped to 7.25. (From Winkler *et al.*, 1982.)

bases causes a shift in the internal pH. The effect of weak acids and weak bases is exerted by the greater egg permeability to the uncharged species than the charged species (Winkler and Grainger, 1978; Boron *et al.*, 1978). The exposure of unfertilized eggs to weak acids causes a fall in the internal pH. The internal pH overshoots the initial pH after exposure to weak acids (Grainger *et al.*, 1979). Exposure of unfertilized eggs to weak bases causes an increase in the internal pH. However, there were two unexpected features in the increase in internal pH with different concentrations of NH$_4$Cl (Shen and Steinhardt, 1978). First, the change in intracellular pH was considerably slower than the rate of penetration of amines into the eggs (Winkler and Grainger, 1978). Second, given enough time, different NH_4Cl concentrations caused similar increases in cytoplasmic pH (Shen and Steinhardt, 1978; Johnson and Epel, 1981). This result is consistent with the earlier observation of Loeb (1913) on the similar effectiveness for egg activation by different concentrations of NH_4OH. The effect of ammonia on cytoplasmic pH of sea urchin eggs might be explained by the presence of an acidic compartment in the egg. This intracellular acidic compartment could then act as a sink for ammonia and delay cytoplasmic alkalinization. Evidence for acidic, lysosomallike vesicles in sea urchin eggs has been reported (Lee *et al.*, 1982). These acidic vesicles are not dissipated after fertilization but ammonia, nigericin, or monensin treatment will discharge the acid stores (Lee *et al.*, 1982). Removal of weak bases causes the internal pH to fall, but the internal pH does not return to the initial value (Shen and Steinhardt, 1978; Whitaker and Steinhardt, 1981). Instead, after exposure to 10 m*M* NH_4Cl, the internal pH of unfertilized eggs stabilizes at the fertilized value, since fertilization of these eggs does not result in further cytoplasmic alkalinization (Shen, 1982).

Although changes of intracellular pH with activation have been studied only in echinoids, other indirect lines of evidence suggest that changes of internal pH may occur during activation in other marine invertebrate eggs. As discussed earlier, exposure to weak acid or weak base activates a variety of marine invertebrate eggs. In addition, acid production following egg activation has been reported for many marine invertebrates. Initially reported by Ashbel (1929) as an evolution of CO_2 upon fertilization of *Arbacia* eggs, Runnstrom (1933) demonstrated that the evolution of CO_2 resulted from the production of an acid that liberates CO_2 from the bicarbonate present in seawater. A decrease in pH (Allen *et al.*, 1958) and in the bicarbonate concentration (Rothschild, 1958) of seawater has been demonstrated during the first few minutes after fertilization. A number of experiments have been reported, which were designed to discern the nature and source of the acid produced at fertilization of sea urchin eggs (Runnstrom, 1935a,b; Rothschild, 1938b; Mehl and Swann, 1961; Aketa, 1963; Ishihara, 1964, 1968; Nakazawa *et al.*, 1970; Paul and Epel, 1975; Paul *et al.*, 1976; Johnson *et al.*, 1976; Nishioka and McGwin, 1980; Gillies *et al.*, 1981; Holland and Gould-Somero, 1982). Although the precise nature of the acid produced is still uncertain, interest has focused on the observations that formation of fertilization acid does not require K^+, Ca^{2+}, or Mg^{2+} ions (Paul and Epel, 1975) but does require Na^+ ions (Johnson *et al.*, 1976) in the seawater.

Two lines of evidence have been presented for a Na^+ requirement for the formation of acid at fertilization of sea urchin eggs. The rate of acid production can be demonstrated to be a function of the external Na^+ concentration with choline-arrested eggs (Johnson *et al.*, 1976). Originally described by Chambers (1976) for demonstrating the Na^+ requirement for egg activation, choline-arrested eggs are prepared by fertilization of eggs in seawater and resuspension of them within 60 seconds after insemination in Na^+-free seawater (choline substituted). Upon addition of Na^+ ions, acid production is observed and the rate of acid production is linearly dependent on the Na^+ concentration (Johnson *et al.*, 1976). Since choline-arrested eggs have undergone a complete cortical exocytosis, the formation of fertilization acid is not a consequence of the cortical reaction. This is further substantiated by the observation that ionophore A23187-activated eggs in normal seawater release acid; however, ionophore-activated eggs in Na^+-free seawater have a greatly reduced acid production (Paul and Epel, 1975; Nishioka and McGwin, 1980). A second line of evidence for a Na^+ requirement utilizes the diuretic drug amiloride. Amiloride is an inhibitor of passive Na^+ flux across many Na^+-transporting epithelial cells (Bentley, 1968; Salako and Smith, 1970). When 40 mM Na^+ is added to choline-arrested eggs in the presence of 10^{-4} M amiloride, acid production is blocked and the eggs remain unactivated (Johnson *et al.*, 1976). Furthermore, acid release is reduced by 80% following fertilization of eggs in choline-substituted seawater containing 50 mM Na^+ and 10^{-4} M amiloride. Since Na^+ influx is also blocked by amiloride following fertilization of eggs in low Na^+ seawater, Johnson *et al.* (1976) proposed that the acid production results from an exchange of extracellular Na^+ ions for intracellular protons.

A direct exchange of extracellular Na^+ ions for intracellular H^+ ions suggests that the increase in intracellular pH following fertilization would be sensitive to both external Na^+ concentration and amiloride. The relationship between external Na^+ concentration and internal pH has been studied during fertilization or ionophore activation of *L. pictus* eggs (Shen and Steinhardt, 1979). As fertilization by sperm is difficult in the complete absence of Na^+ ions (Nishioka and Cross, 1978), unfertilized eggs are activated with the ionophore A23187. Ionophore activation in seawater induces an increase in internal pH similar to that of fertilization. However, when eggs are activated with A23187 in Na^+-free seawater, the rise of the internal pH does not occur until Na^+ ions are added back. Thus, the elevation of cytoplasmic pH associated with fertilization requires external Na^+ ions. Unlike the linear dependence of acid production on Na^+ concentration (Johnson *et al.*, 1976), the rate of cytoplasmic alkalinization is independent of Na^+ concentration between 5 and 485 mM (Shen and Steinhardt, 1979). Amiloride at 10^{-4} M in 25 mM Na^+ seawater does not inhibit the rise of intracellular pH during fertilization. However, 2.5 to 5×10^{-4} M amiloride in 25 mM Na^+ seawater does inhibit reversibly the rate of increase in internal pH, and 1 mM amiloride blocks the rise of internal pH irreversibly (Shen and Steinhardt, 1979). A decreased rate of fertilization acid production by amiloride has been reported for *Psammechinus miliaris* (Cuthbert and Cuthbert, 1978).

Although both acid production and cytoplasmic alkalinization during activation of sea urchin eggs are both Na^+ dependent and amiloride sensitive, acid production and cytoplasmic alkalinization may not be directly coupled for the following reasons. (1) The rate of acid production is linearly dependent on external Na^+ concentration, while the rate of cytoplasmic alkalinization is independent of external Na^+ ions above the minimal concentration necessary for egg activation. (2) Eggs activated with 10 mM NH_4Cl and then washed in fresh seawater release acid upon fertilization (Paul *et al.*, 1976). However, fertilization of ammonia-pulsed eggs does not induce cytoplasmic alkalinization (Shen, 1982). (3) Acid production starts about 30–60 seconds after insemination and is completed by 2–4 minutes (Allen *et al.*, 1958; Nishioka and McGwin, 1980; Tilney and Jaffee, 1980). The rise in intracellular pH starts 60 to 90 seconds after insemination and is completed by 6–8 minutes (Steinhardt *et al.*, 1978). A lack of time correlation is also seen when Na^+ ions are added back to A23187-activated eggs in Na^+-free seawater (Nishioka and McGwin, 1980; Shen and Steinhardt, 1979). (4) The amount of acid production varies with the external pH. At pH 9, acid production is increased; and at pH 7, it is reduced (Mehl and Swann, 1961; Epel, 1978b; Cuthbert and Cuthbert, 1978). If there is more than one source for acid production, such as ionization of groups on the egg surface and exchange reactions with varying pH dependence, then acid production would vary with external pH. Of the normal acid production, nearly 20% is Na^+- and amiloride-insensitive (Johnson *et al.*, 1976). However, a Na^+-independent rise in internal pH has not been observed. Instead, activation of eggs in Na^+-free seawater of 1 mM amiloride causes a gradual acidification of the egg cytoplasm (Shen and Steinhardt, 1979).

Acid production following egg activation has been described for other marine invertebrates. Fertilization or K^+-stimulated activation of the mollusk *Spisula* triggers acid release within 20 seconds and is completed 9 to 15 minutes later (Allen, 1953; Ii and Rebhun, 1979). The acid release induced by K^+-stimulated activation is completely inhibited in Ca^{2+}-free or Na^+-free seawater (Ii and Rebhun, 1979). At least 1 mM Na$^+$ and 0.9 mM Ca^{2+} concentrations are required (Guerrier *et al.*, 1981). The release of acid has been reported at fertilization or ionophore A23187 activation of the echiuroid *Urechis caupo*. Acid production, which is not dependent on the presence of K$^+$ or Ca^{2+} ions, starts 10 seconds after insemination and is completed 6 to 8 minutes later (Paul, 1975). Sperm, protease, or ionophore A23187 activation of prophasic oocytes of the annelid *Sabellaria alveolata* induces a release of acid during the first 15–20 minutes. However, fertilization of matured oocytes is not accompanied by acid production (Peaucellier, 1978). In contrast, fertilization or ionophore A23187 activation of immature and mature oocytes of the starfish *Asterias rubens* or *Marthasterias glacialis* induces acid production, which does not occur during 1-methyladenine-stimulated maturation (Peaucellier and Doree, 1981). The amount of acid released by starfish oocytes is only 20–40% of the acid production reported for other marine invertebrates. While 50% of the acid production by starfish oocytes is suppressed in Na$^+$-free seawater, acid production is significantly stimulated in Ca^{2+}-free seawater during A23187 activation (Peaucellier and Doree, 1981). The observations of acid release from the starfish oocytes is of some interest, since it has been reported that the intracellular pH of starfish oocytes does not change with 1-methyladenine or sperm activation (Johnson and Epel, 1980; Peaucellier and Doree, 1981). Thus, acid production with egg activation does not appear to be directly coupled with an increase in cytoplasmic pH, and the assumption that production of acid with egg activation necessarily means an increase in intracellular pH may be unwarranted. Finally, acid release is not seen following fertilization of the mollusks *Mytilus* and *Acmaea* (Paul, 1975) and of the tunicate *Ascidia* (Lambert and Epel, 1979). However, possible changes in the intracellular pH of these species have not been investigated.

D. Calcium

The importance of calcium for activation of marine invertebrate eggs was recognized by Heilbrunn (1937) and Pasteels (1938). Hellbrunn's view of the role of Ca^{2+} ions in egg activation is generally embodied in his calcium-release theory for cell stimulation. A stimulating agent of egg activation is considered to release Ca^{2+} ions, which are normally bound to proteins localized in the egg cortex, such that at the time of activation, free Ca^{2+} ions are liberated in the egg. Pasteels also considered Ca^{2+} ions to be the true activating agent, such that other parthenogenetic agents acted through the intermediation of calcium.

These other agents were termed sensitizers and could be classified by their action's requiring either the presence or absence of external Ca^{2+} ions. Thus, external sensitizers may be acting by increasing Ca^{2+} entry and internal sensitizers by changing the equilibrium between free and bound Ca^{2+} ions. A large body of evidence has accumulated that supports the general premise of the views of Heilbrunn and Pasteels, namely that an increase in intracellular Ca^{2+} activity occurs during activation of marine invertebrate eggs, and with the exception of weak penetrating bases that most parthenogenetic activating agents trigger a release of intracellular Ca^{2+} ions.

The effectiveness of numerous parthenogenetic activators in the presence or absence of Ca^{2+} ions has been examined. Isotonic Ca^{2+} seawater will activate the eggs of annelid, mollusk, and echinoderm, and the activity of many parthenogenetic agents requires external Ca^{2+} ions (Tyler, 1941). In the mollusk *Barnea candida,* activating treatments, such as butyric acid, isotonic NaCl, hypertonic seawater, heat, or ultraviolet radiation, are ineffective when applied in Ca^{2+}-free condition (Pasteels, 1938). Isotonic KCl, akalinity, and hypertonicity will activate *Barnea* eggs in Ca^{2+}-free conditions, but a prior treatment with citrate will render the eggs unresponsive (Pasteels, 1938). Since addition of Ca^{2+} ions will subsequently activate citrate-treated eggs (Pasteels, 1938), the effect of citrate is not injurious but may be one of removing or binding the internal Ca^{2+} ions (Heilbrunn and Wilbur, 1937). Similarly, activation of the egg of the annelid *Nereis* by ultraviolet irradiation (Just, 1933), isotonic NaCl, or isotonic KCl is blocked by immersion in a citrate solution (Heilbrunn and Wilbur, 1937; Wilbur, 1941). Oxalate block of parthenogenetic activation may be similar to the action of citrate, since the effect of oxalate can be reversed by addition of calcium (Heilbrunn and Young, 1930).

Mazia (1937) provided the first direct demonstration of an increase in free Ca^{2+} ions upon fertilization in the egg of the sea urchin *Arbacia*. Although the Ca^{2+} content is unchanged after fertilization, the concentration of free, ultrafilterable Ca^{2+} ions is increased at the expense of bound Ca^{2+}. More recently, experiments with radioisotopes have shown an increase in the exchangeable Ca^{2+} pool with fertilization (Nigon and Do, 1965). This increase may be due to an increase in the dissociation constant between the Ca^{2+}-binding substance and Ca^{2+} ions (Nakamura and Yasumasu, 1974). Other experiments using ^{45}Ca have shown an increase in the uptake and efflux of Ca^{2+} ions following fertilization of the sea urchin egg (Nakazawa *et al.,* 1970; Azarnia and Chambers, 1969, 1976; Steinhardt and Epel, 1974; Paul and Johnston, 1978). Following a sharp initial 15% rise in Ca^{2+} content, the rate of Ca^{2+} efflux predominates (Azarnia and Chambers, 1976), such that the Ca^{2+} content of fertilized eggs decreases 30–50% by 40 minutes after insemination (Monroy-Oddo, 1946; Azarnia and Chambers, 1976). Increases in ^{45}Ca fluxes following fertilization of the *Urechis* egg have also been reported (Johnston and Paul, 1977; Jaffe *et al.*, 1979). Ca^{2+} entry appears to be primarily by way of the voltage-sensitive calcium channels, activated during the fertilization potential (Jaffe *et al.*, 1979). Since calcium channels are present in other marine invertebrate eggs, these channels may provide a pathway for Ca^{2+} entry during fertilization.

Although Ca^{2+} influx may normally occur during fertilization, the Ca^{2+} influx may not be a prerequisite for the activation of the egg. As noted earlier, some parthenogenetic activators do not require the presence of external Ca^{2+} ions, which suggests that eggs may contain an intracellular store of Ca^{2+} ions. Experiments with the ionophore A23187 demonstrate that in nearly all marine invertebrate eggs tested to date, the presence of exogenous Ca^{2+} ions per se is not necessary for egg activation. An exception is the mollusk *Spisula* (Schuetz, 1975b). Ionophore A23187-stimulated release of intracellular calcium stores of eggs has been demonstrated in a variety of enchinoids (Chambers, 1974; Chambers *et al.*, 1974a; Steinhardt and Epel, 1974; Steinhardt *et al.*, 1974; Schuetz, 1975a; Holland, 1980; Peaucellier and Doree, 1981), mollusk (Steinhardt *et al.*, 1974), annelids (Chambers, 1974; Brachet and Denis-Donini, 1977; Peaucellier, 1978; Meijer, 1979), echiuroid (Paul, 1975), and tunicate (Steinhardt *et al.*, 1974).

Aequorin, the calcium-sensitive photoprotein, has been utilized to characterize the increased intracellular Ca^{2+} activity during egg activation. Injection of unfertilized eggs of the sea urchin *Lytechinus pictus* with aequorin reveals a very low resting level of light emission (Steinhardt *et al.*, 1977). As seen in Fig. 4, fertilization results in a transient increase in Ca^{2+} activity that lasts 2–3 minutes (Steinhardt *et al.*, 1977). Analysis of a single aequorin-filled egg of the sea urchin *L. variegatus* with an image intensifier suggests an increased internal Ca^{2+} activity within 7 seconds of insemination over the entire egg (Kiehart *et al.*, 1977). An increase in intracellular Ca^{2+} activity has also been demonstrated for 1-methyladenine or ionophore A23187 activation of aequorin-injected immature oocytes of the starfish *Marthasterias glacialis* (Moreau *et al.*, 1978; Moreau and Guerrier, 1979). Ca^{2+} release is both a transient and a hormone concentration-dependent process. The addition of 2×10^{-7} M 1-methyladenine, which triggers 100% oocyte maturation, initiates an increase in Ca^{2+} activity in less than 1–2 seconds. The Ca^{2+} release lasts about 30 sec-

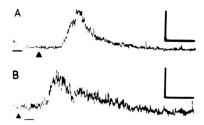

Fig. 4. The increase in internal Ca^{2+} activity during fertilization of eggs of the sea urchin *Lytechinus pictus*. Sperm addition is at the arrow heads and the time base is the right horizontal bar, equal to 1 minute. (A) Best aequorin emission: 25 eggs injected, 12 successfully fertilized. Vertical bar: 2 nA. (B) Typical aequorin emission: 27 eggs injected, seven successfully fertilized. Vertical bar: 1 nA. The lower left horizontal bar is zero light level for each record. (From Steinhardt *et al.*, 1977.)

onds and is estimated to range from 0.5 to 1.5 μM. The hormone-stimulated release differs from that of ionophore stimulation. Ionophore-stimulated light emission is triggered after a lag of 30 to 40 seconds, lasts nearly 4 minutes, and is estimated to be nearly 20-fold greater. Although both 1-methyladenine and ionophore induce a transient increase in Ca^{2+} activity, their effects on the immature oocyte differ. Ionophore A23187 initiates cortical granule exocytosis without nuclear maturation (Schuetz, 1975a), and 1-methyladenine induces meiosis without the cortical reaction (Kanatani, 1973). Moreau *et al.* (1978) suggested the possibility of different sites for Ca^{2+} release. Release of Ca^{2+} ions from different intracellular stores has been demonstrated for the sea urchin egg (Zucker *et al.*, 1978). Ionophore A23187 and nonelectrolyte activators release Ca^{2+} ions from the same store as normal fertilization, while hypertonic treatment appears to release Ca^{2+} ions from a different store. The release of Ca^{2+} ions from the intracellular stores is an all-or-none process, and repeated release is possible only after a period of about 40 mintues, which is required to recharge the store. Evidence for multiple independent Ca^{2+}-regulated pathways has also been found during nuclear maturation and cortical granule exocytosis of *Chaetopterus* eggs (Eckberg and Carroll, 1981).

The nature of the intracellular Ca^{2+} stores is uncertain. Almost all the Ca^{2+}-binding ability of the unfertilized sea urchin egg is found in the microsomal fraction. Because trypsin could decrease the level of the Ca^{2+}-binding substance, it is thought to be protein in nature (Nakamura and Yasumasu, 1974). Precipitation experiments with Ca^{2+}-specific pyroantimonate demonstrate Ca^{2+} deposition on plasma and organelle membranes (Cardasis *et al.*, 1978). The utilization of Ca^{2+}-specific fluorescence of chlorotetracycline suggests that Ca^{2+}

are localized on about one-fourth of the cortical granules, which are lost after fertilization or ionophore A23187 activation (Schatten and Hemmer, 1979). However, nonelectrolyte treatment of fertilized, aequorin-injected eggs causes a transient increase in Ca^{2+} activity long after cortical granule exocytosis (Zucker et al., 1978). The existence of a cortical reticulum, analogous to sarcoplasmic reticulum, has been proposed (Vacquier, 1981). Although structural identification is lacking in marine invertebrate eggs, the Ca^{2+} store of sea urchin eggs may require energy for maintenance (Baker and Whitaker, 1978). Although inhibitors of calcium release from sarcoplasmic reticulum, such as sodium dantrolene, have no effect on sea urchin Ca^{2+} release at fertilization (Steinhardt, 1980), quercetin, an inhibitor of Ca^{2+} sequestration by sarcoplasmic reticulum and other ATPase-dependent activities (Carpenedo et al., 1969), has been reported to induce nuclear maturation in Chaetopterus eggs (Eckberg and Carroll, 1981). Aequorin used as a marker reveals Ca^{2+} release by 1-methyladenine stimulation to be found associated with the plasma membrane fraction in an acellular system of starfish oocytes (Doree et al., 1978). Release of Ca^{2+} ions in the acellular system is sensitive to various agents that block Ca^{2+} release and maturation in the living oocyte.

The amount of Ca^{2+} released at fertilization of the sea urchin egg is uncertain. Since the cortical reaction is dependent on the increase in internal Ca^{2+} concentration (Moser, 1939; Vacquier, 1975, 1976), quantitative estimation of the peak Ca^{2+} activity at fertilization in sea urchin eggs is based upon the free Ca^{2+} concentration required for triggering the cortical reaction in broken egg preparations. Steinhardt et al. (1977) reported 9–18 μM of free Ca^{2+} ions necessary for the discharge of the cortical granules in an isolated cortices preparation. Since aequorin estimation yields 2.5–4.5 μM of peak Ca^{2+} activity during fertilization of the intact egg, they proposed that the transient Ca^{2+} release is confined to the egg cortex. Utilizing eggs made permeable by high-voltage discharge, Baker and Whitaker (1978) estimated free Ca^{2+} concentration of 1–6 μM to be sufficient for the discharge of the cortical granules. The difference between the two quantitative estimates with broken egg preparations may be due to species difference, the EGTA–Ca^{2+} binding constants used, and the concentration of ATP present (Zucker and Steinhardt, 1979; Baker and Whitaker, 1979a). Recent studies of sea urchin egg activation by microinjection of calcium buffers have suggested that even lower free Ca^{2+} concentration may be sufficient (Hamaguchi and Hiramoto, 1981). Cortical reaction is observed in seawater when intracellular Ca^{2+} activity is raised to above 0.2 μM and in Ca^{2+}-free seawater above 0.5 μM. Hyalin formation and monaster are observed in eggs in seawater when injected cytoplasmic Ca^{2+} activity exceeded 0.7 μM and in Ca^{2+}-free seawater above 2 μM. Although the difference in the threshold Ca^{2+} activity between eggs in seawater and those in Ca^{2+}-free seawater is uncertain, the difference in the threshold necessary for the cortical reaction and hyalin formation suggests multiple Ca^{2+}-regulated pathways.

A number of proposals have been presented for the mechanism of Ca^{2+} release triggered during fertilization of the sea urchin egg (Epel, 1980a). Several of these proposals have been experimentally tested. (1) Since the initial events of fertilization are sperm attachment and sperm–egg membrane fusion, the attachment and fusion processes may account for Ca^{2+} release. However, addition of bindin, the sperm protein necessary for attachment, does not activate the egg (Vacquier and Moy, 1977). Furthermore, fusion of egg membranes in 25 mM Ca^{2+} seawater does not cause cortical granule exocytosis (Bennett and Mazia, 1981a,b). (2) The depolarization during the fertilization potential may trigger Ca^{2+} release. Depolarization by direct injection of current does not activate the egg (Jaffe, 1976). Similarly, voltage clamping the egg at -70 mV does not prevent Ca^{2+} release (MacKenzie and Chambers, 1977). (3) The sodium and calcium influxes that occur during fertilization are not necessary for Ca^{2+} release, since the cortical reaction occurs in eggs fertilized in either Na^+-free (Nishioka and Cross, 1978) or Ca^{2+}-free (Chambers, 1980) seawater. (4) Ca^{2+}-induced release of intracellular Ca^{2+} store has been suggested (Gilkey *et al.*, 1978; Schackmann *et al.*, 1978). In essence, the various versions of this hypothesis propose that a small amount of Ca^{2+} ions are released in the egg, which triggers additional Ca^{2+} release. This would result in a self-propagating Ca^{2+} response. Direct evidence with aequorin for a free Ca^{2+} wave from sperm entry point to antipode has been reported for the *Medaka* egg (Gilkey *et al.*, 1978). Furthermore, sea urchin sperm have a rapid, large, and continuous uptake of ^{45}Ca (Schackmann *et al.*, 1978), which could act as a "calcium bomb" for an autocatalytic release of egg Ca^{2+} store (L. F. Jaffe, 1980) in an all-or-none fashion (Steinhardt *et al.*, 1977). However, under special experimental conditions, a partial cortical reaction has been observed in sea urchin eggs following insemination (Sugiyama, 1956). Partial exocytosis is also observed by localized contact of the egg surface with ionophore A23187 (Chambers, 1974; Chambers and Hinkley, 1979). These results suggest that Ca^{2+} release may not be autocatalytic or that the Ca^{2+} ions released in these experimental conditions may be rapidly resequestered. Epel (1980a) has reported complete exocytosis by localized contact of the egg surface with ionophore in 50 mM K$^+$ seawater. Thus, Ca^{2+}-induced release of Ca^{2+} store may require concomitant changes for propagation. Seawater (50 mM K$^+$) would cause membrane depolarization; but the concomitant change is not per se membrane depolarization, since voltage clamping the sea urchin egg does not prevent activation of the egg (MacKenzie and Chambers, 1977). A possible effect of 50 mM K$^+$ seawater is a change in membrane fluidity (Edidin et al., 1980), which normally occurs during fertilization of the sea urchin egg (Campisi and Scandella, 1978, 1980a,b).

E. Magnesium

Aside from the sea urchin, changes in Mg^{2+} content of marine invertebrate eggs have not been examined. Unlike Ca^{2+} ions, 70–80% of the Mg^{2+} content of the unfertilized sea urchin egg is considered to be unbound (Steinhardt and Epel, 1974; Cardasis et al., 1978). Quantitative estimates of Mg^{2+} content in unfertilized sea urchin eggs have ranged from 8.5 to 22 mM (Monroy-Oddo, 1946; Lindvall and Carsjo, 1951; Rothschild and Barnes, 1953; Azarnia and Chambers, 1970, 1976; Steinhardt and Epel, 1974). The intracellular Mg^{2+} concentration is reported to decrease 25–49% by 1 hour after insemination (Monroy-Oddo, 1946; Azarnia and Chambers, 1970, 1976) or remain unchanged (Lindvall and Carsjo, 1951; Hori and Yoshida, 1973). Since Mg^{2+} ions may antagonize the effects of Ca^{2+} ions (Baker et al., 1980), the possible decrease in Mg^{2+} content of eggs after insemination may be of importance. Furthermore, the ability of Mg^{2+} ions to inhibit reversibly the activation of the egg of the annelid Nereis has been reported (Wilbur, 1939). The actual free Mg^{2+} level in sea urchin eggs may be much lower than those reported, since the optimal Mg^{2+} level for protein synthesis in a cell-free system was found to be about 0.5 mM (Winkler and Steinhardt, 1981).

F. Chloride

Although the predominant anion in seawater is chloride ions, studies on Cl$^-$ content and permeability changes with egg activation are extremely limited. The Cl$^-$ content of the unfertilized egg of the sea urchin Echinus esculentus is estimated at 80 mM (Rothschild and Barnes, 1953). More recently, the Cl$^-$ content of the unfertilized egg of another sea urchin, Paracentrotus lividus, is estimated to be near 115 mM (Christen et al., 1979). Similar to cations, the Cl$^-$ uptake of unfertilized eggs is small (Jaffe and Robinson, 1978; Christen *et al.*, 1979) and is increased after fertilization (Christen *et al.*, 1979). The Cl^- content after fertilization is observed to decrease initially and then rise to 140 mM after 4 hours. Since Cl^- ions may be of importance in regulating the cytoplasmic pH of unfertilized sea urchin eggs (Shen, 1982), and the rate of protein synthesis in an *in vitro* sea urchin egg system is Cl^- sensitive (Steinhardt and Winkler, 1979; Winkler and Steinhardt, 1981), further studies of Cl^- content and flux during fertilization are necessary.

VI. IONIC REGULATION OF EARLY DEVELOPMENT

While the varieties of changes in membrane permeability and intracellular ion activity are interesting, their ultimate biological significance lies in their possible roles for regulating early development. The spectrum of morphological, biochemical, and synthetic changes during the early development of marine invertebrate embyros is diverse and multifaceted. This subject is beyond the scope of this review, but has been discussed in several recent reviews (Epel, 1978b; Schuel, 1978; Shapiro *et al.*, 1981; Vacquier, 1981). There is an increasing body of experimental evidence that indicates the importance of ionic changes for activation of the egg. Most of the analyses of ionic changes triggering morphologic and metabolic events of early development have utilized the sea urchin. However, experiments upon other marine invertebrates suggest possible universal, albeit sometimes different, regulatory roles in ionic changes.

In Section V,D, evidence for an increased Ca^{2+} permeability and intracellular activity during both fertilization and parthenogenetic activation was presented. Experiments with ionophore A23187-mediated activation of a variety of marine invertebrate eggs support the idea of an increased intracellular Ca^{2+} activity as a universal factor for triggering early development. Ionophore activation of sea urchin eggs initiates a similar sequence of events that is similar to those seen following fertilization, except cell division and embryogenesis (Steinhardt and Epel, 1974; Chambers *et al.*, 1974a; Brandriff *et al.*, 1975). Since embryogenesis occurs by following the ionophore activation with either a second parthenogenetic treatment of hypertonic seawater (Brandriff *et al.*, 1975) or fertilization (Schuel *et al.*, 1976), the ionophore may be an incomplete parthenogenetic agent because it cannot by itself stimulate the assembly of centrioles by the egg. The apparent source for the increased free Ca^{2+} content of eggs is intracellular, since egg activation by sperm or parthenogenetic agents can occur in Ca^{2+}-free seawater. A noted exception is the egg of the mollusk *Spisula,* which cannot be activated by either sperm or ionophore unless external Ca^{2+} ions are present (Schuetz, 1975b). Since a critical level of Ca^{2+} ions in the seawater was necessary for both methods of egg activation, their action for the reinitiation of meiotic maturation is probably through their effects of Ca^{2+} permeability and content. Further evidence of a causal role for Ca^{2+} ions in fertilization is the induction of sea urchin egg activation by the direct injection of Ca^{2+} buffers (Hamaguchi and Hiramoto, 1981). The clearest evidence for Ca^{2+} involvement in activation of early development comes from experiments using aequorin, which demonstrate a transient increase in free Ca^{2+} level upon activation of the egg (Steinhardt *et al.,* 1977; Moreau *et al.,* 1978; Zucker *et al.,* 1978). The importance of the transient increase in Ca^{2+} activity for egg activation is demonstrated in experiments where the Ca^{2+} rise is blocked by injection of the Ca^{2+}-chelating agent EGTA into the eggs. Sea urchin eggs injected with EGTA do not activate when fertilized (Zucker and Steinhardt, 1978) and starfish oocytes injected with EGTA do not undergo maturation when exposed to 1-methyladenine (Moreau *et al.,* 1978). Since EGTA does not inhibit Ca^{2+} release, the inhibition of activation by EGTA suggests that Ca^{2+} binding by some target is of importance.

The effects of this transient increase in free Ca^{2+} content has been detailed during sea urchin egg activation. The morphologic and metabolic changes effected by Ca^{2+} ions include the cortical reaction (Moser, 1939; Vacquier, 1976, 1981), oxygen consumption linked to the oxidation of unsaturated fatty acids (Perry and Epel, 1977; Epel, 1980b) and the oxidation of echinochrome (Perry and Epel, 1981), the activity of nicotinamide-adenine dinucleotide kinase (Epel, 1978b; Epel *et al.,* 1981), and the phosphorylation of a 40 S ribosomal protein (Hunt and Ballinger, 1981). In the sea urchin egg, Ca^{2+} ions may be acting indirectly through the Ca^{2+}-binding protein calmodulin, which has been identified in sea urchin eggs (Head *et al.,* 1979; Nishida and Kumagal, 1980). Calmodulin may be responsible for the Ca^{2+} sensitivity of the cortical reaction (Baker and Whitaker, 1979b; Steinhardt and Alderton, 1982) and the activation of NAD kinase (Epel *et al.,* 1981).

Exposure of prophase-blocked oocytes of marine invertebrates to the ionophore A23187 will reinitiate meiotic maturation (Masui and Clarke, 1979); however, the ionophore treatment does not induce maturation in the starfish oocyte, despite a 20-fold greater release of Ca^{2+} ions than that released by 1-methyladenine (Schuetz, 1975a;

Moreau *et al.*, 1978). Nonetheless, the transient increase in intracellular Ca^{2+} activity is a major step in 1-methyladenine induction of starfish oocyte maturation. Inhibitors of this process reduce the free Ca^{2+} release, and the effects of inhibitors can be reversed by increasing the concentration of 1-methyladenine, which increases free Ca^{2+} release (Moreau and Guerrier, 1979). Furthermore, iontophoretic injection of Ca^{2+} ions in the starfish oocyte cortex induces maturation (Guerrier *et al.*, 1978). The effect of an increased Ca^{2+} content may be mediated by calmodulin, because inhibitors of calmodulin will inhibit meiosis reinitiation (Meijer and Guerrier, 1981; Doree *et al.*, 1982a). Since exposure to ionophore fails to induce maturation, despite an increase in the Ca^{2+} content, the reinitiation of meiosis may require a level of Ca^{2+} ions within an appropriate range (Masui and Clarke, 1979). Evidence in support of this hypothesis is available. An important effect of 1-methyladenine is the stimulation of protein kinase activity (Guerrier *et al.*, 1977). Ionophore treatment fails to induce stimulation of protein kinase activity, and in a cell-free starfish oocyte system, protein phosphorylation is inhibited by micromolar concentrations of Ca^{2+} ions (Doree and Kishimoto, 1981). This suggests that the Ca^{2+} release stimulated by ionophore is in such excess that the stimulation of protein kinase activity is inhibited.

Another change in intracellular ion activity in eggs of the sea urchin is important for morphologic and metabolic activation—the increase in intracellular pH. Evidence for a causal role in the increase during egg activation derives from several different lines of investigation. As noted earlier in Section V,C, sea urchin eggs can be parthenogenetically activated by either a brief exposure to weak acids or by a more continuous exposure to weak bases. The exposure of unfertilized eggs to ammonia and other weak bases will initiate a number of fertilization reactions, while bypassing earlier events, such as the fertilization potential, the cortical reaction, the Na^+-dependent amino acid transport, and the increased oxygen consumption (Steinhardt and Mazia, 1973; Epel *et al.*, 1974; Vacquier and Brandriff, 1975). Incubation of unfertilized sea urchin eggs in ammonia is reported to initiate increased K^+ conductance, DNA and protein syntheses, chromosome condensation, and cytoplasmic mRNA polyadenylylation (Epel *et al.*, 1974). Since ammonia raises the intracellular pH of the egg (Shen and Steinhardt, 1978), the ammonia-stimulated activation could be attributed to the pH increase. A second line of evidence for pH regulation of egg activation comes from the observation of Chambers (1976) that Na^+ ions are required between 30 seconds and 10 minutes after insemination for metabolic activation. This Na^+ requirement has been

linked to the increase in intracellular pH during fertilization (Johnson
et al., 1976; Shen and Steinhardt, 1979). An alternative approach for
inhibition of cytoplasmic alkalinization during fertilization is the diuretic drug amiloride. If sea urchin eggs are incubated in 25 mM Na$^+$
seawater with 1 mM amiloride, the increase in internal pH, as well as
egg activation, is blocked (Johnson et al., 1976; Shen and Steinhardt,
1979). Since the development of eggs, which have been arrested by
either Na$^+$-free conditions or amiloride, can be rescued by the addition
of ammonia (Nishioka and Cross, 1978; Epel, 1980b), the rise in internal pH, as opposed to a direct participation of Na$^+$ ions, is important
for activation of the sea urchin eggs.

The effects of cytoplasmic alkalinization during fertilization of sea
urchin eggs are extensive and complex. The morphologic and metabolic changes triggered by an increase in internal pH include: protein
synthesis (Epel et al., 1974; Grainger et al., 1979), DNA synthesis and
chromosome condensation (Mazia, 1974), polyadenylylation of mRNA
(Wilt and Mazia, 1974), elongation of microvilli (Mazia et al., 1975),
activation of a Ca^{2+}-ATPase (Petzelt, 1976), increase in bulk membrane fluidity (Campisi and Scandella, 1978, 1980b), activation of
glucose-6-phosphate dehydrogenase (Aune and Epel, 1978), polymerization of actin (Begg and Rebhun, 1979), pronuclear development
(Carron and Longo, 1980), increase in K$^+$ conductance (Shen and
Steinhardt, 1980), enhancement of glycogenolysis (Baginski, 1981),
increase in uptake of thymidine (Nishioka and Magagna, 1981), and
reduction of nicotinamide nucleotides (Whitaker and Steinhardt,
1981). Many of the pH-induced events can be separated from one another. The increase in K$^+$ conductance can be suppressed without
effects on protein synthesis (Epel et al., 1974; Tupper, 1974). If enucleated merogons are used, the polyadenylation of mRNA can be induced
by ammonia, separate from chromosome condensation or DNA synthesis (Wilt and Mazia, 1974). The activation of DNA synthesis can
occur without an increased protein synthesis (Black et al., 1967). On
the other hand, increased protein synthesis can be initiated without
DNA synthesis or chromosome condensation (Epel et al., 1974). Separation of pH-induced events suggests that fertilization induces a single
pervasive change, cytoplasmic alkalinization, which then activates a
series of independent fertilization responses (Epel et al., 1974).

The mechanism by which the increase in intracellular pH initiates
these diverse fertilization responses is not clear. Several possibilities
have been offered, principally, the effects of pH on enzyme activities
and protein-protein interactions (Epel, 1978a, 1980a). One possibility
for pH alteration of enzyme activities is through phosphorylation and

dephosphorylation of specific proteins. Differences in endogenous phosphorylation of specific proteins from unfertilized and fertilized sea urchin eggs have been reported (Keller *et al.*, 1980; Ballinger and Hunt, 1981). The possibility that the pH change during fertilization may be responsible for the altered protein phosphorylation has not been resolved. The effect of increased pH on protein–protein interactions has been tested in the isolated cortex of the unfertilized sea urchin egg (Begg and Rebhun, 1979). The actin of the isolated cortices could be induced to polymerize by an increase in the pH of the isolation medium. If actin polymerization is pH-regulated in the intact egg, then this polymerization may be involved in surface changes seen after fertilization (Mazia *et al.*, 1975; Tilney and Jaffe, 1980).

The effects of the transient increase in Ca^{2+} activity and the permanent rise in pH during fertilization of the sea urchin egg are clearly separable by parthenogenetic agents. Events triggered by Ca^{2+} ions can be demonstrated by activation with the ionophore A23187 in Na^+-free seawater, and events triggered by pH can be demonstrated by activation with ammonia in Ca^{2+}-free seawater. The dissociation of the fertilization responses by ionophore and ammonia points to a dual ionic regulation of activation of sea urchin eggs during fertilization. However, if the maximal metabolic derepression of fertilization with parthenogenetic activation is to be achieved, the combined actions of Ca^{2+} and pH changes are required. The clearest example of the synergistic action of Ca^{2+} ions and pH on metabolic activation is the increase in protein synthesis rate (Winkler *et al.*, 1980).

The sea urchin synthesizes a similar set of proteins before and after fertilization, but fertilization results in a 5- to 30-fold stimulation in the rate of protein synthesis (Epel, 1967; Brandhorst, 1976; Regier and Kafatos, 1977). This stimulation is dependent on stored maternal mRNA (Gross and Cousineau, 1963; Denny and Tyler, 1964); therefore, it is regulated at the translational level. Although protein synthesis in unfertilized eggs is stimulated by exposure to ammonia, the rate of increase and the level of synthesis lag behind those of fertilized controls (Epel *et al.*, 1974; Brandis and Raff, 1979; Grainger *et al.*, 1979). A similar lag between cell-free systems prepared from unfertilized and fertilized eggs at pH 6.9 and 7.4, respectively, has been reported (Winkler and Steinhardt, 1981). As seen in Fig. 5, Ca^{2+} release in the absence of an intracellular pH increase does not stimulate protein synthesis. Increased intracellular pH without Ca^{2+} release stimulated an increase in protein synthesis less than that of fertilized controls, but the combined treatment of ionophore and ammonia of unfertilized eggs stimulated the rate of protein synthesis similar to

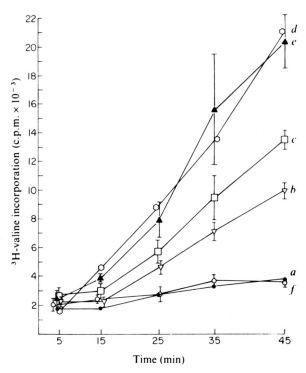

Fig. 5. The total [³H]valine incorporation of preloaded sea urchin eggs in various ionic media. (a) Eggs activated by 2.5 μM A23187 in Na⁺-free seawater: intracellular Ca²⁺ release without an intracellular pH rise. (b) Eggs activated by 10 mM NH₄Cl in Ca²⁺-free seawater: a rise in intracellular pH without a Ca²⁺ release or influx. (c) Eggs activated in 10 mM NH₄Cl in Na⁺-free seawater: an intracellular pH rise with some Ca²⁺ influx. (d) Eggs activated in 10 mM NH₄Cl and 2.5 μM A23187 in Na⁺-free seawater: both an intracellular pH rise and an intracellular Ca²⁺ release. (e) Eggs fertilized in natural seawater. (f) Unfertilized eggs in natural seawater. (From Winkler *et al.,* 1980.)

that of fertilized controls (Winkler *et al.,* 1980). Thus, for the maximal stimulation of protein synthesis, the synergistic action of an intracellular Ca²⁺ release and cytoplasmic alkalinization is required. A current hypothesis to account for the dual ionic regulation of protein synthesis is that the recruitment of maternal mRNA for translation is pH-dependent, whereas the rate of elongation is Ca²⁺-stimulated (Epel, 1980b; Steinhardt, 1980).

Unlike the increase in Ca²⁺ activity, a universal concomitant of fertilization, the rise in intracellular pH may be limited to eggs of marine invertebrates, where a general metabolic arrest has to be overcome at fertilization. In both the occyte of the starfish *Pisaster* (Johnson and Epel, 1980) and the egg of the arthropod *Limulus* (Bannon *et al.*, 1981), amino acid incorporation is sensitive to changes in intracellular pH induced by weak acid or weak base; however, the increased protein synthesis during normal development is not concomitant with cytoplasmic alkalinization. Furthermore, in another starfish, *Asterina,* the addition of weak bases reversibly, supresses meiosis reinitiation induced by 1-methyladenine (Doree *et al.*, 1982b).

VII. CONCLUDING REMARKS

The impression that one could take from the investigations of egg membrane ionic properties and intracellular ionic activities is a central role for electrolytes in the activation of the eggs of marine invertebrates. The parameters of certain ionic changes in egg activation are clear, and the regulatory roles of these changes can be inferred. Yet we are not in a position to propose a unifying account for the role that ions play. Aside from the continuing specifications of ionic changes during activation, we are faced with unraveling the molecular basis of how these apparently nonspecific changes can have such profound effects. The significance of understanding the causal link played by ionic changes exceeds beyond the problem of egg activation. An examination of many cellular and developmental processes reveals a central role played by ionic changes.

ACKNOWLEDGMENTS

I am grateful to Drs. Matthew Winkler and Charles Drewes for their comments and criticisms of this review, to the National Science Foundation (PCM 8003732) for support, and to Ms. Mary Nims for her help in preparing this manuscript.

REFERENCES

Aketa, K. (1963). Studies on the acid production at fertilization of sea urchin eggs. *Exp. Cell Res.* **30,** 93–97.

Allen, R. D. (1953). Fertilization and artificial activation in the egg of the surf-clam, *Spisula solidissima. Biol. Bull. (Woods Hole, Mass.)* **105,** 213–239.

Allen, R. D., and Griffin, J. L. (1958). The time sequence of early events in the fertilization of sea urchin eggs. I. The latent period and the cortical reaction. *Exp. Cell Res.* **15,** 163–173.

Allen, R. D., Markman, B., and Rowe, E. C. (1958). The time sequence of early events in the fertilization of sea urchin eggs. II. The production of acid. *Exp. Cell Res.* **15,** 346–349.

Armstrong, C. M. (1971). Interaction of tetraethylammonium ion derivatives with the potassium channels of giant axons. *J. Gen. Physiol.* **58,** 413–437.

Ashbel, R. (1929). La glicolisi nelle uova di riccio di mare fecondate e non fecondate. *Boll. Soc. Ital. Biol. Sper.* **4,** 492–493.

Aune, T. M., and Epel, D. (1978). Increased intracellular pH shifts the subcellular location of G6PDH. *J. Cell Biol.* **79,** 164a.

Azarnia, R., and Chambers, E. L. (1969). Effect of fertilization on the uptake and efflux of calcium-45 in the eggs of *Arbacia punctulata. Biol. Bull. (Woods Hole, Mass.)* **137,** 391–392.

Azarnia, R., and Chambers, E. L. (1970). Effect of fertilization on the calcium and magnesium content of the eggs of *Arbacia punctulata. Biol. Bull. (Woods Hole, Mass.)* **139,** 413–414.

Azarnia, R., and Chambers, E. L. (1976). The role of divalent cations in activation of the sea urchin egg. I. Effect of fertilization on divalent cation content. *J. Exp. Zool.* **198,** 65–78.

Baginski, R. M. (1981). On the timing and activation of glycogen catabolism in fertilized sea urchin eggs. *J. Exp. Zool.* **216,** 201–203.

Baker, P. F., and Whitaker, M. J. (1978). Influence of ATP and calcium on the cortical reaction in sea urchin eggs. *Nature (London)* **276,** 513–515.

Baker, P. F., and Whitaker, M. J. (1979a). Calcium activation of the cortical reaction in sea urchin eggs. *Nature (London)* **279,** 820–821.

Baker, P. F., and Whitaker, M. J. (1979b). Trifluoroperazine inhibits exocytosis in sea urchin eggs. *J. Physiol. (London)* **298,** 55p.

Baker, P. F., Meves, H., and Ridgeway, E. B. (1973). Effects of manganese and other agents on the calcium uptake that follows depolarization of squid axons. *J. Physiol. (London)* **231,** 511–526.

Baker, P. F., Knight, D. E., and Whitaker, M. J. (1980). The relation between ionized calcium and cortical granule exocytosis in eggs of the sea urchin *Echinus esculentus. Proc. R. Soc. London, Ser. B* **207,** 149–161.

Ballinger, D. G., and Hunt, T. (1981). Fertilization of sea urchin eggs is accompanied by 40S ribosomal subunit phosphorylation. *Dev. Biol.* **87,** 277–285.

Bannon, G. A., Shen, S. S., and Brown, G. G. (1981). Loss of pH sensitivity of amino acid incorporation during early development of the horseshoe crab, *Limulus polyphemus* L. *J. Exp. Zool.* **217,** 447–450.

Begg, D. A., and Rebhun, L. I. (1979). pH regulates the polymerization of actin in the sea urchin egg cortex. *J. Cell Biol.* **83,** 241–248.

Bennett, J., and Mazia, D. (1981a). Interspecific fusion of sea urchin eggs. Surface events and cytoplasmic mixing. *Exp. Cell Res.* **131,** 197–207.

Bennett, J., and Mazia, D. (1981b). Fusion of fertilized and unfertilized sea urchin eggs. Maintenance of cell surface integrity. *Exp. Cell Res.* **134,** 494–498.

Bentley, P. J. (1968). Amiloride: A potent inhibitor of sodium transport across the toad bladder. *J. Physiol. (London)* **195,** 317–330.

Black, R. E., Baptist, E., and Piland, J. (1967). Puromycin and cycloheximide inhibition of thymidine incorporation into DNA of cleaving sea urchin eggs. *Exp. Cell Res.* **48,** 431–439.

Boron, W. F., Roos, A., and De Weer, P. (1978). NH₄Cl and other weak bases in the activation of sea urchin eggs. *Nature (London)* **274,** 190.

Brachet, J. (1938). Oxygen consumption of artificially activated and fertilized *Chaetopterus* eggs. *Biol. Bull. (Woods Hole, Mass.)* **74**, 93–98.

Brachet, J., and Denis-Donini, S. (1977). Effet de divers agents (ionophore du calcium et du potassium organomercuriels, dithiols, colchicine, cytochalasine B) sur la maturation et la différenciation sans clivage chez l'oeuf de *Chaetoptere*. *C.R. Hebd. Seances. Acad. Sci.* **284**, 1091–1096.

Brandhorst, B. P. (1976). Two-dimensional gel patterns of protein synthesis before and after fertilization of sea urchin eggs. *Dev. Biol.* **52**, 310–317.

Brandis, J. W., and Raff, R. A. (1979). Elevation of protein synthesis is a complex response to fertilization. *Nature (London)* **278**, 467–469.

Brandriff, B., Hinegardner, R. T., and Steinhardt, R. (1975). Development and life cycle of the parthenogenetically activated sea urchin embryo. *J. Exp. Zool.* **192**, 13–24.

Brown, K. T., and Flaming, D. G. (1977). New microelectrode techniques for intracellular work in small cells. *Neuroscience* **2**, 813–827.

Byrd, E. W., and Collins, F. D. (1975). Absence of fast block to polyspermy in eggs of sea urchin *Strongylcentrotus purpuratus*. *Nature (London)* **257**, 675–677.

Byrd, E. W., and Perry, G. (1980). Cytochalasin B blocks sperm incorporation but allows activation of the sea urchin egg. *Exp. Cell Res.* **126**, 333–342.

Campisi, J., and Scandella, C. J. (1978). Fertilization induced changes in membrane fluidity of sea urchin eggs. *Science* **199**, 1336–1337.

Campisi, J., and Scandella, C. J. (1980a). Bulk membrane fluidity increases after fertilization or partial activation of sea urchin egg. *J. Biol. Chem.* **255**, 5411–5419.

Campisi, J., and Scandella, C. J. (1980b). Calcium induced decrease in membrane fluidity of sea urchin cortex after fertilization. *Nature (London)* **286**, 185–186.

Cardasis, C. C., Schuel, H., and Herman, L. (1978). Ultrastructural localization of calcium in unfertilized sea urchin eggs. *J. Cell Sci.* **31**, 101–115.

Carpenedo, F., Bortignon, C., Bruni, A., and Santi, R. (1969). Effect of quercetin on membrane-linked activities. *Biochem. Pharmacol.* **18**, 1495–1500.

Carroll, E. J., Jr., and Levitan, H. (1978a). Fertilization in the sea urchin, *Stronglyocentrotus purpuratus* is blocked by fluorescein dyes. *Dev. Biol.* **63**, 432–440.

Carroll, E. J., Jr., and Levitan, H. (1978b). Fertilization is inhibited in five diverse animal phyla by erythrosin B. *Dev. Biol.* **64**, 329–331.

Carron. C. P., and Longo, F. J. (1980). Relation of intracellular pH and pronuclear development in the sea urchin, *Arbacia punctulata*. *Dev. Biol.* **79**, 478–487.

Chambers, E. L. (1949). The uptake and loss of K^{42} in the unfertilized and fertilized eggs of *Strongylocentrotus purpuratus* and *Arbacia punctulata*. *Biol. Bull. (Woods Hole, Mass.)* **97**, 251–252.

Chambers, E. L. (1968). Exchange of sodium following fertilization of sea urchin eggs. *Int. Congr. Ser.—Excerpta Med.* **166**, 42–43.

Chambers, E. L. (1972). Effect of fertilization on the Na^+ and K^+ content, and Na^+ flux in the sea urchin egg. *Physiologist* **15**, 103.

Chambers, E. L. (1974). Effects of ionophores on marine eggs and cation requirements for activation. *Biol. Bull. (Woods Hole, Mass.)* **147**, 471.

Chambers, E. L. (1975a). Potassium exchange in unfertilized sea urchin (*Arbacia punctulata*) eggs. *Biol. Bull. (Woods Hole, Mass.)* **149**, 422–423.

Chambers, E. L. (1975b). Na^+ is required for nuclear and cytoplasmic activation of sea urchin eggs by sperm and divalent ionophores. *J. Cell Biol.* **67**, 60a.

Chambers, E. L. (1976). Na is essential for activation of the inseminated sea urchin egg. *J. Exp. Zool.* **197**, 149–154.

Chambers, E. L. (1980). Fertilization and cleavage of eggs of the sea urchin *Lytechinus variegatus* in Ca^{2+}-free sea water. *Eur. J. Cell Biol.* **22,** 476.

Chambers, E. L., and Chambers, R. (1949). Ion exchanges and fertilization in echinoderm eggs. *Am. Nat.* **83,** 269–284.

Chambers. E. L., and de Armendi, J. (1977a). Electrophysiological studies of fertilization in the sea urchin egg. *J. Gen. Physiol.* **70,** 3a–4a.

Chambers, E. L., and de Armendi, J. (1977b). Membrane potential, activation potential, and activation current of the sea urchin egg. *Physiologist* **20,** 15.

Chambers, E. L., and de Armendi, J. (1979). Membrane potential, activation potential of eggs of the sea urchin, *Lytechinus variegatus. Exp. Cell Res.* **122,** 203–218.

Chambers, E. L., and Hinkley, R. E. (1979). Non-propagated cortical reactions induced by the divalent ionophore A23187 in eggs of the sea urchin, *Lytachinus variegatus. Exp. Cell Res.* **124,** 441–446.

Chambers, E. L., White, W., Jeung, N., and Brooks, S. C. (1948). Penetration and effects of low temperature and cyanide on penetration of radioactive potassium into the eggs of *Strongylocentrotus purpuratus* and *Arbacia punctulata. Biol. Bull. (Woods Hole, Mass.)* **95,** 252–253.

Chambers, E. L., Azarnia, R., and McGowan, W. E. (1970). The effect of temperature on the efflux of ^{45}Ca from the eggs of *Arbacia punctulata. Biol. Bull. (Woods Hole, Mass.)* **139,** 417–418.

Chambers, E. L., Pressman, B. C., and Rose, B. (1974a). The activation of sea urchin eggs by the divalent ionophores A23187 and X-537A. *Biochem. Biophys. Res. Commun.* **60,** 126–132.

Chambers, E. L., Pressman, B. C., and Rose, B. (1974b). Parthenogenetic activation of sea urchin eggs by divalent ionophores. *J. Cell Biol.* **63,** 56a.

Chambers, R. (1922). A micro-injection study on the starfish egg. *J. Gen. Physiol.* **5,** 189–193.

Chambers, R. (1928). Intracellular hydrion concentration studies. I. The relation of the environment to the pH of protoplasm and of its inclusion bodies. *Biol. Bull. (Woods Hole, Mass.)* **55,** 369–376.

Chambers, R., and Chambers, E. L. (1961). "Explorations into the Nature of the Living Cell," pp. 141–174. Harvard Univ. Press, Cambridge, Massachusetts.

Chambers, R., and Pollack, H. (1927). Micrurgical study in cell physiology. IV. Colorimetric determination of the nuclear and cytoplasmic pH in the starfish egg. *J. Gen. Physiol.* **10,** 739–755.

Chandler, D. E., and Heuser, J. (1979). Membrane fusion during secretion. Cortical granule exocytosis in sea urchin eggs studied by quick-freezing and freeze-fracture. *J. Cell Biol.* **83,** 91–108.

Christen, R., Sardet, C., and Lallier, R. (1979). Chloride permeability of sea urchin eggs. *Cell Biol. Int. Rep.* **3,** 121–128.

Conrad, G. W., Krammer, A. E., and Athey, G. F. (1977). Membrane potential of fertilized eggs of *llyanassa obsoleta* during polar lobe formation and cytokinesis. *Dev. Biol.* **57,** 215–220.

Cuthbert, A., and Cuthbert, A. W. (1978). Fertilization acid production in *Psammechinus* eggs under pH clamp conditions, and the effects of some pyrazine derivatives. *Exp. Cell Res.* **114,** 409–415.

Dale, B., and De Santis, A. (1981a). The effect of cytochalasin B and D on the fertilization of sea urchins. *Dev. Biol.* **83,** 232–237.

Dale, B., and De Santis, A. (1981b). Maturation and fertilization of the sea urchin oocyte: an electrophysiological study. *Dev. Biol.* **85,** 474–484.

Dale, B., Denis-Donini, S., De Santis, R., Monroy, A., Rosati, F., and Taglietti, V. (1978a). Sperm-egg interaction in the ascidians. *Biol. Cell.* **32**, 129–133.

Dale, B., De Felice, L. J., and Taglietti, V. (1978b). Membrane noise and conductance increase during single spermatozoon-egg interactions. *Nature (London)* **275**, 217–219.

Dale, S., De Santis, A., and Hoshi, J. (1979). Membrane response to 1-methyladenine requires the presence of the nucleus. *Nature (London)* **282**, 89–90.

DeFelice, L. J., and Dale, B. (1979). Voltage response to fertilization and polyspermy in sea urchin eggs and oocytes. *Dev. Biol.* **72**, 327–341.

Denny, P. C., and Tyler, A. (1964). Activation of protein synthesis in non-nucleated fragments of sea urchin eggs. *Biochem. Biophys. Res. Commun.* **14**, 245–249.

Doree, M. (1981). Hormonal control of meiosis in starfish oocytes. Calcium ion release induced by 1-methyladenine increases membrane permeability to sodium ions. *Exp. Cell Res.* **131**, 115–120.

Doree, M., and Kishimoto, T. (1981). Calcium-mediated transduction of the hormonal message of 1-methyladenine-induced meiosis reinitiation of starfish oocytes. *In* "Metabolism and Molecular Activities of Cytokinins" (J. Guern and C. Peaud-Lenoel, eds.), pp. 338–348. Springer-Verlag, Berlin and New York.

Doree, M., Moreau, M., and Guerrier, P. (1978). Hormonal control of meiosis. *In vitro* induced release of calcium ions from the plasma membrane in starfish oocytes. *Exp. Cell Res.* **115**, 251–260.

Doree, M., Picard, A., Cavadore, J. C., Le Peuch, C., and Demaille, J. G. (1982a). Calmodulin antagonists and hormonal control of meiosis in starfish oocytes. *Exp. Cell Res.* **139**, 135–144.

Doree, M., Sano, K., and Kanatani, H. (1982b). Ammonia and other weak bases applied at any time of the hormone-dependent period inhibit 1-methyladenine-induced meiosis reinitiation of starfish oocyte. *Dev. Biol.* **90**, 13–17.

Dube, F., and Guerrier, P. (1982). Activation of *Barnea candida* (Mollusca, Pelecypoda) oocytes by sperm or KCl, but not by NH₄Cl, requires a calcium influx. *Dev. Biol.* **92**, 408–417.

Eckberg, W. R., and Carroll, A. G. (1981). The effects of chlorpromazine and quercetin on egg maturation and activation in *Chaetopterus pergamentaceus. Biol. Bull. (Woods Hole, Mass.)* **161**, 334–335.

Eddy, E. M., and Shapiro, B. M. (1976). Changes in the topography of the sea urchin egg after fertilization. *J. Cell Biol.* **71**, 35–48.

Edidin, M., Wei, T., and Holmberg, S. (1980). The role of membrane potential in determining rates of lateral diffusion in the plasma membrane of mammalian cells. *Ann. N.Y. Acad. Sci.* **339**, 1–7.

Epel, D. (1967). Protein synthesis in sea urchin eggs: A "late" response to fertilization. *Proc. Natl. Acad. Sci. U.S.A.* **57**, 889–906.

Epel, D. (1978a). Mechanisms of activation of sperm and egg during fertilization of sea urchin gametes. *Curr. Top. Dev. Biol.* **12**, 185–246.

Epel, D. (1978b). Intracellular pH and activation of the sea urchin egg at fertilization. *In* "Cell Reproduction" (E. R. Dirksen, D. Prescott, and C. F. Fox, eds.), pp. 367–378. Academic Press, New York.

Epel, D. (1980a). Ionic triggers in the fertilization of sea urchin eggs. *Ann. N.Y. Acad. Sci.* **339**, 74–85.

Epel, D. (1980b). Experimental analysis of the role of intracellular calcium in the activation of the sea urchin egg at fertilization. *In* "The Cell Surface: Mediator of Developmental Processes" (S. Subtelny and N. K. Wessells, eds.), pp. 169–185. Academic Press, New York.

Epel, D., Steinhardt, R., Humphreys, T., and Mazia, D. (1974). An analysis of the partial derepression of sea urchin eggs by ammonia; the existence of independent pathways. *Dev. Biol.* **40**, 245–255.

Epel, D., Patton, C., Wallace, R. W., and Cheung, W. Y. (1981). Calmodulin activates NAD kinase of sea urchin eggs: An early event of fertilization. *Cell* **23**, 543–549.

Finkel, T., and Wolf, D. P. (1978). Fertilization of surf clam oocytes: The role of membrane potential and internal pH. *Biol. Bull. (Woods Hole, Mass.)* **155**, 437.

Finkel, T., and Wolf, D. P. (1980). Membrane potential, pH and the activation of surf clam oocytes. *Gamete Res.* **3**, 299–304.

Fox, A. P., and Krasne, S. (1981). Two calcium currents in egg cells. *Biophys. J.* **33**, 145a.

Furshpan, E. J. (1955). Electrical measurements of sea urchin eggs. Appendix to thesis, "Studies on Certain Sensory and Motor Systems of Decapod Crustaceans," pp. 130–149. California Institute of Technology, Pasadena.

Gelfan, S. (1931). Electrical potential difference across the nuclear membrane of the starfish egg. *Proc. Soc. Exp. Biol. Med.* **29**, 58–59.

Gilkey, J. C., Jaffe, L. F., Ridgway, E. G., and Reynolds, G. T. (1978). A free calcium wave traverses the activating egg of the medaka, *Oryzias latipes*. *J. Cell Biol.* **76**, 448–466.

Gillies, R. J., and Deamer, D. W. (1979). Intracellular pH; Methods and application. *Curr. Top. Bioenerg.* **9**, 63–89.

Gillies, R. J., Rosenberg, M. P., and Deamer, D. W. (1981). Carbon dioxide efflux accompanies release of fertilization acid from sea urchin eggs. *J. Cell. Physiol.* **108**, 115–122.

Gould-Somero, M. (1981). Localized gating of egg Na^+ channels by sperm. *Nature (London)* **291**, 254–256.

Gould-Somero, M., and Holland, L. (1975). Fine structure investigation of the insemination response in *Urechis caupo*. *Dev. Biol.* **46**, 358–369.

Gould-Somero, M., Holland, L., and Paul, M. (1977). Cytochalasin B inhibits sperm penetration into eggs of *Urechis caupo* (Echiura). *Dev. Biol.* **58**, 11–22.

Gould-Somero, M., Jaffe, L. A., and Holland, L. Z. (1979). Electrically mediated fast polyspermy block in eggs of the marine worm, *Urechis caupo*. *J. Cell Biol.* **82**, 426–440.

Grainger, J. L., Winkler, M. M., Shen, S. S., and Steinhardt, R. A. (1979). Intracellular pH controls protein synthesis rate in the sea urchin egg and early embryo. *Dev. Biol.* **68**, 396–406.

Gross, P. R., and Cousineau, G. H. (1963). Effects of actinomycin D on macromolecule synthesis and early development in sea urchin eggs. *Biochem. Biophys. Res. Commun.* **10**, 321–326.

Guerrier, P., Moreau, M., and Doree, M. (1977). Stimulation of protein phosphorylation induced by 1-methyladenine. *Mol. Cell Endocrinol.* **7**, 137–150.

Guerrier, P., Moreau, M., and Doree, M. (1978). Control of meiosis reinitiation in starfish: Calcium ions as the primary effective trigger. *Ann. Biol. Anim., Biochim., Biophys.* **18**, 441–452.

Guerrier, P., Dube, F., and Moreau, M. (1981). External calcium requirement for oocyte maturation in the surf clam, *Spisula solidissima*. *Biol. Bull. (Woods Hole, Mass.)* **161**, 335–336.

Hagiwara, S., and Jaffe, L. A. (1979). Electrical properties of egg cell membranes. *Annu. Rev. Biophys. Bioeng.* **8**, 385–416.

Hagiwara, S., and Miyasaki, S. (1977). Changes in excitability of the cell membrane during 'Differentiation without Cleavage' in the egg of the annelid, *Chaetopterus pergamentaceus*. *J. Physiol. (London)* **272**, 197–216.

Hagiwara, S., and Takahashi, K. (1974). The anomalous rectification and cation selectivity of the membrane of a starfish egg cell. *J. Membr. Biol.* **18**, 61–80.

Hagiwara, S., and Yoshii, M. (1979). Effects of internal potassium and sodium on the anomalous rectification of the starfish egg as examined by internal perfusion. *J. Physiol. (London)* **292**, 251–265.

Hagiwara, S., Fukuda, J., and Eaton, D. C. (1974). Membrane currents carried by Ca, Sr and Ba in barnacle muscle fiber during voltage clamp. *J. Gen. Physiol.* **63**, 564–578.

Hagiwara, S., Ozawa, S., and Sand, O. (1975). Voltage clamp analysis of two inward current mechanisms in the egg cell membrane of a starfish. *J. Gen. Physiol.* **65**, 617–644.

Hagiwara, S., Yoshida, S., and Yoshii, M. (1981). Transient and delayed potassium currents in the egg cell membrane of the coelenterate, *Renilla koellikeri*. *J. Physiol. (London)* **318**, 123–141.

Hagstrom, B. E., and Lonning, S. (1961). Studies of the species specificity of echinoderms. *Sarsia* **4**, 5–19.

Hamaguchi, Y., and Hiramoto, Y. (1981). Activation of sea urchin eggs by microinjection of calcium buffers. *Exp. Cell Res.* **134**, 171–179.

Harvey, E. B. (1956). "The American Arbacia and Other Sea Urchins." Princeton Univ. Press, Princeton, New Jersey.

Harvey, E. N. (1910). The permeability and cytolysis of eggs. *Science* **32**, 565–567.

Head, J. F., Mader, S., and Kaminer, B. (1979). Calcium-binding modulator protein from the unfertilized egg of the sea urchin, *Arbacia punctulata*. *J. Cell Biol.* **80**, 211–218.

Heilbrunn, L. V. (1937). "An Outline of General Physiology," pp. 428–440. Saunders, Philadelphia, Pennsylvania.

Heilbrunn, L. V., and Wilbur, K. M. (1937). Stimulation and nuclear breakdown in the *Nereis* egg. *Biol. Bull. (Woods Hole, Mass.)* **73**, 557–564.

Heilbrunn, L. V., and Young, R. A. (1930). The action of ultra-violet rays on *Arbacia* egg protoplasm. *Physiol. Zool.* **3**, 330–341.

Higashi, A. (1974). Effects of external ions on the membrane potentials upon fertilization in sea urchin eggs. *Annot. Zool. Jpn.* **47**, 65–73.

Higashi, A., and Kaneko, H. (1971). Membrane potential of sea urchin eggs and effect of external ions. *Annot. Zool. Jpn.* **44**, 65–75.

Hiraiwa, Y. K., and Kawamura, T. (1936). Relation between maturation division and cleavage in artificially activated eggs of *Urechis unicinctus* (von Drasche). *Biol. Bull. (Woods Hole, Mass.)* **70**, 344–351.

Hiramoto, Y. (1959a). Electric properties of echinoderm eggs. *Embryologia* **4**, 219–235.

Hiramoto, Y. (1959b). Changes in electric properties upon fertilization in the sea urchin egg. *Exp. Cell Res.* **16**, 421–424.

Holland, L., and Gould-Somero, M. (1981). Electrophysiological response to insemination in oocytes of *Urechis caupo*. *Dev. Biol.* **83**, 90–100.

Holland, L. Z., and Gould-Somero, M. (1982). Fertilization acid of sea urchin eggs: Evidence that it is H^+, not CO_2. *Dev. Biol.* **92**, 549–552.

Holland, N. D. (1980). Effects of ionophore A23187 on oocytes of *Comanthus japonica* (Echinodermata: Crinoidea). *Dev., Growth Differ.* **22**, 203–207.

Hori, R. (1958). Membrane potential of the sea urchin egg and its change upon fertilization. *Zool. Mag.* **67**, 31.

Hori, R., and Yoshida, T. (1973). On the magnesium content in sea urchin eggs and its changes accompanying fertilization. *Protoplasma* **77**, 137–140.

Hunt, T., and Ballinger, D. (1981). Phosphorylation of the 40S ribosomal protein rp31 in

Arbacia eggs at fertilization requires both Ca^{++} and an increase in intracellular pH. *Biol. Bull. (Woods Hole, Mass.)* **161**, 336.

Ii, I., and Rebhun, L. I. (1979). Acid release following activation of surf clam (*Spisula solidissima*) eggs. *Dev. Biol.* **72**, 195–200.

Ikegami, S., Okada, T. S., and Koide, S. S. (1976). On the role of calcium ions in oocyte maturation in the polychaete *Chaetopterus pergamentaceus. Dev., Growth Differ.* **18**, 33–43.

Inoue, H., and Yoshioka, T. (1980). Measurement of intracellular pH in sea urchin eggs by ^{31}P NMR. *J. Cell Physiol.* **105**, 461–468.

Ishihara, K. (1964). Release of polysaccharides following fertilization of sea urchin eggs. *Exp. Cell Res.* **36**, 354–367.

Ishihara, K. (1968). An analysis of acid polysaccharides produced at fertilization of sea urchin. *Exp. Cell Res.* **51**, 473–484.

Ito, S., and Yoshioka, K. (1972). Real activation potential observed in sea urchin egg during fertilization. *Exp. Cell Res.* **72**, 547–551.

Ito, S., and Yoshioka, K. (1973). Effects of various ionic compositions upon the membrane potentials during activation of sea urchin eggs. *Exp. Cell Res.* **78**, 191–200.

Jacobs, M. H. (1920). The production of intracellular acidity by neutral and alkaline solutions containing carbon dioxide. *Am. J. Physiol.* **53**, 457–563.

Jaffe, L. A. (1976). Fast block to polyspermy in sea urchin eggs is electrically mediated. *Nature (London)* **261**, 68–71.

Jaffe, L. A. (1980). Electrical polyspermy block in sea urchins: Nicotine and low sodium experiments. *Dev., Growth Differ.* **22**, 503–507.

Jaffe, L. A., and Guerrier, P. (1981). Localization of electrical excitability in the early embryo of *Dentalium. Dev. Biol.* **83**, 370–373.

Jaffe, L. A., and Robinson, K. R. (1978). Membrane potential of the unfertilized sea urchin egg. *Dev. Biol.* **62**, 215–228.

Jaffe, L. A., Hagiwara, S., and Kado, R. T. (1978). The time course of cortical vesicle fusion in sea urchin eggs observed as membrane capacitance changes. *Dev. Biol.* **67**, 243–248.

Jaffe, L. A., Gould-Somero, M., and Holland, L. (1979). Ionic mechanism of the fertilization potential of the marine worm, *Urechis caupo* (Echiura). *J. Gen. Physiol.* **73**, 469–492.

Jaffe, L. F. (1980). Calcium explosions as triggers of development. *Ann. N.Y. Acad. Sci.* **339**, 86–101.

Johnson, C. H., and Epel, D. (1980). Intracellular pH does not regulate protein synthesis in starfish oocytes. *J. Cell Biol.* **87**, 142a.

Johnson, C. H., and Epel, D. (1981). Intracellular pH of sea urchin eggs measured by the dimethyloxazolidinedione (DMO) method. *J. Cell Biol.* **89**, 284–291.

Johnson, C. H., and Epel, D. (1982). Starfish oocyte maturation and fertilization: Intracellular pH is not involved in activation. *Dev. Biol.* **92**, 461–469.

Johnson, J. D., Epel, D., and Paul, M. (1976). Intracellular pH and activation of sea urchin eggs after fertilization. *Nature (London)* **262**, 661–664.

Johnston, R. N., and Paul, M. (1977). Calcium influx following fertilization of *Urechis caupo* eggs. *Dev. Biol.* **57**, 364–374.

Just, E. E. (1933). A cytological study of effects of ultra-violet light on the egg of *Nereis limbata. Z. Zellforsch. Mikrosk. Anat.* **17**, 25.

Kamada, T., and Kinosita, H. (1940). Membrane potential of sea urchin eggs. *Proc. Imp. Acad. (Tokyo)* **16**, 149–152.

Kanatani, H. (1973). Maturation-inducing substance in starfishes. *Int. Rev. Cytol.* **35**, 253–298.

Kanatani, H., Kurokawa, T., and Nakanishi, K. (1969). Effects of various adenine derivatives in oocyte maturation and spawning in the starfish. *Biol. Bull. (Woods Hole,
Mass.)* **137**, 384–385.

Keller, C., Gundersen, G., and Shapiro, B. M. (1980). Altered *in vitro* phosphorylation of
specific proteins accompanies fertilization of *Strongylocentrotus purpuratus* eggs.
Dev. Biol. **74**, 86–100.

Kiehart, D. P., Reynolds, G. T., and Eisen, A. (1977). Calcium transients during early
development in echinoderms and teleosts. *Biol. Bull. (Woods Hole, Mass.)* **153**, 432.

Kohlhardt, M., Bauer, B., Krause, H., and Fleckenstein, A. (1972). Differentiation of the
transmembrane Na and Ca channels in mammalian cardiac fibers by the use of
specific inhibitors. *Pfluegers Arch.* **335**, 309–322.

Lambert, C. C., and Epel, D. (1979). Calcium mediated mitochondrial movement in
ascidian sperm during fertilization. *Dev. Biol.* **69**, 296–304.

Lee, H. C., Forte, J. G., and Epel, D. (1982). The use of fluorescent amines for the
measurement of pH_i: Applications in liposomes, gastric microsomes, and sea urchin
gametes. *In* "Intracellular pH: Its Measurement, Regulation and Utilization in
Cellular Functions" (R. Nuccitelli and D. W. Deamer, eds.), pp. 134–160. Alan R.
Liss, Inc., New York.

Lefevre, G. (1907). Artificial parthenogenesis in *Thalassema mellita. J. Exp. Zool.* **4**,
91–150.

Levitan, H., and Carroll, E. J., Jr. (1977). Sea urchin egg membrane properties are
altered by fluorescein dyes. *J. Cell Biol.* **75**, 231a.

Lillie, F. R. (1902). Differentiation without cleavage in the egg of the annelid *Chaetopterus pergamentaceus. Arch. Mikrosk. Anat. Entwicklungsmech.* **14**, 477–499.

Lillie, F. R. (1906). Observations and experiments concerning the elementary phenomenon of embryonic development in *Chaetopterus. J. Exp. Zool.* **3**, 153–
167.

Lillie, R. S. (1911). The physiology of cell division. IV. The action of salt solution followed
by hypertonic sea-water on unfertilized sea urchin eggs and the role of membranes
in mitosis. *J. Morphol.* **22**, 695–730.

Lindvall, S., and Carsjo, A. (1951). On protein fractions and inorganic ions in sea urchin
eggs, unfertilized and fertilized. *Exp. Cell Res.* **2**, 491–498.

Loeb, J. (1910). The prevention of the toxic action of various agencies upon the fertilized
egg through the suppression of oxidation in the cell. *Science* **32**, 411–412.

Loeb, J. (1913). "Artificial Parthenogenesis and Fertilization." Univ. of Chicago Press,
Chicago, Illinois.

Longo, F. J. (1978). Effects of cytochalasin B on sperm-egg interactions. *Dev. Biol.* **67**,
157–173.

Lopo, A., and Vacquier, V. D. (1977). The rise and fall of intracellular pH of sea urchin
eggs after fertilization. *Nature (London)* **269**, 590–592.

Lundberg, A. (1955). Microelectrode experiments on unfertilized sea urchin eggs. *Exp.
Cell Res.* **9**, 393–398.

Lyon, E. P., and Shackell, L. F. (1910). On the increased permeability of sea urchin eggs
following fertilization. *Science* **32**, 249–251.

McClendon, J. F. (1910a). Electrolytic experiments showing increase in permeability of
the egg to ions at the beginning of development. *Science* **32**, 122–124.

McClendon, J. F. (1910b). Further proofs of the increase in permeability of the sea
urchin's egg to electrolytes at the beginning of development. *Science* **32**, 317–
318.

McClendon, J. F. (1910c). On the dynamics of cell division. II. Changes in permeability of
developing eggs to electrolytes. *Am. J. Physiol.* **32**, 240–275.

MacKenzie, D. O., and Chambers, E. L. (1977). Fertilization of voltage clamped sea urchin eggs. *Clin. Res.* **25**, 643A.

Maeno, T. (1959). Electrical characteristics and activation potential of *Bufo* eggs. *J. Gen. Physiol.* **43**, 139–157.

Masui, Y., and Clarke, H. J. (1979). Oocyte maturation. *Int. Rev. Cytol.* **57**, 185–282.

Mazia, D. (1937). The release of calcium in *Arbacia* eggs on fertilization. *J. Cell. Comp. Physiol.* **10**, 291–304.

Mazia, D. (1974). Chromosome cycles turned on in unfertilized sea urchin eggs exposed to NH_4OH. *Proc. Natl. Acad. Sci. U.S.A.* **71**, 690–693.

Mazia, D., Schatten, G., and Steinhardt, R. (1975). Turning on of activities in unfertilized sea urchin eggs: Correlation with changes of the surface. *Proc. Natl. Acad. Sci. U.S.A.* **72**, 4469–4473.

Mehl, J. W., and Swann, M. M. (1961). Acid and base production at fertilization in the sea urchin. *Exp. Cell Res.* **22**, 233–245.

Meijer, L. (1979). Hormonal control of oocyte maturation in *Arenicola marina* (Annelida, Polychaeta). II. Maturation and fertilization. *Dev., Growth Differ.* **21**, 315–329.

Meijer, L., and Guerrier, P. (1981). Calmodulin in starfish oocytes. I. Calmodulin antagonists inhibit meiosis reinitiation. *Dev. Biol.* **88**, 318–324.

Miyazaki, S. (1979). Fast polyspermy block and activation potential. Electrophysiological bases for their changes during oocyte maturation of a starfish. *Dev. Biol.* **70**, 341–354.

Miyazaki, S., and Hirai, S. (1979). Fast polyspermy block and activation potential. Correlated changes during oocyte maturation of a starfish. *Dev. Biol.* **70**, 327–340.

Miyazaki, S., Takahashi, K., and Tsuda, K. (1972). Calcium and sodium contributions to regenerative responses in the embryonic excitable cell membrane. *Science* **176**, 1441–1443.

Miyazaki, S., Takahashi, K., and Tsuda, K. (1974). Electrical excitability in the egg cell membrane of the tunicate. *J. Physiol. (London)* **238**, 37–54.

Miyazaki, S., Ohmori, H., and Sasaki, S. (1975a). Action potential and non-linear current-voltage relation in starfish oocytes. *J. Physiol. (London)* **246**, 37–54.

Miyazaki, S., Ohmori, H., and Sasaki, S. (1975b). Potassium rectifications of the starfish oocyte membrane and their changes during oocyte maturation. *J. Physiol. (London)* **246**, 55–78.

Monroy, A., and Tyler, A. (1958). Changes in efflux and influx of potassium upon fertilization in eggs of *Arbacia punctulata,* measured by use of K^{42}. *Biol. Bull. (Woods Hole, Mass.)* **115**, 339–340.

Monroy-Oddo, A. (1946). Variations in Ca and Mg contents in *Arbacia* eggs as a result of fertilization. *Experientia* **2**, 371–372.

Moreau, M., and Cheval, J. (1976). Electrical properties of the starfish oocyte membranes. *J. Physiol. (Paris)* **72**, 293–300.

Moreau, M., and Guerrier, P. (1979). Free calcium changes associated with hormone action in oocytes. *In* "Detection and Measurement of Free Ca^{2+} in Cells" (C. C. Ashley and A. K. Campbell, eds.), pp. 219–226. Elsevier/North-Holland, Amsterdam.

Moreau, M., and Guerrier, P. (1981). Absence of regional differences in the membrane properties from the embryo of the mud snail *Ilyanassa obsoleta. Biol. Bull. (Woods Hole, Mass.)* **161**, 320–321.

Moreau, M., Guerrier, P., Doree, M., and Ashley, C. C. (1978). Hormone-induced release of intracellular Ca^{2+} triggers meiosis in starfish oocytes. *Nature (London)* **272**, 251–253.

Moser, F. (1939). Studies on a cortical layer response to stimulating agents in the *Arbacia* egg. II. Response to chemical and physical agents. *J. Exp. Zool.* **80**, 447–471.

Nakamura, M., and Yasumasu, I. (1974). Mechanism for increase in intracellular concentration of free calcium in fertilized sea urchin egg. A method for estimating intracellular concentration of free calcium. *J. Gen. Physiol.* **63**, 374–388.

Nakazawa, T., Asami, K., Shogu, R., Fugiwara, A., and Yasumasu, I. (1970). Ca^{2+} uptake, ejection and respiration in sea urchin eggs on fertilization. *Exp. Cell Res.* **63**, 143–146.

Needham, J., and Needham, D. M. (1926). The hydrogen ion concentration and oxidation-reduction potential of the cell-interior before and after fertilization and cleavage: A micro-injection study on marine eggs. *Proc. R. Soc. London, Ser. B* **99**, 173–199.

Nigon, V., and Do, F. (1965). Les mouvements du calcium dans l'oeuf d'*Arbacia lixula* au moment de la fecondation. *C.R. Hebd. Seances Acad. Sci.* **257**, 2178–2180.

Nishida, E., and Kumagai, H. (1980). Calcium sensitivity of sea urchin tubulin in *in vitro* assembly and the effects of calcium-dependent regulator (CDR) proteins isolated from sea urchin eggs and porcine brains. *J. Biochem. (Tokyo)* **87**, 143–151.

Nishioka, D., and Cross, N. (1978). The role of external sodium in sea urchin fertilization. *In* "Cell Reproduction" (E. Dirksen, D. Prescott, and C. F. Fox, eds.), pp. 403–413. Academic Press, New York.

Nishioka, D., and McGwin, N. F. (1980). Relationships between the release of acid, the cortical reaction, and the increase of protein synthesis in sea urchin eggs. *J. Exp. Zool.* **212**, 215–223.

Nishioka, D., and Magagna, L. S. (1981). Increased uptake of thymidine in the activation of sea urchin eggs. Specificity of uptake and dependence on internal pH, the cortical reaction, and external sodium. *Exp. Cell Res.* **133**, 363–372.

Ohmori, H., and Yoshii, M. (1977). Surface potential reflected in both gating and permeation mechanisms of sodium and calcium channels of the tunicate egg cell membrane. *J. Physiol. (London)* **267**, 429–463.

Okamoto, H., Takahashi, K., and Yoshii, M. (1976a). Membrane currents of the tunicate egg under the voltage-clamp condition. *J. Physiol. (London)* **254**, 607–638.

Okamoto, H., Takahashi, K., and Yoshii, M. (1976b). Two components of the calcium current in the egg cell membrane of the tunicate. *J. Physiol. (London)* **255**, 527–561.

Okamoto, H., Takahashi, K., and Yamashita, N. (1977). Ionic currents through the membrane of the mammalian oocyte and their comparison with those in the tunicate and sea urchin. *J. Physiol. (London)* **267**, 465–495.

Pasteels, J. (1938). Sensibilisateurs et réalisateurs dans l'activation de l'oeuf de *Barnea candida*. *Bull. Acad. Belg. Cl. Sci.* **24**, 721–731.

Pasteels, J. J. (1965). Etude au microscope élec ronique de la réaction corticale. *J. Embryol. Exp. Morphol.* **13**, 327–339.

Paul, M. (1975). Release of acid and changes in light-scattering properties following fertilization of *Urechis caupo* eggs. *Dev. Biol.* **43**, 299–312.

Paul, M., and Epel, D. (1971). Fertilization associated light-scattering changes in eggs of the sea urchin, *Strongylocentrotus purpuratus*. *Exp. Cell Res.* **65**, 281–288.

Paul, M., and Epel, D. (1975). Formation of fertilization acid by sea urchin eggs does not require specific cations. *Exp. Cell Res.* **94**, 1–6.

Paul, M., and Johnston, R. N. (1978). Uptake of Ca^{2+} is one of the earliest responses to fertilization of sea urchin eggs. *J. Exp. Zool.* **203**, 143–149.

Paul, M., Johnson, J. D., and Epel, D. (1976). Fertilization acid of sea urchin eggs is not a consequence of cortical granule exocytosis. *J. Exp. Zool.* **197,** 127–133.

Payan, P., Girard, J., Christen, R., and Sardet, C. (1981). Na^+ movements and their oscillations during fertilization and cell cycle in sea urchin eggs. *Exp. Cell Res.* **134,** 339–344.

Peaucellier, G. (1978). Acid release at meiotic maturation of oocytes in the polychaete annelid *Sabellaria alveolata. Experientia* **34,** 789–790.

Peaucellier, G., and Doree, M. (1981). Acid release at activation and fertilization of starfish oocytes. *Dev., Growth Differ.* **23,** 287–296.

Perry, G., and Epel, D. (1977). Calcium stimulation of a lipoxygenase activity accounts for the respiratory burst at fertilization of the sea urchin egg. *J. Cell Biol.* **75,** 40a.

Perry, G., and Epel, D. (1981). Ca^{2+}-stimulated production of H_2O_2 from napthoquinone oxidation in *Arbacia* eggs. *Exp. Cell Res.* **134,** 65–72.

Petzelt, C. (1976). NH_3-treatment of unfertilized sea urchin eggs turns on the Ca^{2+}-ATPase cycle. *Exp. Cell Res.* **102,** 200–204.

Regier, J. C., and Kafatos, F. C. (1977). Absolute rate of protein synthesis in sea urchins with specific activity measurements of radioactive leucine and leucyl t-RNA. *Dev. Biol.* **57,** 270–283.

Robinson, K. R. (1976). Potassium is not compartmentalized within the unfertilized sea urchin egg. *Dev. Biol.* **48,** 466–472.

Rothschild, Lord (1938a). The biophysics of the egg surface of *Echinus esculentus* during fertilization and cytolysis. *J. Exp. Biol.* **15,** 209–216.

Rothschild, Lord (1938b). The effect of phlorizine on the metabolism of cytolysing sea-urchin eggs. *J. Exp. Biol.* **16,** 49–55.

Rothschild, Lord (1956). "Fertilization." Methuen, London.

Rothschild, Lord (1958). Acid production after fertilization of sea-urchin eggs. A re-examination of the lactic acid hypothesis. *J. Exp. Biol.* **35,** 843–849.

Rothschild, Lord, and Barnes, H. (1953). The inorganic constituents of the sea-urchin egg. *J. Exp. Biol.* **30,** 534–544.

Runnstrom, J. (1933). Zur Kenntnis der Stoffwechselvorgänge bei der Entwicklungserregung des Seeigeleies. *Biochem. Z.* **258,** 257–279.

Runnstrom, J. (1935a). Acid formation in frozen and thawed *Arbacia punctulata* eggs and its possible bearing on the problem of activation. *Biol. Bull. (Woods Hole, Mass.)* **69,** 345–350.

Runnstrom, J. (1935b). Influence of iodoacetate on activation and development of the eggs of *Arbacia punctulata. Biol. Bull. (Woods Hole, Mass.)* **69,** 351–355.

Salako, L. A., and Smith, A. J. (1970). Changes in sodium pool and kinetics of sodium transport in frog skin produced by amiloride. *Br. J. Pharmacol.* **39,** 99–109.

Sano, K., and Kanatani, H. (1980). External calcium ions are requisite for fertilization of sea urchin eggs by spermatozoa with reacted acrosomes. *Dev. Biol.* **78,** 242–246.

Sano, K., Usui, N., Ueki, K., Mohri, T., and Mohri, H. (1980). Magnesium ion-requiring step in fertilization of sea urchins. *Dev., Growth Differ.* **22,** 531–541.

Schackmann, R. W., Eddy, E. M., and Shapiro, B. M. (1978). The acrosome reaction of *Strongylocentrotus purpuratus* sperm. Ion requirements and movements. *Dev. Biol.* **65,** 483–495.

Schatten, G., and Hammer, M. (1979). Localization of sequestered calcium in unfertilized sea urchin eggs. *J. Cell Biol.* **83,** 199a.

Schatten, H., and Schatten, G. (1980). Surface activity at the egg plasma membrane during sperm incorporation and its cytochalasin B sensitivity. Scanning electron microscopy and time-lapse video microscopy during fertilization of the sea urchin, *Lytechinus variegatus*. *Dev. Biol.* **78,** 435–449.

Sheer, B. T., Monroy, A., Santangelo, M., and Riccobono, G. (1954). Action potentials in sea urchin eggs at fertilization. *Exp. Cell Res.* **7,** 284–287.

Schuel, H. (1978). Secretory functions of egg cortical granules in fertilization and development: A critical review. *Gamete Res.* **1,** 299–382.

Schuel, H., Troll, W., and Lorand, L. (1976). Physiological response of sea urchin eggs to stimulation by calcium ionophore A23187 analysed with protease inhibitors. *Exp. Cell Res.* **103,** 442–447.

Schuetz, A. W. (1975a). Cytoplasmic activation of starfish oocytes by sperm and ionophore A23187. *J. Cell Biol.* **66,** 86–94.

Schuetz, A. W. (1975b). Induction of nuclear breakdown and meiosis in *Spisula solidissima* oocytes by calcium ionophore. *J. Exp. Zool.* **191,** 433–440.

Scott, J. W. (1903). Periods of susceptibility in the differentiation of unfertilized eggs of *Amphitrite*. *Biol. Bull. (Woods Hole, Mass.)* **5,** 35–41.

Scott, J. W. (1906). Morphology of the parthenogenetic development of *Amphitrite*. *J. Exp. Zool.* **3,** 49–97.

Shapiro, B. M., Schackmann, R. W., and Gabel, C. A. (1981). Molecular approaches to the study of fertilization. *Annu. Rev. Biochem.* **50,** 815–843.

Shen, S. S. (1982). The effect of external ions on pH_i in sea urchin eggs. *In* "Intracellular pH: Its Measurement, Regulation and Utilization in Cellular Functions" (R. Nuccitelli and D. W. Deamer, eds.), pp. 269–282. Alan R. Liss, Inc., New York.

Shen, S. S., and Steinhardt, R. A. (1976). An electrophysiological study of the membrane properties of the immature and mature oocyte of the batstar, *Patiria miniata*. *Dev. Biol.* **48,** 148–162.

Shen, S. S., and Steinhardt, R. A. (1978). Direct measurement of intracellular pH during metabolic derepression of the sea urchin egg. *Nature (London)* **272,** 253–254.

Shen, S. S., and Steinhardt, R. A. (1979). Intracellular pH and the sodium requirement at fertilisation. *Nature (London)* **282,** 87–89.

Shen, S. S., and Steinhardt, R. A. (1980). Intracellular pH controls the development of new potassium conductance after fertilization of the sea urchin egg. *Exp. Cell Res.* **125,** 55–61.

Spitzer, N. C. (1979). Ion channels in development. *Annu. Rev. Neurosci.* **2,** 363–397.

Steinhardt, R. A. (1980). Control of cellular proliferation: Discussion. *Ann. N.Y. Acad. Sci.* **339,** 248–250.

Steinhardt, R. A., and Alderton, J. M. (1982). Calmodulin confers calcium sensitivity on secretory exocytosis. *Nature (London)* **295,** 154–155.

Steinhardt, R. A., and Epel, D. (1974). Activation of sea-urchin eggs by a calcium ionophore. *Proc. Natl. Acad. Sci. U.S.A.* **71,** 1915–1919.

Steinhardt, R. A., and Mazia, D. (1973). Development of K^+-conductance and membrane potentials in unfertilized sea urchin eggs after exposure to NH_4OH. *Nature (London)* **241,** 400–401.

Steinhardt, R. A., and Winkler, M. M. (1979). The ionic hypothesis of cell activation at fertilization. *In* "The Molecular Basis of Immune Cell Function" (J. G. Kaplan, ed.), pp. 11–27. Elsevier/North-Holland, Amsterdam.

Steinhardt, R. A., Lundin, L., and Mazia, D. (1971). Bioelectric responses of the echinoderm egg to fertilization. *Proc. Natl. Acad. Sci. U.S.A.* **68,** 2426–2430.

Steinhardt, R. A., Shen, S., and Mazia, D. (1972). Membrane potential, membrane resistance and an energy requirement for the development of potassium conductance in the fertilization reaction of echinoderm eggs. *Exp. Cell Res.* **72,** 195–203.

Steinhardt, R. A., Epel, D., Carroll, E. J., Jr., and Yanagimachi, R. (1974). Is calcium ionophore a universal activator for unfertilized eggs? *Nature (London)* **252,** 41–43.

Steinhardt, R. A., Zucker, R., and Schatten, G. (1977). Intracellular calcium release at fertilization in the sea urchin egg. *Dev. Biol.* **58,** 185–196.

Steinhardt, R. A., Shen, S. S., and Zucker, R. S. (1978). Direct evidence for ionic messengers in the two phases of metabolic derepression at fertilization in the sea urchin egg. *In* "Cell Reproduction" (E. R. Dirksen, D. Prescott, and C. F. Fox, eds.), pp. 415–424. Academic Press, New York.

Sugiyama, M. (1956). Physiological analysis of the cortical response of the sea urchin eggs. *Exp. Cell Res.* **10,** 364–376.

Taglietti, V. (1979). Early electrical response to fertilization in sea urchin eggs. *Exp. Cell Res.* **120,** 448–451.

Takahashi, K. (1979). Ionic channels in the egg membrane. *In* "Neurobiology of Chemical Transmission" (M. Otsuka and Z. W. Hall, eds.), pp. 103–122. Wiley, New York.

Tasaki, I., and Hagiwara, S. (1957). Demonstration of two stable potential states in the squid giant axon under tetraethylammonium chloride. *J. Gen. Physiol.* **40,** 859–885.

Thomas, R. C. (1974). Intracellular pH of snail neurones measured with a new pH-sensitive glass microelectrode. *J. Physiol. (London)* **238,** 159–180.

Thomas, R. C. (1976). Construction and properties of recessed-tip microelectrodes for sodium and chloride ions and pH. *In* "Ion and Enzyme Electrodes in Biology and Medicine" (M. Kessler, L. C. Clark, Jr., D. W. Lubbers, I. A. Silver, and W. Simon, eds.), pp. 141–148. Urban & Schwarzenberg, Berlin.

Tileny, L. G., and Jaffe, L. A. (1980). Actin, microvilli, and the fertilization cone of sea urchin eggs. *J. Cell Biol.* **87,** 771–782.

Treadwell, A. L. (1902). Notes on the nature of "artificial parthenogenesis" in the egg of *Podarke obscura. Biol. Bull. (Woods Hole, Mass.)* **3,** 235–240.

Tupper, J. T. (1973). Potassium exchangeability, potassium permeability, and membrane potential: Some observations in relation to protein synthesis in the early echinoderm embryo. *Dev. Biol.* **32,** 140–154.

Tupper, J. T. (1974). Inhibition of increased potassium permeability following fertilization of the echinoderm embryo: Its relationship to the initiation of protein synthesis and potassium exchangeability. *Dev. Biol.* **38,** 332–345.

Tyler, A. (1941). Artificial parthenogenesis. *Biol. Rev. Cambridge Philos. Soc.* **16,** 291–336.

Tyler, A. (1958). Changes in efflux and influx of potassium upon fertilization in eggs of *Arbacia punctulata* measured by use of K^{42} *Biol. Bull. (Woods Hole, Mass.)* **115,** 339–340.

Tyler, A., and Bauer, H. (1937). Polar body extrusion and cleavage in artificially activated eggs of *Urechis caupo. Biol. Bull. (Woods Hole, Mass.)* **73,** 164–180.

Tyler, A., and Monroy, A. (1955). Apparent and real micro-injection of echinoderm eggs. *Biol. Bull. (Woods Hole, Mass.)* **109,** 370.

Tyler, A., and Monroy, A. (1956). Change in the release of K^{42} upon fertilization in eggs of *Arbacia punctulata. Biol. Bull. (Woods Hole, Mass.)* **111,** 296.

Tyler, A., and Monroy, A. (1959). Change in rate of transfer of potassium across the membrane upon fertilization of eggs of *Arbacia punctulata. J. Exp. Zool.* **142,** 675–690.

Tyler, A., Monroy, A., Kao, C. Y., and Grundfest, H. (1956). Membrane potential and resistance of the starfish egg before and after fertilization. *Biol. Bull. (Woods Hole, Mass.)* **111,** 153–177.

Vacquier, V. D. (1975). The isolation of intact cortical granules from sea urchin eggs: Calcium ions trigger granule discharge. *Dev. Biol.* **43**, 62–74.

Vacquier, V. D. (1976). Isolated cortical granules: A model system for studying membrane fusion and calcium-mediated exocytosis. *J. Supramol. Struct.* **5**, 27–35.

Vacquier, V. D. (1981). Dynamic changes of the egg cortex. *Dev. Biol.* **84**, 1–26.

Vacquier, V. D., and Brandriff, B. (1975). DNA synthesis in unfertilized sea urchin eggs can be turned on and turned off by the addition and removal of procaine hydrochloride. *Dev. Biol.* **47**, 12–31.

Vacquier, V. D., and Moy, G. W. (1977). Isolation of bindin: The protein responsible for adhesion of sperm to sea urchin egg. *Proc. Natl. Acad. Sci. U.S.A.* **74**, 2456–2460.

Warburg, O. (1910). Über die Oxidationen in lebenden Zellen nach Versuchen am Seeigelei. *Hoppe-Seyler's Physiol. Chem.* **66**, 305–340.

Whitaker, M. J., and Steinhardt, R. A. (1981). The relation between the increase in reduced nicotinamide nucleotides and the initiation of DNA synthesis in sea urchin eggs. *Cell* **25**, 95–103.

Wilbur, K. M. (1939). The relation of the magnesium ion to ultra-violet stimulation in the *Nereis* egg. *Physiol. Zool.* **12**, 102–109.

Wilbur, K. M. (1941). The stimulating action of citrates and oxalates on the *Nereis* egg. *Physiol. Zool.* **14**, 84–95.

Wilt, F. H., and Mazia, D. (1974). The stimulation of cytoplasmic polyadenylation in sea urchin eggs by ammonia. *Dev. Biol.* **37**, 422–424.

Winkler, M. M., and Grainger, J. L. (1978). Mechanism of action of NH_4Cl and other weak bases in the activation of sea urchin eggs. *Nature (London)* **273**, 536–538.

Winkler, M. M., and Steinhardt, R. A. (1981). Activation of protein synthesis in a sea urchin cell-free system. *Dev. Biol.* **84**, 432–439.

Winkler, M. M., Steinhardt, R. A., Grainger, J. L., and Minning, L. (1980). Dual ionic controls for the activation of protein synthesis at fertilization. *Nature (London)* **287**, 558–560.

Winkler, M. M., Matson, G. B., Hershey, J. W., and Bradbury, E. M. (1982). ^{31}P-NMR study of the activation of the sea urchin egg. *Exp. Cell Res.* **139**, 217–222.

Zampetti-Bosseler, F., Huez, G., and Brachet, J. (1973). Effects of several inhibitors of macromolecule synthesis upon maturation of marine invertebrate oocytes. *Exp. Cell Res.* **78**, 383–393.

Zucker, R. S., and Steinhardt, R. A. (1978). Prevention of the cortical reaction in fertilized sea urchin eggs by injection of calcium-chelating ligands. *Biochim. Biophys. Acta* **541**, 459–466.

Zucker, R. S., and Steinhardt, R. A. (1979). Calcium activation of the cortical reaction in sea urchin eggs. *Nature (London)* **279**, 820.

Zucker, R. S., Steinhardt, R. A., and Winkler, M. M. (1978). Intracellular calcium release and the mechanisms of parthenogenetic activation of the sea urchin egg. *Dev. Biol.* **65**, 285–295.

6

Sperm–Egg Interactions in Invertebrates

ALINA C. LOPO

Mechanism and Control of Animal Fertilization
Copyright © 1983 by Academic Press, Inc.
All rights of reproduction in any form reserved.
ISBN 0-12-328520-8

I. INTRODUCTION

From the earliest fertilization studies of the late 1800s, invertebrate organisms have provided a rich source of experimental material. Examination of the contributions from marine laboratories throughout the world reveals that virtually every invertebrate that is readily accessible has been used for analysis of the interaction of sperm and eggs.

The gametes of well over 100 species of invertebrates have been used to study fertilization. The bulk of this work has utilized the eggs and sperm of echinoderms, particularly sea urchins (class Echinoidea). In addition to being plentiful and easy to maintain in the laboratory, sea urchins have many other attractive features that make them particularly useful in a study of the events of fertilization. The sexes are separate, and the gametes are easy to manipulate because fertilization is external. Fertilization and development take place in seawater; thus, the experimental medium has been defined and is simple to replicate. A single adult sea urchin yields generous quantities of pure gametes (5 ml on the average, depending on the species) that, when mixed, interact within seconds and continue development synchronously as far as the larval pluteus stage. The eggs are relatively yolk-free (compared to other organisms) and small enough to facilitate observations with the light microscope. The large quantities of material coupled with the synchrony of development make sea urchin gametes an ideal material in a study of the biochemical aspects of fertilization and early development. Finally, the many features in common with mammalian fertilization make sea urchin fertilization yet more valuable as a model toward an understanding of the molecular details of sperm–egg interaction (Table I).

This chapter examines the early interactions between sperm and egg, from the time of initial recognition of the egg by the sperm to the fusion of the gamete plasma membranes. Because most of this work has been done using the gametes of sea urchins, sand dollars, and sea stars, much of the information presented will deal with echinoderms. Other systems in which detailed study has demonstrated the universality of some of these mechanisms are also discussed in detail. For additional information on invertebrate fertilization, see Giudice (1973), Czihak (1975), Epel and Vacquier (1978), Epel (1978), Vacquier (1980), Lopo and Vacquier (1981), Shapiro (1981), and Shapiro et al. (1981).

TABLE I

Biochemical Events Common to Sea Urchin and Mammalian Fertilization[a]

1. The sperm membranes contain species-specific proteins involved in "recognition" of the egg surface before the acrosome reaction (Lopo and Vacquier, 1980b; Peterson *et al.*, 1980).
2. Occurrence of an acrosome reaction (Dan, 1952; Austin, 1966).
3. Calcium is necessary for the induction of the acrosome reaction (Dan, 1954a,b; Yanagimachi and Usui, 1974; Collins, 1976; Decker *et al.*, 1976; Summers *et al.*, 1976; Talbot *et al.*, 1976).
4. Cyclic nucleotide metabolism is altered in sperm during the acrosome reaction (Garbers and Kopf, 1980).
5. A protease is exposed as a result of the acrosome reaction (Levine *et al.*, 1978; Levine and Walsh, 1979, 1980; Meizel, 1978; Lui and Meizel, 1979; Green and Summers, 1980).
6. Sperm bind to receptors on the extracellular egg coat: the vitelline layer in sea urchins and the zona pellucida in the mammal (Aketa, 1967; Tsuzuki and Aketa, 1969; Aketa *et al.*, 1972; Tsuzuki *et al.*, 1977; Glabe and Vacquier, 1977a, 1978; Glabe and Lennarz, 1979, 1981; Dunbar *et al.*, 1980; Bleil and Wassarman, 1980b).
7. Attachment of sperm to eggs after the acrosome reaction exhibits species specificity (Hanada and Chang, 1972; Yanagimachi, 1972, 1977, 1978; Summers and Hylander, 1976; Kinsey *et al.*, 1980).
8. "Sperm receptor" glycoproteins can be isolated from both the zona pellucida (Bleil and Wassarman, 1980a,b) and the vitelline layer (Schmell *et al.*, 1977; Glabe and Vacquier, 1978).
9. A Ca^{2+} transient in the egg triggers the cortical granule reaction after sperm–egg fusion has occurred (Gilkey *et al.*, 1976; Fulton and Whittingham, 1978; Zucker *et al.*, 1978).
10. A trypsinlike protease released from cortical granules destroys the sperm-binding capacity of the sea urchin vitelline layer (Vacquier *et al.*, 1973; Carroll and Epel, 1975) and the mammalian zona pellucida (Barros and Yanagimachi, 1971; Gwatkin *et al.*, 1973).
11. A peroxidase released from cortical granules hardens the vitelline layer (Foerder and Shapiro, 1977; Hall, 1978) and the zona pellucida (Schmell and Gulyas, 1980) by catalyzing the formation of di- and trityrosine crosslinks between the component proteins.
12. Fusion of sperm and egg results in activation of the new synthetic machinery of the egg and in cell division (Epel, 1978).
13. Sea urchin and mammalian sperm have cross-reacting surface antigens (Lopo and Vacquier, 1980c).

[a] Adapted from Lopo and Vacquier, 1981, with permission of Plenum Press.

II. OVERVIEW OF INVERTEBRATE FERTILIZATION

A. Eggs

The eggs of most invertebrate organisms are spherical cells exhibiting a wide range in size. The eggs are in some stage of meiotic arrest at fertilization, except for those of coelenterates and echinoids, which complete meiosis prior to ovulation.

Most invertebrate eggs have one or more extracellular coats or layers, usually composed of glycoprotein or polysaccharide material. These coats may be fairly simple, as in sea urchins (Kidd, 1978; Chandler and Heuser, 1979, 1981), or fairly complex, as in ascidians (Rosati and De Santis, 1978; Dale *et al.*, 1978; De Santis *et al.*, 1980). The extracellular coats serve a protective function during development as well as play a key role in sperm–egg interaction.

In the sea urchin egg the plasma membrane bears many short microvilli, about 0.2 ×m in length (Tegner and Epel, 1973, 1976; Schroeder, 1978; Mazia *et al.*, 1975). External and tightly apposed to the plasma membrane is the vitelline layer, an extracellular glycoprotein coat 100–300 Å in thickness (Tegner and Epel, 1973, 1976; Glabe and Vacquier, 1977a; Chandler and Heuser, 1979, 1981). Casts or impressions of the plasma membrane microvilli are seen on the vitelline layer (Tegner and Epel, 1973, 1976). Receptors for sperm are found on its external surface (Aketa, 1967; Aketa *et al.*, 1972; Glabe and Vacquier, 1977a, 1978; Glabe and Lennarz, 1979, 1981). Surrounding the egg is a second extracellular coat, the jelly coat. The jelly coat is the first egg substance that the sperm contacts when it approaches the egg. Egg jelly is a transparent, amorphous material composed of both carbohydrate and protein (SeGall and Lennarz, 1979). Its function and biochemistry are considered in gerater detail later in this chapter (Section IV,B,1).

B. Sperm

Sperm are highly specialized cells, with only one function: to fertilize an egg. Their structure and biochemistry reflect this specialization. In sea urchins, sperm have the typical morphology of most animal sperm, and are composed of three parts: a head, a midpiece, and a tail, all limited by a plasma membrane. The dominant structure in the head is the nucleus, containing highly condensed inactive chromatin. At the anterior tip, subjacent to the plasma membrane, is a membrane-bound vesicle, the acrosome. The acrosome contains as a major constituent the protein bindin, which is known to mediate the binding of sperm to egg (Vacquier and Moy, 1977; Glabe and Vacquier, 1978; Glabe and Lennarz, 1979, 1981; Moy and Vacquier, 1979). Immediately posterior to the acrosome is the subacrosomal fossa, which in other echinoderms has been shown to contain unpolymerized G-actin, or profilactin (Tilney *et al.*, 1973). This actin polymerizes to give rise to an acrosome process during initial interaction with the egg (see Section IV,A). Posterior to the nucleus, in the midpiece region, is a single mitochondrion. The tail has the characteristic structure of a eukaryotic flagellum. When sperm are released from the testes they are anoxic and closely packed together ("dry" sperm). Following dilution into seawater, they begin swimming.

Sperm of some other invertebrate show greater or lesser departures from the "typical" morphology. In some species, such as some tunicates and some coelenterates, the acrosome is small or absent (Hinsch, 1974; Woollacott, 1977). In others [e.g., *Mytilus* (the mussel) or *Limulus* (the horseshoe crab; Tilney and Mooseker, 1976; Tilney *et al.*, 1979)], there is a pre-formed acrosome process, poised and ready to extend through the acrosome granule under the correct stimulus. Finally, there are some crustacean sperm that so diverge in structure that they have no trace of the "typical" sperm morphology. These unusual sperm are discussed in more detail later in this chapter (Section VII,B).

C. Overview of Fertilization

Fertilization encompasses the period from initial sperm–egg interaction to fusion of the egg and sperm pronuclei. In sea urchins the entire process requires 20–30 minutes, depending on the species. Initial gamete contact is between the sperm and the egg jelly coat. The egg jelly interacts with the sperm surface to induce the acrosome reaction. The acrosome reaction involves a series of intricate ionic movements that result in the extension of an acrosome process and exposure of the contents of the acrosome. As the acrosome process extends it becomes coated with the acrosome contents, including the sperm-egg binding protein, bindin (Vacquier and Moy, 1977). Sperm attachment to the vitelline layer is mediated by the interaction of bindin with receptors on the vitelline layer. Following attachment, the sperm penetrates the vitelline layer and the plasma membrane of the two cells fuse. The sperm nucleus penetrates into the egg cytoplasm and is transformed into a male pronucleus (Longo, 1976, 1978; Longo and

Kunkel, 1978; Carron and Longo, 1980). The two pronuclei move together, fuse, and DNA synthesis begins in preparation for first cleavage (Mar, 1980; Schatten and Schatten, 1980; Bestor and Schatten, 1981).

III. RECOGNITION OF THE EGG BY THE SPERM— CHEMOTACTIC INTERACTIONS DURING INVERTEBRATE FERTILIZATION

A. Chemotactic Responses of Sperm

Although chemotaxis has been repeatedly demonstrated in plant gamete interaction since Pfeffer's (1884) early work (Rothschild, 1952; Brokaw, 1957; Müller et al., 1979, 1981), the existence of chemotactic phenomena between invertebrate gametes was largely discounted until relatively recently (Monroy, 1965). The first clear-cut demonstration of sperm chemotaxis in invertebrates was made by Richard L. Miller in the cnidarian *Campanularia* (Hydrozoa; Miller, 1966). Since that time, sperm chemotactic behavior has been convincingly demonstrated in over two dozen cnidarians (Miller, 1966, 1977a,b, 1978, 1979a,b, 1980; Miller and Brokaw, 1970; Miller and Tseng, 1974), five species of tunicates (Chordata: Urochordata; Miller, 1975), and six species of chitons (Mollusca: Polyplacophora; Miller, 1977a,b). In all these cases the sperm exhibit gradient-directed turning behavior (i.e., they reorient and swim toward the source of the attractant). In both the cnidaria and tunicates studied so far, the sperm attractant is highly species specific, suggesting that there must be receptors on the sperm that interact with the attractant. However, there is no species specificity seen in the response of chiton sperm to egg attractants (Miller, 1977a).

Does sperm chemotaxis actually have a role in fertilization? Its demonstrated occurrence in only a few unrelated groups suggests that this phenomenon evolved independently on several occasions and is not prerequisite to successful gamete interaction. However, sperm chemotaxis may be more widespread in the animal kingdom than is now known. Miller (1977b) reevaluated evidence from early workers and tentatively proposed the existence of sperm chemotaxis in the Bryozoa, Chaetognatha, and some vertebrates (fish). He also feels that there is circumstantial evidence suggesting sperm chemotactic phenomena are present in the Porifera and Echinoidea (Miller, 1977b). An obvious advantage of chemotaxis in sessile organisms such as hydroids is that, because fertilization is internal, the release of attractant by the female epithelial cells ensures that the sperm will reach an egg. In organisms where fertilization is external, chemotaxis effectively increases the volume of the egg as a target for sperm (Miller, 1980). Although it has not been conclusively shown that sperm are capable of fertilization after exposure to the attractant (Miller, 1980), it seems likely that any sperm that reaches the egg must have been exposed to the attractant and interacted with it. More extensive study of the occurrence of sperm chemotaxis in animal phyla is necessary before the importance of this phenomenon in fertilization can be evaluated.

B. The Swarming Response of Echinoid Sperm

When exposed to solubilized egg jelly, the sperm of many sea urchin species undergo a behavioral response known as "swarming," cluster formation (Loeb, 1916), or isoagglutination (Loeb, 1916; Lillie, 1919; Epel, 1978; Metz, 1978). During swarming, actively swimming sperm aggregate into very dense clumps that may be as large as 2–4 mm (Loeb, 1916; Lillie, 1919; Collins, 1976). After a period of time varying from 30 seconds to 10 minutes, depending on the age of the sperm and the concentration of the jelly, the swarms disperse spontaneously. Sperm that have swarmed lose their fertilizing capacity and fail to swarm again if fresh jelly is added.

The swarming response, which has been known since the early 1900s (Loeb, 1916; Lillie, 1919), formed the basis for the "fertil-izin–antifertilizin" theory of Lillie (later modified by Tyler, 1949). Early workers considered this phenomenon an isoagglutination of the sperm cells (Lillie, 1913a,b, 1915, 1919; Tyler and O'Melveny, 1941; Tyler, 1948, 1949; see also Vacquier, 1979; Vacquier et al. (1979), for a discussion of the Lillie-Loeb controversy). Recently, Collins (1976) investigated swarming and concluded that it is not a true agglutination (see also Loeb, 1916). The cells do not come into actual contact because the clusters cannot be fixed (Collins, 1976). Cluster formation is reversibly inhibited by inclusion of respiratory inhibitors in the medium (Lillie, 1914, 1919; Loeb, 1916; Collins, 1976), showing that the process depends on swimming of the sperm. Sperm mixed with jelly in calcium-free seawater (Dan, 1954a,b; Collins, 1976) will swarm, although they will not undergo the acrosome reaction.

An involvement of chemotaxis in the swarming response of sea urchin sperm has been postulated but never demonstrated (Lillie, 1919; Collins, 1976). Using *Arbacia punctulata,* Lopo et al. (1977) demonstrated the possible existence of a secondary chemoattractant present in the medium, following the initial interaction of sperm with egg jelly that may be responsible for the formation and maintenance of the clusters. Their results suggested that in this species, the swarming sperm release a substance that acts as a secondary chemoattractant. The nature of the signal was investigated but not discovered. Using the same assay system, A. C. Lopo and D. Epel (unpublished results) found that, at least by this procedure, secondary chemotaxis was not demonstrable in *Strongylocentrotus purpuratus* sperm. One possible explanation for this discrepancy is that the chemotactic molecule in *S. purpuratus* is too large to pass through the filters used in the assay.

Another poorly understood aspect of the swarming reaction of sea urchin sperm is its spontaneous reversibility. Tyler (1949) and Metz (1967) suggested that reversibility results from modification of the agglutinating substance of jelly (fertilizin) by sperm from a multivalent form to a univalent form. The multivalent form, in a manner analogous to agglutination by immunoglobins, presumably links cells together into aggregates (Tyler, 1949). During swarming, the sperm somehow break up the multivalent fertilizin (egg jelly) into univalent form. The univalent form binds to the sperm surface, filling all available receptors, but is unable to agglutinate sperm. Hathaway and Metz (1962) presented evidence that ^{35}S-labeled jelly remains bound to sperm that have deagglutinated. However, the recent data of SeGall and Lennarz (1979) and Kopf and Garbers (1980) on isolation of the fucose sulfate-rich fraction from egg jelly show that this material induces the acrosome reaction but not agglutination in sperm, suggesting that the radioactivity is bound to receptors involved in the acrosome reaction but not in swarming. SeGall and Lennarz (1979) have not analyzed the biological activity of the sailoprotein component of egg jelly; however, Isaka *et al.* (1970) reported that swarming in Japanese sea urchins is associated with the sialoprotein fraction from fractionated egg jelly. Further analysis of this phenomenon will require a more complete characterization of the swarm-inducing substance from egg jelly. The agglutinating substance from egg jelly of the starfish *Asterias amurensis* has been isolated and characterized (Uno and Hoshi, 1978). Chemical analysis indicates that the agglutinin is a saponin. However, unlike the case in sea urchins, in starfish the agglutinin is not reversible, and the clusters can be preserved by fixatives, suggesting that the nature of the response is different in asteroids.

Does sperm swarming have a role in fertilization? Lillie (1919) believed that the agglutinating substance, "fertilizin," was modified by the sperm to a form that could induce the activation of the egg. Sperm need not swarm in order to fertilize; sperm of at least one genus, *Lytechinus,* do not swarm at all. However, *S. purpuratus* sperm will swarm in *Lytechinus* egg jelly (Collins, 1976), again suggesting that the swarm-inducing factor is released by sperm. Hagström (1958, 1959) suggested that one role for egg jelly is to keep excess sperm from reaching the egg surface and thus prevent polyspermy. Swarming would thus remove a considerable number from the population of potential fertilizing sperm. It is also possible that the swarming response has the opposite effect, i.e., it allows the attraction of sufficient numbers of sperm to the egg to permit successful fertilization (Epel, 1978). The transient nature of the phenomenon would keep sperm from being attracted to already fertilized eggs. The role of this phenomenon in sperm physiology and fertilization remains unknown.

IV. RECOGNITION OF THE EGG BY THE SPERM—THE ACROSOME REACTION

Whether sperm reach the egg by random motion or by a directed response to a specific stimulus, many additional interactions are required before fertilization is successful and complete. In a large majority of species, the sperm must undergo an acrosome reaction before attachment to the egg and penetration of its extracellular envelope can take place. Because more is known about the acrosome reaction in echinoderm sperm than in any other invertebrate phylum, the following discussion deals primarily with this group.

A. Morphological Events

Echinoderm sperm undergo the acrosome reaction on exposure to egg jelly. The acrosome reaction was first described (although unwittingly) by Herman Fol (1878–1879) in *Asterias.* He observed that the initial contact between gametes was via a thin filament. These observations were later substantiated by Chambers (1930), who termed the filament an "insemination filament." Both authors, however, attributed the filament to the egg and not to the sperm, and presumed that the function was to attach the sperm and draw it toward the egg.

The first observation of a change in sperm during fertilization was made by Popa, who in 1927 described the loss of the acrosome as a response to egg jelly and correctly observed that the material in the granule was responsible for the attachment of sperm to other objects. The significance of these observations, however, was not clearly understood until reinterpreted by Jean Clark Dan in the early 1950s, following her detailed ultrastructural and physiological studies of the acrosome reaction (Dan, 1952, 1956, 1967).

The first visible change in sperm undergoing the acrosome reaction is the formation of several fusion sites between the acrosome membrane and the overlying plasma membrane (Colwin and Colwin, 1967; Summers *et al.*, 1975). This fusion exposes the contents of the acrosome to the extracellular medium. At the same time, unpolymerized G-actin, or profilactin (Tilney *et al.*, 1973; Tilney, 1976a,b, stored in the subacrosomal space (nuclear fossa), begins to polymerize into filamentous F-actin to form a bundle of microfilaments anchored to a specialized region of the outer surface of the nuclear envelope (Tilney, 1976a). Because the polymerization of the actin is toward the apex of the sperm, the microfilament bundle pierces the now-exposed acrosome as it extends. As a result, it becomes coated with the acrosome contents. The result is a rearrangement of the anterior end of the sperm, so that the acrosome-reacted sperm bears a fingerlike process at its anterior end that is composed of a core of microfilaments anchored proximally to the outer nuclear membrane and distally to the plasma membrane overlying the tip of the process.

The length of the acrosome process is species specific: most sea urchins, approximately 1 μm; *Pisaster*, 15 μm; *Asterias*, 25 μm; and *Thyone*, 90 μm (Tilney *et al.*, 1973, 1978). Regardless of the length of the acrosome process, there is a sizable amount of plasma membrane that must appear in a very brief period of time (< 50 msec in *Limulus*; Tilney *et al.*, 1979). There is evidence that in the horseshoe crab (*Limulus*), with an acrosome process > 50 μm in length, the excess membrane is derived from the outer nuclear envelope (Tilney *et al.*, 1979). However, the source of additional membrane in echinoderm sperm is unknown.

An interesting feature of the formation of the acrosome process is the polarity of polymerization. Tilney (1976a,b) has presented evidence for specialization during spermatogenesis of the region of the nuclear envelope around the subacrosomal space. This allows the preferential binding of actin and its associated proteins to the nuclear membrane, resulting in a nonrandom distribution of the g-actin in the developing sperm (Tilney, 1976a). Polarity of polymerization for this actin appears to be provided by the "actomere" (Tilney, 1978), an organelle found in the subacrosomal space (nuclear fossa) of *Thyone* sperm prior to the acrosome reaction. The actomere consists of 20–25 short microfilaments and is believed to act as a nucleating center during polymerization of the profilactin into the microfilaments of the acrosome process.

Levine *et al.* (1978; Levine and Walsh, 1979, 1980) recently demonstrated that a serine protease is exposed during the induction of the acrosome reaction in *S. purpuratus*. Furthermore, they showed that inhibition of the enzyme prior to extension of the acrosome process inhibits its formation (Levine and Walsh, 1979). The enzyme has been localized to the acrosome process in *S. purpuratus* sperm (Green and Summers, 1980). The involvement of sperm proteases and other lytic compounds in penetration of egg envelopes is discussed in Section VI,A.

B. The Induction of the Acrosome Reaction

1. Egg Jelly, the Natural Inducer of the Acrosome Reaction

In sea urchins, the natural inducer of the acrosome reaction is the egg jelly. Egg jelly is a heterogeneous substance composed of about 20% protein and 80% polysaccharide [see Monroy (1965) for a review of the early literature on egg jelly]. There has been disagreement over the kinds and numbers of molecules found in egg jelly (Monroy, 1965; Stern, 1967; Stern and Metz, 1967; Hotta *et al.,* 1970a,b, 1973; Isaka *et al.,* 1970; Ishihara *et al.,* 1973; Lorenzi and Hedrick, 1973). Recently, SeGall and Lennarz (1979, 1981) biochemically characterized the egg jelly from four species of sea urchins, *Strongylocentrotus purpuratus, S. droebachiensis, Arbacia punctulata,* and *Lytechinus variegatus.* They found that the egg jellies of the four species studied were chemically very similar and contained a sialoprotein (20% of the total mass) and a fucose sulfate-rich component (80%; SeGall and Lennarz, 1979; see also Kopf and Garbers, 1980). The acrosome reaction-inducing activity was found to reside in the fucose sulfate-rich fraction, with no detectable activity in the sialoprotein component. In the four species examined, the composition of the fucose sulfate component was strikingly similar (SeGall and Lennarz, 1979). Subsequent structural studies (SeGall and Lennarz, 1981) using proton nuclear magnetic resonance (NMR), periodate oxidation, and infrared analysis have provided evidence that the fucose sulfate molecules from the four species of sea urchin show differences in the position of glycosidic linkages and the position of sulfation. Thus, although the fucose sulfate polysaccharides are compositionally similar, they are structurally different. A fucose-rich factor having similar properties to those isolated by SeGall and Lennarz (1979, 1981) has been purified by Kopf and Garbers (1980) from *S. purpuratus* egg jelly.

Using both soluble egg jelly and the purified fucose-sulfate polysaccharide, SeGall and Lennarz (1979) examined the species specificity of the acrosome reaction-inducing activity. They found that sperm of some species react only when exposed to homologous egg jelly (a fucose–sulfate polysaccharide), but others undergo the acrosome reaction in the presence of heterologous components (SeGall and Lennarz, 1979). For example, sperm of *Arbacia punctulata* or *Strongylocentrotus droebachiensis* undergo the acrosome reaction only when exposed to homologous jelly, while *S. purpuratus* and *Lytechinus variegatus* sperm show less specificity and will react with jelly of other species, but not all (SeGall and Lennarz, 1979). In addition, SeGall and Lennarz (1981) examined the effect of reactive and nonreactive jelly coats on the obligatory Ca^{2+} uptake that occurs during the acrosome reaction (see Section IV,C). Ca^{2+} uptake did not occur in the presence of nonreactive jelly coat. Furthermore, mixing reactive and nonreactive jelly coats did not inhibit Ca^{2+} uptake. This suggests that there is a difference in the ability of the different egg jellies to bind to a given species of sperm and, more importantly, points to the existence of a receptor for egg jelly on the sperm surface (SeGall and Lennarz, 1981; see also Kopf and Garbers, 1980).

The lack of exclusive species specificity in the interaction of sperm with egg jelly correlates well with work of Summers and Hylander (1975). They showed that 9 of 11 heterologous crosses induced the acrosome reaction, although there was no sperm–egg binding or fertilization. These studies (Summers and Hylander, 1975; SeGall and Lennarz, 1979) lend support to the idea that the species specificity of fertilization and, hence, reproductive isolation is not limited to specificity in induction of the acrosome reaction but also resides in the specificity of interaction of the bindin from the acrosome granule with receptors on the vitelline layer of the egg (see Section V,A).

2. The Sperm Surface

The sperm plasma membrane is a prime participant in fertilization, because it is at the level of the plasma membrane that the initial interaction between the two gametes takes place. This is true whether the first recognition event is chemotaxis, capacitation, or the induction of the acrosome reaction. It follows that receptors to the egg substances that elicit initial recognition must exist on the sperm surface. Thus, it is of interest to know the composition of the sperm plasma membrane.

In the last 5 years there has been considerable progress in our understanding of the composition of the mammalian sperm plasma membrane (Friend *et al.*, 1977; Millette, 1979; Oliphant and Singhas, 1979; O'Rand and Porter, 1979; Herr and Eddy, 1980; Millette and Bellvé, 1980; O'Rand and Romrell, 1980a,b, 1981; Primakoff *et al.*, 1980; Bradley *et al.*, 1981; Feuchther *et al.*, 1981; Friend and Heuser, 1981; Ji *et al.*, 1981; Millette and Moulding, 1981). These studies have revealed that there are glycoprotein, protein (Friend and Rudolf, 1974; Friend *et al.*, 1977; Primakoff *et al.*, 1980; Feuchther *et al.*, 1981; Friend and Heuser, 1981), and lipid-restricted domains (Bearer and Friend, 1980, 1981) that correlate with functional regions of the plasma membrane. However, function has not been defined for any of these molecules.

Until recently, information on the composition of the plasma membrane of invertebrate sperm was very limited. Work that used fluorescein-labeled lectins revealed that there is topographic heterogeneity in sea urchin (Aketa, 1975) and ascidian (Rosati *et al.*, 1978) sperm. In the Japanese sea urchin *Anthocidaris crassispina*, fluorescein isothiocyanate-Con A (FITC-Con A) binds primarily to the anterior tip and midpiece of the sperm (Aketa, 1975). In addition, the univalent lectin blocks fertilization. Conversely, *Hemicentrotus pulcherrimus* sperm bind wheat germ agglutinin (WGA), but not Con A, and only univalent WGA blocks fertilization (Aketa, 1975). This suggests that at least in these two species, there are species-specific differences in the surface carbohydrates on the sperm surface and that they may be involved in some initial recognition step between the gametes.

Additional support for sperm surface heterogeneity in invertebrates comes from the work of Gabel *et al.* (1979), in which sea urchin (*S. purpuratus*) sperm were labeled with FITC. This reagent reacts covalently with exposed amino groups. The sperm bind the fluorescent label nonuniformly, with most of the fluorescence associated with the midpiece (Gabel *et al.*, 1979). Because the FITC can be radioiodinated to yield [^{125}I]FITC (Gabel and Shapiro, 1978), the fluorescent molecular components could be identified by gel electrophoresis and autoradiography. Most of the label is associated with a polypeptide of M_r 35,000–37,000 and several low-molecular-weight peptides. Following differential extraction with 3.3% Triton X-100, several polypeptides of higher molecular weight (M_r 55,000, 47,000, 30,000, and 24,000) were also labeled (Gabel *et al.*, 1979). However, because FITC is fairly lipid-soluble in sea urchin sperm [25% of the total label is in chloroform/methanol extractable material (Gabel *et al.*, 1979)], there may have been some labeling of internal proteins.

Lopo and Vacquier (1980a), using standard surface-labeling procedures, approached the problem by radiolabeling the surface of *S. purpuratus* sperm with ^{125}I. Following labeling, the sperm were viable, as evidenced by motility and the ability to undergo the egg jelly-induced acrosome reaction and to fertilize eggs (Lopo and Vacquier, 1980a). When Triton X-100 extracts prepared from ^{125}I-labeled sperm were separated on SDS-polyacrylamide gels, the label was associated with four glycoproteins (by periodic acid-Schiff (PAS) staining; Lopo and Vacquier, 1980a) of $M_r > 250,000$, 84,000, 64,000, and 52,000. Interestingly, 75% of the protein-incorporated radioactivity was associated with the (84K) and (64K) glycoproteins. By this procedure, the 84K and 64K components appeared to be relatively minor constituents of the Triton X-100 extractable material (Lopo and Vacquier, 1980a).

This unusual labeling pattern led to more extensive investigation of the 84K and 64K glycoproteins (Lopo and Vacquier, 1980b). Rabbit antisera against electrophoretically pure 84K and 64K were prepared and used to determine whether these glycoproteins played a role in fertilization. Immunoelectronmicroscopic studies that used the antisera indicated that both 84K and 64K were distributed over the entire sperm surface (Lopo and Vacquier, 1980b). Sperm preincubated with anti-84K Fab fragments were inhibited from undergoing the acrosome reaction when mixed with egg jelly; anti-64K Fab had no effect on the acrosome reaction (Lopo and Vacquier, 1980b). The acrosome reaction could still be induced when the Ca^{2+} ionophore A23187 or pH 9.2 was used, indicating that the mechanism of the reaction was still intact, and that the effect seen was due to blockage of a molecule having a role in the acrosome reaction, either as a jelly receptor or by mediating a later step in the reaction (Lopo and Vacquier, 1980b). The 84K glycoprotein was the first sperm surface component described that may have a role in the acrosome reaction. Although the lack of inhibition by the anti-64K Fab may be because 64K has no role in the induction of the acrosome reaction, an alternative explanation is that the binding of this antiserum did not alter the biological activity of 64K.

N. L. Cross (1983) has also characterized the sea urchin sperm membrane by radioiodination. Following labeling, a fraction containing plasma membrane was isolated (Gray and Drummond, 1976), then separated on SDS-polyacrylamide gels. By autoradiography, radioactivity was associated with five species of M_r 200,000, 149,000, 120,000, 77,000, and 60,000. All proved to be glycoproteins (by PAS staining) and externally disposed (by lactoperoxidase-catalyzed radioiodination. The 200,000, 77,000, and 60,000 components are likely to correspond to the 250,000, 84,000, and 64,000 species described by Lopo and Vacquier (1980a,b). The technique Cross used to isolate the sperm membranes is useful because it enriches the preparation with the molecules of interest.

Recently, Eckberg and Metz (1982) and Saling *et al.* (1982) described from *Arbacia punctulata* sperm two glycoproteins of similar molecular weight to those described by Lopo and Vacquier (1980a). Membrane preparations from sperm extracted with lithium diiodosalicylate revealed two PAS-positive components of M_r 68,000 and 85,000 (Eckberg and Metz, 1982). These authors also used immunological techniques to analyze the role of the sperm surface in the induction of the acrosome reaction. Fab fragments from antisera raised against *Arbacia* sperm homogenates inhibited the acrosome reaction and fertilization (Saling *et al.*, 1982). A23187 could by-pass the inhibition and produce a normal acrosome reaction and fertilization (Saling *et al.*, 1982). Addition of electrophoretically pure 68,000 glycoprotein eliminated the inhibitory activity of the Fab fragments (Eckberg and Metz, 1982), suggesting that this glycoprotein plays a role in the acrosome reaction.

Because the two studies described above were on different species, it is difficult to compare the results unequivocally. The 68,000 and 85,000 glycoproteins from *Arbacia* are likely similar or identical to the 64K and 84K from *S. purpuratus* (Lopo and Vacquier, 1980a,b). The results from these two studies suggest that both 68,000 glycoprotein and 84K may play different, but necessary, roles in the complex series of steps leading to the acrosome reaction.

Lipid analysis of sperm of the sea urchin *Strongylocentrotus intermedius* has been performed (Kozhina *et al.*, 1978). By thin-layer chromatography and gas-lipid chromatography, total membrane lipid was determined as 65.0% phospholipid, 15.5% cholesterol, and a negligible amount of triglyceride. The common membrane phospholipids were identified; among these, diphosphatidylglycerol, a characteristic component of mitochondrial membranes, was unusually high (9% of the total phospholipid content). Nagai and his colleagues (Isono and Nagai, 1966; Nagai and Ohsawa, 1974; Hoshi and Nagai, 1975; Nagai and Hoshi, 1975; Ohsawa and Nagai, 1975) performed careful studies on the glycolipids of gametes of several species of Japanese sea urchins. This work identified gamete- and species-specific sialoglycosphingolipids (Isono and Nagai, 1966; Nagai and Hoshi, 1975) containing sialic acids unique to sea urchin gametes. In addition, using antibodies, Nagai and Ohsawa (1974; Ohsawa and Nagai, 1975) demonstrated that these sialoglycosphingolipids isolated from sea urchin sperm were on the surface of the cell, that the agglutination by the antiserum was partially species specific, and that it could be blocked by specific sugars (100 mM; Ohsawa and Nagai, 1975).

C. Ionic Changes Modulating the Acrosome Reaction

The evidence presented in the preceding sections is consistent with the hypothesis that the acrosome reaction, a necessary prerequisite to successful fertilization, results from the interaction of egg jelly with the sperm surface. Although the molecular nature of this interaction is unknown, in the last few years significant progress has been made in our understanding of the ionic changes modulating the acrosome reaction.

1. Ca^{2+}

The dependence of the acrosome reaction on Ca^{2+} is well documented, not only for echinoderm sperm but for all animal sperm thus far examined (Dan, 1954a,b; Collins, 1976; Gregg and Metz, 1976; Decker *et al.*, 1976; Talbot *et al.*, 1976; Collins and Epel, 1977; Schackmann *et al.*, 1978; Schackmann and Shapiro, 1981). This requirement is for extracellular Ca^{2+}, since addition of the Ca^{2+}-ionophore A23187 to a sperm suspension in calcium-free seawater does not induce the reaction. Thus, there is uptake from the extracellular medium and not a mobilization of Ca^{2+} from intracellular stores (Decker *et al.*, 1976; Talbot *et al.*, 1976; Collins and Epel, 1977; Schackmann *et al.*, 1978). Mg^{2+} does not substitute for Ca^{2+} (Dan, 1956) and actually has an inhibitory effect (Collins and Epel, 1977), suggesting this is not a general divalent cation requirement.

Using ionophores, ion transport inhibitors, and radioactive isotopes, Schackmann *et al.* (1978; Schackmann and Shapiro, 1981) performed an extensive study of the kinds and sequence of ion movements occurring in sea urchin sperm during the acrosome reaction. Their results show that Ca^{2+} uptake occurs by two mechanisms during and following the acrosome reaction. The first is sensitive only to D600 (a calcium-channel blocker) and necessary for the induction of the acrosome reaction. The second is sensitive to respiratory inhibitors, insensitive to D600, and has no role in the acrosome reaction (Schackmann *et al.*, 1978; Schackmann and Shapiro, 1981). The second mechanism accounts for most of the net uptake of Ca^{2+} by the cell, and continues long after the acrosome process has formed, suggesting that is is not required for the generation of the process (Schackmann *et al.*, 1978; Kopf and Garbers, 1980; Schackmann and Shapiro, 1981). Additional analysis of the second, energy-dependent Ca^{2+} uptake supports the hypothesis that it is due to Ca^{2+} accumulation by the sperm mitochondrion (Schackmann and Shapiro, 1981).

2. pH

Loeb (1916) observed that increasing the alkalinity of the medium increased the frequency of cross-fertilization in interspecific crosses. That this was probably the result of a greater frequency of acrosome reactions due to increased extracellular pH was shown by Dan (1956). Sperm will not undergo the acrosome reaction if the pH is lower than 7; increasing the pH to 9 or higher induces the reaction, even in the absence of egg jelly (Loeb, 1916; Dan, 1956; Collins, 1976; Gregg and Metz, 1976; Decker et al., 1976; Collins and Epel, 1977; Tilney et al., 1978). These results suggest that there is H^+ efflux from sperm during the acrosome reaction.

Schackmann et al. (1978; Schackmann and Shapiro, 1981) confirmed and extended the early observations on release of acid from sperm. Following dilution of sperm into seawater, there is a period of acid release. This H^+ efflux has been previously reported (Ohtake, 1976a,b; Nishioka and Cross, 1978) and is likely the result of increased respiration by the sperm upon dilution. Consistent with this conclusion is the cyanide sensitivity of the efflux. Upon addition of egg jelly there is a release of acid that continues for about 10 seconds, followed by a slower release. The acrosome reaction does not take place until the jelly-induced release is complete (Schackmann et al., 1978). The jelly-induced acid release is not sensitive to respiratory inhibitors, but is sensitive to the calcium-channel blockers D600 and verapamil, suggesting that the H^+ release follows Ca^{2+} efflux (Schackmann et al., 1978).

3. Na⁺ and K⁺

The monovalent cations Na^+ and K^+ are also involved in the acrosome reaction (Schackmann et al., 1978; Schackmann and Shapiro, 1981). Exposing sperm to egg jelly results in rapid uptake of Na^+, coincident with the period of filament extension and rapid H^+ release (Schackmann and Shapiro, 1981). Blocking the Na^+ uptake by inhibitors of the acrosome reaction also blocks the H^+ efflux, suggesting Na^+ and H^+ movements are linked. The ratio of Na^+ uptake to acid release is approximately 1:1, so the stoichiometry of the reaction also suggests a coordinated exchange (Schackmann and Shapiro, 1981).

Sperm incubated in seawater lacking Na^+ (choline-substituted seawater) are incapable of undergoing the acrosome reaction (Shapiro et *al.,* 1980; Schackmann and Shapiro, 1981). However, under these conditions, there is some Ca^{2+} influx into sperm (Shapiro *et al.,* 1980; Schackmann and Shapiro, 1981). Increasing the Na^+ concentration to 5 mM causes an influx of Ca^{2+} into sperm even in the absence of egg jelly, but this influx is still apparently not sufficient to trigger the acrosome reaction. If the Na^+ concentration is increased to 20 to 30 mM, the sperm spontaneously undergo the acrosome reaction (low Na^+ trigger; Shapiro *et al.,* 1980; Schackmann and Shapiro, 1981). Increasing the Na^+ concentration to 360 mM, which approximates the level in seawater, suppresses the Ca^{2+} influx. Schackmann and Shapiro (1981) have thus suggested that the extracellular Na^+ concentration may regulate intracellular Ca^{2+} levels. This regulatory mechanism has been demonstrated in squid axon (Dipolo *et al.,* 1976; Blaustein, 1977) and has been suggested for ascidian sperm (Lambert and Epel, 1979).

Potassium ions appears to be released from sperm during the acrosome reaction, since tetraethylammonium chloride (TEA), an inhibitor of K^+ current in the action potential of nerve (Hille, 1967), is also an inhibitor of the acrosome reaction and acid release. Furthermore, the jelly-induced acid release is suppressed as extracellular K^+ levels increase, suggesting the K^+ efflux precedes acid release.

Some of the ionic movements described above have been correlated with specific morphological events of the acrosome reaction by Lewis G. Tilney and co-workers (Tilney, 1978; Tilney *et al.,* 1978). Sperm of three echinoderm species were induced to undergo the acrosome reaction under varying ionic concentrations or pH or in the presence of different ionophores. The sperm were then analyzed ultrastructurally for morphological changes. In the absence of extracellular Ca^{2+}, there is no fusion of the acrosome and plasma membranes and, therefore, no exocytosis (Tilney *et al.,* 1978). Thus, Ca^{2+} appears to be essential for successful membrane fusion and exocytosis of the acrosome contents. However, even in calcium-free medium, the actin in the subacrosomal fossa polymerizes into filamentous material, provided conditions allow H^+ efflux from the sperm (Tilney, 1978; Tilney *et al.,* 1978). This led to the proposal that the H^+ efflux leads to a rise in intracellular pH that allows the actin to polymerize, perhaps by dissociating regulatory proteins (Tilney, 1978; Tilney *et al.,* 1978). These results suggest that each distinct morphological event of the acrosome reaction may have a specific control mechanism. (For a discussion of ionic movements and pH changes in the female gamete at fertilization, see Chapter 5.)

On the basis of the results of their detailed study, Schackmann and Shapiro (1981; Shapiro *et al.,* 1980) have proposed a working model for the sequence of changes occurring during the acrosome reaction (Fig.

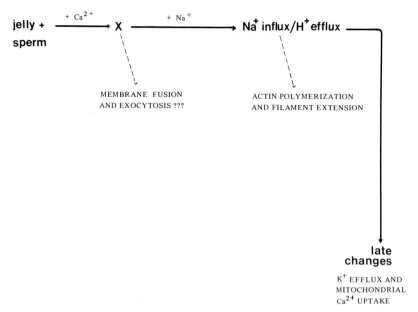

Fig. 1. Working model for ion fluxes during the sea urchin sperm acrosome reaction. See text for further details. (Modified from Schackmann and Shapiro, 1981.)

1). According to the model, Ca^{2+} uptake is an early change in the sequence and results from the interaction of jelly with sperm. This interaction leads to a hypothetical intermediate state X (Fig. 1). The sperm may proceed from X if the proper extracellular ionic conditions are met, as is the case in normal fertilization. Na^+ uptake and acid release follow, and during or immediately following the Na^+ and H^+ movements, actin polymerizes and filament extension occurs. Finally, the late changes take place, including K^+ efflux and an extended, relatively large, mitochondrial Ca^{2+} uptake (Fig. 1). Although these late changes do not have a direct role in the acrosome reaction, they may have a role in other aspects of the fertilization process (Schackmann and Shapiro, 1981).

D. Cyclic Nucleotide Changes during Sperm Activation and the Acrosome Reaction

1. Effects of the Fucose Sulfate Polysaccharide on Cyclic Nucleotide Levels

Garbers and Hardman (1975, 1976) made the initial observation that sperm cyclic AMP (cAMP) levels increase dramatically following exposure of sperm to egg jelly. This has led to a careful analysis of cyclic nucleotide metabolism in sperm and the possible role of changes in cyclic nucleotides in sperm physiology (reviewed in Garbers and Kopf, 1980; Garbers, 1981; Hansborough and Garbers, 1981a,b).

Both crude egg jelly preparations and purified fucose sulfate polysaccharide (SeGall and Lennarz, 1979, 1981; termed FS-1 by Kopf and Garbers, 1980) have been used to analyze the cyclic nucleotide changes seen in sperm during the acrosome reaction. Exposure to FS-1 results in a marked Ca^{2+}-dependent activation of adenylate cyclase activity and an increase in cAMP, but not cGMP, levels (Garbers and Hardman, 1975, 1976; Tubb et al., 1978; Watkins et al., 1978; Kopf and Garbers, 1980; Garbers and Kopf, 1978, 1980; Garbers et al., 1978, 1980a). The frequency of acrosome reactions and the increase in cAMP concentration are tightly correlated, consistent with an involvement of cyclic nucleotide metabolism in the regulation of the acrosome reaction. Artificial inducers of the acrosome reaction induce similar changes in cyclic nucleotide concentrations, again suggesting that cAMP is involved in the acrosome reaction (Garbers and Kopf, 1980). Removal of Ca^{2+} from the extracellular medium or addition of D600 or verapamil blocks these cyclic nucleotide changes (Kopf and Garbers, 1978, 1979, 1980).

Existing evidence suggests that the initial step in the acrosome reaction is an increase in Ca^{2+} permeability (Schackmann and Shapiro, 1981), and all subsequent metabolic changes appear to rest on this initial event. Based on data from other systems (e.g., Wolff and Broström, 1979; Cheung, 1980; Klee et al., 1980; Means and Dedman, 1980), it has been suggested that Ca^{2+} controls change in cyclic nucleotide levels through the formation of Ca^{2+}–calmodulin complexes (Garbers and Kopf, 1980). Calmodulin is present in sea urchin sperm in high concentration (Jones et al., 1978; Garbers et al., 1980b). However, evidence that a Ca^{2+}–calmodulin complex regulates adenylate cyclase activity in sperm of other species has been equivocal (Hyne and Garbers, 1979), since the data are also consistent with a direct Ca^{2+} effect (Hyne and Garbers, 1979). Phosphodiesterase activity, another likely target for calmodulin, is not affected by Ca^{2+} or calmodulin (Wells and Garbers, 1976). Although trifluoroperaxine, a calmodulin inhibitor (Levin and Weiss, 1976), blocks the acrosome reaction, the effect is probably due to effects on the plasma membrane (Seeman, 1972) that results in an inhibition of Ca^{2+} uptake (Kopf and Garbers, 1980).

The mechanism by which changes in cyclic nucleotide metabolism control the acrosome reaction is unknown. Protein phosphorylation is recognized as a major regulatory mechanism in eukaryotes (Green-gard, 1978; Krebs and Beavo, 1979; Weller, 1979) and increases in cAMP levels may result in changes in cAMP-dependent protein kinase activity in sperm. Garbers *et al.* (1980a,b) presented evidence that in sea urchin sperm FS-1 activates a cAMP-dependent protein kinase. The degree of activation of the kinase is dependent on the FS-1 concentration and on extracellular Ca^{2+} (Garbers *et al.*, 1980a).

The suggestion has been made (Garbers and Kopf, 1980) that the protein kinase activation in sperm mediates the polymerization of actin. According to this scheme, phosphorylation of an actin-binding protein would initiate actin polymerization, resulting in extension of the acrosome filament (see, for example, Wallach *et al.*, 1978; Garbers and Kopf, 1980). At this time there is no evidence supporting this interesting hypothesis nor any information on what role, if any, protein kinase activation plays in the induction of the acrosome reaction.

2. Speract

It is well known that egg jelly preparations from many invertebrate species stimulate sperm respiration and motility (Loeb, 1916; Lillie, 1919; Nelson, 1975; Schackmann *et al.*, 1978; Schackmann and Shapiro, 1981). This phenomenon has been studied most extensively in the sea urchin. Although a large literature exists on the subject, until recently there was little information on the nature of the molecule responsible for this activation.

Ohtake (1976a,b), working with three species of Japanese sea urchins, presented evidence that the sperm-activating substance (SAS; Ohtake, 1976b) was a small, dialyzable, pronase-sensitive molecule (Ohtake, 1976b). Analysis of a similar low-molecular-weight factor from *S. purpuratus* showed that it also increased sperm cAMP and cGMP levels (Kopf *et al.*, 1979). The SAS has recently been purified to apparent homogeneity from *S. purpuratus* egg jelly by Hansbrough and Garbers (1981a,b; Garbers *et al.*, 1982) and named speract for its sperm-activating properties (Hansbrough and Garbers, 1981b). Speract is a low-molecular-weight ($M_r < 2000$) peptide, containing only neutral and acidic amino acids, that is particularly rich in glycine (34%; Hansbrough and Garbers, 1981b; Garbers *et al.*, 1982). Purified speract stimulates respiration and motility in a non-species-specific fashion in sea urchin sperm (Hansbrough and Garbers, 1981b) but does not induce the acrosome reaction (Hansbrough and Garbers, 1981a).

Following exposure of sperm to speract, there is both Na^+ uptake and a Na^+-dependent acid release (Hansbrough and Garbers, 1981a). If Na^+ is excluded from the medium, there is no activation of respiration and motility. The effect is K^+- and Ca^{2+}-independent. The ionophore monensin, known to mediate Na^+/H^+ exchange is an early event in the activation process (Hansbrough and Garbers, 1981a). This Na^+ dependency is consistent with earlier results of Nishioka and Cross (1978), demonstrating a requirement for extracellular Na^+ in sperm activation.

Speract also increases cGMP and cAMP levels in sperm (Kopf *et al.*, 1979; Hansbrough *et al.*, 1980; Hansbrough and Garbers, 1981a,b). Similar effects on respiration and motility can be elicited by 8-Br-cGMP (8-bromoguanosine 3′,5′-monophosphate); 8-Br-cAMP and FS-1, which only increase cAMP, have no effect on sperm respiration (Kopf *et al.*, 1979), suggesting that sperm activation may be mediated by a rise in cGMP levels (Kopf *et al.*, 1979; Hansbrough *et al.*, 1980). However, higher concentrations of speract are required for half-maximal elevations of the cyclic nucleotides rather than for stimulation of respiration. The reduced potency of speract in elevating cGMP levels is inconsistent with previous suggestions of cGMP as a second messenger for speract (Kopf *et al.*, 1979; Hansbrough *et al.*, 1980). However, this may only reflect differences in the compartmentalization of cGMP within the sperm (Hansbrough and Garbers, 1981b).

Recently Garbers *et al.* (1982) sequenced and synthesized a peptide (gly-phe-asp-leu-asn-gly-gly-gly-val-gly) having similar properties to speract and have suggested that this new peptide be named speract (Garbers *et al.*, 1982). It may be that a single precursor peptide in the egg gives rise to a variety of peptides having similar properties. The speract peptide sequenced by Garbers *et al.* (1982) is identical to that from *Hemicentrotus pulcherrimus* isolated and sequenced by Suzuki *et al.* (1981).

V. SPERM–EGG BINDING IN ECHINODERMS

A. Bindin as Mediator of Sperm–Egg Adhesion in Sea Urchins

The major consequence of the acrosome reaction is exposure of the contents of the acrosome granule. Popa (1927; Section IV,A) correctly assumed that adhesion of sperm to other objects was mediated by the material in the granule. Later work on the fine structure of sperm–egg interaction showed that the granule contents coated the acrosome process and were localized at the point of adhesion of the sperm to the egg (Dan, 1956, 1967; Summers *et al.*, 1975).

Vacquier and Moy (1977) isolated the insoluble contents from the acrosome granules of *S. purpuratus* sperm. The isolated membraneless granules were similar in size (0.25 μm) and appearance to the granules in intact sperm. Analysis by SDS-polyacrylamide gels showed that the granules primarily contained a single protein of M_r 30,500 (Vacquier and Moy, 1977). There is no detectable carbohydrate by the phenol-sulfuric or anthrone tests (Vacquier and Moy, 1977).

Based on several lines of evidence, bindin has been proposed to be the species-specific mediator of sperm–egg adhesion. First, an antiserum raised against electrophoretically purified bindin showed that bindin is localized at the point of sperm–egg attachment, and is exposed only in acrosome-reacted sperm (Moy and Vacquier, 1979). Second, isolated binding agglutinates intact unfertilized eggs in a fairly species-specific fashion (Glabe and Vacquier, 1977a; Glabe and Lennarz, 1979, 1981). The bindin is localized in the region of contact between the agglutinated eggs (Glabe and Lennarz, 1979). This agglutination may be blocked by a glycopeptide fraction from the egg surface or by trypsinizing the egg surface prior to addition of bindin (Vacquier and Moy, 1977; Glabe and Vacquier, 1977a; Glabe and Lennarz, 1979, 1981), suggesting that bindin interacts specifically with molecules on the vitelline layer. Finally, bindin interacts with a receptor fraction isolated from the vitelline layer of eggs (Glabe and Vacquier 1978; Glabe and Lennarz, 1981).

Preliminary characterization of *S. purpuratus* and *S. franciscanus* bindin showed that the two molecules have a similar amino acid composition that differs only in the number of aspartic acid and proline residues (Bellet *et al.*, 1977). In both cases the terminal residue is tyrosine. In addition, the peptide maps of the two bindins show a large number of coincident spots (Bellet *et al.*, 1977).

The similarities suggested by amino acid analysis and peptide mapping are supported by sequencing studies, which reveal considerable homology in the known segments of the two bindins (Vacquier and Moy, 1978). These studies also established that hydrophobic residues occur with high frequency in the known sequences of *S. purpuratus* and *S. franciscanus* bindins. Although there is no amino acid analysis or sequence information on *Arbacia punctulata* bindin, its behavior indicates that it is even more hydrophobic than *S. purpuratus* bindin. This conclusion is based on the observation that isolated *A. punctulata* bindin exists as lamellar vesicles (Glabe and Lennarz, 1979), containing as many as seven lamellae. Determination of the amount of phospholipid associated with the isolated bindin showed that it accounts for 12% of the total mass (Glabe and Lennarz, 1979). It has been suggested that the extremely hydrophobic character of bindin may allow it to become incorporated into the plasma membrane covering the acrosome process. This insertion may be sufficient to provide the additional membrane surface area required to cover the acrosome process (Moy and Vacquier, 1978; Glabe and Lennarz, 1979).

B. The Interaction of Bindin with Its Receptor

The preceding discussion summarized evidence that bindin is the mediator of species-specific sperm–egg adhesion in sea urchins. It follows that a receptor to bindin must exist on the egg surface. Extensive evidence for the presence of sperm receptors on the egg surface has accumulated over the last 15 years and is summarized in Table II. For a detailed discussion of this evidence see Epel and Vacquier (1978) and Lopo and Vacquier (1981).

A crude receptor fraction was first isolated by Glabe and Vacquier (1978) from *S. purpuratus* eggs, and its *in vitro* interaction with bindin analyzed. When a simple filter assay was used, the bindin-receptor interaction displayed saturation kinetics. Protease-degraded receptor did not interact with the bindin (Glabe and Vacquier, 1978). Since sperm-egg binding is species specific (Summers and Hylander, 1976; Kinsey *et al.*, 1980), the specificity of the *in vitro* interaction was examined (Glabe and Vacquier, 1978). In competition assays the crude re-

TABLE II

Evidence for Sperm Receptors on the Egg Vitelline Layer in Sea Urchins[a]

---

1. Unfertilized eggs treated with trypsin show reduced fertilizability (Aketa *et al.*, 1972; Schmell *et al.*, 1977).
2. Unfertilized eggs incubated in cortical granule protease bind sperm in reduced numbers (Vacquier *et al.*, 1973; Carroll and Epel, 1975).
3. Unfertilized eggs treated with trypsin or cortical granule protease are not agglutinated by bindin (Vacquier and Moy, 1978).
4. Large glycoproteins can be isolated from egg vitelline layers that show species-specific inhibition of fertilization (Aketa, 1973, 1977; Schmell *et al.*, 1977; Glabe and Vacquier, 1978; Glabe and Lennarz, 1979, 1981).
5. Acrosome-reacted sperm exhibit species-specific binding (Summers and Hylander, 1975, 1976; Kinsey *et al.*, 1980).
6. Sperm binding exhibits saturation kinetics (Vacquier and Payne, 1973).
7. Sperm bind only to the external surface of isolated vitelline layers (Glabe and Vacquier, 1977b).
8. Bindin agglutinates eggs in a species-specific fashion (Glabe and Vacquier, 1977a; Vacquier and Moy, 1977; Glabe and Lennarz, 1979).

---

[a] After Lopo and Vacquier, 1981, with permission of Plenum Press.

ceptor preparations interacted with bindin in a species-specific manner.

The nature of the receptor was further investigated by Glabe and Lennarz (1979, 1981). They found that pronase digestion of unfertilized eggs released a glycoconjugate fraction that inhibited bindin-mediated egg agglutination (Glabe and Lennarz, 1979). Further purification of the crude glycoconjugate preparation yielded a fraction with molecular weight in excess of one million (Glabe and Lennarz, 1981) that retained its egg-agglutination inhibition activity and also agglutinated bindin particles. The agglutinated bindin–glycoconjugate complex could be removed by centrifugation, permitting the affinity purification of the glycoconjugates that interacted with the bindin. Exhaustive pronase digestion of the agglutinated bindin particles released the affinity-purified inhibitory activity and permitted compositional analysis (Glabe and Vacquier, 1981). The egg surface glycoconjugate contained fucose, xylose, galactose, glucose, and an unidentified sugar (Glabe and Lennarz, 1981).

The egg surface glycoconjugates isolated by Glabe and Lennarz (1979, 1981) do not interact with bindin in the species-specific fashion in which intact sperm and eggs interact (Summers and Hylander, 1976; Kinsey *et al.*, 1980) or in which bindin agglutinates intact eggs (Vacquier and Moy, 1977; Glabe and Vacquier, 1977a,b; Glabe and Lennarz, 1979). These observations suggest that the species specificity of sperm–egg interaction is a property of another egg surface component, or the result of the precise three-dimensional orientation of the intact glycoconjugate, as has been suggested (Glabe, 1979; Glabe and Lennarz, 1979; 1981).

Rossignol *et al.* (1981), using a cell surface complex preparation (developed by Schmell *et al.*, 1977; Decker and Lennarz, 1979), identified and partially purified a receptor fraction from *S. purpuratus* and *A. punctulata* which interacts with bindin. ^{125}I-labeled proteins from the cell surface complex were found to sediment at specific densities on CsCl-sucrose gradients. A high-density fraction that sediments away from most of the radioactivity was determined to contain bindin receptor activity, based on its ability to interact with the bindin (Rossignol *et al.*, 1981). This receptor fraction also interacted with acrosome-reacted sperm in a species-specific, saturable fashion (Rossignol *et al.*, 1981). In addition, the receptor fraction competed with eggs for sperm binding and, thus, can inhibit fertilization (Rossignol *et al.*, 1981). This evidence indicates that this component of the egg surface complex is involved in the species-specific interaction with sperm bindin during fertilization.

Rossignol *et al.* (1981) further analyzed the putative receptor fraction by preparing a pronase digest. Exhaustive proteolysis yielded soluble glycoconjugates that competed with the receptor fraction for bindin in the same manner as the glycoconjugates prepared by Glabe and Lennarz (1981). Compositional analysis of the glycoconjugates prepared by Rossignol *et al.* (1981) from the receptor fractions has not yet been carried out. However, in view of their reported properties, these glycoconjugates are likely to be similar to those described by Glabe and Lennarz (1981). If this receptor is indeed the species-specific sperm receptor from the egg surface, additional biochemical characterization should reveal the nature of its adhesive and species-specific recognition properties.

VI. POSTBINDING EVENTS DURING FERTILIZATION

A. Penetration of the Vitelline Layer by Sperm

The binding of sperm to the egg vitelline layer must be followed by penetration of the layer to achieve the close proximity between the plasma membranes required for gamete fusion. Two basic mechanisms have been proposed for the unknown process by which the sperm penetrates the vitelline layer. Penetration could be achieved mechanically, with the force of the extending acrosome filament being used to spear an opening through the vitelline layer. As an alternative, the vitelline layer could be digested by lytic substances on the tip of the acrosome process. Evidence for and against these two mechanisms is briefly summarized as follows.

In some organisms, such as starfish (Popa, 1927; Just, 1929; Dan, 1954a; Ikadai and Hoshi, 1981) or horseshoe crabs (Brown, 1976; Tilney and Mooseker, 1976), sperm undergo the acrosome reaction at the outer border of the egg jelly coat. Then a long acrosome filament extends and spans the distance between the border of the jelly coat and the surface of the egg. The membrane at the tip of the acrosome process fuses with the egg plasma membrane, and the sperm is drawn toward the egg surface and incorporated into the egg. Penetration of the jelly coat and vitelline layer is presumably due to the mechanical force generated by filament extension (Brown, 1976; Glabe *et al.*, 1981, 1982). The same mechanism could also operate in organisms like sea urchins, where the acrosome process is shorter. To take advantage of the mechanical force generated during extension of a short filament, the successful sperm would have to undergo the acrosome reaction close to the vitelline layer (Glabe *et al.*, 1982). In support of this idea is the observation that sperm lose their fertilizing ability soon after induction of the acrosome reaction (Vacquier, 1979; Kinsey *et al.*, 1980). In addition, there is evidence that in at least one species of sea urchin (*Pseudocentrotus depressus*) sperm are unable to undergo the acrosome reaction in isolated jelly "hulls," but do so in response to intact eggs (Aketa and Ohta, 1977). This suggests, at least in this species, that an additional factor from the egg surface may be involved in the induction of the acrosome reaction.

Loeb (1919) and Lillie (1919) proposed that penetration of sperm through the extracellular egg investments was facilitated by "lysins" released by the sperm. Evidence that substances with lytic properties exist in sperm has accumulated over the years for a variety of species, including mammals (e.g., Yamane, 1935; Tyler, 1939; Wada *et al.*, 1956; Heller and Raftery, 1973, 1976a,b; Meizel, 1978; Parrish and Polakoski, 1979; Hoshi *et al.*, 1981; Lewis *et al.*, 1982).

As discussed previously (Section IV,A), in the sea urchin *S. purpuratus* a serine protease exposed during the acrosome reaction (Levine *et al.*, 1978) plays a role in the extension of the acrosome process (Levine and Walsh, 1979). In addition, Levine and Walsh (1979) demonstrated that inhibition of the protease following induction of the acrosome reaction inhibits fertilization, although the specific event inhibited is not known. The activity of the enzyme has been localized in the acrosome material exposed during the acrosome reaction (Green and Summers, 1980). Levine *et al.* (1978; Levine and Walsh, 1979, 1980) proposed that this protease is the sea urchin counterpart of mammalian acrosin, the protease implicated in sperm penetration of the zona pellucida (Meizel, 1978; Parrish and Polakoski, 1979). These workers suggested further that a dual role may exist for sea urchin acrosin, first in extension of the acrosome process, and second in a later event in sperm–egg interaction (Levine and Walsh, 1979). The nature of this later event remains unknown at this writing.

Some evidence suggests that chymotrypsin-like activity is exposed following the acrosome reaction in some species of sea urchin. Hoshi *et al.* (1979) reported that in the Japanese sea urchins *Hemicentrotus pulcherrimus* and *S. intermedius* only chymotrypsin inhibitors block fertilization; inhibitors of trypsin-like proteases had no effect. Extracts of *H. pulcherrimus* sperm contain a chymotrypsin-like activity capable of reducing the turbidity of isolated vitelline layer suspensions (Yamada and Aketa, 1981). When isolated vitelline layers are exposed

to the extract and separated by SDS-polyacrylamide gel electrophoresis, there is a loss of high-molecular-weight components in the treated
vitelline layers (Yamada and Aketa, 1981).

Green and Summers (1982) recently presented evidence that a
chymotrypsin-like activity is involved in vitelline layer penetration in
S. purpuratus, S. droebachiensis, and Lytechinus pictus. Sperm binding to either fixed or living eggs proceeded normally in the presence of
TPCK, an inhibitor of chymotrypsin. However, fertilization of living
eggs was reduced in the presence of TPCK. When the vitelline layers
were removed from eggs by trypsinization prior to fertilization, TPCK
was not inhibitory, suggesting an involvement for a sperm chymotrypsin-like protease in penetration of the vitelline layer (Green and Summers, 1982).

Glabe et al. (1981) found that chymostatin, an inhibitor of chymotrypsin, also inhibited fertilization in S. purpuratus and Arbacia punctulata. However, closer examination of the chymostatin-treated sperm
showed that this inhibitor induces an abnormal acrosome reaction
(Glabe et al., 1982). Reduced chymostatin, which is relatively inefficient as a chymotrypsin inhibitor, also induced the abnormal acrosome
reaction, suggesting that the inhibition of fertilization was unrelated
to an inhibition of chymotrypsin activity (Glabe et al., 1981). These
observations led Glabe et al. (1981) to suggest that penetration of the
vitelline layer is achieved mechanically by extension of the acrosome
process, although they did not rule out a role for hydrolases. These
observations were based on the results of experiments in which only
one chymotrypsin inhibitor was used (Glabe et al., 1981). The effects on
sea urchin fertilization of other inhibitors of trypsin- or chymotrypsin-
like activities must be analyzed more carefully before this question can
be resolved. Demonstration of enzymatic activity in sperm by use of
artificial substrates should provide more convincing evidence for a role
for hydrolases in sperm–egg interaction (see, for example, Levine et
al., 1978; Levine and Walsh, 1979).

Recent work on the ascidian Halocynthia roretzi supports the proposed role for proteases in penetration of the extracellular coats (Hoshi
et al., 1981). Three trypsin and two chymotrypsin inhibitors blocked
fertilization of intact eggs. However, if the chorion, the extracellular
egg coat, was removed, the eggs could be fertilized in the presence of
the inhibitors (Hoshi et al., 1981), suggesting that, at least in ascidians, proteases function in penetration of the extracellular egg coats.

An arylsulfatase partially purified from S. intermedius sperm by
Moriya and Hoshi (1980) has been implicated in fertilization in this
species. These workers found that (1) arylsulfatase activity is exposed

following the acrosome reaction; (2) fertilization is blocked in the presence of artificial substrates of arylsulfatase; (3) the vitelline layer is digested by the enzyme; and (4) unfertilized eggs pretreated with the enzyme are fertilizable, but they elevate abnormal fertilization envelopes (Hoshi and Moriya, 1980; Moriya and Hoshi, 1980).

Lewis *et al.* (1980, 1982; Talbot *et al.*, 1980) recently studied the biochemical basis for sperm–egg interactions in the red abalone, *Haliotis rufescens*. Basing their proposal on these studies, they suggested an unusual mechanism of sperm penetration in this species. Abalone sperm have a large bullet-shaped acrosome (Fig. 2a) containing two morphologically distinct components. A microfilament bundle (2.4 μm in length) extends from the nuclear fossa into the acrosomal fossa in the unreacted sperm (cf. Tilney and Mooseker, 1976; Tilney,

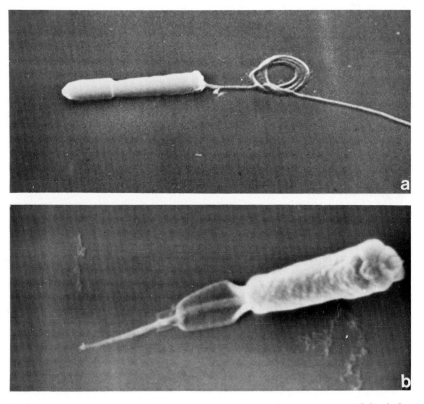

Fig. 2. Scanning electron micrographs of intact (a) and acrosome-reacted (b) abalone sperm (*Haliotis rufescens*). (Reproduced from Lewis *et al.*, 1980, with permission of Academic Press.)

1978). The unfertilized abalone egg is surrounded by a slightly elevated vitelline layer. Sperm bind to the egg surface by the plasma
membrane at the tip of the sperm, then undergo the acrosome reaction.
During the reaction the contents of the acrosome are exposed, and the
acrosome process (7 μm) extends, leaving an empty acrosome vesicle
(Fig. 2b; Lewis *et al.*, 1980).

Lewis *et al.* (1982) analyzed the soluble acrosome contents released
during the acrosome reaction in the red abalone. SDS-polyacrylamide
gel electrophoresis revealed that two major proteins, of M_r 13,000 and
15,000, are released; these two proteins are also the major components
of whole sperm. Additional analysis of the 13,000 protein revealed
that, although it solubilized the egg vitelline layer, it lacked detectable
enzymatic activity in assays for protease, exoglucanase, lipase,
arylsulfatase, carbohydrase, or disulfide bond reduction (Lewis *et al.*,
1982). It was determined that the protein dissolves the vitelline layer
by a stoichiometric, noncatalytic mechanism (Lewis *et al.*, 1982). A
similar conclusion was reached by Haino-Fukushima (1974; Haino and
Kagawa, 1966, 1969) in her study of *Tegula pfeifferi* sperm lysin
(*Tegula* is a member of the same taxonomic order as abalone).

Lysins from other species of mollusks have been described and presumed to be enzymes, although evidence demonstrating enzymatic activity was inconclusive (see, for example, Heller and Raftery, 1973,
1976a,b). Lewis *et al.* (1982) suggested that the mechanism of penetration described for abalone may be more widespread in nature than is
presently acknowledged. This proposed stoichiometric mechanism of
nonenzymatic lysis (Haino-Fukushima, 1974; Lewis *et al.*, 1982) is
attractive for a variety of reasons. A large enzyme concentration in the
acrosome could digest a hole not only in the vitelline layer but also in
the plasma membrane. This could easily be conceived as detrimental to
the egg. A stoichiometric mechanism would be self-limiting and non-
degradative to other egg surface components (Lewis *et al.*, 1982).
Whether this mechanism is restricted to the mollusks or is more widespread in nature is presently unknown.

B. Fusion of the Sperm and Egg

There is practically no information on the molecular basis for
sperm–egg membrane fusion. In most invertebrates the entire egg
surface appears to be available for fusion. In addition, at least in sea
urchins, gamete membrane fusion appears to be non-species specific.
For example, at high sperm concentrations, *S. purpuratus* sperm bind
to *Arbacia punctulata* eggs in the presence of *S. purpuratus* jelly but

few eggs are fertilized (Glabe *et al.*, 1981). If the vitelline layer is removed from *A. punctulata* eggs (Epel *et al.*, 1970), *S. purpuratus* and *A. punctulata* sperm are equally effective at fertilizing the *A. punctulata* eggs (Glabe *et al.*, 1981).

In sea urchins, the plasma membrane covering the tip of the acrosome process is the portion of the sperm that fuses with the egg. Since the process is coated with the acrosome contents, it is possible that the bindin or another acrosomal component has a fusigenic role. The acrosin could modify the bindin into a fusigenic protein, as is the case with the F protein of Sendia virus (Gething *et al.*, 1978).

Conway and Metz (1976) reported that lipase activity is exposed in acrosome-reacted *A. punctulata* sperm. The lipase activity is of two types: an initial phospholipase A activity followed by lysophospholipase activity (Conway and Metz, 1976). These authors presented a model to account for the sequential activity of the two enzymes, suggesting roles for them in the acrosome reaction and sperm–egg fusion (Conway and Metz, 1976). Recent studies make a role for phospholipase in the induction of the acrosome reaction unlikely (SeGall and Lennarz, 1981). However, these same studies showed that phospholipase activity is a consequence, not a prerequisite, of the acrosome reaction, supporting the idea that phospholipases from the sperm have a role in sperm–egg fusion (Conway and Metz, 1976).

VII. SPERM–EGG INTERACTIONS IN OTHER INVERTEBRATES

A. Bindinlike Molecules in Other Phyla

Molecules having properties similar to sea urchin bindin have been isolated from two other invertebrate groups. Brandriff *et al.* (1978) isolated the insoluble material in the acrosome granule of *Crassostrea gigas* (Mollusca: Pelecypoda) sperm. The isolated granules are similar to those of intact sperm in size and appearance and are capable of agglutinating eggs (Brandriff *et al.*, 1978). In addition, a trypsin digest of oyster eggs inhibited the granule-dependent agglutination. Based on this evidence, the oyster bindin has been proposed to function in a manner similar to sea urchin bindin in mediating sperm–egg adhesion at fertilization in oysters (Brandriff *et al.*, 1978).

Analysis of the isolated oyster acrosome granules indicates that the material is 84% protein by dry weight. On SDS-polyacrylamide gels the isolated granules resolve into one to four PAS-positive bands of M_r

65,000, 53,000, 43,000, and 34,000. The 65,000 band is always present, but the presence of the other three components varies from preparation to preparation. Although there is no proteolytic activity in the isolated granules, proteolytic degradation before and during isolation may be responsible for the variability (Brandriff *et al.*, 1978). A preliminary characterization indicated that antiserum against the 65,000 component cross-reacts with the 53,000 and 43,000 bands. Sea urchin anti-bindin does not cross-react with the oyster sperm acrosome material (Moy and Vacquier, 1979).

Using the procedure developed by Brandriff *et al.* (1978), J. Stephano Hornedo and M. Gould-Somero (personal communication) recently isolated the acrosome granules from the worm *Urechis caupo* (Echiuroidea). The material is highly insoluble and agglutinates *Urechis* eggs. However, it also agglutinates sea urchin eggs and *Pelvetia* zygotes, so its adhesive properties are not species-specific (J. Stephano Hornedo and M. Gould-Somero, personal communication). On acid–urea gels the *Urechis* bindin migrates close to calf thymus histone, suggesting a low molecular weight. Although 50% of the amino acid residues are arginine and lysine, the protein is not a histone (J. Stephano Hornedo and M. Gould-Somero, personal communication).

B. Sperm–Egg Interactions in Decapod Crustaceans

The decapod crustaceans include familiar organisms like shrimp and prawns (order Natantia), and lobsters, crabs, and crayfish (order Reptantia). These organisms are of particular interest to reproductive biologists because they possess atypical sperm that are nonmotile, lack flagella, and have uncondensed chromatin. Although these unusual sperm have been known for over a century (Hallez, 1874), a careful analysis of their fertilization interactions has only recently been attempted (Brown, 1971; Hinsch, 1973; Talbot and Summers, 1978; Yudin *et al.*, 1979; Clark *et al.*, 1980, 1981; Kleve *et al.*, 1980; Talbot and Chanmanon, 1980; Lynn and Clark, 1981).

Sperm of these two decapod orders differ in their morphology (Talbot and Summers, 1978). Reptantian sperm are multistellate, i.e., they have multiple spikes extending from the body, while natantian sperm have a single spike (unistellate; Talbot and Summers, 1978; Kleve *et al.*, 1980; Talbot and Chanmanon, 1980). Detailed ultrastructural information of sperm-egg interaction in the Natantia has come from the work of Clark and his colleagues using several species (e.g., *Sicyonia ingentis, Penaeus aztecus, Macrobrachium rosenbergii;* Kleve *et al.*, 1980; Clark *et al.*, 1980, 1981; Lynn and Clark, 1982). In *Sicyonia,*

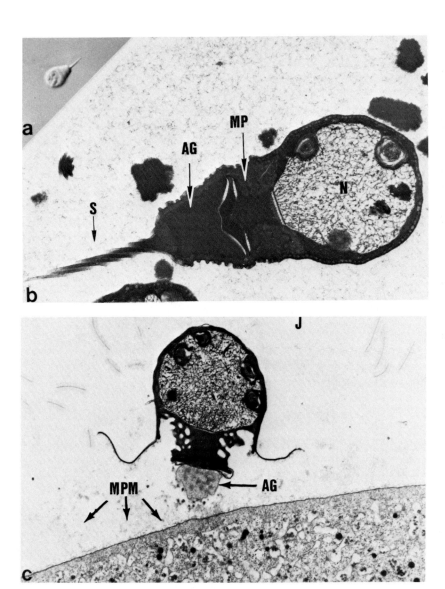

Fig. 3. Intact and acrosome-reacted sperm of the crustacean *Sicyonia ingentis*. (a) Unreacted sperm by phase microscopy. The almost spherical body has a conical cap from which extends the anterior spike (×860). (b) Transmission electron micrograph of a longitudinal section of an unreacted sperm. The acrosome vesicle contains three components: MP, membrane pouches; AG, anterior granule; S, spike. The nucleus (N) is uncondensed (×15,500). (c) Transmission electron micrograph of an acrosome-reacted sperm at the egg surface. The membrane pouches have apparently released a material (MPM) that forms a precipitate between the sperm and egg. The anterior granule (AG) is surrounded by small, spherical electron-dense particles. The egg jelly (J) released from the cortical crypts completely surrounds the sperm. See text and Fig. 4 for additional details (×12,400). (Reproduced from Clark *et al.*, 1981, with permission of the Wistar Institute Press.)

sperm have unistellate natantian morphology (Fig. 3a,b). The posteriorly positioned nucleus contains uncondensed chromatin; anterior to the nucleus is the acrosomal complex, comprising a central cap region, membrane pouches, and a large anterior granule (Fig. 3b; Kleve *et al.*, 1980). A single spiraling spike extends anteriorly from the granule (Fig. 3b). The central cap and spike are limited by a membrane that by transmission electron microscopy appears to be fused to the sperm plasma membrane (Kleve *et al.*, 1980).

The *Sicyonia* egg has large cortical crypts containing a glycoprotein material (Fig. 4a). The material is actually extracellular, so the membrane lining the crypts is continuous with the plasma membrane of the egg. A vitelline envelope can be seen over the material in the crypts (Fig. 4b). At spawning, apparently in response to contact with the seawater, the material in the cortical crypts is extruded and forms a jelly layer on the egg surface (Fig. 4c). Sperm previously stored in the female are released with the eggs into the surrounding seawater. The sperm undergo the acrosome reaction on contact with the eggs and bind to the egg surface (Figs. 3c, 4a–d). The acrosome reaction and initial sperm–egg binding apparently take place prior to the jelly extrusion by the egg (Clark *et al.*, 1981).

Clark *et al.* (1981) have recently performed a detailed study of the changes taking place during the acrosome reaction. The first morphological change is a shortening of the spike accompanied by a swelling of the membrane pouch area at the base of the central cap (Fig. 3a,b; 5a,b). As the membrane pouch material swells, it becomes more flocculent in appearance. At the same time the spike membrane begins to disintegrate and the spike material becomes filamentous and retracts into a spherical mass (Fig. 5b). The membrane around the central cap region continues swelling and retracting, pulling back the remnants of the spike (Fig. 5c). As the spike is pulled back, the large anterior granule becomes the most anterior structure (Fig. 5c,d). It has also swollen to a spherical form and its contents have become less electron-dense than in the unreacted state. Once the membrane of the central cap has completely retracted, the flocculent material within the membrane pouches is totally exposed. This is the way sperm look when they bind to the egg surface (Fig. 3c; 4c,d; 5d; Clark *et al.*, 1981).

Analysis of the physiological requirements of the acrosome reaction in *Sicyonia* indicates that it is dependent on extracellular Ca^{2+}. High pH does not induce the reaction (Clark *et al.*, 1981). The jelly released from the cortical crypts during sperm– egg interaction is also ineffective as an inducer of the acrosome reaction. This is consistent with the observation that sperm interact with eggs prior to jelly release from the crypts (Clark *et al.*, 1981).

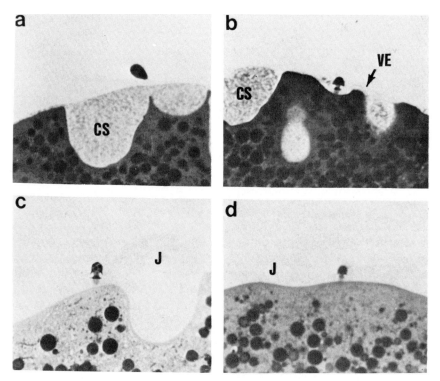

Fig. 4. Light micrograph of sperm–egg interaction in *Sicyonia ingentis* at spawning. (a) An unreacted sperm at the egg surface. Note that the sperm is oriented with the spike toward the egg. The contents of the cortical specializations (CS) have not yet been released (×860). (b) A naturally reacted sperm at the egg surface. The thin vitelline envelope (VE) clearly extends over the cortical crypts (×850). (c) Naturally reacted sperm at the egg surface as the cortical specializations are released to form the jelly (J) (×890). (d) Following a 5-minute exposure to seawater, the sperm is still on the oolemma, and the extruded jelly forms a thick layer around sperm and egg (×840). (Reproduced from Clark *et al.,* 1981, with permission of the Wistar Institute Press.)

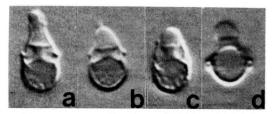

Fig. 5. Phase-contrast micrographs of the acrosome reaction in *Sicyonia ingentis*. (a) As the acrosome reaction begins, the spike retracts and the membrane pouches swell. (b) The completely retracted spike appears as a small spherical mass anterior to the cap. (c) The cap membranes fold back, exposing the anterior granule, which has assumed a spherical shape. The spike remnant (not visible) is carried by the cap membrane and eventually lost. (d) In the fully reacted sperm the membranes have completely retracted (×1600). (Reproduced from Clark *et al.,* 1981, with permission of the Wistar Institute Press.)

Preliminary *in vitro* fertilization studies suggest that initial sperm–egg recognition may be mediated by the interaction of molecules on the spike surface with an extracellular egg material (Yudin *et al.*, 1980). This initial binding is followed by the acrosome reaction, as described above. Clark *et al.* (1981) have proposed that the contraction of the spike during the acrosome reaction pulls the sperm closer to the egg surface. This is supported by work in other species (*Penaeus aztecus* and *Sicyonia brevirostris*) that shows that actin is present in the spike (Brown, 1976). As the spike contracts, the material from the membrane pouches is externalized and is believed to interact with the egg jelly to form a granular precipitate observed between the sperm and egg at fertilization (Fig. 3c; Clark *et al.*, 1981). This granular precipitate has been proposed to be analogous to the sperm–egg binding complex (Yudin *et al.*, 1980; Clark *et al.*, 1981) formed between bindin and the vitelline layer during sea urchin fertilization (Section V,A,B; Epel and Vcaquier, 1978; Lopo and Vacquier, 1981; Lopo *et al.*, 1982). At this time there is no information on the role of the anterior granule material during sperm–egg interaction. The anterior granule is only partially broken down during the early minutes of sperm–egg interaction (Clark *et al.*, 1981).

The studies described above have greatly expanded our knowledge of sperm–egg binding in decapod crustaceans. Isolation of the gamete surface molecules and subsequent *in vitro* analysis of their interaction will be necessary before the nature of gamete interaction in this fascinating system is completely understood.

C. Sperm–Egg Interactions in Ascidians

Ascidians are members of the subphylum Urochordata of the phylum Chordata. Thus, as chordates, they share several characteristics with vertebrates. Although ascidians are hermaphoroditic, most species are self-sterile. There is a large body of knowledge on early development of ascidians; however, only recently have some of the details of sperm–egg interaction come to light.

The ascidian egg is surrounded by a tough extracellular glycoprotein coat called the chorion (1 μm in thickness). Attached to the external surface of the chorion are follicle cells. These are conical cells filled with refractile vacuoles which have been shown to function as flotation devices (Lambert and Lambert, 1978). The space between the chorion and the egg plasma membrane contains test cells. Ascidian sperm are atypical of animal sperm in that there is no midpiece. The single mitochondrion is located alongside the nucleus in the head. The sperm surface binds fluorescein-labeled lectins nonuniformly (Rosati *et al.*, 1978), indicating the presence of restricted domains in the plasma membrane. The presence of an acrosome has been a matter of some controversy (Villa, 1977; Woollacott, 1977). However, there is evidence for the presence of a small acrosome granule at the anterior end of the sperm, at least in several species (Ursprung and Schabtach, 1964; Tuzet *et al.*, 1972, 1974; Rosati *et al.*, 1977; Rosati and De Santis, 1978; Cloney and Abbott, 1980).

Whether an acrosome is present or not, ascidian sperm undergo an ion-controlled, morphological changes during sperm–egg interaction. The morphological and physiological changes taking place during the ascidian sperm reaction have recently been described in *Ascidia ceratodes* (Lambert and Epel, 1979; Lambert and Lambert, 1981). On contact with the chorion the sperm lose their mitochondrion. The mitochondrion first swells, then slides along the length of the tail until it is released from the tip (Lambert and Epel, 1979). The process is completed in about 2 minutes.

Although the natural inducer of the ascidian sperm reaction is chorion-binding by the sperm (Lambert and Epel, 1979), it may also be induced by egg water, high pH, low extracellular Na^+, and the ionophor X537A (Fig. 6). Regardless of the inducer used, the reaction is strictly dependent on extracellular Ca^{2+} (Lambert and Epel, 1979; Lambert and Lambert, 1981). There is a measurable pH drop in extracellular pH during the reaction, indicating there is a release of acid. This is likely due to actual H^+ efflux, since elevating the extracellular pH will induce the reaction (Lambert and Epel, 1979; Lambert and Lambert, 1981). Interestingly, the reaction is also triggered by reducing extracellular Na^+ in a fashion similar to that reported for sea urchins by Schackmann and Shapiro (1981; see also Section IV,C). Although initial studies suggested that there was $H^+:Ca^{2+}$ exchange (Lambert and Epel, 1979), more detailed analysis indicated that the H^+ efflux precedes the Ca^{2+} uptake by 10–13 seconds, and in addition occurs in a ratio of 100 to 1 (Lambert and Lambert, 1981). Lambert and Lambert (1981) have thus proposed that the H^+ efflux induces the Ca^{2+} uptake by increasing Ca^{2+} permeability. In preliminary experiments 10 μM trifluoperazine blocks the movement of the sperm mitochondrion, suggesting a possible role for calmodulin in the ascidian sperm reaction (Lambert, personal communication).

Time-course studies of the mitochondrial reaction have indicated that it is necessary for successful fertilization (Lambert and Epel, 1979); however, the role of this activation phenomenon in sperm–egg interaction has not yet been determined. Steric considerations may

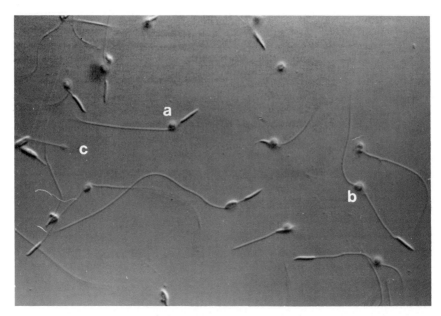

Fig. 6. *Ascidia ceratodes* sperm undergoing the ascidian sperm reaction. The sperm were diluted in pH 9.5 seawater and placed on a slide, then fixed several minutes later. (a) Early reaction. The mitochondrion is immediately behind the head. (b) The reaction has progressed further, and the mitochondrion is about halfway down the tail. (c) Mitochondrion about to be released at the tail terminus. (Unpublished photograph courtesy of Charles Lambert.)

require removal of the mitochondrion prior to penetration of the chorion by the sperm. Another possibility is that the mitochondrial movement provides the mechanical force necessary to push the sperm through the chorion (Lambert and Epel, 1979). The phenomenon does not appear to be limited to *Ascidia ceratodes*. The absence of mitochondrion during sperm–egg interaction has been described for several species (e.g., Ezzell, 1963; Villa, 1977; Lambert and Epel, 1979).

It is intriguing that such different morphological transformations as the ascidian sperm reaction and the echinoderm acrosome reaction are predicated on similar ion requirements, i.e., H^+ efflux and Ca^{2+} uptake. In both cases the morphological changes are necessary prerequisites for successful fertilization. How widespread these similar ionic mechanisms are in the control of sperm reactions during fertilization is uncertain. Extracellular Ca^{2+} is known to be required for the acrosome reaction in species throughout the animal kingdom, including mammals (e.g., Talbot *et al.,* 1976; Meizel, 1978). Although the correlation to changes in pH is less complete, these have also been implicated in the induction of the acrosome reaction in several species (e.g., Schackmann and Shapiro, 1981; Working and Meizel, 1981).

De Santis *et al.* (1980; Rosati *et al.*, 1978; Rosati and De Santis, 1978, 1980) have recently undertaken an analysis of sperm–egg binding in the ascidian *Ciona intestinalis*. In this species, upon reaching the egg, sperm bind to the chorion. Sperm that contact follicle cells swim away from them without binding (Rosati and De Santis, 1978). Binding of sperm to the chorion is restricted to the anterior plasma membrane at the anterior end of the sperm (Rosati and De Santis, 1978). The entire surface of the chorion is available for binding, since sperm will bind to eggs that have had the follicle cells removed and to isolated chorions (De Santis *et al.*, 1980). Although both the external and internal surfaces of isolated chorions bind similar lectins (Rosati *et al.*, 1978), apparently sperm receptors are only externally disposed, because sperm will bind only to the external chorion surface (De Santis *et al.*, 1980). Dechorionated eggs readily accept sperm of other species (Rosati and De Santis, 1978), suggesting that in ascidians, as in sea urchins, there is no species specificity in the membrane fusion event (Section VI,B; Glabe *et al.*, 1981). In addition, the self-sterility barrier is also lost in dechorionated eggs (Rosati and De Santis, 1978), suggesting that the histocompatibility loci responsible for this are expressed on the extracellular coat and not the plasma membrane.

Following attachment, the sperm plasma membrane apparently breaks down, the tip of the sperm blebs, and several tubules form that contact the chorion (De Santis *et al.*, 1980). These changes at the tip of the sperm are considered by De Santis *et al.* (1980) to be an acrosome reaction. Recent evidence suggests that penetration of the chorion may be achieved by proteases from the sperm (Hoshi *et al.*, 1981). Penetration of the chorion is followed by gamete membrane fusion (Rosati and De Santis, 1978).

The studies described above have provided insights into the nature of sperm–egg interaction in ascidians. A complete understanding of the molecular details of fertilization in these organisms will require isolation and characterization of the interacting surface molecules.

VIII. THE UNIVERSALITY OF SURFACE ANTIGENICITY OF ANIMAL SPERM

While studying the surface of sea urchin sperm, Lopo and Vacquier (1980c) developed an antiserum that displayed unusual properties. Their antiserum exhibited a surface cross-reactivity with sperm of 28 species, representing seven animal phyla of the animal kingdom (Lopo and Vacquier, 1980c). To date no negative cross-reaction has been found.

The original antiserum was raised by injecting whole glutaraldehyde-fixed *Strongylocentrotus purpuratus* sperm into a rabbit. The resulting antiserum was absorbed with sea urchin ovary and nongametic male tissues to remove all nonsperm activities. Following absorption, only one precipitin line appeared when the serum was diffused against a Triton X-100 extract of sea urchin sperm. The absorbed antiserum was called "sperm-specific antiserum" or SSA. The SSA agglutinated

TABLE III

Sperm That Reacted with the Sperm-Specific Antiserum (SSA) Prepared against *Strongylocentrotus purpuratus* Sperm[a]

Phylum Coelenterata	Phylum Echinodermata
Class Anthozoa	Class Echinoidea
Metridium senile fibriatum	*Strongylocentrotus purpuratus*
Phylum Annelida	*S. franciscanus*
Class Polychaeta	*S. pallidus*
Family Spionidae (one species)	*S. droebachiensis*
Family Polynoidae (one species)	*Lytechinus pictus*
Phylum Mollusca	*Arbacia punctulata*
Class Amphineura	*Tripneustes gratilla*
Cryptochiton stelleri	*Dendraster excentricus*
Class Gastropoda	Class Ophiuroidea
Acmaea sp.	*Ophioplocus esmarkii*
Class Pelecypoda	Class Asteroidea
Macoma nasuta	*Patiria miniata*
Phylum Echiuroidea	Phylum Chordata
Urechis caupo	Class Urochordata
Phylum Arthropoda	*Styela clava*
Class Crustacea	*S. plicata*
Cancer antennarius	*Ciona intestinalis*
Pinnixa tubicola	Class Osteichthyes
Class Merostomata	*Salmo* sp.
Limulus polyphemus	Class Amphibia
	Rana pipiens
	Class Aves
	Meleagris gallopavo
	Class Mammalia
	Mesocricetus auratus
	Rattus norvegicus

[a] Reactivity of the species-specific antiserum (SSA) was assayed by indirect immunofluorescence or by the immunoperoxidase procedure. The sperm were fixed in either 3% glutaraldehyde or formaldehyde. Preimmune serum did not react. (From Lopo and Vacquier, 1980c, with permission of Macmillan Journals, Ltd.)

intact sperm and the activity could be absorbed out by intact sperm, suggesting surface specificity (Lopo and Vacquier, 1980c).

The immunoperoxidase reaction and indirect immunofluorescence (IIF) were used to test the SSA with sperm of other species. Every species tested gave a positive reactivity (Table III). Phase-contrast and IIF observations of the treated cells indicated that the activity was distributed over the entire sperm surface (Lopo and Vacquier, 1980c). However, light microscopy may not be sensitive enough to detect non-uniform distribution of the reaction product on the sperm surface.

An extensive series of controls was performed to ensure that the observed reactivity was not an artifact. A glutaraldehyde-hapten effect was possible because the initial immunogen was glutaraldehyde-fixed sperm. This was ruled out because (1) the SSA reacted with both living and formaldehyde-fixed sperm; (2) a second antiserum, raised against unfixed, whole sperm had the same specificity; (3) a third antiserum, raised against a Triton X-100 extract of sea urchin sperm, also had similar reactivity; and (4) absorbing the SSA with a membrane extract of whole sperm eliminated the reactivity (Lopo and Vacquier, 1980c).

Other possible sources of artifact were ruled out, including (1) reactivity with carbohydrate sequences in Freund's adjuvant; (2) reactivity with secretions from male accessory glands; (3) reactivity with nervous tissue antigens; (4) recognition of H-Y, the male-specific antigen; (5) recognition of a surface tubulin, and (6) nonspecific binding by the Fc region of antibodies (Lopo and Vacquier, 1980c).

These results suggest that common cross-reactive determinant(s) exist on the surface of all animal sperm. The function of this common sperm surface antigenicity is at this time unknown.

IX. AVENUES FOR FUTURE RESEARCH

The last 10 years have seen exciting advances in our understanding of the molecular nature of sperm–egg interaction. During this time we have made excellent progress in our comprehension of the morphology, physiological control, and biochemical basis for many events of sperm–egg interaction. Invertebrate organisms, particularly sea urchins, have been heavily used as a plentiful source of gametes for these studies. However, there remain countless questions which must be answered before we have a total understanding of these phenomena.

How does the interaction of egg jelly with the sperm surface induce the acrosome reaction? Although the M_r 84,000 glycoprotein from sea urchin sperm described by Lopo and Vacquier (1980b) is implicated in the induction of the acrosome reaction, there is no evidence at this time that it is a receptor for egg jelly. It is possible that jelly acts, not by binding to a specific receptor, but by unmasking ion $(Ca^{2+}??)$ channels or by causing patching or capping of sperm membrane molecules resulting in alterations in membrane permeability (Vacquier, 1979). It is hoped that work in progress in several laboratories will provide an answer in the near future.

Recent work has greatly increased our understanding of the physiological controls of the acrosome reaction; however, much work remains to be done to understand completely not only the sequence of changes but also their significance to physiological conditions. Are the late changes described by Schackmann and Shapiro (1981) artifactual or do they have a physiological role in sperm–egg interaction? Does protein phosphorylation play a role in the control of ion fluxes and/or actin polymerization during the acrosome reaction?

Sea urchin bindin was the first protein isolated from any multicellular animal in fairly pure milligram quantities that mediates a specific multicellular adhesion. The isolation of glycoconjugates from the egg surface that interact with the bindin mark the first time interacting surface components from both egg and sperm have been isolated from any organism. However, much more work is needed to gain a more complete understanding of the nature of these components and their interactions. What is the three-dimensional nature of the egg surface glycoconjugate receptors? Why is it that the crude receptor preparation retains species specificity, yet the glycoconjugate fragments lose it, although they are still capable of interacting with the bindin? Does binding have a role in membrane fusion? What about bindin in other species? Are bindinlike molecules the mediators of sperm–egg adhesion throughout the animal kingdom?

One area of sperm-egg interaction that remains poorly understood is the penetration of extracellular egg envelopes and gamete membrane fusion. Until recently the existence of a sea urchin acrosin was doubted by many. There is still some controversy over the role of these and other sperm proteases in fertilization. Also interesting in this context is the evidence by Haino-Fukushima (1974) and Lewis et al. (1982) for nonenzymatic methods of vitelline layer dissolution in some mollusks. More work is needed to determine how widespread this phenomenon is in the animal kingdom.

In this chapter I have attempted to present an overview of some recent advances in our understanding of the molecular basis of sperm–

egg interaction in invertebrates. Because of limitations in space and the author's data base, many areas of active research were unfortunately omitted. From the work presented it is evident that more questions have been raised than answered. Much work must be done before we can achieve a complete understanding of the molecular details of animal fertilization.

ACKNOWLEDGMENTS

The author would like to thank W. H. Clark, Jr., A. Yudin, J. W. Lynn, D. Clapper, D. Epel, M. Gould-Somero, J. Stephano Hornedo, N. L. Cross, V. D. Vacquier, C. Lewis, and C. Talbot for generously sharing their unpublished results. The author is also grateful to Dr. S. L. Wolfe for reviewing and editing the manuscript and to Ms. Ellen Tani for expert typing.

This chapter was written while the author was a postdoctoral fellow (NIH HD 05894) in the laboratory of Dr. John W. B. Hershey.

REFFERENCES

Aketa, K. (1967). On the sperm-egg bonding as the initial step of fertilization in the sea urchin. *Embryologia* **9**, 238–245.

Aketa, K. (1973). Physiological studies on the sperm surface component responsible for sperm-egg bonding in sea urchin fertilization. *Exp. Cell Res.* **80**, 439–441.

Aketa, K. (1975). Physiological studies on the sperm surface component responsible for sperm-egg bonding in sea urchin fertilization. II. Effect of Concanavalin A on the fertilizing capacity of sperm. *Exp. Cell Res.* **90**, 56–62.

Aketa, K., and Ohta, T. (1977). When do sperm of the sea urchin, *Pseudocentrotus depressus,* undergo the acrosome reaction at fertilization? *Dev. Biol.* **61**, 366–372.

Aketa, K., Onitake, K., and Tsuzuki, H. (1972). Tryptic disruption of sperm-binding site of sea urchin egg surface. *Exp. Cell Res.* **71**, 27–32.

Austin, C. R. (1966). "Fertilization." Prentice-Hall, Englewood Cliffs, New Jersey.

Barros, C., and Yanagimachi, R. (1971). Induction of zona reaction in golden hamster eggs by cortical granule material. *Nature (London)* **233**, 268–269.

Bearer, E. L., and Friend, D. S. (1980). Anionic lipid domains: Correlation with functional topography in a mammalian cell membrane. *Proc. Natl. Acad. Sci. U.S.A.* **77**, 6601–6605.

Bearer, E. L., and Friend, D. S. (1981). Maintenance of lipid domains in the guinea pig sperm membrane. *J. Cell Biol.* **91**, 266a.

Bellet, N. R., Vacquier, J. P., and Vacquier, V. D. (1977). Characterization and comparison of "bindin" isolated from sperm of two species of sea urchins. *Biochem. Biophys. Res. Commun.* **79**, 159–165.

Bestor, T., and Schatten, G. (1981). Anti-tubulin immunofluorescence microscopy of microtubules present during the pronuclear movements of sea urchin fertilization. *Dev. Biol.* **88**, 80–91.

Blaustein, M. P. (1977). Effects of internal and external cations and of ATP on sodium-calcium and calcium-calcium exchange in squid axons. *Biophys. J.* **20**, 79–117.

Bleil, J. D., and Wassarman, P. M. (1980a). Structure and function of the zona pellucida: Identification and characterization of the proteins of the mouse oocyte's zona pellucida. *Dev. Biol.* **76**, 185–202.

Bleil, J. D., and Wassarman, P. M. (1980b). Mammalian sperm-egg interaction: Identification of a glycoprotein in mouse egg zonae pellucidae possessing receptor activity for sperm. *Cell* **20**, 873–882.

Bradley, F. M., Meth, B. N., and Bellvé, A. R. (1981). Structural proteins of the mouse spermatozoan tail: An electrophoretic analysis. *Biol. Reprod.* **24**, 691–701.

Brandriff, B., Moy, G. W., and Vacquier, V. D. (1978). Isolation of sperm bindin from the oyster (*Crassostrea gigas*). *Gamete Res.* **1**, 89–99.

Brokaw, C. J. (1957). "Electro-chemical" orientation of bracken spermatozoids. *Nature (London)* **179**, 525–527.

Brown, G. G. (1976). Scanning electron-microscopical and other observations of sperm fertilization reactions in *Limulus polyphemus* (Merostomata: Xiphosura). *J. Cell Sci.* **22**, 547–562.

Carroll, E. J., and Epel, D. (1975). Isolation and biological activity of the proteases released by sea urchin eggs following fertilization. *Dev. Biol.* **44**, 22–32.

Carron, C. P., and Longo, F. J. (1980). Relation of intracellular pH and pronuclear movement in the sea urchin, *Arbacia punctulata*. *Dev. Biol.* **79**, 478–487.

Chambers, R. (1930). The manner of sperm entry in the starfish egg. *Biol. Bull. (Woods Hole, Mass.)* **58**, 344–369.

Chandler, D. E., and Heuser, J. (1979). The vitelline layer of the sea urchin egg and its modification during fertilization. *J. Cell Biol.* **84**, 618–632.

Chandler, D. E., and Heuser, J. (1981). Postfertilization growth of microvilli in the sea urchin egg: New views from eggs that have been quick-frozen, freeze-fractured, and deeply etched. *Dev. Biol.* **82**, 393–400.

Cheung, W. Y. (1980). Calmodulin plays a pivotal role in cellular regulation. *Science* **207**, 19–27.

Clark, W. H., Jr., Lynn, J. W., Yudin, A. I., and Persyn, H. O. (1980). Morphology of the cortical reaction in the eggs of *Penaeus aztecus*. *Biol. Bull. (Woods Hole, Mass.)* **158**, 175–186.

Clark, W. H., Jr., Kleve, M. G., and Yudin, A. I. (1981). An acrosome reaction in natantian sperm. *J. Exp. Zool.* (in press).

Cloney, R. A., and Abbott, L. C. (1980). The spermatozoa of ascidians: acrosome and nuclear envelope. *Cell Tissue Res.* **206**, 261–270.

Collins, F. (1976). A reevaluation of the fertilizin hypothesis of sperm agglutination and the description of a novel form of sperm adhesion. *Dev. Biol.* **49**, 381–394.

Collins, F., and Epel, D. (1977). The role of calcium ions in the acrosome reaction of sea urchin sperm. *Exp. Cell Res.* **106**, 211–222.

Colwin, L. H., and Colwin, A. L. (1967). Membrane fusion in relation to sperm-egg association. *In* "Fertilization" (C. B. Metz and A. Monroy, eds.), Vol. 1, pp. 295–367. Academic Press, New York.

Conway, A. F., and Metz, C. B. (1976). Phospholipase activity of sea urchin sperm: Its possible involvement in membrane fusion. *J. Exp. Zool.* **198**, 39–48.

Czihak, G. (1975). "The Sea Urchin Embryo. Biochemistry and Morphogenesis." Springer-Verlag, Berlin and New York.

Dale, B., Denis-Donini, S., DeSantis, R., Monroy, A., Rosati, F., and Taglietti, V. (1978). Sperm-egg interaction in the ascidians. *Biol. Cell.* **32**, 129–133.

Dan, J. C. (1952). Studies on the acrosome. I. Reaction to egg-water and other stimuli. *Biol. Bull. (Woods Hole, Mass.)* **103**, 54–61.

Dan, J. C. (1954a). Studies on the acrosome. II. Acrosome reaction in starfish spermatozoa. *Biol. Bull. (Woods Hole, Mass.)* **107**, 203–218.

Dan, J. C. (1954b). Studies on the acrosome. III. Effect of calcium deficiency. *Biol. Bull. (Woods Hole, Mass.)* **107**, 335–349.

Dan, J. C. (1956). The acrosome reaction. *Int. Rev. Cytol.* **5**, 365–393.

Dan, J. C. (1967). Acrosome reaction and lysins. *In* "Fertilization" (C. B. Metz and A. Monroy, eds.), Vol. 1, pp. 237–293. Academic Press, New York.

Decker, G. L., and Lennarz, W. J. (1979). Sperm binding and fertilization envelope formation in a cell surface complex isolated from sea urchin eggs. *J. Cell Biol.* **81**, 92–103.

Decker, G. L., Joseph, D. B., and Lennarz, W. J. (1976). A study of factors involved in induction of the acrosomal reaction in sperm of the sea urchin, *Arbacia punctulata*. *Dev. Biol.* **53**, 115–125.

DeSantis, R., Jammuno, G., and Rosati, F. (1980). A study of the chorion and the follicle cells in relation to the sperm-egg interaction in the ascidian *Ciona intestinalis*. *Dev. Biol.* **74**, 490–499.

Dioplo, R., Requena, J., Brinley, F. J., Mullins, L. J., Scarpa, A., and Tiffert, T. (1976). Ionized calcium concentrations in squid axon. *J. Gen. Physiol.* **67**, 433–467.

Dunbar, B. S., Wardrip, N. J., and Hedrick, J. L. (1980). Isolation, physiochemical properties, and macromolecular composition of zona pellucida from porcine oocytes. *Biochemistry* **19**, 356–365.

Eckberg, W. R., and Metz, C. B. (1982), Isolation of an *Arbacia* sperm fertilization antigen. *J. Exp. Zool.* **221**, 101–105.

Epel, D. (1978). Mechanisms of activation of sperm and egg during fertilization of sea urchin gametes. *Curr. Top. Dev. Biol.* **12**, 185–246.

Epel, D., and Vacquier, V. D. (1978). Membrane fusion events during invertebrate fertilization. *Cell Surf. Rev.* **5**, 1–63.

Epel, D., Weaver, A. M., and Mazia, D. (1970). Methods for removal of the vitelline layer of sea urchin eggs. I. Use of dithiothreitol (Cleland reagent). *Exp. Cell Res.* **61**, 64–68.

Ezzell, S. D. (1963). The lateral body of *Ciona intestinalis* spermatozoa. *Exp. Cell Res.* **30**, 615–617.

Feuchther, F. A., Vernon, R. B., and Eddy, E. M. (1981). Analysis of the sperm surface with monoclonal antibodies: Topographically restricted antigens appearing in the epididymis. *Biol. Reprod.* **24**, 1099–1110.

Foerder, C. A., and Shapiro, B. M. (1977). Release of ovoperoxidase from sea urchin eggs hardens the fertilization membrane with tyrosine cross-links. *Proc. Natl. Acad. Sci. U.S.A.* **74**, 4214–4218.

Fol, H. (1878–1879). Recherches sur la fécondation et le commencement de l'hénogénie chez divers animaux. *Mem. Soc. Phys. Hist. Nat. Geneve* **26**, 89–250.

Friend, D. S., and Heuser, J. E. (1981). Orderly particle arrays on the mitochondrial outer membrane in rapidly-frozen sperm. *Anat. Rec.* **199**, 159–175.

Friend, D. S., and Rudolf, I. (1974). Acrosomal disruption in sperm. *J. Cell Biol.* **63**, 466–479.

Friend, D. S., Orci, L., Perrelet, A., and Yanagimachi, R. (1977). Membrane particle changes attending the acrosome reaction in guinea pig spermatozoa. *J. Cell Biol.* **74**, 561–577.

Fulton, B. P., and Whittingham, D. G. (1978). Activation of mammalian oocytes by intracellular injection of calcium. *Nature (London)* **273**, 149–151.

Gabel, C. A., and Shapiro, B. M. (1978). ^{125}I-diiodofluorescein isothiocyanate: Its synthesis and use as a reagent for labeling proteins and cells to high specific radioactivity. *Anal. Biochem.* **86**, 396–406.

Gabel, C. A., Eddy, E. M., and Shapiro, B. M. (1979). Regional differentiation of the sperm surface as studied with ^{125}I-diiodofluorescein isothiocyanate, an impermeant reagent that allows isolation of the labeled components. *J. Cell Biol.* **82**, 742–754.

Garbers, D. L. (1981). The elevation of cyclic AMP concentrations in flagella-less sea urchin sperm heads. *J. Biol. Chem.* **256**, 620–624.

Garbers, D. L., and Hardman, J. G. (1975). Factors released from sea urchin eggs affect cyclic nucleotide metabolism in sperm. *Nature (London)* **257**, 677–678.

Garbers, D. L., and Hardman, J. G. (1976). Effects of egg factors on cyclic nucleotide metabolism in sea urchin sperm. *J. Cyclic Nucleotide Res.* **2**, 59–70.

Garbers, D. L., and Kopf, G. S. (1978). Effects of factors released from eggs and other agents on cyclic nucleotide concentration of sea urchin spermatozoa. *J. Reprod. Fertil.* **52**, 135–140.

Garbers, D. L., and Kopf, G. S. (1980). The regulation of spermatozoa by cyclic nucleotides. *Adv. Cyclic Nucleotide Res.* **13**, 251–306.

Garbers, D. L., Watkins, H. D., Tubb, D. J., and Kopf, G. S. (1978). Regulation of spermatozoan cyclic nucleotide metabolism by egg factors. *Adv. Cyclic Nucleotide Res.* **9**, 583–595.

Garbers, D. L., Tubb, D. J., and Kopf, G. S. (1980a). Regulation of sea urchin sperm cyclic AMP-dependent protein kinases by an egg associated factor. *Biol. Reprod.* **22**, 526–532.

Garbers, D. L., Hansbrough, J. R., Radany, E. W., Hyne, R. V., and Kopf, G. S. (1980b). Purification and characterization of calmodulin from sea urchin spermatozoa. *J. Reprod. Fertil.* **59**, 377–381.

Garbers, D. L., Watkins, H. D., Hansbrough, J. R., Smith, A., II, Misono, K. S. (1982). The amino acid sequence and chemical synthesis of speract and of speract analogues. *J. Biol. Chem.* **257**, 2734–2737.

Gething, M. J., White, J. M., and Waterfield, N. D. (1978). Purification of the fusion protein of Sendai virus: Analysis of the NH-terminal sequence generated during precursor activation. *Proc. Natl. Acad. Sci. U.S.A.* **75**, 2737–2740.

Gilkey, J. C., Jaffe, L. S., Ridgway, L. S. B., and Reynolds, G. T. (1976). A free calcium wave traverses the activating egg of the medaka *Oryzias latipes. J. Cell Biol.* **76**, 448–466.

Giudice, G. (1973). "Developmental Biology of the Sea Urchin Embryo." Academic Press, New York.

Glabe, C. G., and Lennarz, W. J. (1979). Species-specific sperm adhesion in sea urchins: A quantitative investigation of bindin-mediated egg agglutination. *J. Cell Biol.* **83**, 595–604.

Glabe, C. G., and Lennarz, W. J. (1981). Isolation and partial characterization of a high molecular weight egg surface glycoconjugate implicated in sperm adhesion. *J. Supramol. Struct.* **15**, 387–394.

Glabe, C. G., and Vacquier, V. D. (1977a). Species-specific agglutination of eggs by bindin isolated from sea urchin sperm. *Nature (London)* **267**, 836–838.

Glabe, C. G., and Vacquier, V. D. (1977b). Isolation and characterization of the vitelline layer of sea urchin eggs. *J. Cell Biol.* **75**, 410–421.

Glabe, C. G., and Vacquier, V. D. (1978). Egg surface glycoprotein receptor for sea urchin sperm bindin. *Proc. Natl. Acad. Sci. U.S.A.* **75**, 881–885.

Glabe, C. G., Buchalter, M., and Lennarz, W. J. (1981). Studies on the interactions of sperm with the surface of the sea urchin egg. *Dev. Biol.* **84**, 397–406.

Glabe, C. G., Lennarz, W. J., and Vacquier, V. D. (1982). Sperm surface components involved in sea urchin fertilization. *In* "Cell Recognition" (C. F. Fox, ed.). Academic Press, New York (in press).

Gray, J. P., and Drummond, G. I. (1976). Guanylate cyclase of sea urchin sperm: Subcellular localization. *Arch. Biochem. Biophys.* **172**, 31–38.

Green, J. D., and Summers, R. G. (1980). Ultrastructural demonstration of trypsin-like protease in acrosomes of sea urchin sperm. *Science* **209**, 398–400.

Green, J. D., and Summers, R. G. (1982) Effects of protease inhibitors on sperm-related events in sea urchin fertilization. *Dev. Biol.* **92**, 139–144.

Greengard, P. (1978). Phosphorylated proteins as physiological effectors. *Science* **199**, 146–152.

Gregg, K. W., and Metz, C. B. (1976). Physiological parameters of the sea urchin acrosome reaction. *Biol. Reprod.* **14**, 405–411.

Gwatkin, R. B. L., Williams, D. T., Hartmann, J. F., and Kniazuk, M. (1973). The zona reaction of hamster and mouse eggs: Production *in vitro* by a trypsin-like protease from cortical granules. *J. Reprod. Fertil.* **32**, 259–265.

Hagström, B. E. (1958). The influence of jelly coat solution on sea urchin spermatozoa. *Exp. Cell Res.* **16**, 184–192.

Hagström, B. E. (1959). Further experiments on jelly-free sea urchin eggs. *Exp. Cell Res.* **17**, 256–261.

Haino, K., and Kigawa, M. (1966). Studies on the egg membrane lysin of *Tegula pfeifferi:* Isolation and chemical analysis of the egg membrane. *Exp. Cell Res.* **42**, 625–633.

Haino, K., and Kigawa, M. (1969). Studies on the egg membrane lysin of *Tegula pfeifferi:* Quantitative assay of the lytic activity. *Dev., Growth Differ.* **11**, 203–218.

Haino-Fukushima, D. (1974). Studies on the egg membrane lysin of *Tegula pfeifferi:* The reaction mechanism of the lysin. *Biochim. Biophys. Acta* **352**, 179–191.

Hall, H. G. (1978). Hardening of the sea urchin fertilization envelope by peroxidase-catalyzed phenolic coupling of tyrosines. *Cell* **15**, 343–355.

Hallez, P. (1874). Note sur le développement des spermatozoides des Decapodes Brachyures. *C. R. Hebd. Seances Acad. Sci.* **70**, 243–246.

Hanada, A., and Chang, M. C. (1976). Penetration of hamster and rabbit zona-free eggs by rat and mouse spermatozoa with special reference to sperm capacitation. *J. Reprod. Fertil.* **46**, 239–241.

Hansbrough, J. R., and Garbers, D. L. (1981a). Speract. Purification and characterization of a peptide associated with eggs that activates spermatozoa. *J. Biol. Chem.* **256**, 1447–1452.

Hansbrough, J. R., and Garbers, D. L. (1981b). Sodium-dependent activation of sea urchin spermatozoa by speract and monensin. *J. Biol. Chem.* **256**, 2235–2241.

Hansbrough, J. R., Kopf, G. S., and Garbers, D. L. (1980). The stimulation of sperm metabolism by a factor associated with eggs and by 8-bromoguanosine 3′,5′-monophosphate. *Biochim. Biophys. Acta* **630**, 82–91.

Hathaway, R. R., and Metz, C. B. (1962). Interactions between *Arbacia* sperm and ^{35}S-labeled fertilizin. *Biol. Bull. (Woods Hole, Mass.)* **120**, 360–369.

Heller, E., and Raftery, M. A. (1973). Isolation and purification of three egg-membrane lysins from sperm of the marine invertebrate *Megathura crenulata* (giant keyhole limpet). *Biochemistry* **12**, 4106–4113.

Heller, E., and Raftery, M. A. (1976a). The vitelline envelope of eggs from the giant keyhole limpet *Megathura crenulata*. I. Chemical composition and structural studies. *Biochemistry* **15**, 1194–1198.

Heller, E., and Raftery, M. A. (1976b). The vitelline envelope of eggs from the giant keyhole limpet *Megathura crenulata*. II. Products formed by lysis with sperm enzyme and dithiothreitol. *Biochemistry* **15**, 1199–1203.

Herr, J. C., and Eddy, E. M. (1980). Detection of mouse sperm antigens by a surface labeling and immunoprecipitation approach. *Biol. Reprod.* **22**, 1263–1274.

Hille, B. (1967). The selective inhibition of delayed potassium currents in nerve by tetraethylammonium ion. *J. Gen. Physiol.* **50**, 1287–1302.

Hinsch, G. W. (1973). Comparative fine structure of Cnidaria spermatozoa. *Biol. Reprod.* **8**, 62–73.

Hinsch, G. W. (1974). Comparative ultrastructure of Cnidaria sperm. *A. Zool.* **14**, 457–465.

Hoshi, M., and Moriya, T. (1980). Arylsulfatase of sea urchin sperm. 2. Arylsulfatase as a lysin of sea urchins. *Dev. Biol.* **74**, 343–350.

Hoshi, M., and Nagai, Y. (1975). Novel sialosphingolipids from spermatozoa of the sea urchin *Anthocidaris crassispina*. *Biochim. Biophys. Acta* **388**, 152–162.

Hoshi, M., Moriya, T., Aoyagi, T., Umezawa, H., Mohri, H., and Nagai, Y. (1979). Effects of hydrolase inhibitors on fertilization of sea urchins. I. Protease inhibitors. *Gamete Res.* **2**, 107–119.

Hoshi, M., Numakunai, T., and Sawada, H. (1981). Evidence for participation of sperm proteinases in fertilization of the solitary ascidian, *Halocythia roretzi:* Effects of protease inhibitors. *Dev. Biol.* **86**, 117–121.

Hotta, K., Hamazaki, H., and Kurokawa, M. (1970a). Isolation and properties of a new type of sialopolysaccharide-protein complex from the jelly coat of sea urchin eggs. *J. Biol. Chem.* **245**, 5434–5440.

Hotta, K., Kurokawa, M., and Isaka, S. (1970b). Isolation and identification of two sialic acids from the jelly coat of sea urchin eggs. *J. Biol. Chem.* **245**, 6307–6311.

Hotta, K., Kurokawa, M., and Isaka, S. (1973). A novel sialic acid and fucose-containing disaccharide isolated from the jelly coat of sea urchin eggs. *J. Biol. Chem.* **248**, 629–631.

Hyne, R. V., and Garbers, D. L. (1979). Regulation of guinea pig sperm adenylate cyclase by calcium. *Biol. Reprod.* **21**, 1135–1142.

Ikadai, H., andHoshi, M. (1981). Biochemical studies on the acrosome reaction of the starfish, *Asterias amurensis*. I. Factors participating in the acrosome reaction. *Dev., Growth Differ.* **23**, 73–80.

Isaka, S., Hotta, K., and Kurokawa, M. (1970). Jelly coat substances of sea urchin eggs. *Exp. Cell Res.* **59**, 37–42.

Ishihara, K., Oguri, K., and Taniguchi, H. (1973). Isolation and characterization of fucose sulfate from jelly coat glycoprotein of sea urchin egg. *Biochem. Biophys. Acta* **320**, 628–634.

Ji, I., Yoo, B. Y., and Ji, T. H. (1981). Surface proteins and glycoproteins of ejaculated bovine spermatozoa. I. Iodination and proteolytic digestion. *Biol. Reprod.* **24**, 617–626.

Jones, H. P., Bradford, M. M., McRorie, R. A., and Coxmier, M. J. (1978). High levels of a calcium-dependent modulator protein in spermatozoa and its similarity to brain modulator protein. *Biochem. Biophys. Res. Commun.* **82**, 1264–1272.

Just, E. E. (1929). The production of filaments by echinoderm ova as a response to insemination, with special reference to the phenomena exhibited by ova of the genus *Asterias. Biol. Bull. (Woods Hole, Mass.)* **57,** 311–325.

Kidd, P. (1978). The jelly and vitelline coats of the sea urchin egg: New ultrastructural features. *J. Ultrastruct. Res.* **64,** 204–215.

Kinsey, W. H., Rubin, J. A., and Lennarz, W. J. (1980). Studies on the specificity of sperm binding in echinoderm fertilization. *Dev. Biol.* **74,** 245–250.

Klee, C. B., Crouch, T. H., and Rickman, P. G. (1980). Calmodulin. *Annu. Rev. Biochem.* **49,** 489–515.

Kleve, M. G., Yudin, A. I., and Clark, W. H., Jr. (1980). Fine structure of the unistellate sperm of the shrimp, *Sicyonia ingentis* (Natantia). *Tissue Cell* **12,** 29–45.

Kopf, G. S., and Garbers, D. L. (1978). Correlation between sea urchin sperm respiratory rates and cyclic AMP concentrations as a function of cell dilution. *Biol. Reprod.* **18,** 229–233.

Kopf, G. S., and Garbers, D. L. (1979). A low molecular weight factor from sea urchin eggs elevates sperm cyclic nucleotide concentrations and respiration rates. *J. Reprod. Fertil.* **57,** 353–361.

Kopf, G. S., and Garbers, D. L. (1980). Calcium and fucose-sulfate rich polymer regulate sperm cyclic nucleotide metabolism and the acrosome reaction. *Biol. Reprod.* **22,** 1118–1126.

Kopf, G. S., Tubb, D. J., and Garbers, D. L. (1979). Activation of sperm respiration by a low molecular weight egg factors and by 8-bromoguanosine 3′,5′-monophosphate. *J. Biol. Chem.* **254,** 8554–8560.

Kozhina, V. P., Terekhova, T. A., and Svetashev, V. I. (1978). Lipid composition of gametes and embryos of the sea urchin *Strongylocentrotus intermedius* at early stages of development. *Dev. Biol.* **62,** 512–517.

Krebs, E., and Beavo, J. A. (1979). Phosphorylation-dephosphorylation of enzymes. *Annu. Rev. Biochem.* **48,** 923–959.

Lambert, C. C., and Epel, D. (1979). Calcium-mediated mitochondrial movement in ascidian sperm during fertilization. *Dev. Biol.* **69,** 296–304.

Lambert, C. C., and Lambert, G. (1978). Tunicate eggs utilize ammonium ions for flotation. *Science* **200,** 64–65.

Lambert, C. C., and Lambert, G. (1981). The ascidian sperm reaction: Ca²⁺ uptake in relation to H⁺ efflux. *Dev. Biol.* **88,** 312–317.

Levin, R. M., and Weiss, B. (1976). Mechanisms by which psychotrophic drugs inhibit adenosine cyclic 3′,5′-monophosphate phosphodiesterase of brain. *Mol. Pharmacol.* **12,** 581–589.

Levine, A. E., and Walsh, K. A. (1979). Involvement of an acrosin-like enzyme in the acrosome reaction of sea urchin sperm. *Dev. Biol.* **72,** 126–137.

Levine, A. E., and Walsh, K. A. (1980). Purification of an acrosin-like enzyme from sea urchin sperm. *J. Biol. Chem.* **255,** 4814–4820.

Levine, A. E., Walsh, K. A., and Fodor, E. J. B. (1978). Evidence of an acrosin-like enzyme in the acrosome reaction of sea urchin sperm. *Dev. Biol.* **72,** 126–137.

Lewis, C. A., Leighton, D. L., and Vacquier, V. D. (1980). Morphology of abalone spermatozoa before and after the acrosome reaction. *J. Ulstrastruct. Res.* **72,** 39–46.

Lewis, C. A., Talbot, C. F., and Vacquier, V. D. (1982). A protein from abalone sperm dissolves the egg vitelline layer by a nonenzymatic mechanism. *Dev. Biol.* **92,** 227–239.

Lillie, F. R. (1913a). Mechanism of fertilization. *Science* **38,** 524–528.

Lillie, F. R. (1913b). Studies on fertilization. V. The behavior of the spermatozoa of

Nereis and *Arbacia* with special reference to egg extractives. *J. Exp. Zool.* **14,** 515–574.

Lillie, F. R. (1914). Studies on fertilization. VI. Mechanism of fertilization in *Arbacia. J. Exp. Zool.* **16,** 524–590.

Lillie, F. R. (1915). Sperm agglutinins and fertilization. *Biol. Bull. (Woods Hole, Mass.)* **28,** 18–33.

Lillie, F. R. (1919). "Problems of Fertilization." Univ. of Chicago Press, Chicago, Illinois.

Loeb, J. (1916). "The Organism as a Whole." Univ. of Chicago Press, Chicago, Illinois.

Longo, F. J. (1976) Derivation of the membrane comprising the male pronuclear envelope in inseminated sea urchin eggs. *Dev. Biol.* **49,** 347–368.

Longo, F. J. (1978). Effect of cytochalasin B on sperm–egg interactions. *Dev. Biol.* **67,** 249–265.

Longo, F. J., and Kunkle, M. (1978). Transformations of sperm nuclei upon insemination. *Curr. Top. Dev. Biol.* **12,** 149–184.

Lopo, A. C., and Vacquier, V. D. (1980a). Radioiodination and characterization of the plasma membrane of sea urchin sperm. *Dev. Biol.* **76,** 15–25.

Lopo, A. C., and Vacquier, V. D. (1980b). Antibody to a sperm surface glycoprotein inhibits the egg jelly-induced acrosome reaction of sea urchin sperm. *Dev. Biol.* **79,** 325–333.

Lopo, A. C., and Vacquier, V. D. (1980c). Sperm-specific surface antigenicity common to seven animal phyla. *Nature (London)* **288,** 397–399.

Lopo, A. C., and Vacquier, V. D. (1981). Gamete interaction during sea urchin fertilization: A model for studying the molecular details of animal fertilization. *In* "Fertilization and Early Development" (L. Mastroianni, Jr. and J. D. Biggers, eds.), pp. 199–232. Plenum, New York.

Lopo, A. C., Bean, C. P., and Epel, D. (1977). Studies on sperm-jelly interaction: Is there chemotaxis? *Biol. Bull. (Woods Hole, Mass.)* **153,** 437.

Lopo, A. C., Glabe, C. G., Lennarz, W. J., and Vacquier, V. D. (1982). Sperm-egg interaction in sea urchins. *Ann. N. Y. Acad. Sci.* (in press).

Lui, C. W., and Meizel, S. (1979). Further evidence in support of a role for hamster sperm hydrolytic enzymes in the acrosome reaction. *J. Exp. Zool.* **207,** 173–182.

Lynn, J. W., and Clark, W. H., Jr. (1982). Physiological and biochemical investigations of the egg cortical reaction in *Penaeus aztecus.* (Submitted for publication.)

Mar, H. (1980). Radial cortical fibers and pronuclear migration in fertilized and artificially activated eggs of *Lytechinus pictus. Dev. Biol.* **78,** 1–13.

Mazia, D., Schatten, G., and Steinhardt, R. (1975). Turning on activities in unfertilized sea urchin eggs: Correlation with changes of the surface. *Proc. Natl. Acad. Sci. U.S.A.* **72,** 4469–4473.

Means, A. R., and Dedman, J. R. (1980). Calmodulin—an intracellular calcium receptor. *Nature (London)* **285,** 73–77.

Meizel, S. (1978). The mammalian sperm acrosome reaction, a biochemical approach. *In* "Development in Mammals" (M. H. Johnson, ed.), Vol. 3, 1–64. North-Holland Publ., Amsterdam.

Metz, C. B. (1967). Gamete surface components and their role in fertilization. *In* "Fertilization" (C. B. Metz and A. Monroy, eds.), Vol. 1, pp. 163–236. Academic Press, New York.

Metz, C. B. (1978). Sperm and egg receptors involved in fertilization. *Curr. Top. Dev. Biol.* **12,** 107–147.

Metz, C. B., and Monroy, A., eds. (1967). "Fertilization." Academic Press, New York.

Miller, R. L. (1966). Chemotaxis during fertilization in the hydroid *Campanularia*. *J. Exp. Zool.* **162**, 23–44.

Miller, R. L. (1975). Chemotaxis of the spermatozoa of *Ciona intestinalis*. *Nature (London)* **254**, 244–245.

Miller, R. L. (1977a). Chemotactic behavior of the sperm of chitons (Mollusca: Polyplacophora). *J. Exp. Zool.* **202**, 203–212.

Miller, R. L. (1977b). Distribution of sperm chemotaxis in the animal kingdom. *Adv. Invertebr. Reprod.* **1**, 99–119.

Miller, R. L. (1978). Site-specific sperm agglutination and the timed release of a sperm chemo-attractant by the egg of the leptomedusan, *Orthopyxis caliculata*. *J. Exp. Zool.* **205**, 385–392.

Miller, R. L. (1979a). Sperm chemotaxis in the hydromedusae. I. Species-specificity and sperm behavior. *Mar. Biol.* **53**, 99–114.

Miller, R. L. (1979b). Sperm chemotaxis in the hydromedusae. II. Some chemical properties of the sperm attractants. *Mar. Biol.* **53**, 115–124.

Miller, R. L. (1980). Sperm-egg interactions in hydromedusae. *In* "Advances in Invertebrate Reproduction" (W. H. Clark, Jr. and T. S. Adams, eds.), pp. 289–317. Elsevier North-Holland Publ., Amsterdam.

Miller, R. L., and Brokaw, C. J. (1970). Chemotactic turning behavior of *Tubularia* spermatozoa. *J. Exp. Biol.* **52**, 699–706.

Miller, R. L., and Tseng, C. Y. (1974). Properties and partial purification of the sperm attractant of *Tubularia*. *Am. Zool.* **14**, 467–486.

Millette, C. (1979). Cell surface antigens during mammalian spermatogenesis. *Curr. Top. Dev. Biol.* **13**, 1–32.

Millette, C. F., and Bellvé, A. R. (1980). Selective partitioning of plasma membrane antigens during mouse spermatogenesis. *Dev. Biol.* **79**, 309–324.

Millette, C. F., and Moulding, C. T. (1981). Radio iodination of plasma membrane polypeptides from isolated mouse spermatogenic cells. *Gamete Res.* **4**, 317–331.

Monroy, A. (1965). "Chemistry and Physiology of Fertilization." Holt, New York.

Moriya, T., and Hoshi, M. (1980). Characterization and partial purification of arylsulfatase from the seminal plasma of the sea urchin, *Strongylocentrotus intermedius*. *Arch. Biochem. Biophys.* **201**, 216–223.

Moy, G. W., and Vacquier, V. D. (1979). Immunoperoxidase localization of binding during the adhesion of sperm to sea urchin eggs. *Curr. Top. Dev. Biol.* **13**, 31–44.

Müller, D. G., Gassmann, G., and Leining, K. (1979). Isolation of a spermatozoid-releasing and -attracting substance from female gametophytes of *Laminaria digitata*. *Nature (London)* **279**, 430–431.

Müller, D. G., Gassmann, G., Boland, W., Marner, F., and Jaenicke, L. (1981). *Dictyota dichotoma* (Phaeophyceae): Identification of the sperm attractant. *Science* **212**, 1040–1042.

Nagai, Y., and Hoshi, M. (1975). Sialosphingolipids of sea urchin eggs and spermatozoa showing a characteristic composition for species and gamete. *Biochim. Biophys. Acta* **388**, 146–151.

Nagai, Y., and Ohsawa, T. (1974). Production of high titer antisera against sialoglycosphingolipids and their characterization using sensitized liposome. *Jpn. J. Exp. Med.* **44**, 451–464.

Nelson, L. (1975). Spermatozoa motility. *In* "Handbook of Physiology" (D. W. Hamilton and R. O. Greep, eds.), Sect. 7, Vol. V. pp. 421–435. Am. Physiol. Society, Washington, D. C.

Nishioka, D., and Cross, N. (1978). The role of external sodium in sea urchin fertilization. *In* "Cell Reproduction: Essays in Honor of Daniel Mazia" (E. R. Dirksen, D. M. Prescott, and C. F. Fox, eds.), pp. 403–413. Academic Press, New York.

Ohsawa, T., and Nagai, Y. (1975). Immunological evidence for the localization of sialoglycosphingolipids at the cell surface of sea urchin spermatozoa. *Biochim. Biophys. Acta* **389**, 69–83.

Ohtake, H. (1976a). Respiratory behavior of sea urchin spermatozoa. I. Effect of pH and egg water on the respiratory rate. *J. Exp. Zool.* **198**, 303–312.

Ohtake, H. (1976b). Respiratory behaviour of sea urchin spermatozoa. II. Sperm-activating substances obtained from jelly coat of sea urchin eggs. *J. Exp. Zool.* **198**, 313–322.

Oliphant, G., and Singhas, C. A. (1979). Iodination of rabbit sperm plasma membrane: Relationship of specific surface proteins to epididymal function and sperm capacitation. *Biol. Reprod.* **21**, 937–944.

O'Rand, M. G., and Porter, J. R. (1979). Isolation of a sperm membrane sialoglycoprotein autoantigen from rabbit testes. *J. Immunol.* **122**, 1248–1254.

O'Rand, M. G., and Romrell, L. J. (1980a). Identification of a rabbit sperm autoantigen as a *Ricinus communis* I receptor. *Gamete Res.* **3**, 317–322.

O'Rand, M. G., and Romrell, L. J. (1980b). Appearance of regional surface autoantigens during spermatogenesis: Comparison of anti-testes and anti-sperm autoantisera. *Dev. Biol.* **75**, 431–441.

O'Rand, M. G., and Romrell, L. J. (1981). Localization of a single sperm membrane autoantigen (RSA-1) on spermatogenic cells and spermatozoa. *Dev. Biol.* **84**, 322–331.

Parrish, R. F., and Polakoski, K. L. (1979). Mammalian sperm proacrosin-acrosin system. *Int. J. Biochem.* **10**, 391–395.

Peterson, R. N., Russell, L., Bundman, D., and Freund, M. (1980). Sperm-egg interaction: Evidence for boar sperm plasma membrane receptors for porcine zona pellucida. *Science* **207**, 73–74.

Pfeffer, W. (1984). Locomotorische Richtungsbewegungen durch chemische Reize. *Unters. Bot. Inst. Tübingen* **1**, 304–382.

Popa, G. T. (1927). The distribution of substances in the spermatozoon (*Arbacia* and *Nereis*). *Biol. Bull. (Woods Hole, Mass.)* **52**, 238–257.

Primakoff, P., Myles, D. G., and Bellvé, A. R. (1980). Biochemical analysis of the released products of the mammalian acrosome reaction. *Dev. Biol.* **80**, 324–331.

Rosati, F., and DeSantis, R. (1978). Studies on fertilization in the ascidians. I. Self-sterility and specific recognition between gametes of *Ciona intestinalis*. *Exp. Cell Res.* **112**, 111–119.

Rosati, F., and DeSantis, R. (1980). Role of the surface carbohydrates in sperm-egg interaction in *Ciona intestinalis*. *Nature (London)* **238**, 762–764.

Rosati, F., Monroy, A., and DePrisco, P. (1977). Fine structural study of fertilization in the ascidian, *Ciona intestinalis*. *J. Ultrastruct. Res.* **58**, 261–270.

Rosati, F., De Santis, R., and Monroy, A. (1978). Studies on fertilization in the ascidians. II. Lectin binding to the gametes of *Ciona intestinalis*. *Exp. Cell Res.* **116**, 419–427.

Rossignol, D. P., Roschelle, A. J., and Lennarz, W. J. (1981). Sperm-egg binding: Identification of a species-specific sperm receptor from eggs of *Strongylocentrotus purpuratus*. *J. Supramol. Struct.* **15**, 347–358.

Rothschild, Lord (1952). The behaviour of spermatozoa in the neighborhood of egg. *Int. Rev. Cytol.* **1**, 257–263.

Saling, P. M., Eckberg, W. R., and Metz, C. B. (1982). Mechanism of univalent antisperm antibody inhibition of fertilization in the sea urchin, *Arbacia punctulata. J. Exp. Zool.* **221**, 93–99.

Schackmann, R. W., and Shapiro, B. M. (1981). A partial sequence of ionic changes associated with the acrosome reaction of *Strongylocentrotus purpuratus. Dev. Biol.* **81**, 145–154.

Schackmann, R. W., Eddy, E. M., and Shapiro, B. M. (1978). The acrosome reaction of *Strongylocentrotus purpuratus* sperm. Ion requirements and movements. *Dev. Biol.* **65**, 483–495.

Schatten, H., and Schatten, G. (1980). Surface activity at the egg plasma membrane during sperm incorporation and its cytochalasin B sensitivity. *Dev. Biol.* **78**, 435–449.

Schmell, E. D., and Gulyas, B. J. (1980). Ovoperoxidase activation in ionophore-treated mouse eggs. II. Evidence for the enzyme's role in hardening the zona pellucida. *Gamete Res.* **3**, 279–290.

Schmell, E. D., Earles, B. J., Breaux, C., and Lennarz, W. J. (1977). Identification of a sperm receptor on the surface of the eggs of the sea urchin *Arbacia punctulata. J. Cell Biol.* **72**, 35–46.

Schroeder, T. E. (1978). Microvilli on sea urchin eggs: A second burst of elongation. *Dev. Biol.* **64**, 342–346.

Seeman, P. (1972). The membrane actions of anesthetics and tranquilizers. *Pharmacol. Rev.* **24**, 583–655.

SeGall, G. K., and Lennarz, W. J. (1979). Chemical characterization of the component of the jelly coat from sea urchin eggs responsible for induction of the acrosome reaction. *Dev. Biol.* **71**, 33–48.

SeGall, G. K., and Lennarz, W. J. (1981). Jelly coat and induction of the acrosome reaction in echinoid sperm. *Dev. Biol.* **86**, 87–93.

Shapiro, B. M. (1981). Awakening of the invertebrate egg at fertilization. *In* "Fertilization and Embryonic Development *in Vitro*" (L. Mastroianni, Jr. and J. D. Biggers, eds.), pp. 233–245. Plenum, New York.

Shapiro, B. M., Schackmann, R. W., Gabel, C. A., Foerder, C. A., and Farrance, M. L. (1980). Molecular alterations in gamete surfaces during fertilization and early development. *In* "The Cell Surface: Mediator of Developmental Processes" (S. Subtelney and N. K. Wessells, eds.), pp. 127–149. Academic Press, New York.

Shapiro, B. M., Schackmann, R. W., and Gabel, C. A. (1981). Molecular approaches to the study of fertilization. *Annu. Rev. Biochem.* **50**, 815–843.

Summers, R. G., and Hylander, B. L. (1975). Species-specificity of acrosome reaction and primary gamete binding in echinoids. *Exp. Cell Res.* **96**, 63–68.

Summers, R. G., and Hylander, B. L. (1976). Primary gamete binding. Quantitative determination of its specificity in echinoid fertilization. *Exp. Cell Res.* **100**, 190–194.

Summers, R. G., Hylander, B. L., Colwin, L. H., and Colwin, A. L. (1975). The functional anatomy of the echinoderm spermatozoon and its interaction with the egg at fertilization. *Am. Zool.* **15**, 523–551.

Summers, R. G., Talbot, P., Keough, E. M., Hylander, B. L., and Franklin, L. E. (1976). Ionophore A23187 induces acrosome reactions in sea urchin and guinea pig spermatozoa. *J. Exp. Zool.* **196**, 381–386.

Talbot, C. F., Lewis, C. A., and Vacquier, V. D. (1980). Isolation of an egg vitelline layer lysin from abalone sperm. *J. Cell Biol.* **87**, 138a.

Talbot, P., and Chanmanon, P. (1980). Morphological features of the acrosome reaction of lobster (*Homarus*) sperm and the role of the reaction in generating forward sperm movement. *J. Ultrastruct. Res.* **70**, 287–297.

Talbot, P., and Summers, R. G. (1978). The structure of sperm from *Panulirus,* the spiny lobster, with special regard to the acrosome. *J. Ultrastruct. Res.* **64**, 341– 351.

Talbot, P., Summers, R. G., Hylander, B. L., Keough, E. M., and Franklin, L. E. (1976). The role of calcium in the acrosome reaction: An analysis using ionophore A23187. *J. Exp. Zool.* **198**, 383–392.

Tegner, M. J., and Epel, D. (1973). Sea urchin sperm-egg interactions studied with the scanning electron microscope. *Science* **179**, 685–688.

Tegner, M. J., and Epel, D. (1976). Scanning electron microscope studies of sea urchin fertilization. I. Eggs with vitelline layers. *J. Exp. Zool.* **197**, 31–58.

Tilney, L. G. (1976a). The polymerization of actin. II. How nonfilamentous actin becomes nonrandomly distributed in sperm: Evidence for the association of this actin with membrane. *J. Cell Biol.* **69**, 51–72.

Tilney, L. G. (1976b). The polymerization of actin. III. Aggregates of nonfilamentous actin and its associated proteins: A storage form of actin. *J. Cell Biol.* **69**, 73–89.

Tilney, L. G. (1978) The polymerization of actin. V. A new organelle, the actomere, that initiates the assembly of actin filaments in *Thyone* sperm. *J. Cell Biol.* **77**, 551–564.

Tilney, L. G., and Mooseker, M. S. (1976). Actin in filament-membrane attachment: Are membrane particles involved? *J. Cell Biol.* **71**, 402–416.

Tilney, L. G., Hatano, S., Ishikawa, H., and Mooseker, M. S. (1973). The polymerization of actin: Its role in the generation of the acrosomal process of certain echinoderm sperm. *J. Cell Biol.* **59**, 109–126.

Tilney, L. G., Kiehart, D. P., Sardet, C., and Tilney, M. (1978). Polymerization of actin. IV. Role of Ca^{+2} and H^+ in the assembly of actin and in membrane fusion in the acrosomal reaction of echinoderm sperm. *J. Cell Biol.* **77**, 536–550.

Tilney, L. G., Clain, J. C., and Tilney, M. S. (1979). Membrane events in the acrosomal reaction of *Limulus* sperm. *J. Cell Biol.* **81**, 229–253.

Tsuzuki, H., and Aketa, K. (1969). A study on the possible significance of carbohydrate moiety in the sperm-binding protein from sea urchin egg. *Exp. Cell Res.* **55**, 43–45.

Tsuzuki, H., Yoshida, M., Onitake, K., and Aketa, K. (1977). Purification of the sperm-binding factor from the egg of the sea urchin, *Hemicentrotus pulcherrimus.* *Biochem. Biophys. Res. Commun.* **76**, 502–508.

Tubb, D. J., Kopf, G. S., and Garbers, D. L. (1978). The elevation of sperm adenosine 3′,5′-monophosphate concentrations by factors released from eggs requires calcium. *Biol. Reprod.* **18**, 181–185.

Tuzet, O., Bogoraze, D., and Lafargue, F. (1972). Recherches ultrastructurales sur la spermiogenese de *Diplosoma listerianum* (Milne-Edwards, 1841) and *Lissoclinum pseudoleptoclinum* (Von Drasche, 1833). *Ann. Sci. Nat., Zool., Zool., Biol. Amin.* [12] **14**, 177–190.

Tuzet, O., Bogoraze, D., and Lafargue, F. (1974). La spermatogénèse de *Polysyncration lacazei,* 1872 et *Trididemnum cereum* Giard, 1872. *Bull. Biol. Fr. Belg.* **108**, 151–167.

Tyler, A. (1948). Fertilization and immunity. *Physiol. Rev.* **28**, 180–219.

Tyler, A. (1949). Properties of fertilizin and related substances of eggs and sperm of marine animals. *Am. Nat.* **83**, 195–219.

Tyler, A., and O'Melveny, K. (1941). The role of antifertilizin in the fertilization of sea urchin eggs. *Biol. Bull. (Woods Hole, Mass.)* **81**, 364–374.

Uno, Y., and Hoshi, M. (1978). Separation of the sperm agglutinin and the acrosome-reaction inducing substance in egg jelly of starfish. *Science* **200**, 58–59.

Ursprung, H., and Schabtach, E. (1964). The fine structure of the egg of a tunicate, *Ascidia nigra. J. Exp. Zool.* **156**, 253–268.

Vacquier, V. D. (1979). The fertilizing capacity of sea urchin sperm rapidly decreases after induction of the acrosome reaction. *Dev. Growth Differ.* **21**, 61–69.

Vacquier, V. D. (1980). The adhesion of sperm to sea urchin eggs. *Symp. Soc. Dev. Biol.* **38**, 151–168.

Vacquier, V. D., and Moy, G. W. (1977). Isolation of bindin: The protein responsible for adhesion of sperm to sea urchin eggs. *Proc. Natl. Acad. Sci. U.S.A.* **74**, 2456–2460.

Vacquier, V. D., and Moy, G. W. (1978). Macromolecules mediating sperm–egg recognition and adhesion during sea urchin fertilization. *In* "Cell Reproduction: Essays in Honor of Daniel Mazia" (E. R. Dirksen, D. M. Prescott, and C. F. Fox, eds.), pp. 379–389. Academic Press, New York.

Vacquier, V. D., and Payne, J. E. (1973). Methods for quantitating sea urchin sperm-egg binding. *Exp. Cell Res.* **82**, 227–235.

Vacquier, V. D., Tegner, M. J., and Epel, D. (1973). Protease released from sea urchin eggs at fertilization alters the vitelline layer and aids in preventing polyspermy. *Exp. Cell Res.* **80**, 111–119.

Vacquier, V. D., Brandriff, B., and Glabe, C. G. (1979). The effect of soluble egg jelly on the fertilizability of acid-dejellied sea urchin eggs. *Dev., Growth Differ.* **21**, 47–60.

Villa, L. (1977). An ultrastructural investigation on preliminaries in fertilization of *Ascidia malaca. Acta Embryol. Exp.* pp. 179–193.

Wada, S. K., Collier, J. R., and Dan, J. C. (1956). Studies of the acrosome. V. An egg-membrane lysin from the acrosome of *Mytilus edulis* spermatozoa. *Exp. Cell Res.* **10**, 169–180.

Wallach, D., Davies, P. J. A., and Pastan, I. (1978). Cyclic-AMP-dependent phosphorylation of filamin in mammalian smooth muscle. *J. Biol. Chem.* **253**, 4739–4745.

Watkins, H. D., Kopf, G. S., and Garbers, D. L. (1978). Activation of sperm adenylate cyclase by factors associated with eggs. *Biol. Reprod.* **19**, 890–894.

Weller, M. (1979). "Protein Phosphorylation." Pion Ltd., London.

Wells, J. N., and Garbers, D. L. (1976). Nucleoside 3',5'-monophosphate phosphodiesterase in sea urchin sperm. *Biol. Reprod.* **15**, 46–53.

Wolff, D. J., and Broström, C. D. (1979). Properties and function of the calcium-dependent regulator protein. *Adv. Cyclic Nucleotide Res.* **11**, 27–88.

Woollacott, R. M. (1977). Spermatozoa of *Ciona intestinalis* and analysis of ascidian fertilization. *J. Morphol.* **152**, 77–88.

Working, P. K., and Meizel, S. (1981). Evidence that an ATPase functions in the maintenance of the acidic pH of the hamster sperm acrosome. *J. Biol. Chem.* **256**, 4708–4711.

Yamada, Y., and Aketa, K. (1981). Vitelline layer lytic activity in sperm extracts of sea urchin, *Hemicentrotus pulcherrimus. Gamet Res.* **4**, 193–202.

Yamane, J. (1935). Kausal-analytische Studien über die Befruchtung des Kanincheneies. II. Die Isolierung der auf das Eizyplasma auflösen wirkenden Substanzen aus den Spermatozoen. *Cytologia* **6**, 475–483.

Yanagimachi, R. (1972). Fertilization of guinea pig eggs *in vitro. Anat. Rec.* **174**, 9–20.

Yanagimachi, R. (1977). Specificity of sperm-egg interaction. *In* "Immunobiology of Gametes" (M. H. Johnson and M. Edidin, eds.), pp. 255–296. Cambridge Univ. Press, London and New York.

Yanagimachi, R. (1978). Sperm-egg association in mammals. *Curr. Top. Dev. Biol.* **12,** 83–106.

Yanagimachi, R., and Usui, N. (1974). Calcium dependence of the acrosome reaction and activation of guinea pig spermatozoa. *Exp. Cell Res.* **89,** 161–174.

Yudin, A. I., Clark, W. H., Jr., Kleve, M. G. (1980). Gamete-binding in *Sicyonia ingentis:* Primary and secondary. *Amer. Zool.* **20,** 875.

Zucker, R. S., Steinhardt, R. A., and Winkler, M. M. (1978). Intracellular calcium release and the mechanisms of parthenogenetic activation of the sea urchin egg. *Dev. Biol.* **65,** 285–295.

7

Mammalian Fertilization: Gamete Surface Interactions *in Vitro*

JOHN F. HARTMANN

I. INTRODUCTION

A. Overview

The early contact interactions between mammalian sperm and egg are crucial to the process of fertilization. The binding of sperm, the block to polyspermy in appropriate species, and penetration of the zona pellucida by the sperm are events that require controls at the level of the sperm–zona interface. Mechanistically, these interactions are probably unique. For example, the zona is not a membrane but might more aptly be described as a glycoprotein shell, and the spermatozoon, following capacitation during its remarkable journey through the

325

Mechanism and Control of Animal Fertilization
Copyright © 1983 by Academic Press, Inc.
All rights of reproduction in any form reserved.
ISBN 0-12-328520-8

female reproductive tract to the site of fertilization, the oviduct, must, after interacting with the surface of the zona, penetrate it to consummate fertilization. Thus, the nature of gamete surface interactions can be expected to differ significantly from those which occur between somatic cells.

In the mammal, progress in elucidating the mechanisms of early surface interactions between gametes has been slow, because fertilization occurs within the confines of the female reproductive tract and involves a small number of cells. This places the investigator interested in dissecting molecular events at a considerable disadvantage. Obviously, *in vitro* methods must be employed in order to probe these mechanisms.

The first conclusive demonstration of *in vitro* fertilization was accomplished with rabbit gametes (Chang, 1959). Subsequently, *in vitro* fertilization methods with several other species were devised (summarized by Gwatkin, 1977). Although these techniques are relatively new, this fact has not prevented certain dramatic results from being achieved as the *in vitro* conception of "Baby Louise" (Steptoe and Edwards, 1978) and other similarly conceived progeny of human gamete interactions will testify.

Because of the technical difficulties involved in the study of mammalian gamete interaction there has been a tendency to study one gamete or the other (mainly sperm) and to extrapolate the findings to the fertilization process. This has, I believe, resulted in an oversimplified picture. The conclusions drawn regarding the role of acrosin in fertilization is such an example. Although there is considerable evidence indicating that acrosin is important, it has been assumed by many that it is directly involved in the penetration process (Zaneveld *et al.*, 1975; Fritz *et al.*, 1975a; Stambaugh, 1978). Data supporting this notion are, in fact, not yet convincing. The question of the role of acrosin will be dealt with in a later section of this chapter as well as by others in this volume (see reviews by Dunbar and by Moore and Bedford).

The environment in which mammalian fertilization occurs *in vivo* differs from that *in vitro* (see Bavister, 1981, for discussion of the influence of media components on *in vitro* fertilization). This is reflected, for example, in the different modes of entry of the sperm head into the cytoplasm of the intact egg, reported to occur in these two different environments (Shalgi and Phillips, 1980). In light of this it is remarkable that monospermic fertilization of eggs can be achieved *in vitro* (Wolf and Inoue, 1976; Gwatkin, 1977). It is particularly impressive when one observes the large number of sperm which bind to the zona, far in excess of the quantity which are believed to bind *in vivo* (Braden and Austin, 1954). Thus, there appears to be considerable self-regulation in the interactions between sperm and egg *in vitro*.

B. Brief Description of the Egg

The mammalian egg consists of an egg cell proper or vitellus enveloped by an acellular glycoprotein envelope of several microns thickness, the zona pellucida (see Chapter 3, Table I). The egg is ovulated within a mass of small cells, the cumulus oophorus, which must be traversed by the fertilizing spermatozoon. The presence of the cumulus is not essential for fertilization *in vivo* (Moore and Bedford, 1978) or *in vitro* (Yanagimachi, 1977). Following ovulation, the loosening of the

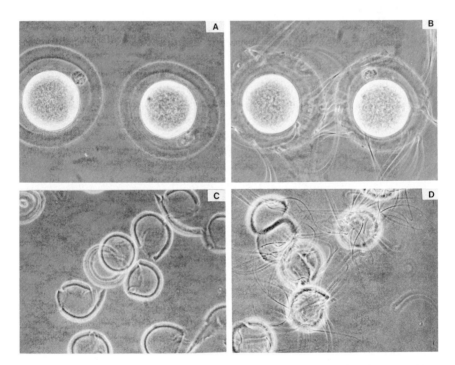

Fig. 1. Eggs (A,B) and isolated zonae pellucidae (C,D) of the golden hamster. Eggs were obtained by superovulation and denuded of cumulus cells with 0.1% hyaluronidase. Zonae pellucidae were isolated when eggs were drawn into a micropipette with an inner diameter of about 60 μm and then the contents were expelled. The zonae were separated from the vitelli and washed three times. Sperm are bound to eggs in (B) and to isolated zonae pellucidae in (D). (D) is reproduced from Hartmann and Gwatkin, 1971. (A,B, approximately × 400; C,D, approximately × 200.)

cumulus cells embedded within a mucoid matrix has an effect on the morphology of the egg. By means of cytoplasmic extensions, the inner cells of the cumulus mass penetrate the matrix of the zona to the vitelline surface. These processes are eventually withdrawn, leaving the zona heavily fenestrated (Phillips and Shalgi, 1980). In addition, after ovulation in many or all species, the vitellus, which has been tightly apposed to the inner surface of the zona, contracts, leaving a gap between the zona and vitellus, the perivitelline "space" (Fig. 1). The first polar body is situated in this region and will be joined by the second polar body, the formation of which occurs following contact between the fertilizing spermatozoon and vitelline surface.

II. ASSESSMENT OF *IN VITRO* METHODS OF CAPACITATION

The development of reliable methods of *in vitro* capacitation has been one of the keys to successful systems of *in vitro* fertilization. Capacitation is defined broadly as the sum total of all changes in sperm that enable them to penetrate the zona pellucida and enter the vitellus. There have been a number of reviews on this subject (Gwatkin, 1977; Rogers, 1978), and these should be consulted for details in technique and historical perspective. Furthermore, it is not our purpose here to describe changes that occur during or following capacitation of spermatozoa (see Chapter 4). Rather, it is our purpose to highlight the commonly used *in vitro* methods and remark on their utility for studying surface interactions between gametes.

A. Capacitation of the Sperm of Laboratory Animals

We will deal only with the sperm of two laboratory species, the hamster and the mouse, since they are the most commonly used and those from which most basic information regarding the surface interactions of mammalian gametes has been obtained thus far. The eggs of both species are readily obtained by hormonally induced superovulation (Gwatkin, 1977).

1. The Golden Hamster

The golden hamster has been a mainstay in the quest for the development of methods of *in vitro* fertilization and has facilitated our understanding of the mechanisms involved in the early steps of fertilization. The hamster sperm cell, compared with that of the mouse, is relatively large, making it possible to count the number of sperm bound to an egg with a dissecting microscope (Hartmann and Hutchison, 1976). This eliminates the need for the gametes to be fixed and mounted on a slide for observation with phase-contrast optics as is commonly practiced in many laboratories in which the mouse is used (Inoue and Wolf, 1975; Saling *et al.*, 1978; Florman and Storey, 1981).

A variety of biological fluids, including follicular fluid, fallopian tube fluid, and blood serum, has been used for capacitating hamster sperm (Rogers, 1978). Fertilization in these fluids is rarely 100% successful and the results vary widely (Mahi and Yanagimachi, 1973). The blood serum method employed by Yanagimachi (1970) also resulted in a high degree of polyspermy. Crude commercial preparations of liver glucuronidase were used by Gwatkin and Hutchison (1971). Here again, penetration of eggs by sperm was not 100% successful and was shown to vary with the enzyme preparation.

For 11 years my laboratory used the cumulus mass to capacitate sperm according to the method described by Gwatkin (1977). A diagram of this method is provided in Fig. 2. It has proved reliable virtually every working day, yielding 100% penetration, and if care is taken to avoid aged eggs, complete monospermic penetration can be consistently achieved. Disadvantages of this system are (1) the additional expense encountered when females are sacrificed to provide cumulus masses for capacitation, and (2) the large number of sperm required (5×10^6/ml) to achieve 100% penetration, possibly because many sperm do not disengage from the cumulus cells. These disadvantages are relatively minor when weighed against the consistency of the method. Nevertheless, it has remained a puzzling fact that the cumulus cell system has not been used more extensively.

In vitro studies employ large numbers of sperm with ratios of sperm to egg of 10^3 to 1 and greater (Talbot *et al.*, 1974; Fraser and Drury, 1976; Hartmann and Hutchison, 1976). The reason for this is not clear, but it appears to be unphysiologic since *in vivo* studies indicate smaller sperm:egg ratios at the site of fertilization (Braden and Austin, 1954). In this regard, the recent report of Bavister's (1979) is of considerable

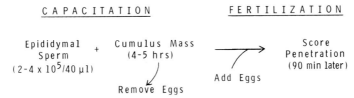

Fig. 2. Protocol for capacitating hamster sperm and *in vitro* fertilization according to updated version described in Gwatkin (1977).

interest. This author has succeeded in fertilizing hamster eggs *in vitro* with sperm:egg ratios approaching unity. The system required supplementation with a "sperm motility factor" derived from hamster adrenal glands and cathecholamine agonists (for a review of this topic, see Chapter 4).

2. The Mouse

An increasing number of *in vitro* studies of surface interaction between mouse gametes has appeared (Wolf and Inoue, 1976; Saling *et al.*, 1978, 1979; Saling and Storey, 1979; Heffner *et al.*, 1980; Bleil and Wassarman, 1980). Sperm can be capacitated merely by incubation in epididymal fluid. The mouse offers the advantage of an extensive armentarium of genetic knowledge which has, to date, only begun to be exploited for *in vitro* fertilization (Olds, 1971; Fraser and Drury, 1976; Olds-Clarke and Carey, 1978). The disadvantage of the mouse system is that penetration of eggs by sperm is rarely 100%, and the small size of the sperm requires observation of fixed preparations with a compound microscope for assessment of binding.

3. The Guinea Pig

Finally, we should not overlook the gametes of the guinea pig; unfortunately, they have been used on a limited basis. This is due, in large measure, to the fact that there is no technique available to induce superovulation in these animals (Rogers *et al.*, 1981). Therefore, immature eggs must be obtained directly from the ovary, then allowed to mature *in vitro* before insemination. Given the large size of the sperm and the relative ease with which binding specificity can be demonstrated (Yanagimachi, 1977; Schmell and Gulyas, 1980), these animals would be an excellent choice for studies of sperm–egg interaction. However, such studies must await an effective method of inducing superovulation in the guinea pig.

B. Capacitation of the Sperm of Farm Animals

In vitro fertilization of the eggs of farm animals has met with little success (Blandau, 1980). The failure to accomplish this is related to a number of factors, not the least of which is the inability to develop a reliable method of *in vitro* capacitation. This is an unfortunate state of affairs since *in vitro* fertilization would be useful in embryo transfer techniques (Seidel, 1981). This method has found commercial application to increase the reproductive capacity of superior ungulate females. It involves the transfer of preimplantation embryos developing within the mother to less valued females acting as incubators. The embryos are usually produced after artificial insemination of superovulated females. The inconvenience associated with *in vivo* inseminations could be circumvented with successful *in vitro* fertilization methods.

The best results to date have been obtained with *in vitro* fertilized cow eggs (Brackett *et al.*, 1980). These eggs were recovered from follicles or from the oviduct and were fertilized with bull sperm which had been capacitated *in vitro* by incubation in high ionic strength medium (Brackett and Oliphant, 1975). More recently, Brackett *et al.* (1981) have transplanted an *in vitro* conceived cow embryo into recipient mothers. The world awaits their results.

The gametes of the pig may prove useful in obtaining basic biochemical knowledge of fertilization. Immature porcine oocytes can be obtained routinely from ovarian minces in quantities of 100–200 per ovary (Dunbar *et al.*, 1980; Dunbar, this volume). Protease treatment of minces yields as many as 500 pig oocytes per ovary (Gwatkin *et al.*, 1980). If such large quantities of oocytes can be matured *in vitro* (Tsafriri and Channing, 1975; McGaughey and Van Blerkom, 1977) and a satisfactory method developed for capacitating porcine sperm *in vitro*, then it may prove possible to conduct biochemical studies on a large scale with a population of mammalian eggs in the process of being synchronously fertilized.

III. GAMETE SURFACE INTERACTIONS

A. The Question of Species Specificity

Penetration is a highly species-specific phenomenon (Yanagimachi, 1977) which prompts the question: are there specific binding sites or receptors on the surfaces of the zonae and capacitated sperm? Unfortunately the answer is not a simple one because a number of conflicting reports exists. With the exceptions of the guinea pig (Yanagimachi, 1977), in which capacitated/acrosome-reacted sperm failed to form a permanent adhesion to hamster zonae and human sperm which do not adhere to the zonae of a variety of species (Bedford, 1977; Swenson and Dunbar, 1982), it is difficult to discern a specific interaction between gamete surfaces of common laboratory species. For example, hamster sperm adhere to hamster, mouse, rat and guinea pig eggs (Hartmann *et al.*, 1972; Yanagimachi, 1977; Schmell and Gulyas, 1980) and capacitated mouse sperm adhere to hamster eggs (Hartmann *et al.*, 1972; Schmell and Gulyas, 1980) but heterologous penetration failed to occur. Mouse sperm also adhere readily to the inner and outer surfaces of porcine and rabbit zona fragments (Swenson and Dunbar, 1982).

A micropipette with a diameter of approximately 140 μm to wash eggs with adhering sperm made it possible to make species-specific distinctions with regard to surface interactions (Hartmann et al., 1972). We found that capacitated hamster sperm adhered only loosely to mouse and rat eggs. This was also true when hamster sperm were combined with homologous eggs. We referred to this loose and non-specific adhesion as attachment. However, a tighter adhesion occurred after hamster gametes had been attached to each other for about 35 minutes. This step, termed binding, failed to occur between hamster sperm and mouse or rat eggs and between mouse sperm and hamster eggs (Hartmann et al., 1972; Hartmann and Hutchison, 1974a). Thus binding is, by definition, species specific. Gwatkin and Williams (1977), using the same in vitro system to capacitate sperm, essentially confirmed the specificity of binding between mouse zona fragments and hamster but observed a very small degree of heterologous binding (approximately 2 sperm/10 zonae). Because no internal controls were run, it was difficult to assess whether this represented attachment or binding. In addition, the zona fragments would be subjected to less shear force in the micropipette than would the intact zona pellucida. Nevertheless, these studies confirm that there is a significant degree of species specificity in the binding interaction between hamster sperm and zona surface.

It was important to establish that attached sperm do eventually bind. Sperm which had attached to eggs did, in fact, bind when removed and added to fresh eggs (Hartmann et al., 1972; Hartmann and Hutchison, 1974b). This demonstrated an obligatory attachment-binding sequence between capacitated hamster sperm and eggs in vitro.

The attachment-binding sequence was confirmed in the hamster (Schmell and Gulyas, 1980) and also observed in the mouse system by another group of investigators (Schmell and Gulyas, 1980; Bleil and Wasserman, 1983). However, Schmell and Gulyas (1980) found that heterologous combinations of gametes bound just as readily as a homologous one. The authors argued that their results differed from those of Hartmann et al. (1972) because of differences in the methods of capacitation and the variation in shear force to which the gametes are subjected during the pipetting procedure. This latter point is a critical one as pointed out by Saling et al. (1979), who resorted to a gradient centrifugation method for measuring binding between mouse gametes. Schmell and Gulyas (1980) observed that binding begins earlier than that reported by us. This difference, at least in part, may well be due to differences in shear forces. It is relevant to point out that in our earlier studies we found the time of binding to vary (cf. Figs. 2 and 3 in Hartmann *et al.,* 1972) but not in subsequent investigations (Hartmann and Hutchison, 1974b, 1976, 1977b). The consistency in our results no doubt simply reflects improvement in our technique. The fertility of the sperm is another point that is not to be overlooked in the report of Schmell and Gulyas (1980), that is, the degree to which they are capacitated. This is difficult to assess in their study due to the absence of penetration controls. Since noncapacitated sperm bind rapidly and with considerable avidity to the zona pellucida (Hartmann *et al.,* 1972; Hartmann and Hutchison, 1976, 1977a; Peterson *et al.,* 1979), one wonders if the bound sperm are adequately capacitated.

Clearly the detection of surface interactions of mammalian gametes *in vitro* depends upon parameters, subjective and otherwise, which include species, media, method of capacitation, and handling procedures. Nevertheless, it is difficult to accept that the specificity of penetration is unrelated to recognition phenomena at the gamete surfaces, especially since it has been demonstrated in invertebrate fertilization systems (Schmell *et al.,* 1977). Possibly at some step after initial contact, but prior to penetration, some specific step occurs that can be detected only in some of the *in vitro* systems.

In terms of species preservation the question arises as to the importance of sperm–egg recognition since, as pointed out by Yanagimachi (1978), the major barriers to hybridization are mediated by reproductive–isolation mechanisms, which include "physiologic and behavioral separation of males and females of different species." From an experimentalist's point of view, however, the ability to detect species-specific binding will prove a useful control to detect nonspecific interactions in, for example, inhibition assays designed to isolate binding components from gametes as proposed by others (Schmell and Gulyas, 1980; Gulyas and Schmell, 1981; Swenson and Dunbar, 1982) for their system. Relevant to this, I shall discuss in a later section the S1 peptides (Hartmann and Hutchison, 1977b, 1980a,b) which are released during the attachment and binding phases. Their detection was the result of the ability to distinguish between various types of surface associations, species specific and otherwise.

B. Status of the Acrosomal Cap during Sperm–Zona Interaction

It is now generally held that capacitation prepares the sperm for the acrosome reaction, an essential prelude to fertilization. Briefly, the acrosome reaction commences when fusion occurs at many points between the outer acrosomal and overlying plasma membrane. Completion of the acrosome reaction results in the exposure of the inner acrosomal membrane. When, in relationship to sperm–egg interaction, does the acrosome reaction occur? More specifically, does it occur prior to or during contact with the surface of the zona surface? In ultrastructural terms, does binding to the zona pellucida involve the plasma or inner acrosomal membrane? The acrosome reaction has been assessed in several laboratories within *in vitro* fertilization systems, that is, with eggs denuded of cumulus cells. However, any relationship between the acrosome reaction and the cumulus mass which might exist *in vivo* must be taken into consideration for a complete evaluation of the changes in the sperm as they approach the egg. This and other above-mentioned phenomena as they occur *in vivo* are discussed in Chapter 10. Because of its relevance to the present chapter, a review of the acrosome reaction as it occurs during *in vitro* fertilization will be presented.

There is ample *in vitro* evidence that capacitated mouse and hamster sperm bind to the zona pellucida by the plasma membrane overlying the acrosome (Franklin *et al.,* 1970; Gwatkin *et al.,* 1976; Saling *et al.,* 1979; Saling and Storey, 1979; Phillips and Shalgi, 1980). Noncapacitated spermatozoa of the boar (Peterson *et al.,* 1981) and hamster (J. F. Hartmann and C. F. Hutchison, unpublished observations), although incapable of penetrating the zona pellucida, also bind to the surface of the zona pellucida by the plasma membrane of the sperm head (see Section III,C,1).

A number of studies appear to indicate that an intact acrosome is essential for binding and penetration *in vitro*. Gwatkin *et al.* (1976) showed that penetration of hamster eggs declined as the proportion of capacitated sperm lacking acrosomal caps increased. Saling and Storey (1979) demonstrated directly the role of an intact acrosome in binding. They were able to distinguish between intact and acrosome-reacted mouse sperm by exposing the sperm to chlorotetracycline, a fluorescent chelator of divalent ions. In the presence of Ca^{2+}, the plasma membrane covering the acrosome became fluorescent. Sperm, including those of the guinea pig which had undergone the acrosome reaction, failed to demonstrate fluorescence. It was then shown that the fluorescent-labeled sperm bound to the zona pellucida, whether or not the vitellus was present, whereas acrosome-reacted sperm, that is, nonfluorescent sperm, failed to bind.

A time-sequence study of mouse gamete interaction *in vitro* revealed that 40 minutes after insemination half of the sperm that bound to the zona pellucida had initiated an acrosome reaction, while the balance remained intact (Saling *et al.,* 1979). Those sperm (12%) which had begun to penetrate after 90 minutes had undergone a full acrosome reaction. Taken together, the following obligatory sequence of events leading to fertilization was postulated: capacitation → binding of sperm via plasma membrane to zona pellucida → acrosome reaction → zona penetration by sperm (Saling *et al.,* 1979; Saling and Storey, 1979).

Scanning electron microscopic studies by Gwatkin *et al.* (1976) of hamster gametes led these authors to conclude that the outer acrosomal and overlying plasma membrane separated from the sperm head as a caplike structure without membrane vesiculation. The cap remained tethered to the sperm until it penetrated the zona pellucida. These observations do not rule out membrane vesiculation in the acrosomal cap, since such a reaction is beyond the resolution of scanning optics. Indeed, vesiculated acrosomes of capacitated hamster sperm, detached from the sperm, have been observed on the zona surface (Franklin *et al.,* 1970; Yanagimachi and Noda, 1970).

The problem of acrosome cap–zona interaction has been pursued further by Florman and Storey (1981). The specific cholinergic antagonist of muscarinic sites, 3-quinuclidinyl benzilate (QNB), inhibited penetration of the zona pellucida of mouse eggs at micromolar concentrations, but without inhibiting the binding of sperm. By means of the fluorescence assay described above (Saling and Storey, 1979), it was concluded that penetration failed to occur because the acrosome reaction was inhibited (Florman and Storey, 1982). Furthermore, QNB inhibited the acrosome reaction of sperm bound to the zona or induced by solubilized zona components but did not inhibit the acrosome reaction of ionophore-treated sperm. Wassarman and Bleil (1981) found that one of the three glycoproteins (ZP3) that make up the zona pellucida of the unfertilized mouse egg induced the acrosome reaction *in vitro*.

In summary, with the possible exception of the guinea pig (Huang *et al.,* 1981; see also Chapter 10, this volume), the balance of evidence indicates that the acrosome reaction occurs while capacitated sperm of the mouse and hamster are associated with the surface of the zona pellucida *in vitro*. The morphological sequence of events, consisting of contact with the zona pellucida via the sperm plasma membrane followed by the acrosome reaction, may parallel the attachment-binding sequence observed in these species.

C. Molecular Participants in the Binding of Sperm to Egg

1. *Binding of Noncapacitated Sperm: A Probe for Studying Sperm–Egg Interactions*

Capacitation alters the plasma membrane of the sperm (see review, Chapter 4). This has been documented by a variety of studies that include ultrastructural (Friend, 1977), lectin binding (reviewed by Koehler, 1978), and membrane influx phenomena (Singh *et al.*, 1978).

Several years ago we observed that capacitated sperm failed to bind to and penetrate trypsin-treated eggs. Noncapacitated epididymal sperm, although incapable of penetrating the zona, bound readily to such eggs even though the enzyme concentration (5 µg/ml) used to treat them was increased 100-fold above that which affected binding of capacitated sperm (Hartmann and Gwatkin, 1971). Thus, capacitation altered sperm binding sites.

In contrast to the 35 minutes that it takes for capacitated sperm to bind to eggs, the binding of noncapacitated sperm occurred rapidly, within 5 to 7 minutes after insemination (Hartmann *et al.*, 1972). Binding of noncapacitated sperm to eggs and to mechanically isolated zonae pellucidae increased in a parallel superimposable way as a function of the concentration of spermatozoa. Capacitated sperm, on the other hand, bound to these structures in a dramatically different fashion (Hartmann and Hutchison, 1976). Binding as a function of sperm concentrations to the isolated zonae was linear, while binding to eggs was sigmoidal. Not only do these results provide evidence for differences in the binding sites of pre- and postcapacitated sperm, but they also implicate the vitellus in sperm–zona interactions. This point will be developed further in a later section of this review.

In addition to the differences in binding, Gwatkin and Williams (1978) have shown that solutions containing heat-dispersed zonae pellucidae of the hamster inhibited the binding and penetration of capacitated sperm but did not interfere with the binding of noncapacitated sperm. Similar results with bovine gametes were also reported. Since no efficient method for bull sperm capacitation was available, these sperm were subjected to hyperosmotic salt solutions which, in other systems (Brackett and Oliphant, 1975), caused sperm surface changes analogous to those observed in capacitated sperm (Talbot and Franklin, 1978). Under these conditions the binding of treated sperm was sharply reduced, while that of untreated sperm was unaffected by solutions of heat-dispersed zonae pellucidae.

In contrast to this, O'Rand (1981) found that the binding of noncapacitated as well as capacitated rabbit sperm to homologous zonae pellucidae was suppressed by Fab antibody fragments against a sperm membrane autoantigen. This antigen may be involved in the binding of both kinds of sperm.

The binding of noncapacitated hamster sperm displays species specificity. Although capable of attaching to heterologous eggs (mouse and rat), noncapacitated hamster sperm will not bind to them (Hartmann and Gwatkin, 1971; Hartmann and Hutchison, 1976). Porcine gametes also show considerable, although not absolute, species-specific binding (Peterson *et al.*, 1980). Noncapacitated boar sperm bind avidly to porcine zonae pellucidae, but human, guinea pig, and rat sperm failed to bind to pig zonae to any significant extent. Noncapacitated bull and hamster sperm bound to porcine eggs 9% and 24% of the controls, respectively. These results indicate that the noncapacitated sperm of several species, although incapable of penetrating the zona pellucida, have specific binding sites on the plasma membrane.

The binding of noncapacitated hamster sperm to the zona pellucida involves glucuronic acid (Hartmann and Hutchison, 1977a). Bound sperm can be dislodged from egg if the gametes are washed in media (Modified Medium 199; Gwatkin *et al.*, 1972) supplemented with micromolar concentrations of glucuronic acid. The sugar acid was probably acting as a haptenlike competitor. The effect appears very specific since galacturonic acid had only a limited effect (20–40% dissociation). Mannose partially dissociated the gametes (50%) but only at relatively high levels (500 μM). Hexosamines were partially effective but failed to demonstrate a clear dose-response (5–500 μM) suggesting nonspecific effects. L-Fucose, D-galactose, and sialic acid had no significant effect on binding. The glucuronide appears to be located on the sperm membrane, since treatment of the male gamete with β-glucuronidase prevented binding. There was no effect on binding when eggs were treated with the enzyme. The dependence of binding on glucuronic acid lasted for only a brief period. After the gametes had been combined for 20 minutes, the media supplemented with the sugar acid lost its effectiveness at reversing binding.

Interestingly, glucuronide has also been implicated in another cell surface-related phenomenon, namely the aggregation-enhancing activity of the cells of the sponge *Microciona prolifera* (Turner and Burger, 1973). One cannot help but wonder if this apparent common component in these two systems, each remote from the other, reflects any underlying functional similarity.

Peterson *et al.* (1980) found no evidence for glucuronide involvement in the binding of porcine noncapacitated sperm. However, they assayed for binding 45–60 minutes after insemination of eggs, a period of time during which the interaction became insensitive to glucuronic acid-mediated dissociation in the hamster system (Hartmann and Hutchison, 1977a).

Removal of terminal glucuronic acid and possibly other sugars from the sperm surface may be an important step in the capacitation of hamster spermatozoa, since crude preparations of β-glucuronidase are capable of capacitating sperm (Gwatkin and Hutchison, 1971). The removal of surface receptors on rabbit (Gordon *et al.*, 1974) and hamster sperm (Kinsey and Koehler, 1978) for lectins by *in vitro* capacitating conditions is consistent with this conclusion.

The binding of noncapacitated hamster sperm to homologous eggs required a supernatant factor (Hartmann and Hutchison, 1977a). This factor was unnecessary for the binding of capacitated hamster sperm to eggs. The activity of the factor was resistant to pronase and appeared to be an oligosaccharide, possibly the glycopeptide portions of an epididymal fluid glycoprotein. The requirement for the supernatant fraction was not specific, since a number of fractions derived from pronase digests of epididymal fluid and the plasma glycoprotein fetuin were effective in inducing binding of washed sperm to homologous eggs. None of these substances induced the binding of washed hamster sperm to mouse egg.

Peterson and his co-workers have used a novel approach in an attempt to assess the nature of the binding of noncapacitated boar sperm to the zona pellucida (Peterson *et al.*, 1980, 1981). The binding of boar sperm was blocked by antisera or a univalent antibody (Fab) prepared against sperm plasma membrane vesicles. However, binding occurred when the Fab antibody preparation was absorbed with the membrane vesicles prior to exposure to the sperm. Peterson *et al.* (1981) exploited this absorption technique to probe the nature of the noncapacitated sperm binding site. Prior to the absorption step, the membrane vesicles were treated by various means and then tested for their ability to neutralize the inhibitory activity of the antibody on binding of boar sperm to homologous eggs. Only boiling and trichloracetic acid treatment interfered with receptor activity, that is, the ability to absorb (neutralize) the Fab antibody preparations. None of the enzymatic treatments, which included trypsin, pronase, a variety of glycosidases and polysaccharidases, blocked receptor activity. Unfortunately, given the nonspecific nature of the effective treatments, little can be concluded as to the chemistry of the binding site of noncapacitated porcine sperm.

In summary, noncapacitated sperm bind to homologous eggs of the hamster, rabbit, and pig *in vitro;* apparently such binding does not occur in the mouse (Inoue and Wolf, 1975). Whether the binding of noncapacitated sperm has any physiological significance, for example, as a precursor step to the acrosome reaction (Peterson *et al.*, 1981), remains to be seen. Clearly this idea would be at odds with the gamete contact sequence proposed by Saling *et al.* (1979) (see Section III,B). Those of us who have studied the binding of noncapacitated sperm would do well to prepare ourselves for the possibility that this phenomenon may turn out to be the kind of scientific question classified by Max Planck (1949) in his autobiography as a "phantom problem," that is, interesting but, interpreted in biological terms, of no physiological significance.

2. Interaction between Capacitated Hamster Sperm and Egg in Vitro

a. Significance of and Relationship between "Early" Binding, Attachment, and "Late" Binding. Whether physiologic or not, knowledge of the mechanism of noncapacitated sperm binding, at the very least, is valuable for assessment of the capacitation-induced changes in the sperm that are relevant to sperm–egg interaction. Such comparative studies have only been conducted extensively with the hamster. For example, as already stated, one of the most prominent differences between the binding of noncapacitated and capacitated hamster sperm to eggs is the lengthy attachment period (Hartmann *et al.*, 1972; Hartmann and Hutchison, 1974a; Schmell and Gulyas, 1980), which occurs after hamster sperm are capacitated but not before (Hartmann *et al.*, 1972; Hartmann and Hutchison, 1976). One might argue that this change is of little physiological significance, since capacitation could have made the surface of the sperm less "sticky," necessitating a lengthy period of looser attachment prior to the establishment of a tighter binding. Clearly this is not the case as shown by the observation that capacitated hamster sperm bind very rapidly to mechanically isolated zonae pellucidae with essentially no significant interval of attachment. Thus, capacitated sperm *are* capable of binding rapidly to the zona pellucida but after the vitellus has been removed. A summary of the various sperm–egg interactions that we have encountered in the hamster *in vitro* system is shown in Fig. 3.

We sought to determine if a rapid binding component could also be detected between sperm and egg and discovered that it was. Early binding was detected by assaying at 1- to 2-minute intervals after hamster eggs had been inseminated with homologous sperm. Mouse eggs included in the same drop and to which hamster sperm attached

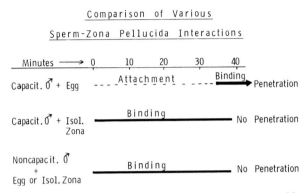

Fig. 3. Comparison of various sperm–zona interactions of the golden hamster *in vitro.*

were washed simultaneously with the hamster gametes as an internal control for binding. No binding was detected in the heterologous association at any time (Hartmann and Hutchison, 1974a). However, an early binding component was detected between a small proportion of hamster eggs (usually three to four) and a very small number of homologous sperm (see Fig. 7A,B). After 5 minutes, however, only attachment was detected, which was followed by the final binding step, 30 minutes later. Additional analysis revealed that the extent of early binding between sperm and egg was a function of the concentration of spermatozoa. Most of the early binding was prevented, presumably by a vitelline-related mechanism (Hartmann and Hutchison, 1976). The residual early binding per se that was observed between sperm and egg is probably physiologically insignificant, being nothing more that the vestige of the nonfunctional binding that occurs between sperm and isolated zona. However, these early events are of considerable heuristic value since they reflect a change at the sperm–zona interface that occurs almost immediately after contact is made and in which the vitellus, several microns distant from this interaction, participates in some manner.

Finally, it is important to establish that attached sperm do subsequently bind. This was demonstrated in experiments in which attached hamster sperm were removed and added to fresh eggs (Hartmann *et al.*, 1972; Hartmann and Hutchison, 1974a). Such sperm did bind, thereby demonstrating an obligatory attachment-binding sequence between capacitated hamster sperm and egg. Bleil and Wassarman (1983) have recently confirmed this observation in another species, the mouse.

b. The Vitelline Factor: Summary of Early Evidence. Several pieces of evidence suggest that the vitellus is involved in the prepenetration interaction between the surfaces of the gametes (Hartmann *et al.*, 1972; Hartmann and Hutchison, 1974a, 1976). (1) The time of binding to isolated zonae (rapid) and eggs (slow) differ from each other. (2) Binding to eggs as a function of the concentrations of capacitated sperm was sigmoidal, while that to isolated zonae pellucidae was linear. Binding of noncapacitated sperm under the same conditions was essentially linear and identical for both eggs and isolated zonae. (3) Binding was blocked when sperm were pretreated with a synthetic trypsin inhibitor, while binding to the zona pellucida was unaffected by such treatment. (4) Sperm, although capable of burrowing into the zona matrix (unpublished observations) rarely, if ever, penetrate the isolated zona pellucida (see also Gwatkin *et al.*, 1976). In those few instances when sperm were observed curled within the isolated zonae, it appeared that they may have gained entrance through the tear created by the pipette used in the isolation procedure. The assumption has been made, in a comparison of the interaction of sperm with eggs and with isolated zonae, that the binding components of the zona have been unaltered by the isolation procedure. In support of this we have observed monospermic penetration of eggs with single tears in the zona created by micropipetting of eggs (Fig. 4). Thus, an apparently normal interaction is possible between spermatozoa and eggs with a torn zona.

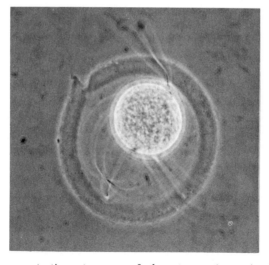

Fig. 4. Sperm penetrating a torn zona of a hamster egg (approximately × 400).

c. Events during the Attachment Phase: Triggering of Soluble Factor Release. Several years ago in a study intended as a control, we found that the addition of isolated zonae pellucidae to a drop containing capacitated sperm and eggs resulted in a delay of the normal binding between the gametes (Hartmann and Hutchison, 1974b). This change appeared to reflect a specific phenomenon, since replacement of hamster isolated zonae with those of the mouse failed to affect sperm–egg binding. Furthermore, the media in which hamster sperm and homologous isolated zonae had been incubated together also delayed binding when added to interacting hamster gametes. However, media in which isolated hamster zonae had been incubated alone or media in which hamster sperm had been combined with mouse zonae pellucidae were ineffective. Thus the binding delay was caused by the action of a substance, released when hamster sperm made contact with homologous zonae.

An assay was developed which took advantage of the soluble character of this substance. Briefly, a small aliquot (1–2 μl) of the medium in which sperm were interacting with eggs or isolated zonae pellucidae (experimental drop) was transferred to a second drop (assay drop) of interacting gametes (Hartmann and Hutchison, 1977b). This induced early binding between the gametes in the assay drop when the aliquot was added 20 minutes after the gametes had been combined. The significance of this early binding is not known, since it does not lead to early penetration. However, it proved to be a valuable tool in our hands for detecting and measuring the relative quantity of this material. We have termed this substance, S1.

Having this assay in hand we posed a number of questions. First, is the vitellus required for factor release? The answer is no. As much activity, if not slightly more, was detected when eggs were replaced with homologous isolated zonae pellucidae to which hamster sperm bind but do not attach (see Fig. 3). However, more recent studies indicate that the vitellus appears to interact with at least some of these factors (Hartmann et al., 1982). This question will be dealt with in a later section. Second, is the S1 factor released when hamster sperm are combined with mouse eggs? Although there is contact between these gametes, significant S1 activity could not be detected. Thus, it would appear that homology of the sperm and zona surfaces is more critical to the mechanism of release than the tightness of their association. A negative response was also obtained when noncapacitated hamster sperm were combined with homologous eggs. Taken together, these results indicate, at the very least, that a specific contact reaction between sperm and zona pellucida is required to release the S1 factor.

The S1 factor was not detected when isolated zonae were pretreated with nanogram quantities of trypsin (Hartmann and Hutchison, 1977b). Glycosidase treatment of the zonae failed to block release. Inhibition occurred at concentrations of trypsin which also blocked the penetration of eggs by sperm. Thus, a relationship between the release of the factors and fertilization is, at least, implied.

In view of the relatively lengthy period of attachment that precedes binding to and penetration of the zona pellucida, it was important to determine the time of factor release relative to these events. The question was answered by an assay of the supernatant at various times after the gametes had been combined. Four major peaks of activity were detected at 2, 20–25, 31, and 50 minutes. The activity declined sharply after each peak before the appearance of the next one. The final peak at 50 minutes coincided with the completion of binding, just at the time the earliest penetration can be detected (Hartmann and Hutchison, 1977b).

The quantities of each of the released factors were all a function of sperm concentration (Fig. 5). It is assumed that the quantity of factor released is related to the number of sperm bound to the zona, since our earlier studies (Hartmann and Hutchison, 1976) and those conducted with mouse gametes (Wolf and Inoue, 1976) showed that the extent of binding was a function of sperm concentration.

d. Nature of the S1 Factors. The identification of these factors was simplified when it was discovered that they were relatively small in size and that three of the four were stable after separation from the gametes (Hartmann and Hutchison, 1980a,b). The 2-minute factor had

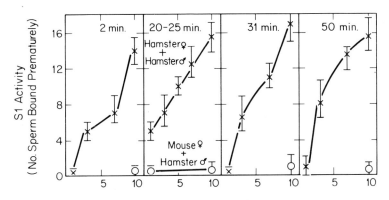

Fig. 5. Release of S1 factors as a function of sperm concentration in the experimental drop. (Reproduced from Hartmann and Hutchinson, 1980a,b.)

only limited stability (Hartmann and Hutchison, 1980b) but was stabilized when it was separated by ultrafiltration from macromolecular components in the supernatant (J. F. Hartmann, unpublished results). Thus, simply by separation of the supernatant from the cells at the appropriate time, each of the S1 factors could be studied.

It was possible to obtain an estimate of the molecular weights of these factors by assay of the supernatant for early binding activity before and after ultrafiltration. Table I summarizes these experiments. There was a striking difference between the first and second pairs of S1 factors. The 2- and 20- to 25-minute factors were partially retained by filters with cutoffs of M_r 1000 but passed unimpeded through the M_r 5000 cutoff filter. In contrast to these results, those S1 factors released at 31 and 50 minutes passed unimpeded through the M_r 1000 filter.

A more accurate picture of the size of the S1 factors was obtained when they were fractionated on gel filtration columns. Figure 6 shows the elution profile of the 2-, 31- and 50-minute S1 factors. The 2-minute factor eluted in two regions of activity from a Biogel P-6 column. The first peak appeared in the void volume ($V_0 = M_r$ 6000), and the second, just in advance of the phenol red marker ($M_r = 356$). Preliminary results obtained with the 20- to 25-minute S1 factor also revealed a complex elution profile after fractionation on Biogel P-6 (J. F. Hartmann, unpublished results).

In contrast to these profiles, those obtained with the 31- and 50-minute factors were simpler. Because the ultrafiltration data indicated that these factors were smaller, they were fractionated on Biogel P-2 ($V_0 = M_r$ 1800). The 30-minute factors eluted as a single peak in the

TABLE I

Molecular Weights (M_r) of S1 Factors Determined by Ultrafiltration

S1 factor (minutes)[a]	Filter[b]	M_r cutoff	S1 activity (% change)
2	UM2	1000	−37.5
	YM5	5000	+2.5
20–25	UM2	1000	−49.0
	YM5	5000	0
31	UM2	1000	+2.0
50	UM2	1000	+5.0

[a] S1 factors were isolated and stabilized according to Hartmann and Hutchison (1980a). S1 activity was compared to an unfiltered control.

[b] Amicon Corp., Lexington, Massachusetts.

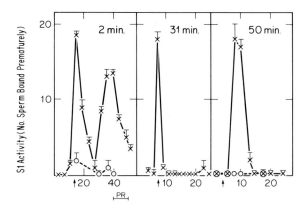

Fraction Number

Fig. 6. Gel chromatography elution profiles of S1 factors. Two-minute factor was eluted from Biogel P-6 and the 31- and 50-minute factors were chromatographed on Biogel P-2. X———X, S1 factors; O———O, sperm ultrafiltrate control. Arrows indicate void volume. (Reproduced from Hartmann and Hutchison, 1980a, 1982.)

void volume, while the 50-minute factor appeared as a slightly re-tarded broad region of activity.

Because the quantities of the S1 factors are so minute, the question of their nature can be approached at this time only through enzymatic sensitivity studies. Their small size proved to be advantageous because it was possible to treat the S1 factors and separate them from the enzymes by ultrafiltration before an assay was made. The filtration step was necessitated by the interference with the assay by some of the enzymes. All of the S1 factors were sensitive to nanogram quantities of at least two or more different proteases (Hartmann and Hutchison, 1980a,b). The 2- and 20- to 25-minute S1 factors were sensitive to trypsin, subtilisin, and aminopeptidase (heavily contaminated with endopeptidases), while the 31- and 50-minute factors were inactivated by subtilisin and aminopeptidase. The most sensitive factor was the 2 minute, while the 20- to 25-minute factor was the least sensitive. Glycosidases failed to affect significantly the activity of any of these factors. These results indicate that all of the S1 factors are peptides.

e. S1 Peptides and Prepenetration Protease Activity. Several years ago we observed that binding between hamster gametes *in vitro* was inhibited by a trypsin inhibitor (Hartmann and Hutchison, 1974a). This observation has been confirmed with a number of such inhibitors in the mouse system (Saling, 1981). These results suggest that proteolytic activity, very likely that of sperm acrosin, plays a critical role in fertilization prior to penetration of the zona pellucida. Indeed, Saling (1981) showed that once binding had occurred the application of an inhibitor was without an effect on penetration. (For a discussion of the mechanism of penetration, see Chapter 10.)

We posed the question as to whether the release of any of the S1 peptides was triggered by a trypsinlike protease (Hartmann and Hutchison, 1980a,b). When gametes were combined in the presence of soybean- or lima bean-trypsin inhibitors, the release of 2- and 31-minute peptides was inhibited significantly (48% and 74%, respectively) at levels which also inhibited completely the penetration of eggs by sperm. The release of the 20–25 minute peptide failed to display any significant sensitivity to the presence of moderate levels of soybean inhibitor; the 50-minute S1 factor was only slightly affected (18% inhibition) by lima bean inhibitor.These results indicate that of the four populations of peptides detected after hamster sperm made contact with homologous zonae pellucidae *in vitro,* the release of at least two of them appears to have been mediated by a trypsin-inhibitor-sensitive protease(s).

There is additional evidence of another nature in support of the involvement of a trypsinlike enzyme in the release of the 2-minute peptide (Hartmann and Hutchison, 1974a). As mentioned above, the period of attachment that precedes binding occurs only between capacitated sperm and egg, but not between capacitated sperm and isolated zonae, in which case binding begins almost immediately after contact has been made. Binding, which mimicked that which occurs between sperm and isolated zonae, was induced when eggs were inseminated in the presence of either of two potent synthetic trypsin inhibitors, either *p*-aminobenzamidine (Mares-Guia and Shaw, 1965) or propamadine diisethionate (Geratz, 1969) (Fig. 7A,B). The eggs, in other words, were apparently "chemically devitellized" by the compounds.*

After the early, inhibitor-induced binding between sperm and egg reached a maximum value, it began to decline more or less sharply until no sperm were bound after 60 minutes. The reason for the decline is not known. In contrast to these results, neither inhibitor had a significant effect on the binding between sperm and isolated zonae pellucidae, and binding did not decline (Fig. 7C,D). The decline was not caused by a toxic effect on the sperm since binding to the isolated zona was not affected by these compounds; rather the decline appears to have been a vitelline-mediated phenomenon.

These observations are interpreted as follows: (1) Within 2 minutes

---

*I thank R. B. L. Gwatkin for suggesting this expression.

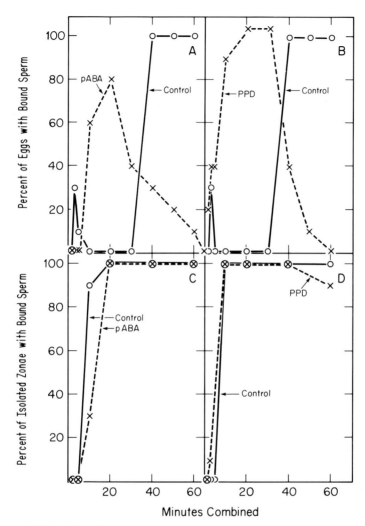

Fig. 7. Effect of synthetic trypsin inhibitors on the surface interactions between hamster sperm and eggs or isolated zonae pellucidae. pABA, *p*-aminobenzamidine; PPD, propamidine diisethionate. Compounds were added to a final concentration of 5×10^{-4} *M* at the time eggs and isolated zonae were inseminated. A, B, sperm plus eggs; C, D, sperm plus isolated zonae. (A and C reproduced from Hartmann and Hutchison, 1974b.)

after hamster sperm make contact with the zona pellucida, the first of several sets of peptides is released. (2) Coincident with the release of the 2-minute peptide or immediately thereafter, the attachment phase is induced between sperm and egg but not between sperm and isolated zonae. (3) Based upon the effects of trypsin inhibitors, both peptide release and the induction of the attachment phase involve the activity of a trypsinlike protease. Since natural trypsin inhibitors and the synthetic ones used are potent inhibitors of sperm acrosin (reviewed by Fritz *et al.*, 1975b; Bhattacharyya *et al.*, 1976), this enzyme may be involved in the triggering of these events.

Evidence implicating the vitellus in these early events will be reviewed in the next section.

f. Consequences of the Interaction between the S1 Peptide and Vitellus. Although the S1 peptides have all been detected by means of the same assay, it is likely, given their apparent diversity, that each one has a different function. However, it was recently shown that the ultrafiltrate containing the 2- and 50-minute S1 peptides were both capable of inhibiting penetration of the zona pellucida by the sperm (Hartmann and Hutchison, 1981). The inhibition was transient and the inhibitors were sensitive to the protease, subtilisin. We concluded that the inhibitory activity resided in the peptides, which may operate to prevent polyspermy. We have also found that this property is shared by the 20- to 25- and 31-minute peptides as well (J. F. Hartmann, unpublished observations). Thus, despite their diversity, the S1 peptides appear to have a collective property in that they all are capable of inhibiting penetration to varying extents. The relative potency of each of the S1 peptides cannot yet be assessed because of our inability to measure the peptides in quantitative terms. It is not known which of the components of those S1 peptides which are obviously heterogeneous (2- and 20- to 25-minute peptides) possess inhibitory activity.

Further analysis of the 2- minute peptides revealed that their ability to inhibit penetration of the zona pellucida by sperm was dependent upon the presence of the vitellus (Hartmann *et al.*, 1982). As mentioned earlier (Section III,C,2,c), the S1 peptides, as measured by the early binding assay, were also released when sperm were combined with homologous isolated zonae pellucidae. However, the 2-minute peptides resulting from sperm–zona (isolated zona) contact had little or no effect on penetration (Fig. 8).

The differences in the effectiveness of sperm–egg versus the sperm–zona S1 peptides in inhibiting the penetration of the zona pellucida were also reflected in their elution profiles from Biogel P-6 (Hartmann *et al.*, 1982). The sperm–zona S1 peptides eluted in three regions of activity but that obtained with sperm–egg eluted in two regions. Furthermore, incubation of sperm–zona peptides with eggs resulted in the disappearance of one of the components and the acquisition of the ability to inhibit penetration by the resulting peptides. These results

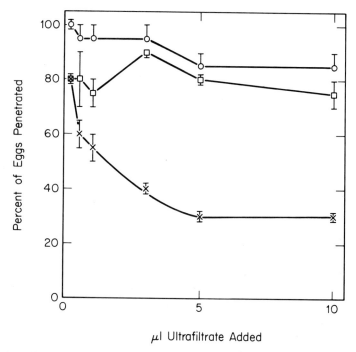

Fig. 8. Effect of 2-minute ultrafiltrates (5000 M_r cutoff) on penetration of egg by sperm. X———X, sperm–egg ultrafiltrate; □———□, sperm–zona ultrafiltrate; ○———○, medium control (Hartman *et al.*, 1982).

suggest that one or more components of the 2-minute S1 peptides interact with the vitellus, resulting in (1) the apparent removal or alteration of this component and (2) the generation of a potent peptide inhibitor of zona penetration by sperm.

Finally, there is no *a priori* reason to expect that the zona would be impervious to the S1 peptides. The fenestrated architecture of the zona pellucida is now well documented (Gwatkin *et al.*, 1976; Phillips and Shalgi, 1980), and both viruses (Gwatkin, 1967) and proteins as large as immunoglobulins ($M_r = 2 \times 10^5$) and ferritin ($M_r = 5 \times 10^5$) are capable of penetrating the zona of a variety of species (Sellens and Jenkinson, 1975; Hastings *et al.*, 1972).

To summarize, within the initial 2–3 minutes after hamster sperm have interacted with the surface of homologous zonae pellucidae *in vitro*, a number of interactions are set into motion that involve gamete surfaces, proteases, and peptide mediators. Contact with the zona triggers the release of at least some peptides by means of a trypsinlike protease, long before binding and penetration occur. At least one of these peptides interacts with the vitellus, followed by the generation of a peptide which affects the ability of the sperm to penetrate the zona pellucida. All of these data will be incorporated into a model of pre-penetration gamete interactions (Section III,C,5), a partial version of which has been presented (Hartmann *et al.*, 1982).

3. Probing the Nature of Binding between Capacitated Sperm and Egg

a. The Effect of Temperature on Binding. Given the dynamic nature of the early interactions between hamster sperm and egg, it is not surprising that binding is temperature-sensitive (Hartmann *et al.*, 1972). More recently, an analysis of the restoration of the ability to bind to the zona pellucida of cold-exposed mouse sperm indicated that membrane fluidity, an important phenomenon in various membrane-related functions of somatic cells (e.g., Edidin and Weiss, 1972), is not a factor in the binding reaction between sperm and zona (Heffner and Storey, 1982). Rather the authors suggest that the results may reflect an effect of temperature on enzymatic activity involved in the estab-lishment of binding. This idea is not without precedent since binding between hamster gametes was shown several years ago to be sensitive to a trypsin inhibitor (Hartmann and Hutchison, 1974b); more re-cently, a number of such inhibitors were used to confirm these findings with mouse gametes (Saling, 1981).

b. Calcium and Binding. Calcium ions play a critical role in mam-malian fertilization. Their requirement has been demonstrated in some species for motility (Morton *et al.*, 1974, 1978, cited in Heffner *et al.*, 1980), the acrosome reaction in the guinea pig (Yanagimachi and Usui, 1974) and hamster (Talbot *et al.*, 1976), and fertilization in the rat and mouse (Miyamoto and Ishibashi, 1975). Saling *et al.* (1978) have shown, in the mouse system, that Ca^{2+} is required for binding between sperm and egg *in vitro*. This requirement can be reversed with EGTA; binding can be largely restored by the addition of Ca^{2+}. Cal-cium ions are apparently bound to the plasma membrane, since lan-thanide cations, potent inhibitors of transmembrane Ca^{2+} transport, failed to affect the binding reaction. The dependence of binding on Ca^{2+} exhibited some specificity. Neither Mg^{2+} (Saling *et al.*, 1978) nor Sr^{2+} (Heffner *et al.*, 1980) supported the binding of mouse sperm to eggs. The effects of these cations were different: Mg^{2+} appeared to compete with Ca^{2+} while Sr^{2+} did not.

Lanthanide ions and the polyamine spermine were good substitutes for the Ca^{2+} in the binding reaction (Heffner *et al.*, 1980). However, since penetration was not assessed, it is not known if lanthanide and spermine induced a physiological binding, that is, one that leads to penetration. This is an important consideration since various non-physiologic bindings have been demonstrated in the hamster system (Hartmann *et al.*, 1972; Hartmann and Hutchison, 1976). At any rate, the manipulation of cations in the mouse system used by Storey and his co-workers (Saling *et al.*, 1978; Heffner *et al.*, 1980) has enabled them to make distinctions between Ca^{2+}-dependent processes controlling binding and motility. This approach should prove to be useful for probing these phenomena, independently of each other (Heffner *et al.*, 1980).

c. **Immunological-Mediated Inhibition.** The zona pellucida is a strong immunogen. A number of investigations have demonstrated that antisera to the zona pellucida will block the binding to and penetration of the zona pellucida *in vitro* by sperm. This has been shown for the gametes of the hamster (Shivers *et al.*, 1972; Oikawa and Yanagimachi, 1975; Dunbar and Shivers, 1976) and mouse (Glass and Hanson, 1974; Aitken and Richardson, 1981). Similarly, the binding of hamster (Tzartos, 1979) and rabbit (O'Rand, 1981) sperm to homologous zonae pellucidae was suppressed by Fab antibodies to whole sperm and sperm membrane autoantigen, respectively. Aitken and Richardson (1981) have argued that antisera against the zona pellucida blocked binding and penetration by masking the receptor site for the sperm and not necessarily reacting with it. This conclusion was based on the observation that a precipitate formed on the outer surface of the zona pellucida after reacting with an antiserum to it which suppressed binding. Neither binding of sperm nor formation of a precipitate occurred on the inner surface of zona fragments. It was concluded that inhibition of binding was produced by the precipitate, resulting in a "steric-hindrance" masking of the zona receptor for sperm.

This conclusion is supported by the findings of Ahuja and Tzartos (1981) who found that antizona Fab fragments derived from papain digests of immune globulins, although capable of reacting with the zona as shown by immune fluorescence and an indirect precipitation assay, failed to form a precipitate on the zona pellucida or inhibit *in vitro* fertilization of hamster eggs. Furthermore, it was shown that the ability of heat-solubilized zonae to inhibit binding to and penetration of the zona pellucida (Gwatkin and Williams, 1977) was unaffected by antizona Fab fragments. Ahuja and Tzartos (1981) concluded that the binding site on the zona for capacitated sperm has little or no anti-genicity. It is unfortunate that the authors did not determine the effects of intact immune γglobulins on the penetration-inhibitory properties of the solubilized zonae. Assuming that the antigen–antibody complex would remain in solution, this experiment might have shown whether the precipitate on the zona *per se* blocks binding and penetration (see Chapter 3 for additional comments on these studies).

One can anticipate that specific antibodies will continue to be useful tools for the study of the mechanism of mammalian sperm–egg interaction. In particular, the generation of monoclonal antibodies by hybridoma technology against gamete- and associated antigens will be, as early work already suggests (Schmell *et al.*, 1982), a boon to these studies.

d. Effects of Enzymes. Treatment of cumulus-denuded hamster eggs with nanogram levels of trypsin in phosphate-buffered saline blocked the binding to and penetration of zonae pellucidae by hamster sperm *in vitro* (Hartmann and Gwatkin, 1971; Oikawa *et al.*, 1975). Chymotrypsin at higher levels (0.7–0.1 µg/ml) also suppressed binding (Hartmann and Gwatkin, 1971), but the enzyme preparation was contaminated with trypsin which could be responsible for the inhibition. Wolf and Inoue (1976) reported that trypsin treatment of mouse eggs at very high concentrations (200 µg/ml) failed to inhibit significantly the binding of sperm to eggs. This treatment, unlike that conducted by Hartmann and Gwatkin (1971) and Oikawa *et al.* (1975), was done in the presence of albumin which may have inhibited trypsin. In contrast to the sensitivity of zona binding sites of the hamster egg, those of the rabbit are insensitive to trypsin and chymotrypsin (Overstreet and Bedford, 1975).

Treatment of hamster eggs with acrosin, the sperm protease, purified from hamster and ram sperm, inhibited penetration of eggs by sperm (Gwatkin *et al.*, 1977). Acrosin may be affecting the zona binding sites in a manner identical to that of trypsin with which it shares similar cleavage specificities.

The binding of hamster sperm was unaffected when eggs were treated with a variety of glycosidases (Gwatkin *et al.*, 1973). Whether the enzyme affected the carbohydrate-rich outer zona surfaces (Oikawa *et al.*, 1974; Nicolson *et al.*, 1975) was, however, not determined.

e. Effects of Lectins. Wheat germ agglutinin blocked *in vitro* fertilization of hamster eggs (Oikawa *et al.*, 1973), but, as cautioned by

Gwatkin (1977), some lectins are capable of triggering the cortical granules to release their contents, a possibility that was not assessed by Oikawa *et al.* (1973). Alternatively, the lectins could be masking the sperm receptors on the zona by binding to an adjoining site.

f. Inhibition of Binding by Soluble "Receptor." Cholewa-Stewart and Massaro (1972) observed that heating of mouse eggs to 68°–70°C resulted in the apparent dissolution of the zona pellucida. Gwatkin and Williams (1977) obtained similar results with the isolated zona pellucida of the hamster; moreover, the zonae remained in an apparent state of dissolution even after cooling. The addition of such heat-dispersed zonae to suspensions of capacitated hamster sperm blocked their ability to bind to and fertilize eggs *in vitro*. This was interpreted by Gwatkin and Williams (1977) as evidence that receptor-for-sperm activity had been demonstrated in the melted zonae. More recently Bleil and Wassarman (1980) reported that binding between mouse gametes was suppressed when sperm were pretreated with one of the three major glycoproteins (ZP3) that make up the mouse zona pellucida. On the other hand, the ZP3 component from two-cell embryos failed to block binding. The authors concluded that the ZP3 component possessed the "receptor" for sperm which upon fertilization was modified in a manner such that it became incapable of functioning in that role.

Although these results are of considerable interest, it may be premature to conclude that the inhibition assay employed by Gwatkin (1977) and Bleil and Wassarman (1980) has demonstrated binding site "receptors." In the hamster system (Hartmann *et al.*, 1972; Schmell and Gulyas, 1980) and in the mouse and guinea pig (Schmell and Gulyas, 1980), it has been shown that binding is preceded by a lengthy interval of attachment. As we have already discussed (see Section III,C,2a), the attachment phase appears to be more than a passive one during which sperm merely "feel" their way for the binding receptor on the zona surface; rather, it is a dynamic period reflected, for example, in the existence of mechanisms which are sensitive to protease inhibitors and upon which binding is dependent (Hartmann and Hutchison, 1974b; Saling, 1981). Such a phase, preliminary to and necessary for the establishment of stable binding, has also been reported to occur between aggregating neural retina and liver cells of the chicken embryo (Umbreit and Roseman, 1975). Therefore, if a cause–effect relationship is assumed between those events which are triggered during sperm-egg attachment and subsequent binding, the results of Gwatkin (1977) and Bleil and Wassarman (1980) could just as readily be accounted for by the inhibition of one or more of these steps and not necessarily of the binding site per se.

4. Proteases and Penetration

During the past 12 years considerable attention has been focused on acrosin, a protease located in the sperm acrosome which can exist as an inactive zymogen (Meizel and Mukerji, 1975) and with a trypsinlike cleavage specificity (Fritz *et al.*, 1975a; Hartree, 1977). This interest was generated by the concept of a "zona lysin" located in the sperm and which was assumed to play a role in the penetration of the zona pellucida (Austin and Bishop, 1958). The reader is referred to Chapter 10 for a thorough discussion of the mechanism of zona penetration.

Suffice it to say that there is now reason at least to doubt that sperm proteases are directly involved in producing a penetration channel. In view of the sensitivity of binding (Hartmann and Hutchison, 1974b; Saling, 1981), the acrosome reaction (Lui and Meizel, 1979), and the release of some of the S1 peptides (Hartmann and Hutchison, 1980a,b) to trypsin inhibitors, consideration should be given to alternate roles for trypsinlike proteases in the fertilization process.

5. A Model of Prepenetration Interactions between Hamster Gametes

There are three major components of this model: (1) the capacitated sperm–zona pellucida surface interface, (2) the S1 peptides, and (3) the vitellus. The model will attempt to explain how these three interact by integrating the data accumulated in our laboratory and reviewed in Section III,C,2c–f. Primarily because there are more data dealing with the first 5 minutes of sperm–zona interaction, I will confine my interpretation largely to this period. Where no data exist for any aspect of the model, mention will be made of this.

The interaction between capacitated hamster sperm and egg is unique among all of the surface contact interactions in the *in vitro* fertilization system used by us (Fig. 3). It is the only one in which a relatively lengthy period of readily reversible attachment precedes binding. This sequence appears to be essential for penetration of the zona by the sperm to occur. The discovery of the S1 peptides, released by sperm–zona contact during these stages, provided the needed component through which events at the zona surface could communicate with the vitellus, the participation of which was suspected but which has been difficult to visualize because of its distance (several microns) from the outer surface of the zona.

A flow diagram depicting the essential features of the model is

Early Stages of Sperm-Zona Contact

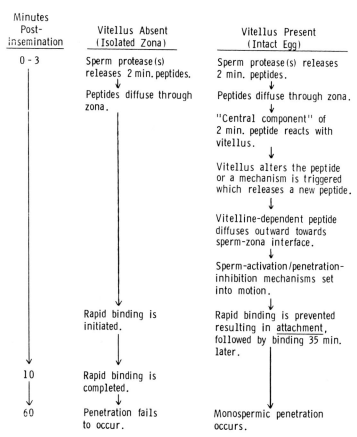

Minutes Post-insemination	Vitellus Absent (Isolated Zona)	Vitellus Present (Intact Egg)
0 - 3	Sperm protease(s) releases 2 min. peptides. ↓ Peptides diffuse through zona.	Sperm protease(s) releases 2 min. peptides. ↓ Peptides diffuse through zona. ↓ "Central component" of 2 min. peptide reacts with vitellus. ↓ Vitellus alters the peptide or a mechanism is triggered which releases a new peptide. ↓ Vitelline-dependent peptide diffuses outward towards sperm-zona interface. ↓ Sperm-activation/penetration-inhibition mechanisms set into motion. ↓
	Rapid binding is initiated.	Rapid binding is prevented resulting in attachment, followed by binding 35 min. later.
10	Rapid binding is completed. ↓	
60	Penetration fails to occur.	Monospermic penetration occurs.

Fig. 9. Flow diagram model depicting earliest events during sperm–egg interaction between hamster sperm and homologous egg and hamster isolated zona pellucida. (Modified from Hartmann *et al.*, 1982.)

shown in Fig. 9. The role of the vitellus is accented by comparing sperm–egg interaction with events that occur between sperm and isolated zonae pellucidae. The first set of peptides are released, at least in part, through the action of a trypsinlike protease. Because the peptides were not detected when heterologous gametes were combined, a specific signal(s) must trigger their release. Thus, homologous contact activates a protease(s) which then cleaves an appropriate protein substrate. Sperm acrosin may be the protease. The origin of the 2-minute peptide(s), whether from the zona or the sperm, is at this time unknown, but the vitellus is not involved in contributing to those factors released initially. After their release, the peptides diffuse and some enter the pores of the zona pellucida, eventually reaching the vitelline surface. At least one of the 2-minute peptides is altered by contact with the vitellus. Alternatively, this peptide may trigger the release of another peptide from the vitellus. The altered or new peptide then diffuses in the opposite direction, within the zona pores, toward the sperm–zona interface. The peptide(s) may act directly on the sperm, or indirectly by affecting the zona which, in turn, alters the sperm. Instead of the spermatozoa beginning to engage in early binding as they would in the absence of the vitellus, they are prevented from doing so by the action of outward diffusing peptide, and instead are altered to enter the attachment stage.

These early interactions set into motion those events that lead to penetration, that is, the activation of the sperm to bind to and subsequently penetrate the zona pellucida in a controlled "monospermic manner." It should be emphasized that there is no direct evidence for a vitelline-mediated activation of sperm. This is inferred from the observation that sperm fail to penetrate the isolated zona pellucida, a phenomenon apparently unrelated to the tear in the zona (Fig. 4). The activation of the sperm must be complemented by a mechanism which inhibits polyspermic penetration of the zona, shown to be a property of the vitelline-dependent peptide. The need to postulate a precortical granule block to polyspermy is evident when one observes the large number of hamster sperm which bind to the surface of eggs *in vitro* but which are penetrated, in most cases, only by a single sperm. Unlike the cortical granule-mediated block to polyspermy, however, the S1 peptide-mediated inhibition is transient. The degree of S1 peptide-mediated inhibition of sperm penetration is dose-related. The dose is determined by the quantity of peptide released, which in turn is proportional to the number of bound sperm. This ability to adjust, in a quantitative way, to the number of sperm bound to the zona reflects the self-regulating property of the system.

At this time little can be suggested as to the role of those peptides released subsequently during the balance of the attachment phase and during the binding stage, that is, those detected at 20–25, 31, and 50 minutes after insemination. At any rate the demonstrated ability of both the first and last peptides, released at the beginning and end of a considerable span of time, to inhibit penetration may reflect the operation of a "vigilante"-like system, evolved to monitor the possibility of polyspermy and prevent its occurrence during the lengthy prepenetration contact phase.

As indicated earlier the S1 peptides can affect certain changes at the sperm–zona interface only after their interaction with the vitellus. The resulting peptide, whether a modified S1 peptide or one released anew from the vitellus, would diffuse outward and, therefore, be directed toward those sperm adhering to the zona. It may be interesting to note that a vitelline-mediated mechanism of sperm activation would ensure the activation of zona-penetrating mechanisms at the crucial time, and not before the sperm reaches the egg. Others have shown that the acrosome reaction, an essential prelude to fertilization, can be induced by solubilized zonae (Florman and Storey, 1982) or a protein component of it (Wassarman and Bleil, 1981). Clearly then the vitellus is not a requirement for the induction of the acrosome reaction. The vitellus may play, in addition to its demonstrated involvement in the slowing of penetration, a subtle and, as yet, undefined role in the penetration-inducing mechanism, while acting in cooperation with the acrosome reaction.

Trypsin inhibitor studies have implicated sperm acrosin in one component of the acrosome reaction (membrane vesiculation of hamster sperm; Lui and Meizel, 1979) or another (acrosomal matrix dispersion of guinea pig sperm; Perrault *et al.*, 1982). This suggests a relationship between those S1 peptides sensitive to the presence of trypsin inhibitors (2 and 31 minutes) and the acrosome reaction.

IV. EPILOGUE AND SUGGESTED FUTURE APPROACHES

In vitro methods of fertilization have become useful tools for probing the mechanism of mammalian fertilization. An understanding of this phenomenon has bearly begun. To date major emphases have been placed on morphological and "preliminary" biochemical aspects of sperm–egg interaction, a state of affairs imposed by the small quantities of interacting cells. However, much of this difficulty will be circumvented through the exploitation of new sources of gametes and new methods. For example, large quantities of eggs, adequate for biochemical analysis, can be obtained from porcine ovaries (see Chapter 3). Furthermore, as mentioned earlier (II,B), the successful application of methods for capacitating large quantities of swine sperm combined with techniques for maturing large numbers of porcine ovarian oocytes *in vitro* will permit studies on fertilization in quantities on a scale heretofore unanticipated in the mammal.

On the other side of the coin, new information has been obtained through the application of highly sensitive radiochemical and electrophoretic techniques to the interaction of small quantities of cells, as demonstrated for example, by Bleil *et al.* (1981) (see also Chapter 1). Ultrasensitive methods that employ fluorescent substrates are now also available for the detection and measurement of proteolytic activity (Zimmerman *et al.*, 1977). This method has found ready applications for measurement of protease activity in mammalian eggs (Mumford *et al.*, 1981). The continued application of these methods should help shed light, for example, on the role of egg proteases following penetration of the egg by the sperm.

Additional suggestions will be provided below. They are not meant to be particularly broad and all inclusive but, obviously, reflect the prejudices of the author.

Clearly the issue of the species specificity of binding remains unresolved, possibly because it depends upon a variety of subjective factors. In order to minimize these variables, I recommend that future research into sperm–egg interaction take into account the following minimal considerations: (1) demonstration that sperm are adequately capacitated by conducting penetration controls; (2) select *in vitro* systems and species in which 100% penetration can be achieved; (3) select conditions in which penetration is monospermic or very close to it.

Efforts have been made to standardize the binding assay by centrifugation (Saling *et al.*, 1979). However, such methods are experimentally restrictive and others have found that measurement of the binding of gametes of other species by centrifugation is less reproducible than if they are washed with a micropipette (Peterson *et al.*, 1980). Certainly the approach of Schmell and Gulyas (1980), which employs the guinea pig egg to which mouse and hamster sperm fail to form a permanent association, would be a convenient specificity check.

The existence of the S1 peptides must be confirmed in other species if their importance is to be established, since ubiquity and significance go hand-in-hand in biological mechanisms. This will require the development of new assays, biochemical in nature, which are based on the functions of the S1 peptides. Only then will their existence be demonstrated convincingly. Such studies will also lead to a determination of the gamete of origin of these factors.

Finally, convincing evidence for the "activation" of the sperm by the mechanism proposed herein can be provided by induction of penetration of the isolated zona pellucida after all of the proposed interacting components (isolated zonae, capacitated sperm, S1 peptides and vitelli) have been combined in the correct reconstructed sequence. This kind of experimental protocol would, all or in part, confirm the model or perhaps, less dramatically, refute it. Time and effort will tell.

ACKNOWLEDGMENT

I am most grateful to Mr. Cameron Hutchison for many years of superb technical assistance and to Mr. Richard Mumford for his comments on this review. My thanks go to Ms. Donna Sloan for her assistance in preparing the manuscript and to Ms. Patricia Levan for editorial assistance.

REFERENCES

Ahuja, K. K., and Tzartos, S. J. (1981). Investigation of sperm receptors in the hamster zona pellucida by using univalent (Fab) antibodies to hamster ovary. *J. Reprod. Fertil.* **61,** 257–264.

Aitken, R. J., and Richardson, D. W. (1981). Mechanism of sperm-binding inhibition by anti-zona antisera. *Gamete Res.* **4,** 41–47.

Austin, C. R., and Bishop, A. W. H. (1958). Some features of the acrosome and perforatorium in mammalian spermatozoa. *Proc. Royal Soc. Ser. B.* **149,** 234–240.

Bavister, B. D. (1979). Fertilization of hamster eggs in vitro at sperm: egg ratios close to unity. *J. Exp. Zool.* **210,** 259–264.

Bavister, B. D. (1981). Analysis of culture media for *in vitro* fertilization and criteria for success. *In* "Fertilization and Embryonic Development *in Vitro*" (J. D. Biggers and L. Mastroianni, Jr., eds.), pp. 41–60. Plenum, New York.

Bedford, J. M. (1977). Sperm/egg interaction: The specificity of human spermatozoa. *Anat. Rec.* **188,** 477–488.

Bhattacharyya, A. K., Zaneveld, L. J. D., Dragoje, B. M., Schumacher, G. F. B., and Travis, J. (1976). Inhibition of human sperm acrosin by synthetic agents. *J. Reprod. Fertil.* **47,** 97–100.

Blandau, R. J. (1980). *In vitro* fertilization and embryo transfer. *Fertil. Steril.* **33,** 3–11.

Bleil, J. D., and Wassarman, P. M. (1980). Mammalian sperm-egg interaction: Identification of a glycoprotein in mouse zonae pellucidae possessing receptor activity for sperm. *Cell* **20,** 873–882.

Bleil, J. D., Beall, C. F., and Wassarman, P. M. (1981). Mammalian sperm–egg interaction: Fertilization of mouse eggs triggers modification of the major zona pellucida glycoprotein, ZP2. *Dev. Biol.* **86,** 189–197.

Bleil, J. D., and Wassarman, P. M. (1983). Sperm–egg interactions in the mouse: Sequence of events and induction of the acrosome reaction by a zona pellucida glycoprotein. *Dev. Biol.* (in press).

Brackett, B. G., and Oliphant, G. (1975). Capacitation of rabbit spermatozoa in vitro. *Biol. Reprod.* **12,** 260–274.

Brackett, B. G., Oh, Y. K., Evans, J. F., and Donawick, W. J. (1980). Fertilization and early development of cow ova. *Biol. Reprod.* **23,** 189–205.

Brackett, B. G., Bousquet, D., Boice, M. L., Donawick, W. J., and Evans, J. F. (1981). Pregnancy following cow in vitro fertilization. *Biol. Reprod.* **24,** Suppl. 1, 109A.

Braden, A. W. H., and Austin, C. R. (1954). The number of sperms about the eggs in mammals and its significance for normal fertilization. *Aust. J. Biol. Sci.* **7,** 543–551.

Chang, M. C. (1959). Fertilization of rabbit ova *in vitro*. *Nature (London)* **184,** 466–467.

Cholewa-Stewart, J., and Massaro, E. J. (1972). Thermally-induced dissolution of the murine zona pellucida. *Biol. Reprod.* **7,** 166–169.

Dunbar, B. S., and Shivers, C. A. (1976). Immunological aspects of sperm receptors on the zona pellucida of mammalian eggs. *Immunol. Commun.* **5,** 375–385.

Dunbar, B. S., Wardrip, N. J., and Hedrick, J. L. (1980). Isolation, physiocochemical properties and the macromolecular composition of the zona pellucida from porcine oocytes. *Biochemistry* **19,** 356–365.

Edidin, M., and Weiss, A. (1972). Antigen cap formation in cultured fibroblasts: A reflection of membrane fluidity and of cell motility. *Proc. Natl. Acad. Sci. U.S.A.* **69,** 2456–2459.

Florman, H. M., and Storey, B. T. (1981). Inhibition of in vitro fertilization of mouse eggs: 3-quinuclidinyl benzilate specifically blocks penetration of zonae pellucidae by mouse spermatozoa. *J. Exp. Zool.* **216,** 159–167.

Florman, H. M., and Storey, B. T. (1982). Mouse gamete interactions: The zona pellucida is the site of the acrosome reaction leading to fertilization in vitro. *Dev. Biol.* **91,** 121–130.

Franklin, L. E., Barros, C., and Fussell, E. N. (1970). The acrosomal region and the acrosome reaction in sperm of the golden hamster. *Biol. Reprod.* **3,** 180–200.

Fraser, L. R., and Drury, L. M. (1975). The relationship between sperm concentration and fertilization in vitro of mouse eggs. *Biol. Reprod.* **13,** 513–518.

Fraser, L. R., and Drury, L. M. (1976). Mouse sperm genotype and the rate of egg penetration in vitro. *J. Exp. Zool.* **197,** 13–20.

Friend, D. S. (1977). The organization of the spermatozoal membrane. *In* "Immunobiology of Gametes" (M. Edidin and M. H. Johnson, eds.), pp. 5–30. Cambridge Univ. Press, London and New York.

Fritz, H., Schleuning, W.-D., Schiessler, H., Schill, W.-B., Wendt, V., and Winkler, G. (1975a). Boar, bull and human acrosin. *Cold Spring Harbor Conf. Cell Proliferation* **2,** 715–736.

Fritz, H., Schiessler, H., Schill, W.-B., Tschesche, H., Heimburger, N., and Wallner, O. (1975b). Low molecular weight proteinase (acrosin) inhibitors from human and boar seminal plasma and spermatozoa and human cervical mucus-isolation, properties and biological aspects. *Cold Spring Harbor Conf. Cell Proliferation* **2,** 737–766.

Geratz, J. D. (1969). Inhibitory effect of aromatic diamidines on trypsin and enterokinase. *Experientia* **25,** 1254–1255.

Glass, L. E., and Hanson, J. E. (1974). An immunologic approach to contraception: Localization of antiembryo and antizona pellucida serum during mouse preimplantation development. *Fertil. Steril.* **25,** 484–493.

Gordon, M., Dandekar, P. V., and Bartoszewiez, W. (1974). Ultrastructural localization of surface receptors for concanavalin A on rabbit spermatozoa. *J. Reprod. Fertil.* **36,** 211–214.

Gulyas, B. J., and Schmell, E. D. (1981). Sperm-egg recognition and binding in mammals. *In* "Bioregulators of Reproduction" (G. Jagiello and H. J. Vogel, eds.), pp. 499–519. Academic Press, New York.

Gwatkin, R. B. L. (1967). Passage of mengovirus through the zona pellucida of the mouse morula. *J. Reprod. Fertil.* **13,** 577–578.

Gwatkin, R. B. L. (1977). "Fertilization Mechanisms in Man and Mammals." Plenum, New York.

Gwatkin, R. B. L., and Hutchison, C. F. (1971). Capacitation of hamster spermatozoa by β glucuronidase. *Nature (London)* **229,** 343–344.

Gwatkin, R. B. L., and Williams, D. T. (1977). Receptor activity of the hamster and mouse solubilized zona pellucida before and after the zona reactions. *J. Reprod. Fertil.* **49,** 55–59.

Gwatkin, R. B. L., and Williams, D. T. (1978). Bovine and hamster zona solutions exhibit receptor activity for capacitated but not for noncapacitated sperm. *Gamete Res.* **1,** 259–263.

Gwatkin, R. B. L., Andersen, O. F., and Williams, D. T. (1972). Capacitation of hamster spermatozoa in vitro: The role of cumulus components. *J. Reprod. Fertil.* **30,** 389–394.

Gwatkin, R. B. L., Williams, D. T., and Anderson, O. F. (1973). Zona reaction of mammalian eggs: Properties of the cortical granule protease (cortin) and its receptor substrate in hamster eggs. *J. Cell Biol.* **59,** 128a.

Gwatkin, R. B. L., Carter, H. W., and Patterson, H. (1976). Association of mammalian sperm with the cumulus cells and the zona pellucida studied by scanning electron microscopy. *Scanning Electron Microsc.,* pp. 379–384.

Gwatkin, R. B. L., Wudl, L., Hartree, E. F., and Fink, E. (1977). Prevention of fertilization by exposure of hamster eggs to soluble acrosin. *J. Reprod. Fertil.* **50,** 359–361.

Gwatkin, R. B. L., Andersen, O. F., and Williams, D. T. (1980). Large scale isolation of bovine and pig zonae pellucidae: Chemical, immunological and receptor properties. *Gamete Res.* **3,** 217–231.

Hartmann, J. F., and Gwatkin, R. B. L. (1971). Alteration of sites on the mammalian sperm surface following capacitation. *Nature (London)* **234,** 479–481.

Hartmann, J. F., and Hutchison, C. F. (1974a). Nature of the pre-penetration contact interactions between hamster gametes in vitro. *J. Reprod. Fertil.* **36,** 49–57.

Hartmann, J. F., and Hutchison, C. F. (1974b). Contact between hamster spermatozoa and the zona pellucida releases a factor which influences early binding stages. *J. Reprod. Fertil.* **37,** 61–66.

Hartmann, J. F., and Hutchison, C. F. (1976). Surface interactions between mammalian sperm and egg: Variation of spermatozoa concentration as a probe for the study of binding in vitro. *J. Cell. Physiol.* **88,** 219–226.

Hartmann, J. F., and Hutchison, C. F. (1977a). Involvement of two carbohydrate-containing components in the binding of uncapacitated spermatozoa to eggs of the golden hamster in vitro. *J. Exp. Zool.* **201,** 383–390.

Hartmann, J. F., and Hutchison, C. F. (1977b). Release of a factor during early stages of contact between hamster sperm and eggs in vitro. *J. Cell. Physiol.* **93,** 41–48.

Hartmann, J. F., and Hutchison, C. F. (1980a). Nature and fate of the factors released during early contact interactions between hamster sperm and egg prior to fertilization in vitro. *Dev. Biol.* **78,** 380–393.

Hartmann, J. F., and Hutchison, C. F. (1980b). Properties of the first and second factors released after hamster sperm make contact with the zona pellucida prior to fertilization in vitro. *Gamete Res.* **3,** 395–403.

Hartmann, J. F., and Hutchison, C. F. (1981). Modulation of fertilization in vitro by peptides released during hamster sperm-zona pellucida interaction. *Proc. Natl. Acad. Sci. U.S.A.* **78,** 1690–1694.

Hartmann, J. F., Gwatkin, R. B. L., and Hutchison, C. F. (1972). Early contact interactions between mammalian gametes in vitro: Evidence that the vitellus influences adherence between sperm and zona pellucida. *Proc. Natl. Acad. Sci. U.S.A.* **69,** 2767–2769.

Hartmann, J. F., Hutchison, C. F., and Vandlen, R. L. (1982). Modulation of fertilization by the vitellus after apparent interaction with peptides released by hamster sperm–zona pellucida contact. *Dev. Biol.* **93,** 145–151.

Hartree, E. F. (1977). Spermatozoa, eggs and proteinases. *Biochem. Soc. Trans.* **5,** 375–394.

Hastings, R. A., Enders, A. C., and Schlafke, S. (1972). Permeability of the zona pellucida to protein tracers. *Biol. Reprod.* **7**, 288–296.

Heffner, L. S., and Storey, B. T. (1982). Cold lability of mouse sperm binding to zona pellucida. *J. Exp. Zool.* **219**, 155–161.

Heffner, L. J., Saling, P. M., and Storey, B. T. (1980). Separation of calcium effects on motility and zona binding ability in mouse spermatozoa. *J. Exp. Zool.* **212**, 53–59.

Huang, T. T. F., Fleming, A. D., and Yanagimachi, R. (1981). Only acrosome-reacted spermatozoa can bind to and penetrate zona pellucida: A study using the guinea pig. *J. Exp. Zool.* **217**, 287–290.

Inoue, M., and Wolf, D. P. (1975). Sperm binding characteristics of the murine zona pellucida. *Biol. Reprod.* **13**, 340–346.

Kinsey, W. H., and Koehler, J. K. (1978). Cell surface changes associated with in vitro capacitation of hamster sperm. *J. Ultrastruct, Res.* **64**, 1–13.

Koehler, J. K. (1978). The mammalian sperm surface: Studies with specific labelling techniques. *Int. Rev. Cytol.* **54**, 73–108.

Lui, C. W., and Meizel, S. (1979). Further evidence in support of a role for hamster sperm hydrolytic enzymes in the acrosome reaction. *J. Exp. Zool.* **207**, 173–182.

McGaughey, R. W., and Van Blerkom, J. (1977). Patterns of polypeptide synthesis of procine oocytes during maturation in vitro. *Dev. Biol.* **56**, 241–254.

Mahi, C. A., and Yanagimachi, R. (1973). The effect of temperature, osmolarity and hydrogen ion concentration on the activation and acrosome reaction of golden hamster spermatozoa. *J. Reprod. Fertil.* **35**, 55–56.

Mares-Guia, M., and Shaw, E. (1965). Studies on the active center of trypsin: The binding of amidines and guanidines as models of the substrate side chain. *J. Biol. Chem.* **240**, 1579–1585.

Meizel, S., and MuKerji, S. K. (1975). Proacrosin from rabbit epididymal spermatozoa: Partial purification and initial biochemical characterization. *Biol. Reprod.* **13**, 83–93.

Miyamoto, H., and Ishibashi, T. (1975). The role of calcium ions in fertilization of mouse and rat eggs in vitro. *J. Reprod. Fertil.* **45**, 523–526.

Moore, H. D. M., and Bedford, J. M. (1978). An in vivo analysis of factors influencing the fertilization of hamster eggs. *Biol. Reprod.* **19**, 879–885.

Mumford, R., Hartmann, J. F., Ashe, B. M., and Zimmerman, M. (1981). Proteinase activities of the golden hamster eggs and cells of the cumulus oophorus. *Dev. Biol.* **81**, 332–335.

Nicolson, G. L., Yanagimachi, R., and Yanagimachi, H. (1975). Ultrastructural localization of lectin binding sites on the zona pellucida and plasma membranes of mammalian eggs. *J. Cell Biol.* **66**, 263–274.

Oikawa, T., and Yanagimachi, R. (1975). Block of hamster fertilization by anti-ovary antibody. *J. Reprod. Fertil.* **45**, 487–494.

Oikawa, T., Yanagimachi, R., and Nicolson, G. L. (1973). Wheat germ agglutinin blocks mammalian fertilization. *Nature (London)* **241**, 256–259.

Oikawa, T., Nicolson, G. L., and Yanagimachi, R. (1974). Inhibition of hamster fertilization by phytoagglutinins. *Exp. Cell Res.* **83**, 239–246.

Oikawa, T., Nicolson, G. L., and Yanagimachi, R. (1975). Trypsin-mediated modification of the zona pellucida glycopeptide structure of hamster eggs. *J. Reprod. Fertil.* **43**, 133–136.

Olds, P. (1971). Effect of the T locus on fertilization in the house mouse. *J. Exp. Zool.* **177**, 417–434.

Olds-Clarke, P., and Carey, J. E. (1978). Rate of egg penetration in vitro accelerated by T/t locus in the mouse. *J. Exp. Zool.* **206**, 323–332.

O'Rand, M. (1981). Inhibition of fertility and sperm-zona binding by antiserum to the rabbit sperm membrane autoantigen RSA-1. *Biol. Reprod.* **25**, 621–628.

Overstreet, J. W., and Bedford, J. M. (1975). The penetrability of rabbit ova treated with enzymes or anti-progesterone antibody: A probe into the nature of a mammalian fertilizin. *J. Reprod. Fertil.* **44**, 273–284.

Perrault, S. D., Zirkin, B. R., and Rogers, B. J. (1982). Effect of trypsin inhibitors on acrosome reaction of guinea pig spermatozoa. *Biol. Reprod.* **26**, 343–351.

Peterson, R. N., Russell, L., Bundman, D., and Freund, M. (1980). Sperm-egg interaction: Evidence for boar sperm plasma membrane receptors for porcine zona pellucida. *Science* **207**, 73–74.

Peterson, R. N., Russell, L. D., Bundman, D., Conway, M., and Freund, M. (1981). The interaction of living boar sperm and sperm plasma membrane vesicles with the porcine zona pellucida. *Dev. Biol.* **84**, 144–156.

Phillips, D. M., and Shalgi, R. M. (1980). Surface properties of the zona pellucida. *J. Exp. Zool.* **213**, 1–8.

Planck, M. (1949). "Scientific Autobiography and Other Papers." Philosophical Library, New York.

Rogers, B. J. (1978). Mammalian sperm capacitation and fertilization in vitro: a critique of methodology. *Gamete Res.* **1**, 165–223.

Rogers, B. J., Ueno, M , and Yanagimachi, R. (1981). Fertilization by guinea pig spermatozoa requires potassium ions. *Biol. Reprod.* **25**, 639–648.

Saling, P. M. (1981). Involvement of trypsin-like activity in binding of mouse spermatozoa to zonae pellucidae. *Proc. Natl. Acad. Sci. U.S.A.* **78**, 1690–1694.

Saling, P. M., and Storey, B. T. (1979). Mouse gamete interactions during fertilization in vitro: Chlorotetracycline as a fluorescent probe for the mouse sperm acrosome reaction. *J. Cell Biol.* **83**, 541–555.

Saling, P. M., Storey, B. T., and Wolf, D. P. (1978). Calcium-dependent binding of mouse epididymal spermatozoa to the zona pellucida. *Dev. Biol.* **65**, 515–525.

Saling, P. M., Sowinski, J., and Storey, B. T. (1979). An ultrastructural study of epididymal mouse spermatozoa binding to zonae pellucidae in vitro: Sequential relationship to the acrosome reaction. *J. Exp. Zool.* **209**, 229–238.

Schmell, E. D., and Gulyas, B. J. (1980). Mammalian sperm-egg recognition and binding in vitro. I. Specificity of sperm interactions with live and fixed eggs in homologous and heterologous inseminations of hamster, mouse and guinea pig oocytes. *Biol. Reprod.* **23**, 1075–1085.

Schmell, E. D., Earles, B. J., Breaux, C., and Lennarz, W. J. (1977). Identification of a sperm receptor on the surface of the eggs of the sea urchin *Arbacia punctulata*. *J. Cell Biol.* **72**, 35–46.

Schmell, E. D.,Yuan, L. C., Gulyas, B. J., and August, J. T. (1982). Identification of mammalian sperm surface antigens. I. Production of monoclonal anti-mouse sperm antibodies. *Fertil. Steril.* **37**, 249–257.

Seidel, G. E., Jr. (1981). Superovulation and embyro transfer in cattle. *Science* **211**, 351–358.

Sellens, M. H., and Jenkinson, E. J. (1975). Permeability of the mouse zona pellucida to immunoglobulin. *J. Reprod. Fertil.* **42**, 153–157.

Shalgi, R., and Phillips, D. M. (1980). Mechanics of in vitro fertilization in the hamster. *Biol. Reprod.* **23**, 433–444.

Shivers, C. A., Dudkiewicz, A. B., Franklin, L. E., and Fussel, E. N. (1972). Inhibition of sperm-egg interaction by specific antibody. *Science* **178**, 1211–1213.

Singh, J. P., Babcock, D. F., and Lardy, H. A. (1978). Increased calcium-ion influx is a component of capacitation of spermatozoa. *Biochem. J.* **172**, 549–556.

Stambaugh, R. (1978). Enzymatic and morphological events in mammalian fertilization. *Gamete Res.* **1,** 65–85.

Steptoe, P. C., and Edwards, R. G. (1978). Birth after the reimplantation of a human embryo. *Lancet* **2,** 366.

Swenson, C. E., and Dunbar, B. S. (1982). Specificity of sperm-zona interaction. *J. Exp. Zool.* **219,** 97–104.

Talbot, P., and Franklin, L. E. (1978). Surface modification of guinea pig sperm during in vitro capacitation: An assessment using lectin-induced agglutination of living sperm. *J. Exp. Zool.* **203,** 1–14.

Talbot, P., Franklin, L. E., and Fussell, E. N. (1974). The effect of the concentration of golden hamster spermatozoa on the acrosome reaction and egg penetration in vitro. *J. Reprod. Fertil.* **36,** 429–432.

Talbot, P., Summers, R. G., Hylander, B. L., Keogh, E. M., and Franklin, L. E. (1976). The role of calcium in the acrosome reaction: An analysis using ionophore A23187. *J. Exp. Zool.* **198,** 383–392.

Tsafriri, A., and Channing, C. P. (1975). Influence of follicular maturation and culture conditions on the meiosis of pig oocytes in vitro. *J. Reprod. Fertil.* **43,** 149–152.

Turner, R. S., and Burger, M. M. (1973). Involvement of a carbohydrate group in the active site for surface guided reassociation of animal cells. *Nature (London)* **244,** 509–510.

Tzartos, S. J. (1979). Inhibition of *in vitro* fertilization of intact and denuded hamster eggs by univalent anti-sperm antibodies. *J. Reprod. Fertil.* **55,** 447–455.

Umbreit, J., and Roseman, S. (1975). A requirement for reversible binding between aggregating embryonic cells before stable adhesion. *J. Biol. Chem.* **250,** 9360–9368.

Wassarman, P. M., and Bleil, J. D. (1981). The role of zona pellucida glycoproteins as regulators of sperm-egg interactions in the mouse. *J. Supramol. Struct. Cell. Biochem. Suppl.* **5,** 245 (abstr.).

Wolf, D. P., and Inoue, M. (1976). Sperm concentration dependency in the fertilization and zonae sperm binding properties of mouse eggs inseminated in vitro. *J. Exp. Zool.* **196,** 27–38.

Yanagimachi, R. (1970). In vitro capacitation of golden hamster spermatozoa by homologous and heterologous blood sera. *Biol. Reprod.* **3,** 147–153.

Yanagimachi, R. (1977). Specificity of sperm-egg interaction. *In* "Immunobiology of Gametes" (M. Edidin and M. H. Johnson, eds.), pp. 255–289. Cambridge Univ. Press, London and New York.

Yanagimachi, R. (1978). Sperm-egg association in mammals. *Curr. Top. Dev. Biol.* **12,** 83–105.

Yanagimachi, R., and Noda, Y. D. (1970). Ultrastructural changes in the hamster sperm head during fertilization. *J. Ultrastructure Res.* **31,** 465–485.

Yanagimachi, R., and Usui, N. (1974). Calcium dependence of the acrosome reaction and activation of guinea pig spermatozoa. *Exp. Cell Res.* **89,** 161–174.

Zaneveld, L. J. D., Polakoski, K. L., and Schumacher, G. F. B. (1975). The proteolytic enzyme systems of mammalian genital tract secretions and spermatozoa. *Cold Spring Harbor Conf. Cell Proliferation* **2,** 683–706.

Zimmerman, M., Ashe, B., Yurewicz, E. C., and Patel, G. (1977). Sensitive assays for trypsin, elastase, and chymotrypsin using new fluorogenic substrates. *Anal. Biochem.* **78,** 47–51.

8

Egg Surface Changes during Fertilization and the Molecular Mechanism of the Block to Polyspermy

ELI D. SCHMELL, BELA J. GULYAS, AND JERRY L. HEDRICK

I. INTRODUCTION

There are striking similarities throughout the animal kingdom in the biology of the reproductive process. For example, with the exception of some species, fertilization of animal eggs is generally monosper-

Mechanism and Control of Animal Fertilization
Copyright © 1983 by Academic Press, Inc.
All rights of reproduction in any form reserved.
ISBN 0-12-328520-8

mic. That is to say, in most animal species cellular and molecular mechanisms exist to ensure that only one sperm cell penetrates the plasma membrane of the ovum. In this manner normal syngamy, that is, the combination of only one male pronucleus with the female pronucleus, is assured. This is crucial for survival of the species since polyspermic fertilization is pathological in most species and results in abnormal development and early embryonic death. Thus, through the process of natural selection, defense mechanisms against polyspermy have evolved, inherent in the activation process of many animal eggs.

It should be noted that eggs of some species (including selachians, urodeles, reptiles, birds, some mollusks, and many insects) are normally polyspermic, or demonstrate physiologic polyspermy, in that many sperm penetrate the egg at fertilization (see review by Rothschild, 1956; Austin, 1978). In these systems normal development still occurs because only one male pronucleus subsequently fuses with the female pronucleus. The remaining male pronuclei degenerate at the periphery of the egg cytoplasm. The mechanism whereby fusion of more than one male pronucleus with the female pronucleus is prevented in these systems remains unknown. In still other species polyspermic fertilization is blocked by limitation of the possibility of sperm access and entry to specific regions of the egg surface. An extreme example of this case is the medaka fish (*Oryzias latipes*). In this system only one site is available for sperm fusion, which is accessible through a single micropyle, or tunnel, in the outer egg investments. The diameter of the micropyle is just wide enough to accommodate the passage of one sperm. Fertilization in this system results in a sealing off of the micropyle, making multiple sperm entry impossible (Iwamatsu and Ohta, 1978).

In many animal eggs, however, such as those of the sea urchin, frog, and mammal, multiple sites apparently exist at the egg surface for sperm attachment, binding, and subsequent fusion; yet only one sperm will usually penetrate the ovum. Thus, in the context of this chapter, the term "block to polyspermy" means the prevention of penetration or entry of more than one sperm into the egg cytoplasm. This chapter will review the state of knowledge concerning the cellular and molecular aspects of the block to polyspermy that are operative at the surface of animal eggs. The information available will be reviewed in a comparative fashion for the following three members of the animal kingdom: (1) the marine invertebrates, primarily the sea urchin (Echinodermata); (2) the lower, nonmammalian vertebrates, principally the anuran *Xenopus laevis;* and (3) mammals, primarily small laboratory animals.

II. SURFACE MORPHOLOGY OF UNFERTILIZED AND FERTILIZED EGGS

In order to understand the details of the mechanism of the block to polyspermy in animal eggs, one needs a description of the morphology of the unfertilized egg, as well as a summary of the morphological changes that occur at the surface of the egg upon successful fusion with the sperm cell. The surface of both the fertilized and unfertilized egg is a rather complex structure, being composed of several distinct extra-cellular investments. The various surface components of both unfer-tilized and fertilized eggs are presented schematically in Fig. 1 for sea urchin, anuran, and mammalian cells. In each species the surface structures contribute to the overall process of fertilization and the block to polyspermy and require at least limited description if the surface mechanism involved in the block to polyspermy is to be appreciated.

A. Sea Urchin

1. The Surface Morphology of Unfertilized Eggs

As shown schematically in Fig. 1, the outermost investment of the sea urchin egg is a gelatinous matrix called the jelly coat (JC). This transparent coating is added to the egg surface during the later stages of oogenesis; however, its site of synthesis remains unknown (Giudice, 1973). It is composed of at least two separable, macromolecular compo-nents: a fucose-sulfate polysaccharide and a sialoprotein (SeGall and Lennarz, 1979). Early studies with sea urchins (Lillie, 1914; Tyler, 1941) suggested that the JC may function as a receptor for sperm; thus, it was subsequently referred to as "fertilizin" (Lillie, 1919). However, more recent investigations indicate that this role is unlikely (Kinsey *et al.*, 1979). It is clear from numerous studies that the JC induces the acrosome reaction in the sperm of a number of species, as first reported by Dan (1952). The ability to induce the acrosome reaction apparently resides in the fucose-sulfate polymer portion of the JC (SeGall and Lennarz, 1979).

Beneath the JC and closely opposed to the extracellular face of the egg plasma membrane (PM) lies the vitelline envelope (VE). The VE of sea urchin eggs is less visible than the VE of frog oocytes, for example, and, in fact, the existence of the VE in sea urchin eggs was debated in the earlier literature (for a review, see Giudice, 1973, and references therein). Although it remains to be extensively characterized, the VE

Echinoderm

Unfertilized   Fertilized

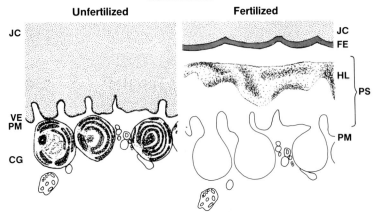

Anuran

Unfertilized   Fertilized

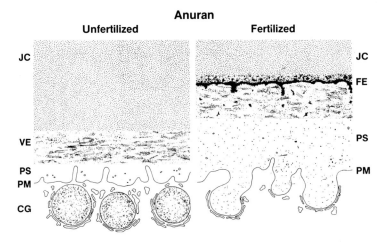

Mammal

Unfertilized   Fertilized

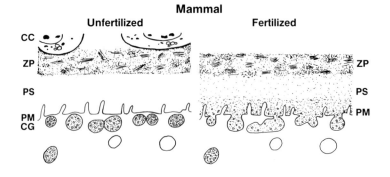

has since been unequivocally observed by both transmission electron microscopy (TEM) and scanning electron microscopy (SEM) by numerous investigators. In the TEM the VE appears to be a fluffy amorphous layer which surrounds and follows the contour of the PM. Studies of the VE using SEM reveal a surface composed of numerous short papillae about 0.2 μm in length (Hagström and Lonning, 1976; Schatten and Mazia, 1976). Functionally, the VE is apparently the site of species-specific receptors for sperm–egg binding (Aketa *et al.*, 1972; Schmell *et al.*, 1977; Glabe and Vacquier, 1978).

The limiting PM of the sea urchin egg is 60–80 nm thick and exhibits the usual trilamellar structure characteristic of cellular membranes when observed in the TEM. Also apparent in the TEM are numerous microvilli (MV), as many as 134,000 per egg, which are about 0.35 μm in length (Schroeder, 1978). These MV appear as fingerlike projections of the PM, when observed in the SEM following treatments that remove the VE. The papillae of the VE mentioned above are apparently castings or reflections of the numerous MV formed by these projections of the PM.

Within the egg cell and closely associated with the PM is a layer of highly specialized, secretory vesicles, each about 1 μm in diameter, known as the cortical granules (CG) (for a recent review, see Schuel, 1978). The entire layer of cytoplasm ∼ 5 μm thick just beneath the PM, including the CG, has been referred to as the cortex or cortical layer The structure and function of the cortex and its dynamic role in fertilization and development has recently been reviewed at length by Vacquier (1981).

In general the numerous CG are evenly spaced within the cortex along the cytoplasmic face of the egg PM. Eggs of the sea urchin *Strongylocentrotus purpuratus* for example contain about 18,000 CG (Schroeder, 1979). The fine structure of echinoderm cortical granules varies from genus to genus (Runnström, 1966). The CG of *Arbacia punctulata* eggs, for example, exhibit a characteristically electron-

---

Fig. 1. Diagrams of unfertilized and fertilized egg surfaces. Schematic representation of the surface structures of echinoderm (top), anuran (middle), and mammalian (bottom) eggs. Abbreviations: CC, cumulus cell; CG, cortical granule; FE, fertilization envelope; HL, hyaline layer; JC, jelly coat; PM, plasma membrane; PS, perivitelline space; VE, vitelline envelope; ZP, zona pellucida. [Diagrams were adopted from the following micrographs as follows: echinoderm (*Strongylocentrotus purpuratus*), Chandler and Heuser, 1979, 1980; anuran (*Xenopus laevis*), Wyrick *et al.*, 1974; mammal (mouse), Nicosia *et al.*, 1977; Thompson *et al.*, 1974; Zamboni, 1974. The diagrams are not to scale; the references cited should be consulted for the dimensions of the cell structures depicted.]

dense stellate core, whereas *Strongylocentrotus purpuratus* CG contain spiral-shaped lamellae. Studies by Anderson (1968) have shown that the CG are produced in the Golgi complex of the oocyte and subsequently migrate toward and apparently attach to the cytoplasmic face of the egg surface. The structure, composition, and physiological function of CG have recently been reviewed at length by Schuel (1978).

2. Morphological Alterations following Sperm–Egg Interactions

Upon fertilization, the surface of the sea urchin egg cell undergoes a series of striking morphological changes resulting in formation of the hyaline layer, elevation of the VE, and subsequent transformation of the VE into the fertilization envelope (FE). These alterations, for the most part, are the result of the cortical reaction or CG exocytosis which occurs at fertilization. During this process the numerous CG fuse with the PM and secrete their contents, the fertilization product, into the perivitelline space (PVS)—the space between the PM and the rising VE. The process begins about 20–30 seconds postinsemination, in most species of sea urchins, and ends about 30–40 seconds later. The cortical reaction initiates from the point of fusion of the fertilizing sperm and propagates in a wavelike fashion around the egg. Evidence recently reviewed by Epel (1980) and by Vacquier (1981) indicates that initiation of the cortical reaction apparently involves a transient rise of free calcium ions in the egg cortex. The secretory components of CG interact with and modify the VE, resulting in formation of the FE. Thus the surface of the newly fertilized egg is radically different than that of the oocyte (Fig. 1).

The outermost extracellular layer of the egg is now the FE. This structure, in contrast to the VE, is readily observed even in the light microscope, surrounding the entire egg. During VE conversion to the FE, a distinct morphological alteration in the VE surface can be observed in the TEM. The shape of the papillae of the VE is altered. In the unfertilized egg these structures are igloolike or an inverted U shape, and are converted to a tentlike or inverted V shape during elevation and hardening of the FE (Veron *et al.*, 1977). Sperm do not bind to the FE and apparently cannot penetrate this structure.

Within the FE and filling the PVS is a highly birefringent gel-like structure, called the hyaline layer. The hyaline material apparently originates in the CG (Endo, 1961) and has reportedly been isolated and characterized (for a review, see Schuel, 1978, and references therein). The apparent function of the hyaline layer is to act as an extracellular cement to maintain the relative positions and proximity of the blastomeres as they are formed and migrate during embryogenesis.

The PM of the newly fertilized egg is a dynamic or mosaic structure in that several alterations occur in its composition and morphology following sperm–egg interaction. First, during the cortical reaction the limiting membranes of the CG are incorporated into the PM. This addition of membranous material, of course, greatly increases the surface area of the egg PM. This results in a transient extension of the egg surface MV (0.35 μm to 1.0 μm) in the first few minutes following fertilization. The MV subsequently shorten once again to about 0.5 μm soon after (Shroeder, 1978). A second dynamic PM modification occurs at the site of sperm–egg fusion. Several investigators have described extension of MV to engulf the fertilizing sperm in a transitory structure called the "fertilization cone" (Schatten and Schatten, 1980; Tilney and Jaffe, 1980). This process apparently involves F-actin and is sensitive to cytochalasin B. Thus, the egg plasma membrane is a dynamic mosaic of membranous material just subsequent to fertilization.

Another striking morphological event observed at the egg surface following fertilization is the contraction of the egg cortex. This process has been most extensively studied in frog eggs as described in Section II,B. Schatten (1979) has described this phenomenon in the sea urchin *Lytechinus variegatus*. Time-lapse cinematography reveals a rapid surface contraction, radiating from the point of sperm fusion. This contraction is cytochalasin B-sensitive and apparently distinct from the cortical reaction itself, which is not inhibited by cytochalasin.

B. Frog

1. Surface Morphology of an Unfertilized Anuran Egg

The outer surface of anuran eggs, as shown in Fig. 1, is covered by several layers of investments that can be subdivided into JC layers and a VE (for review of the older literature, see Wischnitzer, 1966). The JC layers are secretory products of different regions of the oviduct. The cellular site of VE biosynthesis has not been unequivocally established; the VE may be a secretory product of the oocyte itself, the follicle cells, or both. The number of JC layers surrounding the egg is variable and often controversial, being three–six in *Rana pipiens* (Steinke and Benson, 1970; Pereda, 1970; Shivers and James, 1969), three in *Xenopus laevis* (Freeman, 1968), and four in *Bufo arenarum* (Barbieri and Budequer de Atenor, 1973). The chemistry and macromolecular composition of the jelly coat layers have been investigated in a number of anurans (Katagiri, 1973; Yurewicz et al., 1975; Seshadri and Reddy, 1980).

The VE is bounded on the outside by a JC while its innermost aspect forms the outer boundary of the PVS. The VE is generally constructed of filaments or fibers arranged parallel to the egg surface (*Rana temporaria*, Wartenburg and Schmidt, 1961; *Rana pipiens*, Kemp and Istock, 1967). The VE has been most completely described in *Xenopus laevis* (Grey et al., 1974). In this species the VE is approximately 1 μm thick. Its inner surface is often in contact with glycocalyx-covered tips of the MV, and its outer surface is juxtaposed to the JC layer, designated J_1. The fibers composing the VE are 40–70 Å in diameter, and are loosely and evenly arranged in bundles. The bundles are positioned parallel to the egg surface and are organized into layers oriented at an angle to one another. The morphology of the VE of the oviposited egg is generated by the action of oviducal secretions on the envelope of the newly ovulated coelomic egg.

The egg envelope recovered from the coelom has a distinctly different morphology in eggs from *Rana pipiens, Rana japonica,* and *Xenopus laevis*. The distinguishing features of the coelomic egg envelope (CE) are: (1) The fibers of the envelope are tightly bundled or arranged into fasicles, 50–120 nm in diameter, which give the envelope a very netlike appearance, and (2) the fasicles are randomly arranged relative to the egg surface. The morphological transformation of the CE to the VE is effected physiologically by substances released from the first 1–2 cm of the oviduct or it can be effected *in vitro* by alteration of the pH of the medium away from neutrality, e.g., pH 5 or 9 (Grey et al., 1976; Yoshizaki and Katagiri, 1981). This morphological difference is matched by a functional difference in the envelope; the CE cannot be penetrated by sperm while the VE can. As will be mentioned later, macromolecular differences between CE and VE have recently been determined. The PM of the anuran egg typically has MV that project into the PVS (for references, see Elinson, 1980). The size and shape of the MV vary from the animal to the vegetal pole of the egg. Moreover, the MV change in length and surface density when the egg is fertilized (Elinson, 1980).

The PM and a thin layer of the underlying cytoplasm are organized into what is referred to as the egg cortex. The egg cortex has a distinct morphological structure which changes at fertilization; the cortex can be isolated as a subcellular fraction (Richter, 1980). A layer of membrane bound granules, CG, lay under the PM and, in many instances, in intimate contact with it (Grey et al., 1974, for references). The CG are 1.5–2.5 μm in diameter, are of a featureless uniform density as determined by ultrastructural studies, and contain protein and carbohydrate as determined by cytochemical methods as well as chemical analyses of the isolated contents of the CG. The size and ultrastructural appearance of the CG differ between the animal and vegetal halves in *Xenopus laevis* (Grey *et al.,* 1974; Campanella, 1975). The functional significance of this difference is unknown.

The cortex-embedded cortical granules appear to be interconnected with a reticulum or cisternae in the case of *Xenopus laevis* (Grey *et al.,* 1974; Campanella and Andreucetti, 1977). Campanella and Andreucetti (1977) suggest that this CG interconnecting reticulum may function in the propagation phase of the sperm-induced cortical reaction (fusion of CG with the PM). This is a provocative suggestion that up to the present time has not been dealt with experimentally. The cortex of the egg also contains actin (Franke *et al.,* 1976). The form of the actin (G- or F-actin) and its specific function in the numerous cortical movements that take place at fertilization have yet to be defined.

2. Surface Morphology of a Fertilized Anuran Egg

Compared with the information we have on the morphological events involved in sperm–egg fusion in sea urchins or mammals, that available on sperm-egg fusion in anurans is less complete. Anuran sperm have acrosomes (Burgos and Fawcett, 1956; Buongiorno-Nardelli and Bertolini, 1967; Poirier and Spink, 1971; Reed and Stanley, 1972) and, by analogy with sea urchins and mammals, must necessarily undergo the acrosome reaction in order to penetrate the egg investments and successfully fuse with the egg PM. However, the sperm of only one anuran, *Leptodactylus chaguensis* (Raisman and Cabada, 1977), and one urodele, *Pleurodeles waltlii* (Picheral, 1977a), have been ultrastructurally characterized in terms of the acrosome reaction. Ultrastructural studies on sperm–jelly coat layer interaction (jelly is required for fertilization), sperm–VE interaction, and sperm–egg fusion have not been reported. This deficiency should be corrected so that a more accurate comparison with other organisms can be made of the morphological events in anuran fertilization.

The site of sperm–egg fusion, i.e., the sperm entry site, is limited to the pigmented animal hemisphere in *Rana pipiens,* although sperm may penetrate the egg integuments at any point at the egg surface (see Elinson, 1975, for references). In *Discoglossus pictus,* sperm entry is limited to a specialized cell surface structure termed the animal dimple (Campanella, 1975).

The sperm entry sites in *Rana pipiens* and *Xenopus laevis* are readily discernable as the microvillar pattern on the PM and the underlying pigmentation pattern is altered (Elinson and Manes, 1978; Palacek *et al.*, 1978). The ultimate fate of the sperm entry site on the plasmalemma is unknown, although Picheral (1977b) observed that this area was pinched off much like a polar body in the urodele egg of *Pleurodeles waltlii*. It is also clear that the sperm entry site does dictate the plane of the first cleavage (see Palecek *et al.*, 1978, for references).

Following the interaction of the sperm and the egg PM, the cortex of the anuran egg undergoes many morphological changes (Fig. 1). Fusion of the CG membrane with the PM results in exocytosis of the CG contents in the classical cortical reaction. The cortical reaction starts at the point of entry and is propagated as a wave over the egg surface. The rate at which the wave is propagated is 10 μm/sec at 21° in *Xenopus laevis* (Hara and Tydeman, 1979), 20–30 μm/sec in *Rana pipens* (Kemp and Istock, 1967), and 12–24 μm/sec at 15° in *Rana temporaria* (Kas'yanov *et al.*, 1971). Assuming that an anuran egg is 1000 μm in diameter, that the sperm entry site is 45° from the animal pole, and that the propagation rate is 10–30 μm/second, the cortical wave completely covers the animal hemisphere in 39–117 seconds.

In anurans, as in the sea urchin, the cortical reaction produces a change in the surface MV in that they are more elongated after the cortical wave has past (Grey *et al.*, 1974; Wolf, 1974a; Elinson, 1980). The cortex itself is also altered after the cortical reaction. In *Xenopus laevis*, the cytoplasm of the cortex appears more dense, and organelles, such as pigment granules and mitochondria, are displaced toward the interior of the egg (Grey *et al.*, 1974; Campanella and Andreucetti, 1977). The reticulum or cisterna that formerly interconnected the CG is rearranged and undercuts the dense cytoplasm.

After the cortical reaction, the cortex of the egg contracts symmetrically around the animal pole, displacing the pigment granules poleward. This contraction has been observed in many anurans and is referred to as the activaton contraction (for a recent review, see Elinson, 1980). It begins some 3–5 minutes after sperm–egg fusion or artificial activation and reaches its maximum by 12–15 minutes (see Palacek *et al.*, 1978, for references). The area of pigmented cortex is greatly reduced as a result of the activation contraction. The MV on the surface of the PM are correspondingly rearranged, becoming more tightly packed in the animal hemipshere and more dispersed in the vegetal hemisphere. The cortical contraction involves Ca^{2+}, as treatment with the divalent cation binding ionophore A23187 (Schroeder and Strickland, 1974) or injection of Ca^{2+} into the egg (Gingell, 1970) will induce cortical contraction. The cortex gradually relaxes and the pigment granules are redistributed in the egg cortex.

The function of the cortical contraction has not been unequivocally established. Elinson (1975) has suggested that the contraction can act as an "elevator" for the male pronucleus embedded in the egg cortex, moving it closer to the female pronucleus which is located beneath the animal pole. The pronuclei subsequently migrate into the egg cytoplasm and fuse (syngamy) deep within the cytoplasm of the animal hemisphere (Ancel and Vintemberger, 1948; Graham, 1966).

The VE is altered morphologically at fertilization in the case of *Xenopus laevis* (Grey *et al.*, 1974) and *Rana temporaria* (Wartenberg and Schmidt, 1961) by formation of a dense layer on the jelly side of the envelope. This layer is termed the fertilization (F) layer and, together with the modified vitelline envelope, VE*, constitute the FE. As will be discussed later, the F layer is formed by the interaction of a CG lectin released by the cortical reaction and a JC ligand. Morphological alteration of the VE at fertilization does not seem to be a general phenomenon as it has not been reported for anurans other than the two mentioned.

The FE is elevated or raised from the egg surface by the cortical reaction, thereby increasing the volume of the PVS (see Palacek *et al.*, 1978, for references). The envelope elevation permits rotation and gravitational orientation of the egg, a developmentally important event. As will be discussed later, in *Xenopus laevis* the FE elevation is osmotically driven due to the macromolecular impermeability of the F layer.

C. Mammal

1. Surface and Cortical Structure of Unpenetrated Ova

The outer surface of the unfertilized mammalian oocyte is surrounded by several layers of granulosa cells which cover the zona pellucida (ZP). Numerous cytoplasmic processes emanate from the cells of the innermost layer of granulosa cells. These processes traverse through the zona and communicate with the oocyte. Just prior to ovulation, in most, but not all, species, these processes are retracted, enabling the subsequent shedding of granulosa cells and exposure of the outer surface of the ZP (Fig. 1).

Scanning electron microscopic observations of Phillips and Shalgi (1980a) have shown the outer zona surface of recently ovulated mouse and hamster ova to be a laminated structure with numerous fenestrations of irregular size and shape, giving it a somewhat spongelike appearance. In the mouse, thick bands of material traverse the ZP surface in an undefined pattern. A similar, but not identical, description of the outer zona surface has been reported by several other investigators (Zamboni, 1971; Gwatkin et al., 1976a; Jackowski and Dumont, 1979). The internal surface of the hamster ZP is structurally dissimilar from the external surface in that it lacks fenestrations and exhibits a particulate appearance (Phillips and Shalgi, 1980b). The two surfaces also appear to differ in their sperm-binding properties. That is, only the outer surface binds spermatozoa, the inner one fails to bind sperm cells. Transmission electron microscopic observations reaffirm the structural differences between the inner and outer portions of the zona. In unfertilized pig and mouse ova, the ZP is composed of two distinct layers. Of the two, the inner is thicker and denser and consists mostly of fibrillar elements oriented perpendicular to the oocyte PM (Baranska et al., 1975; Dunbar et al., 1980; Hedrick and Fry, 1980). The thinner external layer appears less dense and the fibrillar components run circumferentially.

In terms of molecular composition and structure, an asymetrical distribution of glycoproteins in the ZP has been suggested as a result of lectin-binding experiments (for references, see Wolf, 1981). Recently Bleil and Wassarman (1980a) have shown that the ZP of the mouse egg is composed of three major glycoproteins designated ZP1, ZP2, and ZP3, with apparent molecular weights (MW_{app}) of 200,000, 120,000, and 83,000, respectively. It was suggested that ZP3 may be a sperm-binding site in ZP of unfertilized eggs (Bleil and Wassarman 1980b).

The PMs of unfertilized mammalian ova (mouse, rat, rabbit, and hamster) are extensively covered by short, slender MV about 0.3–1.0 μm in length (Calarco and Epstein, 1973; Gould, 1973; Burgos et al., 1976; Nicosia et al., 1978; Wabik-Sliz and Kujat, 1979; Phillips and Shalgi, 1980a). However, several investigators have reported that the area overlying the second meiotic spindle is relatively smooth and devoid of MV (Zamboni, 1971; Gulyas, 1976; Nicosia et al., 1977, 1978; Phillips and Shalgi, 1980a). The significance of this polarity in MV distribution at the oocyte surface is not entirely clear. However, Johnson et al. (1975) point out that sperm attachment to this area is rarely observed. This is not unreasonable, since incorporation of sperm over the meiotic spindle might interfere with extrusion of the second polar body. A filamentous band or layer is present mostly, but not exclusively, beneath this smooth area of the PM which lacks MV (Szollosi, 1967; Zamboni, 1970; Gulyas, 1976). The composition, origin, and functional significance of the microfilament bundle also remain unclear.

capacitated spermatozoa which cannot fuse with the egg membrane fail to elicit a cortical reaction, it has been suggested that gamete fusion, rather than contact, is essential for the cortical reaction (Yanagimachi and Noda, 1970). However, this does not disprove that contact, rather than fusion, of capacitated and/or acrosome-reacted sperm with the oolemma is incapable of eliciting a cortical reaction. It is conceivable that the acrosome-reacted sperm triggers cortical reaction upon attachment by initiating minor changes in the oolemma. However, it is clear that numerous membrane-active agents such as neuraminidase, positively charged polystyrene microbeads, lectins, and ionophores such as boromycin and guanidine (Gwatkin et al., 1976b), as well as the Ca^{2+} ionophore A23187 (Steinhardt et al., 1978; Wolf et al., 1979; Gulyas and Schmell, 1980) can trigger CG breakdown. Initiation of the cortical reaction by Ca^{2+} ionophores suggests that a general trigger mechanism may exist for sea urchins, frogs, and mammals.

Several observations concerning the morphology of the ZP following fertilization have been reported. Phillips and Shalgi (1980a) observed no obvious alterations in the outer zona surface following fertilization of mouse and hamster eggs. In contrast, Jackowski and Dumont (1979) reported distinct alterations in the ZP of the fertilized mouse ova. The zona becomes smoother and lacks deep furrows following fertilization, whereas the zonae of zygotes appear ropy and porous. Thus, according to Jackowski and Dumont (1979), the highly textured zona of the unfertilized ovum is transformed into a less textured structure. These striking differences in morphology may arise as a result of variations in fixation, artifacts introduced during critical point drying and coating, extent of enzyme treatment to expose the egg surface, or because of other physical manipulations.

Similarly, differing descriptions have also been reported concerning alterations of the PM following fertilization. As in case of the zona, Phillips and Shalgi (1980a) observed no changes in the surface microvilli although they reported that the bulging over the meiotic spindle disappears. Szollosi (1967) reported that in recently penetrated eggs there is a decrease in density and size of microvilli. Nicosia et al. (1978), however, observed, following insemination of mouse eggs, a conversion of the predominantly microvillar surface into a smoother configuration, with subsequent reappearance of MV. These modulations in cell surface topography can be correlated with different phases of the cell cycle of the fertilized mouse ovum (Jackowski and Dumont, 1979). Careful kinetic studies of MV appearance, disappearance, and reappearance might resolve these observations.

III. POTENTIAL SITES FOR AND TYPES OF BLOCKS TO POLYSPERMY

Early investigators of sea urchin fertilization realized that some cellular mechanism was responsible for the low levels of polyspermy or multiple sperm entry, normally observed in sea urchin eggs, even when eggs were exposed to relatively high titers of sperm. They attributed this low level of polyspermy to the CG exocytosis or cortical reation and subsequent elevation of the FE (Fol, 1877, 1879). However, as Lillie (1919) noted, FE formation is too slow to account for the block to polyspermy completely, since it begins about 20 seconds postinsemination and is completed only 30–40 seconds later. In contrast, multiple sperm entry was apparently blocked almost immediately following insemination. He proposed, therefore, that the actual block to polyspermy occurred earlier. Rothschild and Swann (1952) were the first to suggest "that there are two separate or separable blocks to polyspermy." This idea was based on the fact that a complete block to polyspermy requires more than 60 seconds to develop, whereas eggs become less penetrable by sperm much earlier. These conclusions were based on quantitative investigations of sperm attachment and fusion relative to the incidence of polyspermy (Rothschild and Swann, 1952). Similarly, Allen and Griffin (1958) noted that about a 20-second latent period exists between sperm attachment ($\sim$ 2 seconds postinsemination) and the beginning of the cortical reaction ($\sim$ 20 seconds postinsemination). Therefore, they too suggested that another mechanism other than that of the cortical reaction must exist to protect the egg against polyspermy during this early latent period. Rothschild (1956) thus suggested "that the block to polyspermy is probably diphasic, in the sense that a partial block to polyspermy sweeps over the egg surface in a second or so, and is followed by a slower mopping-up process which makes the egg completely impermeable to sperm."

Today these two blocks to polyspermy are commonly referred to as the rapid block and slow block to polyspermy. It has become apparent, however, that the overall process of excluding supernumerary sperm, or the block to polyspermy, is a composite process consisting of elegantly coordinated events. The initial phase, or early block, is a rapid but transient modification at the level of the PM. This alteration remains in effect only long enough to allow the cortical reaction to complete a slower but permanent block to sperm entry which involves removal of sperm receptors from the VE. Thus, the block to polyspermy can be viewed as a single event composed of more than one subcomponent. A great deal has been learned at both the cellular and molecular

level concerning the mechanisms of the components involved in the
block to polyspermy in sea urchins, these will be described in detail
below.

In anurans, as in sea urchins, the block to polyspermy is also composed of multiple, coordinated surface events. A rapid but transient
PM-mediated block precedes a slower more permanent VE-level block.
It also appears that other minor—albeit functional—mechanisms exist
to reduce sperm access to the egg surface.

As with the eggs of the lower animal species, those of mammals also
demonstrate more than one distinct component of the block to polyspermy. It is commonly thought that in mammals a block to polyspermy exists to varying degrees either at the level of the PM, in such
animals as the rabbit, mole, and pocket gopher (for references, see Wolf
1981; Braden et al., 1954); or at the level of the ZP in the form of a zona
modification termed the zona reaction, in sheep, pig, dog, and hamster
(Austin, 1965; Gwatkin, 1976). In the rat and the mouse the block is
thought to be attained by a combination of both processes (Austin,
1965). The relationship, temporal and spatial, between the PM and ZP-
mediated block to polyspermy, however, remains unclear. Indeed, the
molecular aspects of the mammalian block to polyspermy, at both the
level of the PM and ZP, remain to be elucidated.

IV. CELLULAR AND MOLECULAR MECHANISM OF THE
BLOCK TO POLYSPERMY

A. Sea Urchin

1. A Plasma Membrane Block Mediated by Membrane
Potential Changes

As mentioned above, early investigators of fertilization appreciated
the necessity for an initial, rapid block (1–2 seconds) to polyspermy
(Lillie, 1919). More than 50 years later, in experiments with the sea
urchin *Strongylocentrotus purpuratus,* Jaffe (1976) demonstrated that
this initial phase of the block to polyspermy is caused by an electrical
depolarization of egg cell PM which occurs following entrance of the
fertilizing sperm (for a recent and more detailed review, see Hagiwara
and Jaffe, 1979).

It is clear that the resting potential of the unfertilized egg is lower
than that of the external medium, although there is some controversy
concerning its absolute value. Some investigators report that it is
about −10 to −15 mV (Steinhardt *et al.,* 1971; De Felice and Dale,

1979; Taglietti, 1979), while others report it to be −60 to −80 mV (Jaffe, 1976). It has been argued that the true resting potential is −60 to −80 mV. More positive values (∼ 10 mV) have been observed by some investigators, apparently as a result of membrane damage by the measuring electrode (Hagiwara and Jaffe, 1979). Regardless of the absolute value of the resting potential, upon fertilization, a rapid depolarization of the PM is observed (net positive change in membrane potential). This change in potential is known as the fertilization potential or activation potential (see Chapter 5). Within 3 seconds of sperm addition, the membrane potential rises to about 20 mV in the sea urchin *Strongylocentrotus purpuratus;* remains positive for about 1 minute, and then slowly repolarizes (Jaffe, 1976). This membrane depolarization had been reported earlier by other investigators as well (see references in Hagiwara and Jaffe, 1979).

Identification of membrane depolarization as the mechanism of the rapid block to polyspermy is based on the following observations reported by Jaffe (1976): (1) Eggs which reached a plateau activation potential more positive than 0 mV were not polyspermic, whereas eggs with more negative plateau potential were often polyspermic. (2) If current was applied to an unfertilized egg to hold the membrane potential more positive than +5 mV, sperm did not fertilize the egg even though sperm attachment to the VE was observed and untreated eggs in the same sample were fertilized. (3) When the current was subsequently removed from such eggs, the potential returned to resting levels, and fertilization occurred with a normal activation potential and FE formation. (4) Application of a current to eggs, which reduced the plateau level of the activation potential to below −30 mV following fertilization, resulted in polyspermic fertilization of such eggs. It is also of interest to note that in the case of the medaka fish no indication of a membrane depolarization at fertilization has been observed (Nuccitelli, 1980a,b). As mentioned earlier this species apparently would not require a rapid phase of the block to polyspermy, since the sealed micropyle precludes multiple sperm entry.

In the experiments reported by Jaffe (1976), the time course of the electrical events and the correlation with sperm attachment are also significant. First, the initial rise in potential was observed as quickly as 3 seconds postinsemination and the membrane remained depolarized for about 1 minute. Therefore, the rapid phase of the block to polyspermy mediated by membrane potential change is established on the order of 1–2 seconds following sperm attachment to the egg, and the block endures until the cortical reaction has occurred. Thus, this phase of the block would cover the latent period discussed by earlier investigators.

These experiments strongly suggest that an initial, rapid phase of the block to polyspermy is mediated by the electrical depolarization of the egg cell PM at fertilization. Despite the identification of this cellular or physiological block to sperm entry, the molecular mechanism by which sperm are excluded from the egg cell as a result of this membrane depolarization remains to be elucidated.

More information is available, however, pertaining to the molecular aspects or ionic requirements of the electrical depolarization. At least three cations are involved in the fertilization potential, Na^+, Ca^{2+}, and K^+ (for recent review, see Hagiwara and Jaffee, 1979). The initial increase in membrane potential is apparently Na^+ dependent (Steinhardt et al., 1971; Chambers and de Armendi, 1978) and involves opening of Ca^{2+} channels as well (Jaffe, 1976; Chambers and de Armendi, 1978). The net negative phase of the potential shift involves a large increase in K^+ permeability (Chambers et al., 1974; Steinhardt et al., 1971; Tupper, 1973; Jaffe and Robinson, 1978).

In conclusion, it seems clear that the fertilizing sea urchin sperm initiates, in an unknown fashion, electrical potential changes in the egg plasma membrane. The potential changes are dependent on changes in Na^+, Ca^{2+}, and K^+ permeabilities and the initial depolarization of the PM constitutes the rapid but transient phase of the block to polyspermy. The question remains, however, how the membrane depolarization prevents sperm penetration, since sperm attachment and binding to the VE are obviously not impeded.

Quite recently this electrical phase of the block to polyspermy has been questioned (Dale and Monroy, 1981) as a result of experiments reported using the eggs of the sea urchins *Paracentrotus lividus* and *Psammechinus microtuberculatus* (Dale et al., 1978; De Felice and Dale, 1979; Dale and De Santis, 1981). In these species the details and kinetics of membrane depolarization are apparently somewhat different than the results described above. A small, 1–2 mV, membrane depolarization during initial sperm–egg interaction is observed in these species (Dale et al., 1978). The large depolarization or activation potential is not observed until 10–15 seconds later, i.e., at the same time that the cortical reaction begins (Dale and De Santis, 1981). Moreover it was shown that each sperm entering an egg causes a 1–2 μV depolarization, and the number of sperm entering an egg is proportional to sperm concentration (De Felice and Dale, 1979). Thus, in these species, no evidence for an electrically mediated, rapid phase block exists. Whether this reflects species variation or some subtle differences in experimental technique can only be resolved by investigation of both observations by both groups.

2. Polyspermy Block Mediated by Alterations in the Vitelline Envelope

The slower, more permanent phase of the block to polyspermy in the sea urchin, in contrast to the initial, transient phase, involves permanent modifications of the egg surface including enzymatic removal of sperm receptors from the vitelline layer, as well as elevation and hardening of the FE. These alterations preclude sperm attachment to and penetration through the vitelline layer. In turn, access of supernumerary sperm to the egg plasma membrane is prevented. Thus, fusion and penetration by supernumerary sperm are impossible. These modifications of the egg surface are the result of cortical granule exocytosis or the cortical reaction.

As mentioned above, the cortical reaction involves fusion of the numerous cortical granules with the egg plasma membrane and secretion of the granules' contents, i.e., the fertilization product. The immediate, observable consequences of the cortical reaction are, of course, elevation of the VE, its transformation to the FE, and formation of the hyaline layer. A more subtle element of the cortical reaction, however, is secretion of several enzymes into the PVS including: (1) a β-1,3-glucanase (Epel et al., 1969); (2) at least two proteases (Vacquier et al., 1972, 1973a,b; Carroll and Epel, 1975); and (3) a peroxidase termed the ovoperoxidase (Foerder and Shapiro, 1977; Hall, 1978). The physiological function of the glucanase remains unknown. However, much more is known concerning the proteases and ovoperoxidase, which are apparently involved in the slower phase of the block to polyspermy and hardening of the FE, respectively.

Secretion of a protease (proteoesterase) by sea urchin eggs upon fertilization was first reported by Vacquier et al. (1972). In subsequent publications (Vacquier et al., 1973a,b) the enzyme was implicated in the block to polyspermy. Ultimately Carrol and Epel (1975) demonstrated the presence of two protease activities in the fertilization product, with distinct physiological functions. Both enzymes were reported to be sensitive to soybean trypsin inhibitor. The proteases were purified from the fertilization product and partially separated from one another by affinity chromatography. One of the proteases, termed vitelline delaminase, has been shown to cleave the linkages between the VE and the PM, allowing elevation of the VE for its subsequent conversion to the FE (see Section V,A). The second protease, called sperm receptor hydrolase, was shown to cleave the sperm receptors from the VE, thus preventing subsequent attachment of sperm to the egg. As such the CG proteases contribute to the block to polyspermy at the molecular level in two ways. First, the physical separation of the VE from the egg PM reduces the possibility of sperm access to and potential fusion with the egg PM. Second, by removing sperm receptors from the VE, not only is the attachment of more sperm to the egg surface prevented, but also the removal of sperm already attached to the VE, the supernumerary sperm, is accomplished.

3. Other Processes That May Reduce Sperm–Egg Interactions and Sperm Penetration

Currently, as reviewed above, there are two popularly accepted components or phases of the block to polyspermy in sea urchins; the early portion or reversible phase due to the membrane potential change and the later more permanent phase of the block caused by the removal of sperm receptors by the CG proteases. Another less universally accepted mechanism is the FE hardening process and possible inactivation of sperm by the CG ovoperoxidase. This concept, which has been suggested by Foerder and Shapiro (1977), will be discussed in Section V,A.

Of course, as suggested earlier, it is conceivable that there are numerous processes any or all of which may constitute or contribute to the overall blocking of multiple sperm entry. For example, Hagström (1956, 1959) suggested that the JC may contribute to the early block to polyspermy. This conclusion was based on two observations. First, jelly-free eggs are much more susceptible to polyspermy than jelly-intact eggs (Hagström, 1956). Second, by comparing the rates of fertilization of jelly-free and jelly-intact eggs, he calculated that 80–90% of the sperm available for fertilization are inactivated or rendered incapable of fertilizing the egg, apparently because of the presence of the JC. It would seem that both observations are easily explained in light of current knowledge of the effect of JC on inducing the acrosomal reaction and the fact that sperm are capable of fertilizing eggs for only a short period following the acrosome reaction (Kinsey et al., 1979). However, the fact remains that the presence of jelly does indeed reduce polyspermy. Thus, JC, by virtue of its ability to induce the acrosome reaction, may also aid in the block to polyspermy.

It should also be noted that in a recent review Dale and Monroy (1981) assert that under normal spawing conditions sperm–egg ratios may be low enough to insure that the rate of gamete collisions is probably less than one in every 100 seconds. Such a low collision ratio would mean that no sperm collisions occur between the time of fusion of the fertilizing sperm and the conclusion of CG exocytosis. Thus, under normal mating conditions the rapid phase of the block to poly-spermy may be unnecessary to ensure monospermic fertilization, since the permanent VE modifications would be manifested prior to any possibility of a second sperm cell colliding with the egg surface.

B. Frog

1. A Plasma Membrane Block Mediated by Membrane Potential Changes

As first interpreted by Jaffe (1976) in the sea urchin, membrane potential changes in the egg affect the early phase of the block to polyspermy at the level of the PM. In anurans, such potential changes were first observed by Maéno (1959) in artificially activated eggs in *Bufo vulgaris formosus*. The potential change observed by Maéno was due to a Cl^- efflux from the egg. Ito (1972) and Iwao et al., 1981) observed potential changes associated with fertilization in eggs from *Bufo vulgaris formosus* (now *Bufo bufo japonicus*) and verified that the potential change was due to a Cl^- gradient. In anurans, it is a gener-ality that the potential changes caused by fertilization or by activation are due to Cl^- flux. This conclusion was predated by Bataillon's (1919) observations that alteration of the extracellular concentration of halide ions induced polyspermy in *Rana fusca* eggs. The involve-ment of Cl^- ions in generating potential changes at fertilization that function as a block to polyspermy has been established for *Rana pi-piens* and *Bufo americanus* (Cross and Elinson, 1980; Schlichter and Elinson, 1981) and *Xenopus laevis* (Grey et al., 1982). The resting egg potential is altered by interaction of the fertilizing sperm with the egg PM to a maximum value that is reached within 1–2 seconds (*Bufo americanus*, −9 to +21 mV; *Bufo bufo japonicus*, −2 to +33 mV; *Rana pipiens*, −28 to +8 mV; *Xeonpus laevis*, −19 to +9 mV). These poten-tial measurements were not made in identical media so the absolute values and differences between the resting and activated states in different anurans are only approximately comparable. The sperm-in-duced depolarization decays over the subsequent 20–30 minutes to a more negative potential. If the membrane potential of the unfertilized egg is brought to positive values (+1 to +22 mV) by passing outward current through the membrane, fertilization is prevented (Cross and Elinson, 1980). Eggs can be made polyspermic if the hyperpolarization is prevented either by injection of current through a second implanted electrode (*Rana pipiens*) or by adding halide ions to the medium (*Rana pipiens, Bufo americanus,* and *Xenopus laevis*). Of the halide ions, the order of effectiveness in reducing the membrane potential as well as permitting polyspermy was $I^- > Br^- > Cl^- > F^-$. A concentration of 20–40 mM NaI resulted in high levels of polyspermy. The order of effectiveness of the halide ions observed in these contemporary experiments was the same as that originally reported by Bataillion (1919) more than 60 years ago.

When natural mating of *Xenopus laevis* was performed in media containing 20 mM NaI, polyspermic fertilization occurred in 65% of the fertilized eggs, thus indicating that the membrane potential changes are operative and physiologically relevant under "natural" conditions (as well as under the experimental conditions of the laboratory vessel; Grey *et al.*, 1982).

As in the sea urchin, the molecular mechanism by which a change in membrane potential alters sperm attachment/fusion remains unknown. Presumably the molecular topography of the membrane is altered, but identification of the molecules in the membranes of the sperm and egg and how an electrical potential change alters their interaction remain goals for future research.

The kinetics and duration of the membrane potential changes in anurans, as in sea urchins, optimally fit with the kinetics and duration of the cortical reaction and the subsequent changes in the egg envelope. The membrane potential change is rapid (1–2 seconds) but transitory (20–30 minutes), while the cortical reaction is slower (39–117 seconds) but alteration of the envelope by the contents of the cortical granules (VE → FE) is permanent. Thus, a block to polyspermy in anurans also consists of two elegantly coordinated events at different cellular sites. An initial, but transitory, block is established at the PM; the block function is subsequently and permanently transferred to the extracellular fertilization envelope. Presumably this transfer of function frees the PM for performance of other vital functions for the now activated and developmentally directed cell.

2. The Cortical Granule Lectin Hypothesis

The CG lectin hypothesis for establishing a late phase of the block to polyspermy in *Xenopus laevis* is depicted in Fig. 2. The fertilizing sperm triggers the cortical granule exocytosis which dumps the contents of the CG into the perivitelline space. The CG lectin diffuses through the VE and interacts with its JC ligand which interfaces with the VE. This interaction (heteropolymerization), which requires Ca^{2+}, results in the formation of a microscopically observable "precipitin" line, the F layer, on the outer surface of the VE. Another CG compo-

Unfertilized

Fertilized

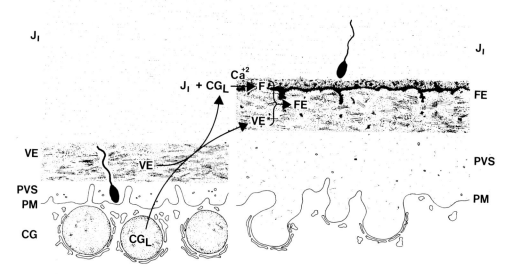

Fig. 2. Diagrammatic representation of the structural changes in an *Xenopus laevis* egg at fertilization and the CG lectin hypothesis for F-layer formation. Abbreviations are as in Fig. 1 except for: CG_L, cortical granule lectin; F, fertilization layer; J_1, jelly coat layer J_1; PVS, perivitelline space; VE*, vitelline envelope component of the FE. (From Greve and Hedrick, 1978.)

nent, X (enzyme), acts on two VE components (69,000 and 64,000) via limited hydrolysis to form an altered VE, VE*. The combination of the F layer and VE* produce the fertilization envelope, FE, which is impenetrable to sperm, thereby providing a block to polyspermy to the fertilized egg (Grey *et al.*, 1976). The following observations support this hypothesis:

1. A CG lectin has been purified to homogeneity from the eggs of *Xenopus laevis* (Wyrick *et al.*, 1974; Wolf, 1974b; Nishihara *et al.*, 1982). This lectin is a metalloglycoprotein existing in two-size isomeric forms with MW_{app} of 539,000 and 655,000. It is composed of several dissimilar subunits with MW_{app} between 38,000 and 45,000, has a galactosyl sugar specificity, and requires a divalent metal cation (Ca^{2+} preferred) for ligand binding.

2. Using antibodies prepared against the purified CG lectin, immu-

nocytochemical studies showed the CG lectin to be localized in the CG before fertilization and in the F layer and the PVS after fertilization (Greve and Hedrick, 1978).

3. A radioimmunoassay for the CG lectin showed that the kinetics of the release of CG lectin into the medium in A23187-activated and dejellied eggs were consistent with the kinetics of the cortical reaction (Monk and Hedrick, 1982; Grey *et al.*, 1974).

4. The isolated FE contained the CG lectin line as shown by immunological and gel electrophoretic analyses (T. Nishihara and J. L. Hedrick, unpublished observations).

5. The isolated FE could be dissociated into solubilized F material (CG lectin plus J_1 ligand) and particulate VE* by treatment with a mixture of galactose and EDTA (Gal/EDTA) and the two moieties could be separated by centrifugation. The FE structure was reconstituted when solubilized F material (Gal/EDTA removed), VE*, and $CaCl_2$ were added together (Nishihara and Hedrick, 1977b).

6. Treatment of jellied unfertilized eggs with CG lectin produced a precipitin line in jelly layer J_1 that could be dissociated with Gal/EDTA. Such a CG lectin-treated egg was unfertilizable. When the lectin–ligand precipitin line was dissolved with Gal/EDTA and the jellied egg washed to remove the Gal/EDTA and the CG lectin, the egg could be fertilized by addition of a fresh sperm suspension (T. Nishihara and J. L. Hedrick, unpublished observations).

As mentioned earlier, the FE elevates away from the egg PM at fertilization. The mechanism for envelope elevation was long ago postulated as being osmotic in nature (Bialaszewicz, 1912). A suggestion as to what structure specifically acts as a selective permeability barrier to effect such a condition has been missing, until the present. In *Xenopus laevis,* the F layer of the FE acts not only as a cellular block (polyspermy) but also as a molecular block to macromolecules released into the PVS from the CG (Nishihara and Hedrick, 1977a). The permeability to ferritin of the envelopes around unfertilized eggs (VE) and fertilized eggs (FE) was determined with electron microscopy (the size of ferritin approximates that of the CG lectin). Ferritin freely penetrated into the PVS in an unfertilized egg but was excluded by the F layer in a fertilized egg. In addition, when an egg was pretreated with ferritin and fertilized, the ferritin within the PVS was trapped by the F layer and could not be washed away. As previously mentioned, a significant portion of the CG lectin is also found within the PVS after the cortical reaction (Greve and Hedrick, 1978). Since the CG lectin is the major protein constituent (78%) of the CG, it not only produces the permeability barrier via formation of the F layer, but also appears to be the major macromolecular constituent of the PVS that generates the osmotic pressure differential which causes an influx of water and thus elevates the envelope.

The CG lectin hypothesis has sufficient experimental support that it can, perhaps, be considered a theory. However, there are many incomplete aspects to this theory yet to be understood. For instance, the structure–function relations of the CG lectin are not completely defined. We know that the CG lectin quaternary structure is dependent on metal–protein interactions and intrachain–disulfide bonds (Nishihara and Hedrick, 1982) but nothing is known of its primary structure in terms of protein or carbohydrate or of the affinity and stoichiometry of carbohydrate binding. The jelly ligand bound by the CG lectin has yet to be isolated. The jelly ligand is very large, is predominantly carbohydrate, and is sulfated, but has yet to be isolated; its structure and, thus, the biological specificity of the CG lectin remain undetermined (Yurewicz et al., 1975; Wyrick et al., 1974; Y. H. Chen and J. L. Hedrick, unpublished observations). Isolation of the CGL ligand could provide the first instance of isolation of a ligand for a lectin with a known biological function. The VE → VE* transformation has only been defined in terms of the molecules being modified, e.g., conversion of substrates to products. The chemical nature of the modification and the CG component(s) responsible for this change have yet to be identified and isolated. The VE* itself is not penetrable by sperm (Grey et al., 1976). This alteration constitutes a separate and distinct (from the F layer) block to polyspermy in Xenopus laevis. The relatively subtle chemical change from VE → VE* (limited hydrolysis of two envelope components) results in substantial physical changes in the envelope, as will be discussed in a later section. The cooperative conformational changes at the molecular level which must occur to alter the properties of the entire envelope are totally undefined. How does the F layer, in molecular terms, prevent penetration of the envelope by sperm? Does it block sperm binding sites or interfere with the access of sperm enzymes (acrosin?) to their substrates, thereby preventing envelope penetration? The possible involvement of a lectin in establishing a block to polyspermy at fertilization needs to be examined in other animal gametes; the theory needs to be tested as to its potential universality.

3. Processes That Reduce the Frequency of Sperm–Egg Interaction in Anurans

As mentioned earlier, Rothschild and Swann (1952) pointed out that the speed with which an egg must establish a block to polyspermy to protect itself from supernumerary sperm is a function of the collision frequency of sperm and eggs. Processes which reduce this frequency contribute to decreasing the possibility of polyspermy.

In anurans, the jelly coat is required for fertilization but also acts as a filter or screen to reduce the number of sperm that arrive at the egg PM (Morgan, 1897; Cross and Elinson, 1980). Many sperm become "embedded" in various JC layers of anuran eggs or are greatly slowed down by the JC layer in terms of their movement toward the eggs. In the case of *Rana pipiens,* under normal experimental conditions, e.g., sperm: egg ratios of 10^4–10^6:1, less than 10 sperm are in the vicinity of the egg surface at the time of fertilization (Norton, 1976). This JC filtration process reduces the number of sperm arriving at the egg surface by orders of magnitude and, hence, reduces the sperm–egg collision frequency. Functionally, the jelly coat of an anuran egg, therefore, may serve in analogy to the uterotubal junction in mammals. This junction serves as a control point that regulates the number of sperm entering the oviduct, thereby controlling the sperm–egg collision frequency (Gaddum-Rosse, 1981).

After oviposition in solutions of low ionic strength, e.g., pond water, jellied anuran eggs rapidly lose their ability to be fertilized. This loss of fertilizability can be correlated with jelly hydration (Bataillion and Tchou-Su, 1930; Katagiri, 1962; Wolf and Hedrick, 1971; del Pino, 1973). In addition, jelly substances required by the sperm for fertilization may diffuse from the jelly (Barbieri and Cabada, 1969; Katagiri, 1973). Thus, hydration of the jelly or loss of essential jelly components prevents sperm penetration of the egg integuments and, thereby, functions to protect the egg from polyspermy.

As mentioned earlier, sperm can fuse only with the PM in the animal hemisphere of anuran eggs (see Elinson, 1975, for references). Thus, sperm which successfully traverse the egg integuments but approach the PM of the vegetal hemisphere do not produce effective sperm–egg collisions. This process is more highly developed in the case of *Discoglossus pictus* where effective sperm–egg interaction is restricted not only to the animal hemisphere but to a specialized portion of the animal hemisphere, the animal dimple (Campanella, 1975). The most highly specialized example of this process is found perhaps in fish eggs where sperm penetration is restricted to the micropyle in the egg envelope (chorion) (see Section I). Thus, restriction of the area of the egg surface with which sperm can interact effectively lowers the frequency of sperm–egg collision and contributes to the rate at which an egg must effect a block to polyspermy.

The developmentally essential process of establishing a block to polyspermy in anurans is a multifaceted phenomenon involving the timely coordination of a number of events. The mechanisms that contribute in total to the block to polyspermy in anuran eggs are strikingly efficient as sperm:egg ratios of 10^7:1 do not result in polyspermic fertilization. It is meaningless and potentially misleading to refer to any one of these events as more essential or more important than any other event. Each particular event, or phase of the block, is a part of the overall process that contributes to the cell's vital defense against supernumerary sperm penetration and assurance of the cell's chance to divide and subsequently develop into a new organism.

C. Mammal

1. Plasma Membrane-Mediated Block

Direct experimental evidence demonstrating a block to polyspermy at the level of the PM in mammalian eggs is limited. Few data are available regarding a block mediated by membrane potential changes. In fact the characteristic electrical properties of the PM of sperm receptive mammalian eggs are not well established. Measurements of the membrane resting potential are available only for mouse eggs at metaphase of the second meiotic division (Powers and Tupper, 1974; Miyazaki and Igusa, 1981). Membrane potential changes in mammalian oocytes upon sperm entry have been reported only for the golden hamster (Miyazaki and Igusa, 1981). Unlike echinoderm and anuran eggs, where the membrane potential shifts transiently to positive values, the fertilization potential in hamster eggs consists of recurring hyperpolarizations beginning at about the time of sperm entry. Whether the hyperpolarization response in hamster eggs reflects changes in ion flux has not been demonstrated. Furthermore, whether such recurring hyperpolarizations are in any way related to prevention of polyspermy *in vivo* has yet to be clarified. Recent direct measurements in mouse oocytes have shown a series of oscillatory Ca^{2+} transients preceding an exponential rise in free Ca^{2+} during fertilization, but not artificial activation, of mouse oocytes (Cuthbertson *et al.*, 1981). Again, the relationship of these observations to a block to polyspermy or membrane potential changes is unknown. Thus, in mammals definitive correlation between the block to polyspermy and membrane potential changes has not yet been demonstrated. Depending on the nature of the block to polyspermy, membrane potential changes, if any, may differ considerably among species.

In the rabbit, it is believed that a block to polyspermy occurs at the level of the PM since fertilization is monospermic even though supplementary spermatozoa freely penetrate the ZP. The mechanism of this block, however, remains to be elucidated. Indeed, only one PM alteration following fertilization has been reported in the rabbit. Utilizing positive, electron-dense, ferric, colloid particles, Cooper and Bedford (1971) demonstrated that at pH 1.8 the PM of fertilized eggs invariably binds a greater number of particles per unit area than unfertilized eggs, presumably because of an increase in the number of sialic acid residues on the PM. These observations would suggest a shift in the net surface charges after fertilization in this species; however, this change has not been correlated with the PM block to polyspermy.

Some indirect evidence exists indicating that the cortical reaction may be necessary for the PM block in the rabbit. This conclusion is based on the observation that polyspermic rabbit zygotes, obtained from natural matings, retain numerous cortical granules beneath the PM (Gulyas, 1974), indicating that the failure of normal CG dehiscence results in polyspermy. It is possible, in the case of these polyspermic rabbit eggs, that the cortical reaction was defective and failed to occur to its fullest extent after entry of the first spermatozoon. Under these conditions it is assumed that the changes in the PM could not reach the threshold point necessary to prevent polyspermy.

The notion that a PM component or phase of the block to polyspermy exists in the mouse (Pavlok and McLaren, 1972) and the rat (Toyoda and Chang, 1968) was initially derived from the observation that polyspermy levels are comparable in zona-free and zona-intact eggs in these species. However, whether the proteolytic enzymes used to remove the zonae in these experiments reduced or altered the fertilizability of zona-free oocytes is of concern. Indeed, Wolf (1978) has reported somewhat increased levels of polyspermy in mouse eggs, dependent on sperm concentrations, in mechanically denuded eggs. However, even in this system it is probable that some PM block is established, since only about two to three sperm enter such denuded eggs. Total absence of a PM block would presumably result in numerous sperm cells entering the cell. High levels of polyspermy can also be obtained under different experimental conditions in the rat (Niwa and Chang, 1975), hamster (Yanagimachi and Noda, 1970), and human (Soupart and Strong, 1975), among others.

As in the case of rabbit eggs, the role of the CG exudate, if any, in the establishment of the PM block in the mouse is based on indirect observations. For example, in certain inbred strains of mice, low CG complements have been associated with low fertility (Wabik-Sliz, 1979). Moreover, premature CG release apparently results in subsequent fertility impairment (Kaleta, 1979). These observations would be consistent with a CG role in prevention of polyspermy. On the other hand, Wolf *et al.* (1979) suggested that premature CG loss by itself does not result in a PM block to polyspermy, nor does it prevent a sperm-induced block from being established. For these reasons they argued that, in mammals, CG are not invovled in the establishment of the PM phase of the block to polyspermy. Instead, these investigators suggest an electrically mediated block at the level of the PM, although evidence for such a mechanism is not available, as indicated above.

In conclusion, although some experimental evidence indicates a PM block to polyspermy in some mammalian species, the mechanism of such a block remains completely unknown. Moreover, the role of the CG and the CG exudate, if any, in such a block remains to be established.

2. Block to Polyspermy Mediated by Alterations of the Zona Pellucida

A relationship between the cortical reaction and fertilization-dependent changes in the ZP has been known for some time. Braden and Austin (1954), working with hamster eggs, were the first to suggest that the CG exudate, which is released into the perivitelline space, could modify the ZP, rendering it less permeable or totally impermeable to supernumerary sperm. This modification of the ZP was termed the "zona reaction." Later, a temporal correlation between CG dehiscence and the establishment of a zona block to sperm penetration was suggested (Szollosi, 1967). Experimental evidence for direct involvement of CG exudate in establishing the ZP-mediated block to polyspermy comes from two separate laboratories. Barros and Yanagimachi (1971, 1972) demonstrated that sperm-penetrated hamster eggs, which have undergone a cortical reaction, fail to bind sperm to the outer zona. Furthermore, they showed that incubation of unfertilized eggs with CG exudate collected from fertilized, zona-free oocytes prevented sperm attachment to the zonae of the unfertilized eggs. From these two observations they concluded that the ZP-mediated block in hamster eggs is elicited by a CG component. Subsequently, in similar experiments with hamster eggs, Gwatkin *et al.* (1973) demonstrated that CG exudate released by electrical stimulation induced the ZP-mediated block in unfertilized eggs pretreated with the exudate. It is uncertain whether, in addition to the CG exudate, some ooplasmic components may have been released after electrical stimulation (see Gulyas, 1976) that may have caused the changes in the zona pellucida. This effect is not species specific since CG exudate from hamster eggs is effective on the zonae of mouse oocytes (Gwatkin and Williams, 1974). Soybean trypsin inhibitor blocks the action of the CG material in both mouse and hamster eggs, and the activity is also heat sensitive (Gwatkin and Williams, 1974). It was proposed, therefore, that in the mouse and the hamster, a trypsinlike protease induces the zona reaction (Wolf and Hamada, 1977) by removing sperm receptors from the ZP. This proposal, in large part, is analogous to the observations made earlier in sea urchins (see Section IV,A). However, it should be noted that although direct demonstration of a CG protease, or a secreted protease following fertilization has not been reported, at least one ZP protein is modified, following fertilization (Bleil *et al.*, 1981).

The temporal relationships between penetration of the fertilizing sperm and establishment of the ZP-mediated block to polyspermy varies significantly, depending not only on the species but also on experimental conditions utilized in different laboratories. Whereas in the marine invertebrates there is a rapid but incomplete phase of the block to polyspermy within seconds after insemination, in mammals such a rapid phase has not been established unequivocally. Reconstructing the time course of fertilization-related changes in the ZP and relating these to the establishment of the block to polyspermy in such species as the mouse and hamster, one is confronted with some unexplained time gaps. For instance, the CG exudate can become involved in the blocking process only after sperm contact and/or fusion with the egg PM. The shortest recorded time needed in any species for the zona reaction to occur is 8–10 minutes following insemination (Table I). Yet, normally only one spermatozoon penetrates the ZP during this time period. What is to stop numerous sperm from penetrating either partially or fully through the zona during this time period?

One possible explanation could be that oocytes in the oviduct are challenged by considerably fewer spermatozoa (see below). This would

TABLE I

Time Required for Establishment of Zona Reaction and PM Block to Polyspermy in Mammalian Eggs

Species	Zona reaction time (minutes)	PM block (minutes)	References
Hamster	17–35	120–210	Barros and Yanagimachi, 1972
	8	–	Gwatkin *et al.*, 1973
Mouse	–	40	Wolf, 1978
	60–120	–	Inoue and Wolf, 1975a
Rat	10–120	–	Braden *et al.*, 1954

mean that only one sperm is available per oocyte for the duration of 8–10 minutes, and that the chances of a penetrated oocyte being challenged again during this period are unlikely. Alternatively, yet-unknown mechanisms of preventing polyspermy may prevail in mammals. For example, recent *in vitro* studies of Hartmann and Hutchison (1980, 1981) with hamster oocytes have shown that after a large number of sperm make contact with the outer surface of the ZP, several factors are released into the supernatant during the first 50 minutes following first contact. The release of factors is highly regulated. It occurs only after contact of homologous gametes, and the activity of these factors declines rapidly after they have made their appearance; thus, their action becomes reversible. At least two of these factors inhibit penetration of the ZP, one of which is released within 2 minutes of insemination. Thus, it has been suggested that one of the functions of these factors may be the prevention of polyspermic penetration under physiological conditions, until the zona reaction develops to its fullest. The source of these factors has not yet been identified.

3. Other Processes That Reduce Sperm–Egg Interactions

In mammals large numbers of spermatozoa are produced and deposited in the female reproductive tract (see reviews by Gwatkin, 1977; Dale and Monroy, 1981). It appears that the female reproductive tract acts as a filter and selects a few highly competent sperm that can reach the oocytes (Overstreet and Cooper, 1978). Indeed, sperm wastage is very high in mammals, as indicated by the marked dilution that occurs by the time they have reached the ampulla. Of the 50–3000 million ejaculated mammalian sperm, only a maximum of 700 have been recorded in the ampulla, although in most species it is less than 100 (Gwatkin, 1977). In the mouse only a 1:1 sperm–egg ratio has been reported (see Dale and Monroy, 1981). The question arises, what happens when this low ratio becomes unbalanced in favor of the spermatozoa? Would large numbers of spermatozoa alone at the site of fertilization result in a higher frequency of polyspermy? The results of some experimental work at first site indicate that the answer is yes. Instilling whole boar semen into the tubal isthmus of the estrous gilts increased the number of zona-attached sperm as well as the incidence of polyspermy to 33%, as compared to 3% when the semen was deposited into the uterine lumen (Hunter, 1973). Similarly, the incidence of polyspermy was increased significantly following resection of the isthmus in pig (Hunter and Leglise, 1971a) and rabbit (Hunter and Leglise, 1971b). These observations indicate that the occurrance of polyspermy in some eggs increases significantly when large numbers of sperm confront the oocyte *in vivo*.

With *in vitro* systems, where most often fertilization is observed with cumulus-free oocytes, the incidence of polyspermy is significantly elevated, although significant variation is observed, depending on the systems used (see reviews by Gwatkin, 1976; Gulyas, 1980). Indeed, earlier investigators considered the cumulus to be a selective barrier, important for preventing polyspermy (Austin, 1961). However, more recent ovum transfer experiments in hamster suggest that the state of the ovum itself, not the cumulus, is critical for establishment of an efficient block when there is an excess of sperm present (Moore and Bedford, 1978).

V. HARDENING REACTIONS IN THE OUTER INVESTMENTS OF THE EGG

A. Elevation and Hardening of the Fertilization Envelope in Sea Urchins

1. The Cortical Granule Ovoperoxidase

In a series of papers Shapiro and co-workers have described a peroxidase activity or ovoperoxidase localized in the CG of unfertilized sea urchin eggs, which is responsible for hardening of the FE (see reviews by Shapiro *et al.*, 1980, 1981). Hardening of the FE, defined as the stability of the FE to numerous disruptive agents such as mercaptans and detergents, has been recognized for many years (see reviews by Giudice, 1973; Czihak, 1975; Veron *et al.*, 1977; Harvey, 1910). The hardening is now attributed, at least in part, to dityrosine cross-links catalyzed by the CG ovoperoxidase (Foerder and Shapiro, 1977; Hall, 1978). The sequence of events involved can be summarized as follows: An ovoperoxidase resides in the CG of unfertilized eggs (Katsura and Tominga, 1974; Klebanoff *et al.*, 1979). Upon fertilization it is secreted into the PVS in the fertilization product (Foerder *et al.*, 1978; Hall, 1978) along with the CG proteases. The VE is released from the PM by the protease vitelline delaminase (see above) and converted into the "soft" fertilization envelope. Cross-links are introduced between proteins in the VE by the ovoperoxidase, which, following fertilization, is secreted into the perivitelline space and later is found localized in the FE itself (Klebanoff *et al.*, 1979). The oxidizing substrate hydrogen peroxide, necessary for catalysis, is synthesized by the egg (Foerder *et al.*, 1978).

It has been argued that cross-linking alone may not account entirely for FE hardening in sea urchins. Indeed, Shapiro and Eddy (1980) have suggested that a lectin-mediated mechanism similar to that observed in the frog *Xenopus* (see Section V,B) may also occur in sea urchins. The basis for this suggestion is twofold. First, the bulk of the protein in the FE is not cross-linked by the ovoperoxidase, since most (70%) of the FE protein can be extracted and separated into five polypeptides ranging in MW_{app} from 18,000–92,000 (Carroll and Baginski, 1978). Secondly, Ca^{2+}-insoluble components of the CG exudate (Bryan, 1970a,b) may also contribute to the observed hardening or insolubility of the altered FE. For this reason, Shapiro and Eddy (1980) conclude that further investigation of the complete mechanism of FE hardening is required.

2. The Ovoperoxidase and Envelope Hardening and the Block to Polyspermy

In the context of the block to polyspermy it should be noted that a hardened FE constitutes a physical barrier to sperm penetration or access to the PM (Foerder and Shapiro, 1977). In this regard the early refertilization experiments of Sugiyama (1951) are of interest. In these experiments it was shown that sperm are capable of penetrating fertilized sea urchin eggs upon removal of the FE, even up to the two-cell stage. These supernumerary sperm participated in the mitotic process and caused abnormal cleavage. Thus, a more permanent barrier to sperm, such as a hardened FE would indeed help to assure that sperm would not fuse with the PM and penetrate the fertilized egg. However, in general, such a component of the block is unnecessary since sperm cannot bind to the elevated VE, whether it has been hardened or not, since the sperm receptors have been removed by the CG sperm receptor hydrolase. Moreover, elevation of VE virtually precludes the sperms' access to the PM even if binding were to occur.

It has also been suggested that the ovoperoxidase, along with the peroxidase-generating system, may aid in or contribute to the block to polyspermy by a second mechanism (Foerder and Shapiro, 1977); that is, hydrogen peroxide is known to be toxic to echinoderm sperm (Evans, 1947; Boldt *et al.,* 1981) and peroxidases are toxic to both sea urchin sperm (E. D. Schmell and W. J. Lennarz, unpublished) and mammalian sperm (Smith and Klebanoff, 1970). Thus, secretion of the ovoperoxidase and production of hydrogen peroxide following fertilization would expose sperm in the immediate vicinity of the newly activated egg to toxic conditions. In this regard, Boldt *et al.* (1981) have suggested, based on experiments with peroxidase inhibitors, that a sperm peroxidase, not the ovoperoxidase, may act in concert with the peroxide produced at fertilization to block polyspermy. This conclusion was based on the results of measurments of the level of polyspermy observed in the presence of various peroxidase and catalase inhibitors. It should be noted, however, that in these experiments no sperm peroxidase activity was demonstrated. Regardless of the details, it is clear that the timing of peroxide generation and its adverse effects on sperm, particularly in the presence of peroxidase, may indeed be another mechanism by which supernumerary sperm are inactivated.

B. Egg Envelope Modifications in Anurans

1. Chemical and Physical Differences in Egg Envelopes

The envelopes from coelomic eggs, CE, oviposited eggs, VE, and fertilized eggs, FE, have been isolated and characterized most extensively in *Xenopus laevis* (Wolf *et al.*, 1976; Gerton, 1980; Gerton and Hedrick, unpublished). The VE and FE from eggs of *Bufo arenarum* have also been isolated and compared on a more limited basis (Miceli *et al.*, 1977), as have the CE and VE from eggs of *Rana japonica* (Yoshizaki and Katagiri, 1981) and the VE from *Bufo vulgaris* (Uchiyama *et al.*, 1971). In general, the envelopes are composed of glycoproteins which interact and assemble through noncovalent forces to form the intact morphologically distinct envelopes characteristic of a given type, e.g., CE and VE.

In the case of *Xenopus laevis,* the macromolecular compositions of the CE, VE, and FE has been determined by SDS gel electrophoresis (Wolf *et al.*, 1976; Gerton, 1980; Gerton and Hedrick, unpublished). Three glycoprotein components with MW_{app} 120,000, 112,000, and 37,000 are common to the three forms of the envelope. When the CE is converted to the VE in the oviduct, a new component is added with a MW_{app} of 57,000 and a 43,000 component is altered to a glycoprotein with a MW_{app} of 41,000. Yoshizaki and Katagiri (1981), using *Rana japonica,* reported somewhat analogous results in a preliminary note. They found two additional macromolecules in VE compared with CE. A protease from the oviduct of *Bufo arenarum* which can alter the sperm penetrability of a coelomic egg to that of an oviposited egg, i.e., CE to VE transformation, has been reported (Micelli *et al.*, 1978a,b). A working hypothesis that incorporates and unifies the observations from these different anurans is the following. As the coelomic egg enters the oviduct, a secreted protease (57,000) is added to the CE which acts upon a major envelope component (43,000) via limited hydrolysis [proteolytic (?) loss of a 2000 peptide equivalent]. The limited hydrolytic event results in a conformational change of the 41,000 component which in turn alters the supramolecular structure and the ultrastructure of the envelope (randomly oriented and tightly packed filament bundles of the CE expand to form the loosely packed and oriented filament bundles of the VE). The limited hydrolysis and/or the resulting conformational change of the envelope components alters the interaction of the envelope with sperm, either in terms of sperm binding or of envelope susceptibility to sperm enzymes (acrosin). This hypothesis provides a molecular basis for alteration of the function of the envelope by modulation of its molecular structure and ultrastructure. Since the components involved have been isolated, or can be isolated, this hypothesis is testable.

Comparison of the macromolecular composition of VE and FE indicated that upon fertilization, two envelope components are modified ($69,000 \rightarrow 66,000$ and $64,000 \rightarrow 61,000$), and new glycoproteins are added to the envelope (undefined high molecular weight, 87,000 and 43,000 components). The altered envelope components are thought to result from limited proteolysis of VE glycoproteins by CG proteases released by the cortical reaction (Gerton, 1980; Gerton and Hedrick, unpublished). However, the action of a carbohydrase(s) on the envelope components is also possible and cannot be eliminated at this time. The high-molecular-weight component is due to a jelly coat glycoprotein and the 88,000 and 43,000 components are derived from a CG lectin. The interaction of this lectin and its jelly coat ligand provides the basis for the CGL hypothesis for a block to polyspermy in *Xenopus laevis*.

2. Envelope Hardening in Anurans

The altered properties of the VE when it is converted to the FE (F layer plus VE*), which constitute what has been called hardening, are perhaps best described in the case of *Xenopus laevis*. These altered physiochemical properties of the envelopes are the following.

1. The envelopes have different optical properties such that under the light microscope the VE is more translucent and less light-scattering than the FE (D. P. Wolf and J. L. Hedrick, unpublished observations).

2. The envelopes are differently affected by temperature in terms of their dissolution in aqueous solutions. The temperature at which the process is 50% complete, T_m, is 43° C for VE and 63° C for FE (pH 9.5, low ionic strength) (Wyrick, 1974). The melting process appears to be cooperative in nature and the T_m of the envelopes are differentially affected by solution conditions, e.g., pH and ionic strength (at pH 8, VE has a T_m of 65° C whereas the FE will not dissolve up to 100° C).

3. Chemical reactivity of the envelopes, in terms of reduction of disulfide bonds, is markedly different. The disulfide bonds of VE are

readily reduced by mercaptoethanol solutions at room temperature (which also solubilizes the envelope), whereas the disulfide bonds of FE are not reduced nor is the FE soluble under these conditions (Wyrick, 1974). The FE disulfide bonds can be reduced when the structural integrity of the FE is destroyed by denaturing agents, e.g., urea, guanidine salts, or SDS.

4. The envelopes have very different susceptibilities to proteases. The VE is more readily hydrolyzed by trypsin than is the FE (Wolf, 1974b), and the same is true in terms of hydrolysis by the hatching enzyme (Urch and Hedrick, 1981).

Only two chemical differences between VE and FE which can explain the above results have been observed. Two components in the VE undergo limited hydrolysis and the loss of approximately 3000 mass units each to convert the envelope to VE* (Gerton, 1980; Gerton and Hedrick, unpublished). The F layer is bound to the outer surface of the VE* (evidence cited earlier). In the case of observations 2–4, the F layer makes no contribution or a minor contribution to the observed differences between VE and FE (Wolf, 1974b; Wyrick, 1974). Thus, the physical properties of FE are largely determined by those of the VE* moiety. The simplest chemical explanation which incorporates the current set of observations is that limited hydrolysis of two envelope components (69,000 and 64,000) results in a cooperative conformational change of some or all of the glycoproteins composing the VE moiety (VE*), such that the physiochemical properties of the envelope as a whole are altered. Additional experimental evidence for such a hypothesis for hardening in anurans should be sought.

FE hardening in sea urchins clearly involves an ovoperoxidase (see Section V,A above), and such a mechanism has been proposed for zona hardening in mammals (see Section V,C). However in *Xenopus laevis* eggs, a peroxidatic reaction is apparently not involved as supported by the following observations.

1. Cytochemical and enzymatic attempts to demonstrate a CG-associated ovoperoxidase have been negative (L. C. Greve, G. L. Gerton, and J. L. Hedrick, unpublished observations).

2. The FE can be totally solubilized in the case of *Xenopus laevis* as contrasted to *Strongylocentrotus purpuratus* (Wolf et al., 1976).

3. No polymerization or increase in the molecular weight of FE components has been detected (Wolf et al., 1976; Gerton, 1980).

4. No di- or triiodotyrosine residues have been detected in the FE (G. L. Gerton and J. L. Hedrick, unpublished observations).

C. Zona Hardening in Mammalian Eggs

In addition to changes in the sperm binding properties of the ZP following fertilization, the physical properties of the ZP are also altered. This is shown by an increased resistance of the ZP to enzymatic and chemical dissolution. This physical modification has been termed "zona hardening." Increased resistance of the zona to proteolytic dissolution has been reported in the mouse (Smithberg, 1953; Gwatkin, 1964), rat (Chang and Hunt, 1956), and rabbit (Chang and Hunt, 1956; Conrad *et al.*, 1971) but not in hamster eggs (Gwatkin, 1977). Inoue and Wolf (1974, 1975a), using 2-mercaptoethanol to dissolve zonae, reported similar observations on zona hardening in mouse, rat, and hamster eggs.

The mechanism of zona hardening in mammals has not been unequivocally demonstrated. Recently a cross-linking mechanism for zona hardening in mouse eggs, analogous to that demonstrated for FE hardening in sea urchin eggs has been suggested (Gulyas and Schmell, 1980; Schmell and Gulyas, 1980). This conclusion is based on the following observations: (1) TEM histochemical demonstration of an ovoperoxidase in intact CG of unfertilized eggs and on the surface of fertilized eggs; (2) inhibition of zona hardening by peroxidase inhibitors and tyrosine analogs; and (3) limited hardening of ZP in unfertilized mouse eggs by exogenous peroxidase.

It should be noted, however, that this conclusion, concerning a cross-linking mechanism for zona hardening, is based on indirect observations. First, only histochemical data are available for the mammalian ovoperoxidase. Second, cross-linking of zona proteins is implied only from inhibition experiments. Indeed, the only direct observations concerning changes in the proteins of the ZP indicate proteolysis and a decrease in MW_{app}, not an increase which would be expected if cross-linking occurred (Bleil *et al.*, 1981). However, even in the sea urchin, where strong evidence exists for a cross-linking mechanism for VE hardening (see Section V,A), limited proteolysis is observed at the cell surface following fertilization (Shapiro, 1975). At any rate, a definitive conclusion of such a cross-linking mechanism in mammals would require more direct results such as demonstration of enzyme activity and the formation of tyrosine cross-links with subsequent increase in the apparent molecular weight of ZP proteins. Moreover, since electron-dense material of CG origin is readily observed in ZP of activated eggs, a lectin-mediated process, as in anurans, should not be overlooked.

The function of zona hardening in the fertilization process is poorly understood. In terms of a block to polyspermy no direct function for zona hardening has been elucidated. Indeed, caution must be exercised in correlating zona hardening with the block to polyspermy. For example, zona hardening occurs in rabbit eggs but these cells do not demonstrate a block to polyspermy at the level of the ZP. The opposite is true in hamster eggs. However, if sperm penetration of the ZP does involve the protease acrosin, as has been suggested, increased resistance of the zona to dissolution by proteases would reduce sperm penetration of ZP. This conclusion remains to be shown unequivocally.

VI. SUMMARY AND CONCLUSIONS

This chapter reviews the available information concerning cellular and molecular changes evident at the surface of the egg upon fertilization. Morphological and molecular alterations are reviewed at both the cellular and subcellular levels. The major emphasis has been an attempt to present these surface modifications in an integrated fashion for each species, particularly within the context of an understanding of the overall process of the block to polyspermy—or the egg's ability to screen out all sperm save the fertilizing spermatozoon. In the case of the sea urchin and mammal much of this information has been reviewed previously, as indicated throughout the chapter; however, it has not been reviewed from the viewpoint of the block to polyspermy per se. For the anuran, this chapter represents the first comprehensive review of the subject matter.

It seems clear that, despite some differences at the molecular level, the overall cellular process of the block to polyspermy is quite similar in both the sea urchin and anuran. The block is composed of at least two major subcomponents or phases. One component is a relatively rapid but transient modification mediated at the level of the plasma membrane via a qualitative change in the membrane potential. In time this phase of the block dissipates but a more permanent modification is manifest involving elevation and/or modification of the vitelline envelope following the cortical reaction. This slower vitelline envelope alteration ensures permanent resistance to multiple sperm entry.

In contrast to the information available regarding the block to polyspermy in the sea urchin and anuran, much less is known in the mammalian systems, particularly at the molecular level. Limitations in these systems are clearly due to the limited amounts of material available as well as to the variations presented from species to species. Some indirect experiments, however, indicate that the block may indeed be bimodal in the mammal as well, with both a plasma membrane and a zona pellucida-mediated component. However, the kinetics of and temporal relationship between the two components is unknown. Clearly, much more experimentation is necessary in these higher organisms.

ACKNOWLEDGMENTS

Preparation of this chapter was supported in part by a U.S. Public Health Service grant HD-4906 awarded to JLH.

REFERENCES

Aketa, K., Onitake, K., and Tsuzuki, H. (1972). Tryptic disruption of sperm-binding site of sea urchin egg surface. *Exp. Cell Res.* **71**, 27–32.

Allen, R. D., and Griffin, J. L. (1958). The time sequence of early events in the fertilization of sea urchin eggs. 1. The latent period and the cortical reaction. *Exp. Cell Res.* **15**, 163–173.

Ancel, P., and Vintemberger, P. (1948). Recherches sur le déterminisme de la symetrie bilaterale dans l'oeuf des amphibiens. *Bull. Biol. Fr. Belg., Suppl.* **31**, 1–182.

Anderson, E. (1968). Oocyte differentiation in the sea urchin, *Arbacia punctulata,* with particular reference to the origin of cortical granules and their participation in the cortical reaction. *J. Cell Biol.* **37**, 514–539.

Austin, C. R. (1961). "The Mammalian Egg." Blackwell, Oxford.

Austin, C. R. (1965). "Fertilization." Prentice-Hall, Englewood Cliffs, New Jersey.

Austin, C. R. (1978). Patterns in metazoan fertilization. *Curr. Top. Dev. Biol.* **12**, 1–9.

Baranska, W., Konwinski, M., and Kujawa, M. (1975). Fine structure of the zona pellucida of unfertilized egg cells and embryos. *J. Exp. Zool.* **192**, 193–202.

Barbieri, F. D., and Budequer de Atenor, M. S. (1973). Role of oviducal secretions in the fertilization of *Bufo arenarum* oocytes. *Arch. Biol.* **84**, 501–511.

Barbieri, F. D., and Cabada, M. O. (1969). The role of the diffusible factor released by the egg jelly in fertilization of the toad egg. *Experientia* **25**, 1312–1313.

Barros, C., and Yanagimachi, R. (1971). Induction of zona reaction in golden hamster eggs by cortical granule material. *Nature (London)* **233**, 268–269.

Barros, C., and Yanagimachi, R. (1972). Polyspermy-preventing mechanisms in the golden hamster egg. *J. Exp. Zool.* **180**, 251–266.

Bataillion, E., and Tchou-Su. (1930). Etudes analytiques et expérimentales sur les rythmes cinétiques dan l'oeuf *(Hyla arborea, Paracentrotus lividus, Bombyx mori).* *Arch. Biol.* **40**, 439–540.

Bialaszewicz, K. (1912). Über das Verhalten des osmotishen Druckes wahrend der Entwicklung der Wirbeltierembryonen. *Wilhelm Roux' Arch. Entwicklungsmech. Org.* **34**, 489–540.

Bleil, J. D., and Wassarman, P. M. (1980a). Structure and function of the zona pellucida: Identification and characterization of the proteins of the mouse oocyte's zona pellucida. *Dev., Biol.* **76**, 185–202.

Bleil, J. D., and Wassarman, P. M. (1980b). Mammalian sperm–egg interaction: Identification of a glycoprotein in mouse egg zonae pellucidae possessing receptor activity for sperm. *Cell* **20,** 873–882.

Bleil, J. D., Beall, C. F., and Wassarman, P. M. (1981). Mammalian sperm–egg interaction: Fertilization of mouse eggs triggers modification of the major zona pellucida glycoprotein, ZP2. *Dev. Biol.* **86,** 189–197.

Boldt, J., Schuel, H., Schuel, R., Dandekar, P. V., and Troll, W. (1981). Reaction of sperm with egg-derived hydrogen peroxide helps prevent polyspermy during fertilization in the sea urchin egg. *Gamete Res.* **4,** 365–377.

Braden, A. W. H., and Austin, C. R. (1954). The number of sperm about the eggs in mammals and its significance for normal fertilization. *Aust. J. Biol. Sci.* **7,** 543–551.

Braden, A. W. H., Austin, C. R., and David, H. A. (1954). The reaction of zona pellucida to sperm penetration. *Aust. J. Biol. Sci.* **7,** 391–409.

Bryan, J. (1970a). The isolation of a major structural element of the sea urchin fertilization membrane. *J. Cell Biol.* **44,** 635–644.

Bryan, J. (1970b). On the reconstitution of the crystalline components of the sea urchin fertilization membrane. *J. Cell Biol.* **45,** 606–614.

Buongiorno-Nardelli, M., and Bertolini, B. (1967). Subcellular localization of some acid hydrolases in *Triturus cristatus* spermatozoa. *Histochemie* **8,** 34–44.

Burgos, M. H., and Fawcett, D. W. (1956). An electron microscopic study of spermatid differentiation in the toad, *Bufo arenarum* Hensel. *J. Biophys. Biochem. Cytol.* **3,** 223–240.

Burgos, M. H., Segal, S. J., and Passantino, T. (1976). Surface changes of the rat embryo before implantation. *Fertil. Steril.* **27,** 1085–1094.

Calarco, P. G., and Epstein, C. J. (1973). Cell surface changes during preimplantation development in the mouse. *Dev. Biol.* **32,** 208–213.

Campanella, C. (1975). The site of spermatozoon entrance in the unfertilized egg of *Discoglossus pictus* (Anura): An electron microscopy study. *Biol. Reprod.* **12,** 439–447.

Campanella, C., and Andreuccetti, P. (1977). Ultrastructural observations on cortical endoplasmic reticulum and on residual cortical granules in the egg of *Xenopus laevis. Dev. Biol.* **56,** 1–10.

Carroll, E. J., and Baginski, R. M. (1978). Sea urchin fertilization envelope: Isolation, extraction, and characterization of a major protein fraction from *Strongylocentrotus purpuratus* embryos. *Biochemistry* **17,** 2605–2612.

Carroll, E. J., and Epel, D. (1975). Isolation and biological activity of the proteases released by sea urchin eggs following fertilization. *Dev. Biol.* **44,** 22–32.

Chambers, E. L., and de Armendi, J. (1978). Components of the activation potential in eggs of the sea urchin, *Lytechinus variegatus. J. Gen. Physiol.* **72,** 3a.

Chambers, E. L., Pressman, B. C., and Rose, B. (1974). The activation of sea urchin eggs by the divalent ionophores A23187 and X537A. *Biochem. Biophys. Res. Commun.* **60,** 126–132.

Chandler, D. E., and Heuser, J. (1979). Membrane fusion during secretion. *J. Cell Biol.* **83,** 91–108.

Chandler, D. E., and Heuser, J. (1980). The vitelline layer of the sea urchin egg. *J. Cell Biol.* **84,** 618–632.

Chang, M. C., and Hunt, D. M. (1956). Effects of proteolytic enzymes on the zona pellucida of fertilized and unfertilized mammalian eggs. *Exp. Cell Res.* **11,** 497–499.

Conrad, K., Buckley, J., and Stambaugh, R. (1971). Studies on the nature of the block to polyspermy in rabbit ova. *J. Reprod. Fertil.* **27,** 133–135.

Cooper, G. W., and Bedford, J. M. (1971). Charge density change in the vitelline surface following fertilization of the rabbit egg. *J. Reprod. Fertil.* **25,** 431–436.

Cross, N. L., and Elinson, R. P. (1980). A fast block to polyspermy in frogs mediated by changes in the membrane potential. *Dev. Biol.* **75,** 187–198.

Cuthbertson, K. S. R., Whittingham, D. G., and Cobbold, P. M. (1981). Free Ca^{2+} increases in exponential phases during mouse oocyte activation. *Nature (London)* **294,** 254–257.

Czihak, G. (1975). "The Sea Urchin Embryo. Biochemistry and Morphogenesis." Springer-Verlag, Berlin and New York.

Dale, B., and De Santis, A. (1981). Maturation and fertilization of the sea urchin oocyte; an electrophysiological study. *Dev. Biol.* **85,** 474–484.

Dale, B., and Monroy, A. (1981). How is polyspermy prevented? *Gamete Res.* **4,** 151–164.

Dale, B., De Felice, L. J., and Taglietti, V. (1978). Membrane noise and conductance increase during single spermatozoon-egg interactions. *Nature (London)* **275,** 217–219.

Dan, J. C. (1952). Studies on the acrosome. I. Reaction to egg-water and other stimuli. *Biol. Bull. (Woods Hole, Mass.)* **103,** 54–66.

De Felice, L. J., and Dale, B. (1979). Voltage response to fertilization and polyspermy in sea urchin eggs and oocytes. *Dev. Biol.* **72,** 327–341.

del Pino, E. M. (1973). Interactions between gametes and environment in the toad *Xenopus laevis* (Daudin) and their relationship to fertilization. *J. Exp. Zool.* **185,** 121–132.

Dunbar, B. S., Wardrip, N. J., and Hedrick, J. L. (1980). Isolation, physicochemical properties, and macromolecular composition of zona pellucida from procine oocytes. *Biochemistry* **19,** 356–365.

Elinson, R. P. (1975). Site of sperm entry and a cortical contraction associated with egg activation in the frog *Rana pipiens. Dev. Biol.* **47,** 257–268.

Elinson, R. P. (1980). The amphibian egg cortex in fertilization and early development. *In* "The Cell Surface: Mediator of Developmental Processes" (S. Subtelny and N. K. Wessels, eds.), pp. 217–234. Academic Press, New York.

Elinson, R. P., and Manes, M. E. (1978). Morphology of the site of sperm entry on the frog egg. *Dev. Biol.* **63,** 67–75.

Endo, Y. (1961). Changes in the cortical layer of sea urchin eggs at fertilization studied with the electron microscope. *Exp. Cell Res.* **25,** 383–397.

Epel, D. (1980). Experimental analysis of the role of intercellular calcium in the activation of the sea urchin egg. *In* "The Cell Surface: Mediator of Developmental Processes" (S. Subtelny and N. K. Wessels, eds.), pp. 169–183. Academic Press, New York.

Epel, D., Weaver, A. M., Muchmore, A. V., and Schimke, R. T. (1969). Betaglucanase of sea urchin eggs: Release from particles at fertilization. *Science* **163,** 294–296.

Evans, T. C. (1947). Effects of hydrogen peroxide produced in the medium by radiation on spermatozoa and fertilized eggs of *Arbacia punctualata. Biol. Bull. (Woods Hole, Mass.)* **92,** 99–109.

Foerder, C. A., and Shapiro, B. M. (1977). Release of ovoperoxidase from sea urchin eggs hardens the fertilization membrane with tyrosine cross-links. *Proc. Natl. Acad. Sci. U.S.A.* **74,** 4214–4218.

Foerder, C. A., Klebanoff, S. J., and Shapiro, B. M. (1978). Hydrogen peroxide production, chemiluminescence and the respiratory burst of fertilization. Interrelated events in early sea urchin development. *Proc. Natl. Acad. Sci. U.S.A.* **75**, 3183–3187.

Fol, H. (1877). Sur le commencement de l'hénogenie chez divers ammaux. *Arch. Zool. Exp. Gen.* **6**, 145–169.

Fol, H. (1879). Recherches sur la fécondation et le commencement de l'hénogenie chez divers animaux. *Geneve Soc. Phys. Mem.* **26**, 89–397.

Franke, W. W., Rathke, P. C., Seib, E., Trendelenburg, M. F., Osborn, M., and Weber, K. (1976). Distribution and mode of arrangement of microfilamentous structures and actin in the cortex of the amphibian oocyte. *Cytobiologie* **14**, 111–130.

Freeman, S. B. (1968). A study of the jelly envelopes surrounding the egg of the amphibian, *Xenopus laevis*. *Biol. Bull. (Woods Hole, Mass.)* **135**, 501–513.

Gaddum-Rosse, P. (1981). Some observations on sperm transport through the uterotubal junction of the rat. *Am. J. Anat.* **160**, 333–341.

Gerton, G. L. (1980). Glycoprotein and protein changes in envelopes from *Xenopus laevis* eggs. Ph.D. Thesis, University of California, Davis.

Gingell, D. (1970). Contractile responses at the surface of the amphibian egg. *J. Embryol. Exp. Morphol.* **23**, 583–609.

Giudice, G. (1973). "Developmental Biology of the Sea Urchin Embryo." Academic Press, New York.

Glabe, C. G., and Vacqiuer, V. D. (1978). Egg surface glycoprotein receptor for sea urchin sperm binding. *Proc. Natl. Acad. Sci. U.S.A.* **75**, 881–885.

Gould, K. G., (1973). Preparation of mammalian gametes and reproductive tract tissues for scanning electron microscopy. *Fertil. Steril.* **24**, 448–456.

Graham, C. F. (1966). The regulation of DNA synthesis and mitosis in multinucleate frog eggs. *J. Cell Sci.* **1**, 363–374.

Greve, L. C., and Hedrick, J. L. (1978). An immunocytochemical localization of the cortical granule lectin in fertilized and unfertilized eggs of *Xenopus laevis*. *Gamete Res.* **1**, 13–18.

Grey, R. D., Wolf, D. P., and Hedrick, J. L. (1974). Formation and structure of the fertilization envelope in *Xenopus laevis*. *Dev. Biol.* **36**, 44–61.

Grey, R. D., Working, P. K., and Hedrick, J. L. (1976). Evidence that the fertilization envelope blocks sperm entry in eggs of *Xenopus laevis*: Interaction of sperm with isolated envelopes. *Dev. Biol.* **54**, 52–60.

Grey, R. D., Bastiani, M. J., Webb, D. J., and Schertel, E. R. (1982). An electrical block is required to prevent polyspermy in eggs fertilized by natural mating of *Xenopus laevis*. *Dev. Biol.* **89**, 475–484.

Gulyas, B. J. (1974). Electron microscopic observations on advanced stages of spontaneous polyspermy in rabbit zygotes. *Anat. Rec.* **179**, 285–296.

Gulyas, B.J. (1976). Ultrastructural observations on rabbit, hamster and mouse eggs following electrical stimulation in vitro. *Am. J. Anat.* **147**, 203–218.

Gulyas, B. J. (1980). Cortical granules of mammalian eggs. *Int. Rev. Cytol.* **63**, 357–392.

Gulyas, B. J., and Schmell, E. D. (1980). Ovoperoxidase activity in ionophore treated mouse eggs. I. Electron microscopic localization. *Gamete Res.* **3**, 267–277.

Gulyas, B. J., and Schmell, E. D. (1981). Sperm-egg recognition and binding in mammals. *In* "Bioregulators of Reproduction" (G. Jagiello and H. J. Vogel, eds.), pp. 499–519. Academic Press, New York.

Gwatkin, R. B. L. (1964). Effect of enzymes and acidity on the zona pellucida of the mouse egg before and after fertilization. *J. Reprod. Fertil.* **7**, 99–105.

Gwatkin, R. B. L. (1976). Fertilization. *In* "The Cell Surface in Animal Embryogenesis and Development" (G. Poste and G. L. Nicolson, eds.), pp. 1–54. Elsevier/North-Holland Biomedical Press, Amsterdam.

Gwatkin, R. B. L. (1977). "Fertilization Mechanisms in Man and Mammals." Plenum, New York.

Gwatkin, R. B. L., and Williams, D. T. (1974). Heat sensitivity of the cortical granule protease from hamster eggs. *J. Reprod. Fertil.* **39**, 153–155.

Gwatkin, R. B. L., Williams, D. T., Hartmann, J. F., and Kniazuk, M. (1973). The zona reaction of hamster and mouse eggs: Production in vitro by a trypsin-like protease from cortical granules. *J. Reprod. Fertil.* **32**, 259–265.

Gwatkin, R. B. L., Carter, H. W., and Patterson, H. (1976a). Association of mammalian sperm with cumulus cells and the zona pellucida studied by scanning electron microscopy. *Scanning Electron Microsc.* pp. 379–384.

Gwatkin, R. B. L., Rasmusson, G. H., and Williams, D. T. (1976b). Induction of the cortical reaction in hamster eggs by membrane active agents. *J. Reprod. Fertil.* **47**, 299–303.

Hagiwara, S., and Jaffe, L. A. (1979). Electrical properties of egg cell membranes. *Annu. Rev. Biophys. Bioeng.* **8**, 385–416.

Hagström, B. E. (1956). Effect of removal of the jelly coat on fertilization in sea urchins. *Exp. Cell Res.* **10**, 740–743.

Hagström, B. E. (1959). Further experiments on jelly-free sea urchin eggs. *Exp. Cell Res.* **17**, 256–261.

Hagström, B. E., and Lonning, S. (1976). Scanning electron microscope studies of the surface of the sea urchin egg. *Protoplasma* **87**, 281–290.

Hall, H. G. (1978). Hardening of the sea urchin fertilization envelope by peroxidase catalyzed phenolic coupling of tyrosines. *Cell* **15**, 343–355.

Hara, K., and Tydeman, P. (1979). Cinematographic observation of an "activation wave" (AW) on the locally inseminated egg of *Xenopus laevis*. *Wilhelm Roux's Arch. Dev. Biol.* **186**, 91–94.

Hartmann, J. F., and Hutchison, C. F. (1980). Nature and fate of the factors released during early contact interactions between hamster sperm and egg prior to fertilization in vitro. *Dev. Biol.* **78**, 380–393.

Hartmann, J. F., and Hutchison, C. F. (1981). Modulation of fertilization in vitro by peptides released during hamster sperm-zona pellucida interaction. *Proc. Natl. Acad. Sci. U.S.A.* **78**, 1690–1694.

Harvey, E. N. (1910). The mechanism of membrane formation and other early changes in developing sea urchin eggs as bearing upon the problem of artificial parthenogenesis. *J. Exp. Zool.* **8**, 355–376.

Hedrick, J. L., and Fry, G. N. (1980). Immunocytochemical studies on the porcine zona pellucida. *J. Cell Biol.* **87**, 136a.

Hunter, R. H. F. (1973). Polyspermic fertilization in pigs after deposition of excessive numbers of spermatozoa. *J. Exp. Zool.* **183**, 57–64.

Hunter, R. H. F., and Leglise, P. C. (1971a). Polyspermic fertilization following tubal surgery in pigs, with particular reference to the role of the isthmus. *J. Reprod. Fertil.* **24**, 233–246.

Hunter, R. H. F., and Leglise, P. C. (1971b). Tubal surgery in the rabbit: fertilization and polyspermy after resection of the isthmus. *Am. J. Anat.* **132**, 45–52.

Inoue, M., and Wolf, D. P. (1974). Comparative solubility properties of the zonae pellucidae of unfertilized and fertilized mouse ova. *Biol. Reprod.* **11**, 558–565.

Inoue, M., and Wolf, D. P. (1975a). Comparative solubility properties of rat and hamster zonae pellucidae. *Biol. Reprod.* **12,** 535–540.

Inoue, M., and Wolf, D. P. (1975b). Fertilization-associated changes in the murine zona pellucida: A time sequence study. *Biol. Reprod.* **13,** 546–551.

Ito, S. (1972). Effects of media of different ionic composition on the activation potential of anuran egg cells. *Dev, Growth Differ.* **14,** 217–227.

Iwamatsu, T., and Ohta, T. (1978). Electron microscopic observation on sperm penetration and pronuclear formation in the fish egg. *J. Exp. Zool.* **205,** 157–180.

Iwao, Y., Ito, S., and Katagiri, C. (1981). Electrical properties of toad oocytes during maturation and activation. *Dev. Growth Differ.* **23,** 89–100.

Jackowski, S., and Dumont, J. N. (1979). Surface alterations of the mouse zona pellucida and ovum following in vivo fertilization: Correlation with the cell cycle. *Biol. Reprod.* **20,** 150–161.

Jaffe, L. A. (1976). Fast block to polyspermy in sea urchin eggs is electrically mediated. *Nature (London)* **261,** 68–71.

Jaffe, L. A., and Robinson, K. R. (1978). Membrane potential of the unfertilized sea urchin egg. *Dev. Biol.* **62,** 215–228.

Johnson, M. H., Eager, D. Muggleton-Harris, A., and Grave, H. M. (1975). Mosaicism in organisation of concanavalin A-receptors on surface membrane of mouse egg. *Nature (London)* **257,** 321–322.

Kaleta, E. (1979). Sperm penetration in vitro into ovarian and tubal oocytes from mice of the inbred KE and C57 strains. *Gamete Res.* **2,** 99–104.

Kas'yanov, V. L., Svyatogor, G. P., and Drozdov, A. L. (1971). Cortical reaction of frog eggs. *Ontaogenez* **2,** 507–511 transl. by Consultants Bureau, 1972.

Katagiri, C. (1962). On the fertilizability of the frog egg. II. Change of the jelly envelopes in water. *Jpn. J. Zool.* **13,** 365–373.

Katagiri, C. (1973). Chemical analysis of toad egg-jelly in relation to its "sperm-capacitating" activity. *Dev. Growth Differ.* **15,** 81–92.

Katsura, S., and Tominga, A. (1974). Peroxidatic activity of catalase in the cortical granules of sea urchin eggs. *Dev. Biol.* **40,** 292–297.

Kemp, N. E., and Istock, N. L. (1967). Cortical changes in growing and in fertilized or pricked eggs of *Rana pipiens. J. Cell Biol.* **34,** 111–122.

Kinsey, W. H., SeGall, G. K., and Lennarz, W. J. (1979). The effect of the acrosome reaction on respiratory activity and fertilizing capacity of echinoid sperm. *Dev. Biol.* **71,** 49–59.

Klebanoff, S. J., Foerder, C. A., Eddy, E. M., and Shapiro, B. M. (1979). Metabolic similarities between fertilization and phagocytosis. *J. Exp. Med.* **149,** 938–953.

Lillie, F. R. (1914). Studies on fertilization. V. The behavior of the spermatozoa of *Nereis* and *Arbacia* with special reference to egg-extractives. *J. Exp. Zool.* **14,** 515–574.

Lillie, F. R. (1919). "Problems of Fertilization." Univ. of Chicago Press, Chicago, Illinois.

Maeno, T. (1959). Electrical characteristics and activation potential of *Bufo* eggs. *J. Gen. Physiol.* **43,** 139–157.

Miceli, D. C., del Pino, E. J., Barbieri, F. D., Mariano, M. I., and Raisman, J. S. (1977). The vitelline envelope-to-fertilization envelope transformation in the toad *Bufo arenarum. Dev. Biol.* **59,** 101–110.

Miceli, D. C., Fernandez, S. N., Raisman, J. S., and Barbieri, F. D. (1978a). A trypsin-like oviducal proteinase involved in *Bufo arenarum* fertilization. *J. Embryol. Exp. Morphol.* **48,** 79–91.

Miceli, D. C., Fernandez, S. N., and del Pino, E. J. (1978b). An oviducal enzyme isolated by affinity chromatography which acts upon the vitelline envelope of *Bufo arenarum* coelomic oocytes. *Biochim Biophys. Acta* **526**, 289–292.

Miyazaki, S., and Igusa, Y. (1981). Fertilization potential in golden hamster eggs consists of recurring hyperpolarizations. *Nature (London)* **290**, 702–704.

Monk, B. C., and Hedrick, J. L. (1982). The cortical reaction in *Xenopus laevis* oocytes: A radiommuneassay to measure the exocytotic release of the cortical granule lectin. *Dev. Biol.* (in press).

Moore, H. D. M., and Bedford, J. M. (1978). An in vivo analysis of factors influencing the fertilization of hamster eggs. *Biol. Reprod.* **19**, 879–885.

Morgan, T. H. (1897). "The Development of the Frog's Egg. An Introduction to Experimental Embryology." Macmillian, New York.

Nicosia, S. V., Wolf, D. P., and Inoue, M. (1977). Cortical granule distribution and cell surface characteristics in mouse eggs. *Dev. Biol.* **57**, 56–74.

Nicosia, S. V., Wolf, D. P., and Mastroianni, L., Jr. (1978). Surface topography of mouse eggs before and after insemination. *Gamete Res.* **1**, 145–155.

Nishihara, T., and Hedrick, J. L. (1977a). A molecular mechanism for envelope elevation at fertilization. *Fed. Proc., Fed. Am. Soc. Exp. Biol.* **36**, 811.

Nishihara, T., and Hedrick, J. L. (1977b). Reconstruction of the fertilization envelope from its component parts. *J. Cell Biol.* **75**, 172a.

Nishihara, T., Wyrick, R. E., Working, P. K., Chen, Y., and Hedrick, J. L. (1982). Isolation and characterization of a lectin from the cortical granules of *Xenopus laevis* eggs. *J. Biol. Chem.* (submitted for publication).

Niwa, K., and Chang, M. C. (1975). Requirement of capacitation for sperm penetration of zona-free rat eggs. *J. Reprod. Fertil.* **44**, 305–308.

Norton, J. G. (1976). Parameters of the block to polyspermy in *Rana pipiens*. M.Sc. Thesis, University of Toronto.

Nuccitelli, R. (1980a). The electrical changes accompanying fertilization and cortical vesicle secretion in the medaka egg. *Dev. Biol.* **76**, 483–498.

Nuccitelli, R. (1980b). The fertilization potential is not necessary for the block to polyspermy or the activation of development in the medaka egg. *Dev. Biol.* **76**, 499–504.

Overstreet, J. W., and Cooper, G. W. (1978). Sperm transport in the reproductive tract of the female rabbit. II. The sustained phase of transport. *Biol. Reprod.* **19**, 115–132.

Palacek, J., Ubbels, G. A., and Rzehak, K. (1978). Changes of the external and internal pigment pattern upon fertilization in the egg of *Xenopus laevis*. *J. Embryol. Exp. Morphol.* **45**, 203–214.

Pavlok, A., and McLaren, A. (1972). The role of cumulus cells and the zona pellucida in fertilization of mouse eggs in vitro. *J. Reprod. Fertil.* **29**, 91–97.

Pereda, J. (1970). Etude histochimique des mucopolysaccharides de l'oviducte et des gangues muqueuses des ovocytes de *Rana pipiens:* Incorporation du $^{35}SO_4 2-$. *Dev. Biol.* **21**, 318–330.

Phillips, D. M., and Shalgi, R. (1980a). Surface architecture of the mouse and hamster zona pellucida and oocyte. *J. Ultrastruct. Res.* **72**, 1–12.

Phillips, D. M., and Shalgi, R. M. (1980b). Surface properties of the zona pellucida. *J. Exp. Zool.* **213**, 1–8.

Picheral, B. (1977a). La fécondation chez le Triton Pleurodele. 1. La traversée des envelopes de l'oeuf par les spermatozoides. *J. Ultrastruct. Res.* **60**, 106–120.

Picheral, B. (1977b). La fécondation chez le triton pleurodele. 2. La pénétration des spermatozoides et la réaction locale de l'oeuf. *J. Ultrastruct. Res.* **60**, 181–202.

Poirier, G. R., and Spink, G. C. (1971). The ultrastructure of testicular spermatozoa in two species of *Rana*. *J. Ultrastruct. Res.* **36**, 455–465.

Powers, R. D., and Tupper, J. T. (1974). Some electrophysiological and permeability properties of the mouse egg. *Dev. Biol.* **38**, 320–331.

Raisman, J. S., and Cabada, M. O. (1977). Acrosomic reaction and proteolytic activity in the spermatozoa of an anuran amphibian, *Leptodactylus chaquensis* (Cei). *Dev., Growth Differ.* **19**, 227–232.

Reed, S. C., and Stanley, H. P. (1972). Fine structure of spermatogenesis in the South African clawed toad *Xenopus laevis* Daudin. *J. Ultrastruct. Res.* **41**, 277–295.

Richter, H. (1980). SDS-polyacrylamide gel electrophoresis of isolated cortices of *Xenopus laevis* eggs. *Cell Biol. Int. Rep.* **4**, 985–995.

Rothschild, Lord (1956). "Fertilization." Methuen, London.

Rothschild, Lord, and Swann, M. M. (1952). The fertilization reaction in the sea urchin. The block to polyspermy. *J. Exp. Biol.* **29**, 469–483.

Runnström, J. (1966). The vitelline membrane and cortical particles in sea urchin eggs and their function in maturation and fertilization. *Adv. Morphog.* **5**, 221–325.

Saling, P. M., and Storey, B. T. (1979). Mouse gamete interactions during fertilization in vitro. *J. Cell Biol.* **83**, 544–555.

Schatten, G. (1979). Pronuclear movements and fusion at fertilization. *J. Cell Biol.* **83**, 198a.

Schatten, G., and Mazia, D. (1976). The penetration of the spermatozoan through the sea urchin egg surface at fertilization. *Exp. Cell Res.* **98**, 325–337.

Schatten, H., and Schatten, G. (1980). Surface activity at the egg plasma membrane during sperm incorporation and its cytochalasin B sensitivity. *Dev. Biol.* **78**, 435–449.

Schlichter, L. C., and Elinson, R. P. (1981). Electrical responses of immature and mature *Rana pipiens* oocytes to sperm and other activating stimuli. *Dev. Biol.* **83**, 33–41.

Schmell, E. D., and Gulyas, B. J. (1980). Ovoperoxidase activity in ionophore treated mouse eggs. II. Evidence for the enzyme's role in hardening the zona pellucida. *Gamete Res.* **3**, 279–290.

Schmell, E. D., Earles, B. J., Breaux, C., and Lennarz, W. J. (1977). Identification of a sperm receptor on the surface of sea urchin eggs. *J. Cell Biol.* **72**, 35–46.

Schroeder, T. E. (1978). Microvilli on sea urchin eggs: A second burst of elongation. *Dev. Biol.* **64**, 342–346.

Schroeder, T. E. (1979). Surface area change at fertilization: Resorption of the mosaic membrane. *Dev. Biol.* **70**, 306–326.

Schroeder, T. E., and Strickland, D. L. (1974). Ionophore A23187, calcium and contractility in frog eggs. *Exp. Cell Res.* **83**, 139–142.

Schuel, H. (1978). Secretory functions of egg cortical granules in fertilization and development: A critical review. *Gamete Res.* **1**, 299–382.

SeGall, G. K., and Lennarz, W. J. (1979). Chemical characterization of the component of the jelly coat from sea urchin eggs responsible for induction of the acrosome reaction. *Dev. Biol.* **71**, 33–48.

Seshadri, H. S., and Reddy, M. S. (1980). Studies on toad egg jelly glycoproteins. Part 2. Isolation of glycopeptide and investigation on structure of carbohydrate moiety. *Indian J. Biochem. Biophys.* **17**, 24–31.

Shapiro, B. M. (1975). Limited proteolysis of some egg surface components is an early event following fertilization of the sea urchin, *Strongylocentrotus purpuratus*. *Dev. Biol.* **46**, 88–102.

Shapiro, B. M., and Eddy, E. M. (1980). When sperm meets eggs: Biochemical mechanisms of gamete interactions. *Int. Rev. Cytol.* **66**, 257–302.

Shapiro, B. M., Schackmann, R. W., Gabel, C. A., Foerder, C. A., Farrance, M. L., Eddy, E. M., and Klebanoff, S. J. (1980). Molecular alterations in gamete surfaces during fertilization and early development. *In* "The Cell Surface: Mediator of Developmental Processes" (S. Subtelny and N. K. Wessells, eds.), pp. 127–150. Academic Press, New York.

Shapiro, B. M., Schackmann, R. W., and Gabel, C. A. (1981). Molecular approaches to the study of fertilization. *Annu. Rev. Biochem.* **50**, 815–843.

Shivers, C. A., and James, J. M. (1969). Morphology and histochemistry of the oviduct and egg-jelly layers in the frog, *Rana pipiens. Anat. Rec.* **166**, 541–556.

Smith, D. C., and Klebanoff, S. J. (1970). A uterine fluid-mediated sperm-inhibitory system. *Biol. Reprod.* **3**, 229–235.

Smithberg, M. (1953). The effect of different proteolytic enzymes on the zona pellucida of mouse ova. *Anat. Rec.* **117**, 554–555.

Soupart, P., and Strong, P. A. (1975). Ultrastructural observations on polyspermic penetration of zona pellucida-free human oocytes inseminated in vitro. *Fertil. Steril.* **26**, 523–537.

Steinhardt, R. A., Londin, L., and Mazia, D. (1971). Bioelectric response of the echinoderm egg to fertilization. *Proc. Natl. Acad. Sci. U.S.A.* **68**, 2426–2430.

Steinhardt, R. A., Epel, D., and Carroll, E. J. (1978). Is calcium ionophore a universal activator for unfertilized eggs? *Nature (London)* **252**, 41–43.

Steinke, J. H., and Benson, D. G. (1970). The structure and polysaccharide cytochemistry of the jelly envelopes of the egg of the frog *Rana pipiens. J. Morphol.* **130**, 57–66.

Sugiyama, M. (1951). Re-fertilization of fertilized eggs of the sea urchin. *Biol. Bull. (Woods Hole, Mass.)* **101**, 335–344.

Szollosi, D. (1967). Development of cortical granules and the cortical reaction in rat and hamster eggs. *Anat. Rec.* **159**, 431–446.

Taglietti, V. (1979). Early electrical responses to fertilization in sea urchin eggs. *Exp. Cell Res.* **120**, 448–452.

Thompson, R. S., Smith, D. M., and Zamboni, L. (1974). Fertilization of mouse ova in vitro: An electron microscopic study. *Fertil. Steril.* **25**, 222–249.

Tilney, L. G., Jaffe, L. A. (1980). Actin, microvilli, and the fertilization cone of sea urchin eggs. *J. Cell Biol.* **87**, 771–782.

Toyoda, Y., and Chang, M. C. (1968). Sperm penetration of rat eggs in vitro after dissolution of zona pellucida by chymotrypsin. *Nature (London)* **220**, 589–591.

Tupper, J. T. (1973). Potassium exchangeability, potassium permeability and membrane potential: Some observations in relation to protein synthesis in the early echinoderm embryo. *Dev. Biol.* **32**, 140–154.

Tyler, A. (1941). The role of fertilizin in the fertilization of the sea urchin and other animals. *Biol. Bull. (Woods Hole, Mass.)* **81**, 190–204.

Uchiyama, S., Ishihara, K., and Ishida, J. (1971). Chemical composition of the egg membrane of the toad. *Annot. Zool. Jpn.* **44**, 1–7.

Urch, U. A., and Hedrick, J. L. (1981). The hatching enzyme from *Xenopus laevis:* Limited proteolysis of the fertilization envelope. *J. Supramol. Struct. Cell. Biochem.* **15**, 111–117.

Vacquier, V. D. (1981). Dynamic changes of the egg cortex. *Dev. Biol.* **84**, 1–26.

Vacquier, V. D., Epel, D., and Douglas, L. A. (1972). Sea urchin eggs release a protease activity at fertilization. *Nature (London)* **237**, 34–36.

Vacquier, V. D., Tegner, M. J., and Epel, D. (1973a). Protease activity establishes block against polyspermy in sea urchin eggs. *Nature (London)* **240**, 352–353.

Vacquier, V. D., Tegner, M. J., and Epel, D. (1973b). Protease released from sea urchin eggs at fertilization alters the vitelline layer and aids in preventing polyspermy. *Exp. Cell Res.* **80**, 111–119.

Veron, M., Foerder, C., Eddy, E. M., and Shapiro, B. M. (1977). Sequential biochemical and morphological events during assembly of the fertilization membrane of the sea urchin. *Cell* **10**, 321–328.

Wabik-Sliz, B. (1979). Number of cortical granules in mouse oocytes from inbred strains differing in efficiency of fertilization. *Biol. Reprod.* **21**, 89–97.

Wabik-Sliz, B., and Kujat, R. (1979). The surface of mouse oocytes from two inbred strains differing in efficiency of fertilization, as revealed by scanning electron microscopy. *Biol. Reprod.* **20**, 405–408.

Wartenberg, H., and Schmidt, W. (1961). Elektronenmikroskopische Untersuchungen der strukturellen Veranderungen im Rindenbereich des Amphibieneies im ovar und nach der Befruchtung. *Z. Zellforsch. Mikrosk. Anat.* **54**, 118–146.

Wischnitzer, S. (1966). The ultrastructure of the cytoplasm of the developing amphibian egg. *Adv. Morphog.* **5**, 131–179.

Wolf, D. P. (1974a). The cortical granule reaction in living eggs of the toad *Xenopus laevis. Dev. Biol.* **36**, 62–71.

Wolf, D. P. (1974b). On the contents of the cortical granules from *Xenopus laevis* eggs. *Dev. Biol.* **38**, 14–29.

Wolf, D. P. (1978). The block to sperm penetration in zona-free mouse eggs. *Dev. Biol.* **64**, 1–10.

Wolf, D. P. (1981). The mammalian egg's block to polyspermy. *In* "Fertilization and Embryonic Development In Vitro" (L. Mastroianni, Jr. and J. D. Biggers, eds.), pp. 183–197. Plenum, New York.

Wolf, D. P., and Hamada, M. (1977). Induction of zonal and egg plasma membrane blocks to sperm penetration in mouse eggs with cortical granule exudate. *Biol. Reprod.* **17**, 350–354.

Wolf, D. P., and Hedrick, J. L. (1971). A molecular approach to fertilization. II. Viability and artificial fertilization of *Xenopus laevis* gametes. *Dev. Biol.* **25**, 348–395.

Wolf, D. P., Nishihara, T., West, D. M., Wyrick, R. E., and Hendrick, J. L. (1976). Isolation, physicochemical properties, and the macromolecular composition of the vitelline and fertilization envelopes from *Xenopus laevis* eggs. *Biochemistry* **15**, 3671–3678.

Wolf, D. P., Nicosia, S. V., and Hamada, M. (1979). Premature cortical granule loss does not prevent sperm penetration of mouse eggs. *Dev. Biol.* **71**, 22–32.

Wyrick, R. E. (1974). Molecular and ultrastructural studies of the vitelline-to-fertilization envelope conversion in *Xenopus laevis*. Ph.D. Thesis, University of California, Davis.

Wyrick, R. E., Nishihara, T., and Hedrick, J. L. (1974). Agglutination of jelly coat and cortical granule components and the block to polyspermy in the amphibian *Xenopus laevis. Proc. Natl. Acad. Sci. U.S.A.* **71**, 2067–2071.

Yanagimachi, R. (1981). Mechanisms of fertilization. *In* "Fertilization and Embryonic Development In Vitro" (L. Mastroianni, Jr. and J. D. Biggers, eds.), pp. 81–182. Plenum, New York.

Yanagimachi, R., and Noda, Y. D. (1970). Physiological changes in the postnuclear cap region of the mammalian sperm: A necessary preliminary to the membrane fusion between sperm cells. *J. Ultrastruct. Res.* **31**, 486–493.

Yoshizaki, N., and Katagiri, C. H. (1981). Oviducal contribution to alteration of the vitelline coat (VC) of frog eggs. *Dev., Growth Differ.* **23**, 495–506.

Yurewicz, E. C., Oliphant, G., and Hedrick, J. L. (1975). The macromolecular composition of *Xenopus laevis* egg jelly coat. *Biochemistry* **14**, 3101–3107.

Zamboni, L. (1970). Ultrastructure of mammalian oocytes and ova. *Biol. Reprod., Suppl.* **2**, 44–63.

Zamboni, L. (1971). Differentation and maturation of the egg. *In* "Fine Morphology of Mammalian Fertilization" (L. Zamboni, ed.), pp. 68–116. Harper, New York.

Zamboni, L. (1974). Fine morphology of the follicle wall and follicle cell-oocyte association. *Biol. Reprod.* **10**, 125–149.

9

Synthetic Activities of the Mammalian Early Embryo: Molecular and Genetic Alterations following Fertilization

DEBRA J. WOLGEMUTH

I. INTRODUCTION

Our understanding of the molecular mechanisms of fertilization in mammals has been limited severely by the difficulty in obtaining sufficient quantities of female gametes and embryos for biochemical studies. Even in species where superovulation can be employed to increase the number of fertilizable ova, hundreds rather than millions of cells are available for analysis. Thus, the majority of available information on the events of mammalian fertilization and early embryonic develop-

Mechanism and Control of Animal Fertilization
Copyright © 1983 by Academic Press, Inc.
All rights of reproduction in any form reserved.
ISBN 0-12-328520-8

ment is primarily morphological and descriptive. Several excellent reviews of this body of information have been written, including those by Longo (1973), Longo and Kunkle (1978), and Yanagimachi (1978).

Recently, the development of increasingly sensitive techniques for detecting and quantitating macromolecular synthesis has opened up new avenues of experimental approaches; that is, it is becoming feasible to perform biochemical studies of the fertilization process and of early embryogenesis in mammals. Such studies are absolutely critical for elucidating the mechanisms responsible for the activation of development and are of particular importance in light of current interest in mammalian *in vitro* fertilization.

This chapter will attempt to describe this newly obtained body of information, set into the context of previous morphological and cellular observations on the fertilization process. The scope of this review is restricted on several levels and is biased in certain directions. First, there is an emphasis on the changes in cellular macromolecular synthetic activities rather than on, for example, physiological changes such as ion fluxes or morphological alterations. Second, an assessment of the contribution of genetic activity of the male and female gametes in these synthetic processes is considered important. Third, the majority of studies presented examine animal model systems most suitable to the laboratory setting, notably the mouse and rabbit. However, the belief that there are certain important differences in even the most basic biological phenomena among species dictates consideration of the use of other mammalian models whenever possible. Finally, the time period of development that will be discussed is narrow: emphasis is on that period after gametogenesis is complete and before the completion of the second cell division by the embryo. More detailed descriptions of the biochemistry of male and female gametogenesis are provided in Chapters 1 and 2 of this volume. The biochemistry and molecular biology of early mammalian embryogenesis has received the attention of several reviewers and among the excellent recent reviews are those of Sherman (1979), McLaren (1979), Magnuson and Epstein (1981), and Johnson (1981).

II. PROPERTIES OF THE GAMETES AT THE TIME OF FERTILIZATION

The process of gametogenesis in mammals yields two very different cell types as mature gametes. The oocyte has undergone tremendous growth and has stockpiled proteins and other molecules, presumably for use during the period of time following fertilization and before the embryonic genome has become functional. At ovulation, the oocyte is arrested at the second metaphase stage, awaiting an as yet unidentified stimulus from the fertilization process. In contrast, the spermatozoon is an extremely streamlined cell, containing only elements for essential functions such as motility and a few critical enzymes. Genetically, meiosis is complete and the haploid genome is packaged quite differently than the usual somatic cell nucleus. It is the condition of the genome at the moment of fertilization, with respect to both structure and genetic activity, that will be emphasized in this discussion.

A. The Sperm Nucleus

DNA of the mature mammalian sperm nucleus is found in association with highly basic protamine-like proteins. These proteins are laid down during terminal stages of spermiogenesis in all the mammalian species in which they have been identified and characterized (e.g., Bloch, 1969; Coelingh and Rozijn, 1975; Bellvé, 1979). The majority of studies in which sperm nuclei have been analyzed for their protein composition suggests that protamine-like proteins essentially replace the somatic histones as the primary component of chromatin (Bloch, 1969; Calvin, 1976; Bellvé, 1979).

It had been generally accepted that this substitution was complete and that the spermatozoon was devoid of histones—whether somatic or testis-specific. A few recent studies suggest that this may not be the case, at least in mouse and human sperm. Electrophoretic analysis of rigorously purified sperm heads revealed the presence of small amounts of proteins that comigrate with histones H2B and H4 in mouse epididymal spermatozoa (O'Brien and Bellvé, 1980). Both electrophoretic and immunohistochemical analyses have been used to examine the basic nuclear protein composition of ejaculated human spermatozoa. All somatic histones have been detected (Samuel et al., 1976; Puwaravutipanich and Panyim, 1975; Kolk and Samuel, 1975; Tanphaichitr et al., 1978, 1981; van Meel and Pearson, 1979). TH2B, a testis-specific variant of H2B, was shown to be the major species of histone present (Tanphaichitr et al., 1978). These results are in contrast to earlier studies on human sperm chromatin in which no histones were detected (Calvin, 1976). This may have been due to loss of such proteins in the $8M$ urea-DTT extraction procedures (Tanphaichitr et al., 1981). It is known that human ejaculated sperm are heterogeneous morphologically with respect to their extent of chromatin con-

As in lower species, CG are located beneath the PM of unfertilized mammalian ova. In the unfertilized oocyte, most of the CG are spaced irregularly in a monolayer just beneath the PM, although some are observed deeper in the cytoplasm (for further details, see Gulyas, 1980). In the area overlying the meiotic spindle, CG are completely absent (Szollosi, 1967; Zamboni, 1970, 1971; Gulyas, 1976). The polarity of the CG distribution in recently ovulated ova has been best demonstrated in the mouse (Nicosia *et al.*, 1977), CG density being the greatest in the vegetal hemisphere of the ovum. Furthermore, although mammalian CG lack any fine structure, two distinct classes of CG, light and dark granules, have been observed in unpenetrated ova.

2. Morphological Alterations with Sperm Penetration

Detailed *in vitro* studies in the mouse indicate that only intact spermatozoa can bind to the ZP (Saling and Storey, 1979). Following contact and attachment of intact sperm, the acrosome reaction occurs. Ultimately sperm penetration through the ZP is observed (for recent reviews, see Moore and Bedford, 1978; Gulyas and Schmell, 1981; Yanagimachi, 1981; this volume, Chapter 10). The interactions of the fertilizing spermatozoan with the egg surface result in extensive reorganization of the egg cortex, the PM, and the ZP. However, in contrast to observations in lower species (sea urchins and anurans), the changes in mammalian eggs can be resolved only at the level of the electron microscope.

The most obvious surface alteration at fertilization, aside from sperm–egg fusion, is the cortical reaction. In this process the limiting membrane of the CG and the adjacent PM fuse. The PM becomes a mosiac consisting of the original PM and the limiting membrane of the CG. Channels are created between the internal position of the CG and the PVS, enabling the dehiscence of the CG content (for a recent review, see Gulyas, 1980). This is thought to be a rapid process, although kinetic studies are unavailable. The CG exudate is recognizable in the PVS for a short time before it disperses onto the egg surface or into the ZP.

It is unclear whether the cortical reaction is initiated by sperm–egg contact, fusion of gamete membranes, or penetration of the spermatozoon into the ooplasm. Indications are that sperm penetration into the cytoplasm is not required to elicit a cortical reaction, since frozen-thawed hamster spermatozoa which fail to penetrate, although they do attach to the egg, do elicit a cortical reaction (Gwatkin *et al.*, 1976b). No experimental results have clearly distinguished between the need of membrane contact versus membrane fusion. Because un-

densation, both within a single nucleus and among different nuclei (Bedford *et al.*, 1973; Evenson *et al.*, 1980). Whether such heterogeneity is a result of a heterogeneity in chromatin composition is not known. However, the possibility that the minor histone components identified in the cells from human ejaculates might not originate from mature, normally condensed spermatozoa but rather from a small number of contaminating somatic cells should also be considered.

The possible function of these trace amounts of histones is difficult to imagine. Although it is generally believed that sperm nuclei in which protamine-like proteins are the major components lack a nucleosomal chromatin structure (Kierszenbaum and Très, 1975, 1978; Young and Sweeney, 1979), the subunit and higher order structure of sperm chromatin remain to be determined (Sipski and Wagner, 1977; Wagner *et al.*, 1978; Gusse and Chevaillier, 1980; Tanphaichitr *et al.*, 1981). Indeed, the role of protamine-like proteins themselves in the sperm nucleus remains an enigma. Various functions have been attributed to these proteins: from a purely structural, protective role to a removal of previous regulatory information from the sperm nucleus so as to provide the early embryo with a clean slate upon which to deposit regulatory signals for developmental stage-specific gene expression (discussed in Bellvè, 1979). Whether because of the presence of protamine-like proteins or not, it is clear that the sperm nucleus is inert with respect to gene expression at the time of fertilization. Transcriptional, replicative, and protein synthetic activities have been demonstrated to be quiescent (Bellvé, 1979). Interestingly, however, such inactivity is apparently not due to the lack of necessary synthetic machinery. For example, the capabilities exist for nuclear DNA polymerase activities (Witkin *et al.*, 1975; Witkin and Bendich, 1977; Richards and Witkin, 1978; Chevaillier and Philippe, 1976). These DNA polymerases appear to be distinct from nonnuclear apparently mitochondrial DNA-synthesizing activities (Hecht, 1974).

B. Oocyte Nucleus at Fertilization

In contrast to the growing body of information available detailing the protein composition of sperm nuclei, little is known about the composition of oocyte nuclei at corresponding stages. It should be recalled that meiosis itself is chronologically quite different in the two gametes. At the time of fertilization the oocyte is arrested at metaphase of the second meiotic division. The biochemical properties of the proteins associated with the oocyte chromosomes and the chromosomes of the first polar body are not known. Evidence has been presented that suggests that female meiotic chromosomes are differentially sensitive to trypsin digestion at different stages of meiosis (Rodman and Barth, 1979). Some arginine-containing proteins synthesized prior to germinal vesicle breakdown appear to remain associated with the meiotic chromosomes of mouse through metaphase I (Rodman and Barth, 1979). Proteins that label with [³H]lysine and [³⁵S]methionine are retained on metaphase II chromosomes in the rabbit but only through metaphase I in the pig (Motlik et al., 1978). A very lysine-rich protein synthesized during meiotic maturation in mouse was shown to be associated with condensing chromosomes (Wassarman and LeTourneau, 1976a). In addition, a protein synthesized and phosphorylated at this same time is highly enriched in the nucleus; whether it remains in stable association during ensuing meiotic divisions has not been reported (Wassarman et al., 1979). Studies demonstrating mammalian-oocyte-specific histone variants or unique oocyte-specific basic proteins are lacking. One recent report noted the presence of a substance cross-reacting with antibodies to mouse protamines in the metaphase II chromosome complement of the mouse oocyte (Rodman et al., 1981). Although this raises the intriguing possibility that there are similarities among the proteins associated with the male and female genetic complements, direct biochemical analysis is needed.

Transcriptional activity is present until the time of germinal vesicle breakdown in oocytes from all mammals thus far studied (Wassarman and Letourneau, 1976b; Rodman and Bachvarova, 1976; Wolgemuth-Jarashow and Jagiello, 1979). In contrast, protein synthesis appears to continue throughout all meiotic stages, although the level of synthesis varies (reviewed by Wassarman et al., 1981; this volume, Chapter 1). Apart from the association of some proteins with condensing chromosomes as described above, the functions of the proteins synthesized at this time are unknown. Thus, the overall picture of the two gametes at the time of fertilization is one of genetic inactivity. The process of fertilization, by mechanisms as yet unidentified, provides the trigger for the onset of genetic activity by the early embryo.

III. ALTERATIONS IN THE GAMETES AT FERTILIZATION

Each of the events of fertilization, from release of the cortical granules to extrusion of the second polar body to formation of the pronuclei could itself form the subject of a review. This discussion will focus on what is known about alterations of the nuclear components of the gametes as they reflect or subsequently affect genetic activity.

TABLE I

Timing of Postfertilization Events in Mouse[a]

Source of ova	Insemination	Sperm within vitellus	PB[II]	Female pronucleus	Sperm decondensation	Male pronucleus	DNA synthesis	Reference
Superovulated Swiss Webster	In vivo; 1.5 hours after ovulation (13.5 hours post-HCG)	1.5–4 hours pi	1.5–4 hr pi	>4 hours pi	1–4 hours pi	>4 hours pi	—	McGaughey and Chang, 1969
Superovulated CF1	In vivo; placed with females at time of HCG; plugs 2–12 hours later	—	—	~4–12 hours pi[b] (16–24 hours post-HCG)	—	~4–12 hours pi[b] (16–24 hours post-HCG)	Inferred to have occurred before metaphase of first cleavage; thus before 16–22 hours pi[b]	Donahue, 1972
Superovulated CF1	In vivo; placed with females at time of HCG; plugs 13 hours post-HCG	—	(DNA synthesis in PB[II] detected 9–19 hours pi; 23–33 hours post-HCG)	~3–9 hours pi (17–23 hours post-HCG)	—	~3–9 hours pi (17–23 hours post-HCG)	From 7–9 hours to 17 hours pi (21–31 hours post-HCG); peak at 25 hours post-HCG; S estimated as 4.0 hours	Luthardt and Donahue, 1973
Superovulated Swiss (CD-1)	In vivo; placed with females 9.5 hours post-HCG; plugs checked every 30 minutes until 23.5 hours	—	(DNA synthesis in PB[I] detected from 10 up to 20+ hours pi)	by 8 hours pi[b]	—	by 8 hours pi[b]	10–18 hours pi; peak from 12–16 hours pi; S estimated as 5.5 hours	Siracusa et al., 1975

Treatment							Reference
Superovulated Swiss *In vivo*; placed with females 12.5 hours post-HCG; plugs 13.5 and 15 hours post-HCG	—	1–10 hours pi; peak at 3 hours pi; (DNA synthesis 10–22 hours pi)	2–13 hours pi	—	2–13 hours pi	4–13 hours pi; male pronucleus ahead of female; S estimated as 3.5–4.0 hours	Abramczuk and Sawicki, 1975
Superovulated Swiss *In vitro*; cultured for 1 to 2 hours prior to insemination	0.5–1.5 hours pi	—	—	—	—	—	Wolf *et al.*, 1977
Naturally ovulated F₁ (C3H × C57BL) (estimated time of arrival in ampulla within 60 to 90 minutes after end of dark period) *In vivo*; placed with female 2 hours after end of dark period	1.5–2.0 to 6.5–7.0 hours pi; peak at 3.0–5.0 hours pi	— (DNA synthesis in PB_{II} detected at 8–17 hours pi)	4.5–9.5 hours pi (male pronucleus slightly ahead of female)	—	4.5–9.5 hours pi	8–16 hours pi; peak at 12.5 hours pi	Krishna and Generoso, 1977
Superovulated Swiss *In vitro*; cultured for 2 to 3 hours prior to insemination	0.5–1.5 hours pi	1.5–3.0 hours pi	2 hours pi	—	—	—	Sato and Blandau, 1979
Superovulated F₁ (C57BL/10 × CBA/H) *In vitro*; zona-free ova; 15–19 hours post-HCG; sperm cultured 1 hour prior to insemination	—	by 4.5 hours pi	by 4.5–5 hours pi	—	by 4.5–5 hours pi; all at stage III or stage IV[c]	—	Witkowska, 1981

[a] pi, Postinsemination; HCG, human chorionic gonadotrophin; S, length of DNA synthesis period; PB, polar body; dash indicates data not provided by authors.
[b] Calculated from data provided.
[c] Only monospermic fertilizations tabulated; Stage III (sperm head round or oval; occasional nucleoli); Stage IV (pronucleus large; one or a few nucleoli).

A. Chronology of Nuclear Events after Fertilization

During the last 10 years, a fairly detailed description of the sequence of postfertilization changes at the light microscopic, electron microscopic, and cinematographic levels, especially in the mouse, has emerged. Both *in vivo* and *in vitro* fertilization have been compared, as has fertilization of naturally ovulated versus superovulated ova. The timing of these events in the mouse, as revealed from investigations from several different laboratories, is summarized in Table I. It would appear that the assessment of the time of appearance of gross cytological changes is remarkably constant, in spite of differences in methods of timing the moment of insemination. The greatest differences lie in the estimation of time of onset of pronuclear DNA synthesis. This may indicate true biological variation, for example, among strains of mice. More likely, however, is that this variation reflects the sensitivity of detection of incorporation of radioactive precursors. It is interesting to note that incorporation of DNA precursors into the second polar body was a common observation (Table I).

Analogous but far less detailed studies have been carried out on other species, for example, rat (Shalgi and Kraicer, 1978). rabbit (Szollosi, 1965; Longo and Anderson, 1969), pig (Hunter, 1972; Szollosi and Hunter, 1973), cow (Brackett *et al.,* 1980), and human (Lopata *et al.,* 1980). Although there is obvious variation in the intervals in timing of the events, the order of events appears universal.

B. Changes in the Sperm Nucleus and Formation of the Male Pronucleus

A detailed examination of the events in male pronucleus formation would seem to be of particular relevance on several levels. First, the unique protamine-like proteins laid down during spermiogenesis are removed during the process of pronuclear formation. Second, one critical aspect of this process, decondensation of the sperm nucleus, has been investigated under *in vitro* conditions (e.g., Mahi and Yanagimachi, 1975). The ability to mimic some of the *in vivo* events may provide the means for more biochemical studies. Finally, the successful formation of a male pronucleus is apparently dependent upon developmental stage-specific oocyte factors. This provides a potential endpoint for studies that examine the role of the oocyte's cytoplasm in the progression of events after fertilization.

1. Morphological and Molecular Aspects of Male Pronucleus Formation in Vivo

The sequence of the critical events in the formation of the male pronucleus is as follows: (1) breakdown of the sperm nuclear membrane, (2) decondensation of the tightly compacted sperm chromatin, (3) turnover of protamine-like proteins, (4) deposition of histones, (5) formation of the pronuclear membrane, and (6) onset of DNA synthesis. As will become evident in the following discussion, each of the events, with the possible exception of some degree of decondensation (Berrios and Bedford, 1979), appears to be dependent upon completion of the preceding event.

Studies in which staining procedures have been used to monitor the species of nuclear proteins in association with the sperm nucleus have suggested that the protamine-like proteins are lost from the sperm nucleus shortly after entry into the oocyte cytoplasm (Alfert, 1958). The fate of sperm proteins has been assessed directly in the mouse by several experimental approaches. Mice whose sperm were labeled *in vivo* with [³H]arginine were used to fertilize superovulated females *in vivo* (Ecklund and Levine, 1975) and *in vitro* (Kopecny and Pavlok, 1975a). The arginine-labeled proteins in the nucleus of the fertilizing sperm were detected by light microscopic autoradiography. After completion of anaphase II of the second meiotic division, before extrusion of the second polar body, no radioactivity was observed in association with the sperm nucleus. Similarly, antibodies to mouse sperm basic proteins failed to detect antigenic sites in swollen sperm heads in the cytoplasm of ova at telophase II (Rodman *et al.*, 1981). It is impossible to infer when removal of the protamine-like proteins is complete, however, in light of the low sensitivity of detection of these methods.

It appears reasonably well established that, at the one-cell stage in the mouse, the embryonic genome is complexed with histones in a nucleosomal organization (Hughes *et al.*, 1979; Petrov *et al.*, 1980). It has not been resolved how and when histones are deposited upon the DNA of the male genome. [³H]Arginine has been shown to be incorporated into proteins that associate with both swollen sperm heads and female chromosomes at anaphase and telophase of the second meiotic division (Kopecny and Pavlok, 1975b). This implies an association of newly synthesized basic proteins with the decondensing sperm nucleus at approximately the time that the protamine-like proteins have been removed (Kopecny and Pavlok, 1975b). It is not known if these proteins are histones. Using antisera containing antibodies to protamines (and to other sperm nuclear components) and to histones H2B and H4, Rod-man *et al.* (1981) reported that there is an interval between the removal of protamines and the appearance of histones in the sperm component of the mouse zygote. The investigators proposed that this indicates the existence of a period of time when the chromatin is devoid of basic nuclear proteins. If true, this would seem to represent a most unique situation, since even in rapidly dividing cells, histones are deposited almost immediately upon the DNA (e.g., McKnight and Miller, 1977, 1979; Laird *et al.*, 1976; Jackson and Chalkley, 1981). Since the antisera used in these studies have not been well characterized immunologically, it cannot be inferred to what extent this unusual staining pattern reflects protamine turnover.

The origin and time of synthesis of the histones that associate with the developing male pronucleus has not been established unequivocally. The experimental approaches used to examine this question have involved a determination of the incorporation of lysine or arginine into proteins before and after fertilization. Studies examining the fate of proteins labeled with [^{3}H]lysine during various stages of meiotic maturation in rabbit oocytes revealed that the labeled proteins were retained in the ooplasm during early pronuclear development and became associated with male and female pronuclei that were fully developed (Motlik *et al.*, 1980). In the previously discussed studies on mouse (Kopecny and Pavlok, 1975b), labeling of pronuclei was seen when the radioactive precursors were added after fertilization. The problem with these studies is that it was not possible to demonstrate that the labeling seen over the pronuclei represented histone molecules.

Biochemical studies examining directly the synthesis of histones throughout late meiotic stages and at fertilization in the rabbit indicated that histones are synthesized at all stages thus far studied (Matheson and Schultz, 1980). In mouse, although the rate of histone H4 synthesis decreases during meiotic prophase and sufficient histones are present to support two or three cell divisions (Wassarman and Mrozak, 1981), there is clear evidence for synthesis of histones at all stages (Kaye and Wales, 1981). The possibility is thus raised that the histones deposited on the forming pronuclei could be newly synthesized. This should be considered in light of the observation in amphibian eggs where stored histones associate with the developing pronuclei (Woodland and Adamson, 1977). Although it has not been demonstrated definitively, it is likely that the histones associated with the developing pronuclei are of oocyte origin, since, as discussed in greater detail in later sections, the deposition of histones appears to precede the onset of transcription of the embryonic genomes in mammalian zygotes.

2. In Vitro Analysis of Events of Male Pronuclear Formation

The one aspect of pronuclear formation that has been accessible to *in vitro* analysis is that of sperm decondensation. The properties of *in vitro* decondensation of sperm nuclei have been explored in a wide variety of chemical and enzymatic conditions. These experiments have emphasized two aspects of the structure and function of mammalian sperm chromatin. In the first, there is an emphasis on examination of the properties of sperm chromatin during spermiogenesis and epididymal maturation as reflected by biochemically detectable changes in relative resistance to experimentally induced decondensation and chromatin dispersion. The second goal has been to elucidate the biochemical mechanisms of the decondensation and protein turnover that occur *in vivo* after fertilization. While the results have provided a reasonably extensive background of information regarding methods for experimentally decondensing sperm nuclei, the extent to which any of these methods reflect the *in vivo* situation remains to be determined.

It is believed that the extensive disulfide bonding of the cysteine residues of mammalian sperm chromatin provides an almost keratin-like quality quite resistant to the effects of outside agents (Calvin and Bedford, 1971). A summary of the various methods utilized in sperm decondensation *in vitro* is presented in Table II. The species listed therein—mouse, hamster, rat, rabbit, and human—were selected either because they are most frequently used in fertilization experiments or, as in the case of the human, because they are of obvious importance. It is interesting to note that the ease with which decondensation is accomplished varies among species. A recurrent feature is the combination of a reducing agent, such as dithiothreitol or 2-mercaptoethanol, and a displacing agent, whether chemical (urea) or enzymatic (trypsin).

Clearly, the extreme conditions of most of the *in vitro* chemical decondensation methodologies, such as 8 M urea or 1% SDS with 5 mM DTT (Table II), may mimic but could not possibly reflect the biology of *in vivo* decondensation. In an effort to circumvent such obviously nonphysiological conditions, a series of studies was undertaken to examine the possible involvement of endogeneous proteolytic enzymes in protamine breakdown (Marushige and Marushige, 1975, 1978; Chang and Zirkin, 1978; Zirkin *et al.*, 1980). Proteolytic degradation of protamines

TABLE II

In Vitro Decondensation of Sperm Nuclei from Five Mammalian Species[a]

Species	Starting condition of nuclei	Treatment	Observations	Reference
Mouse	Heads with acrosome intact	Hanks BSS; 10 mM Tris-HCl, pH 7.4; RT	No decondensation	Gall and Ohsumi, 1976
Mouse	Heads with acrosome intact	+20 mM DTT	Intact up to 8 hours	Gall and Ohsumi, 1976
Mouse	Heads with acrosome intact	+100 µg/ml trypsin	Intact up to 8 hours	Gall and Ohsumi, 1976
Mouse	Heads with acrosome intact	+20 mM DTT; 100 µg/ml trypsin	Decondensation by 30 minutes	Gall and Ohsumi, 1976
Mouse	Heads with acrosome intact	+1–10 mM 2-mercaptoethanol; then 100 µg/ml trypsin	Decondensation by 30 minutes	Gall and Ohsumi, 1976
Mouse	Heads with acrosome intact	+0.5–10 mM reduced glutathione; then 100 µg/ml trypsin	Decondensation by 30 minutes	Gall and Ohsumi, 1976
Mouse	Heads with acrosome intact	+20 mM DTT; then 200 µg/ml pronase, chymotrypsin, or papain	Decondensation by 30 minutes	Gall and Ohsumi, 1976
Mouse	Heads with acrosome intact	+20 mM DTT; then MNase, DNase I, β-glucuronidase, neuraminidase or phospholipase A and C	No decondensation	Gall and Ohsumi, 1976
Mouse	Heads with acrosome intact	+20 mM DTT; then 1% NP40, 1% Triton X-100, or 3 M guanidine hydrochloride	Decondensation by 30 minutes	Gall and Ohsumi, 1976
Mouse	Heads with acrosome intact	+20 mM DTT; then 2 M KCl	Decondensation by 30 minutes	Gall and Ohsumi, 1976

Mouse	Heads with acrosome intact	+20 mM DTT; then 0.5 M KCl	No decondensation	Gall and Ohsumi, 1976
Rat	"Acrosome-free" sperm heads	8M Urea; 5 mM DTT; 10 mM Tris-HCl, pH 7.4; 1 mM PMSF; 8 hours; 26° C	70% of nuclei decondensed	Sobhon et al., 1981
Rat	"Acrosome-free" sperm heads	As above, then digestion in 25 mM sucrose; 1 mM CaCl$_2$; 10 mM tri-ethanolamine-HCl, pH 7.4; 1 mM PMSF; 125 units/ml MNase; 6 hours; 37° C	70% of nuclei decondensed	Sobhon et al., 1981
Rat	Intact spermatozoa	0.045% NaCl; 30 minutes; 37° C	No decondensation	Mahi and Yanagimachi, 1976
Rat	Intact spermatozoa	+0.2 M DTT; 0.5% SDS	Extensive decondensation by 30 minutes	Mahi and Yanagimachi, 1976
Rat	Intact spermatozoa	+100 mM 2-mercaptoethanol; 0.5% SDS	Extensive decondensation by 30 minutes	Mahi and Yanagimachi, 1976
Rat	Intact spermatozoa	+1 M L-cysteine; 0.5% SDS	Extensive decondensation by 30 minutes	Mahi and Yanagimachi, 1976
Rat	Intact spermatozoa	+0.8 M thioglycolate, pH 9.0	Extensive decondensation by 30 minutes	Mahi and Yanagimachi, 1976
Rat	Intact spermatozoa	+0.5 M (NH$_4$)$_2$S	Extensive decondensation by 30 minutes	Mahi and Yanagimachi, 1976
Rat	Intact spermatozoa	+0.5 M K$_2$S	Extensive decondensation by 30 minutes	Mahi and Yanagimachi, 1976
Rat	Intact spermatozoa	+0.1 M Na$_2$S	Extensive decondensation by 30 minutes	Mahi and Yanagimachi, 1976

(continued)

TABLE II—*Continued*

Species	Starting condition of nuclei	Treatment	Observations	Reference
Rat	Intact spermatozoa	+1 M KOH	Extensive decondensation by 30 minutes	Mahi and Yanagimachi, 1976
Rat	Intact spermatozoa	+0.8 M NaOH	Extensive decondensation by 30 minutes	Mahi and Yanagimachi, 1976
Rat	Intact spermatozoa	+2 M KCN	Extensive decondensation by 30 minutes	Mahi and Yanagimachi, 1976
Rat	Intact spermatozoa	+7 M NH$_4$OH	No decondensation	Mahi and Yanagimachi, 1976
Hamster	Intact spermatozoa	0.045% NaCl; 30 minutes 37° C	No decondensation	Mahi and Yanagimachi, 1976
Hamster	Intact spermatozoa	+ 2 mM DTT; 0.5% SDS	Extensive decondensation by 30 minutes	Mahi and Yanagimachi, 1976
Hamster	Intact spermatozoa	+0.1 M 2-mercaptoethanol; 0.5% SDS	Extensive decondensation by 30 minutes	Mahi and Yanagimachi, 1976
Hamster	Intact spermatozoa	+1 M L-cysteine; 0.5% SDS	Extensive decondensation by 30 minutes	Mahi and Yanagimachi, 1976
Hamster	Intact spermatozoa	+0.8 M thioglycolate	Extensive decondensation by 30 minutes	Mahi and Yanagimachi, 1976
Hamster	Intact spermatozoa	+0.5 M (NH$_4$)$_2$S	Extensive decondensation by 30 minutes	Mahi and Yanagimachi, 1976
Hamster	Intact spermatozoa	+0.1 M K$_2$S	Extensive decondensation by 30 minutes	Mahi and Yanagimachi, 1976
Hamster	Intact spermatozoa	+0.1 M Na$_2$S	Extensive decondensation by 30 minutes	Mahi and Yanagimachi, 1976
Hamster	Intact spermatozoa	+1 M KOH	Extensive decondensation by 30 minutes	Mahi and Yanagimachi, 1976
Hamster	Intact spermatozoa	+1 M NaOH	Extensive decondensation by 30 minutes	Mahi and Yanagimachi, 1976

Species	Material	Treatment	Result	Reference
Hamster	Intact spermatozoa	+2 M KCN	Extensive decondensation by 30 minutes	Mahi and Yanagimachi, 1976
Hamster	Intact spermatozoa	+7 M NH$_4$OH	Slight decondensation	Mahi and Yanagimachi, 1976
Hamster	"Denuded" sperm heads (stripped of "greater part" of acrosomal contents)	20 mM Tris-HCl, pH 8.0; 0.1 M 2-mercaptoethanol; 0–60 minutes; 37° C	Decondensation complete by 60 minutes as assayed by proteolysis of protamines	Marushige and Marushige, 1978
Rabbit	Intact spermatozoa	0.9% SDS; 50 mM Na borate, pH 9.0; 0.27 mg/ml DTT; 15–60 minutes; RT	Uniform decondensation among nuclei; complete by 45 minutes	Bedford et al., 1973
Rabbit	Nuclei (heads treated with 1% Triton X-100)	50 mM Tris-HCl, pH 7.4; 0–90 minutes; 37° C	No decondensation by 90 minutes	Chang and Zirkin, 1978; Zirkin et al., 1980
Rabbit	Nuclei (heads treated with 1% Triton X-100)	+5 mM DTT; 1% Triton X-100	Decondensation 95% complete by 90 minutes	Chang and Zirkin, 1978; Zirkin et al., 1980
Rabbit	Nuclei (heads treated with 1% Triton X-100)	50 mM Tris-HCl, pH 7.4; 0–90 minutes; 37° C; 5 mM DTT; 1% Triton X-100; trypsin inhibitors	No decondensation by 90 minutes	Chang and Zirkin, 1978; Zirkin et al., 1980
Rabbit	Intact spermatozoa	0.045% NaCl; 30 minutes; 37° C	No decondensation	Mahi and Yanagimachi, 1976
Rabbit	Intact spermatozoa	+20 mM DTT; 0.5% SDS	Complete decondensation by 30 minutes	Mahi and Yanagimachi, 1976
Rabbit	Intact spermatozoa	+0.1 M 2-mercaptoethanol; 0.5% SDS	Complete decondensation by 30 minutes	Mahi and Yanagimachi, 1976
Rabbit	Intact spermatozoa	+1 M L-cysteine; 0.5% SDS	Complete decondensation by 30 minutes	Mahi and Yanagimachi, 1976
Rabbit	Intact spermatozoa	+0.8 M thioglycolate	Complete decondensation by 30 minutes	Mahi and Yanagimachi, 1976
Rabbit	Intact spermatozoa	+0.5 M (NH$_4$)$_2$S	Complete decondensation by 30 minutes	Mahi and Yanagimachi, 1976
Rabbit	Intact spermatozoa	+0.25 M K$_2$S	Complete decondensation by 30 minutes	Mahi and Yanagimachi, 1976

(continued)

TABLE II—*Continued*

Species	Starting condition of nuclei	Treatment	Observations	Reference
Rabbit	Intact spermatozoa	+0.05 M Na$_2$S	Complete decondensation by 30 minutes	Mahi and Yanagimachi, 1976
Rabbit	Intact spermatozoa	+0.8 M KOH	Complete decondensation by 30 minutes	Mahi and Yanagimachi, 1976
Rabbit	Intact spermatozoa	+0.8 M NaOH	Complete decondensation by 30 minutes	Mahi and Yanagimachi, 1976
Rabbit	Intact spermatozoa	+1 M KCN	Complete decondensation by 30 minutes	Mahi and Yanagimachi, 1976
Rabbit	Intact spermatozoa	+4 M NH$_4$OH	Slight decondensation	Mahi and Yanagimachi, 1976
Rabbit	"Denuded" sperm heads (stripped of "greater part of acrosomal contents")	20 mM Tris-HCl, pH 8.0; 0.1 M 2-mercaptoethanol; 0–2 hours; 37° C	Decondensation complete by 60 minutes as assayed by proteolysis of protamines	Marushige and Marushige, 1978
Rabbit	Intact heads	50 mM Tris-HCl, pH 7.4; 1% Triton X-100; 24 hours; RT	No decondensation	Young, 1979
Rabbit	Intact heads	+5 mM DDT	Decondensation by 60 minutes	Young, 1979
Rabbit	Acrosome-free nuclei	+5 mM DTT	No decondensation	Young, 1979
Human	Intact sperm	0.2–0.4 M alkaline thioglycolate (pH 9.0); 1–5 minutes; RT	Decondensation by 5 minutes	Lung, 1972

Human	Intact sperm	0.9% SDS; 50 mM Na borate, pH 9.0; 0.27 mg/ml DTT; 15–60 minutes; RT	Highly heterogeneous decondensation among sperm in sample and between samples; complete by 60 minutes	Bedford et al., 1973
Human	Nuclei (stripped of acrosome by treatment with 1.5% Sarkosyl; 60 minutes; RT)	Nuclei pelleted through 60% sucrose	Peripheral boundaries intact; "some swelling"	Evenson et al., 1978
Human	Nuclei (stripped of acrosome by treatment with 1.5% Sarkosyl; 60 minutes; RT)	+50 mM Tris-HCl, pH 7.5; 20 mM DTT; 20′-2 hours; RT	Majority partially decondensed by 20 minutes; most by 2 hours; presence of "chromatin bodies" in both	Evenson et al., 1978
Human	Nuclei (stripped of acrosome by treatment with 1.5% Sarkosyl; 60 minutes; RT)	Nuclei pelleted through 60% sucrose; then 50 mM Tris-HCl, pH 7.5; 20 mM DTT; 20 minutes to 2 hours; RT; 100 μg/ml trypsin	Mostly decondensed; "chromatin bodies" disrupted by 20 minutes	Evenson et al., 1978
Human	Nuclei (stripped of acrosome)	8 M urea; 1% 2-mercaptoethanol; 10 mM Tris-HCl, pH 7.4; 1 mM PMSF; 15 minutes; RT	Majority of nuclei retain shape with only patches of decondensation	Tanphaichitr et al., 1981
Human	Nuclei (stripped of acrosome)	+0.2 M NaCl	Nuclei heavily swollen	Tanphaichitr et al., 1981

[a] Abbreviations: PMSF, phenylmethylsulfonyl fluoride; SDS, sodium dodecyl sulfate; DTT, dithiothreitol; RT, room temperature (22°–25° C); MNase, micrococcal nuclease.

by an enzyme has been detected in the sperm head fraction of both bull and rabbit spermatozoa (Chang and Zirkin, 1978; Marushige and Marushige, 1978). In the bull, the morphological pattern of dispersion of sperm chromatin resembled the pattern of decondensation of the fertilizing sperm within the egg cytoplasm: dispersion commenced in the periphery of the posterior half of the sperm nucleus and proceeded to anterior and core regions (Marushige and Marushige, 1978). Biochemically, the degradation process yielded a heterogeneous series of arginine-rich peptides of molecular weights ranging from 400 to 1500 D. The degradative enzyme activity was ascribed to a component of acrosin which is located close to the nuclear surface and which becomes associated with nuclear chromatin during structural alterations of the sperm nucleus. Under similar conditions of thiol-induced proteolysis, analagous results were obtained with rabbit, hamster, and guinea pig sperm (Chang and Zirkin, 1978; Marushige and Marushige, 1978) but not with rat sperm (Marushige and Marushige, 1978).

An important feature, if such an enzymatic activity is to be considered of biological relevance at fertilization, is that the activity be associated with the sperm nucleus; that is, it is unlikely that components of the acrosome, for example, would be involved in turnover of sperm chromatin within the fertilized ovum since the acrosome does not enter the egg cytoplasm (see discussion in Young, 1979). By altering the washing conditions of sperm heads, Young (1979) obtained completely "denuded" sperm heads (acrosome fragment-free). These sperm nuclei did not decondense in the presence of a reducing agent alone as had been reported previously (Chang and Zirkin, 1978; Marushige and Marushige, 1978; Table II). This raises the possibility that the proteolytic degradation of sperm nuclear components was due to contaminating acrosin of extranuclear origin. Subsequent studies have not resolved this question in that further characterization of this enzymatic activity revealed that it is quite similar to acrosin (Zirkin *et al.*, 1980). Indeed, purified acrosin digestion of rabbit protamines produced a pattern of digestion products that are similar to the putative decondensation enzyme products. Demonstration of the presence of such an activity in the intact sperm nucleus is thus required before any role can be ascribed to this enzyme during fertilization.

An important prediction obtained from the *in vitro* studies summarized in Table II is that there exists a source of sulfhydryl groups at the time of fertilization. The question of whether the ovum might provide the source for both the reducing and proteolytic activities probably required for decondensation is important and has received very little attention in mammalian systems. Even in amphibia, where the existence of cytoplasmic "factors" responsible for decondensation and male pronucleus formation have been described extensively (reviewed in Masui and Clarke, 1979), the biochemical nature of such factors remains undetermined. Given the paucity of mammalian ova that can be obtained at the appropriate stages, it is likely that it will be some time before sperm decondensation factors will be identified. Important steps in this direction were made recently by the direct demonstration of the capacity of ovulated rabbit ova to generate a reducing agent (Wiesel and Schultz, 1981). However, direct proof of the involvement of these molecules in pronuclear formation *in vivo* is lacking. A recent study of Miller and Masui (1982) would suggest that, at least in mouse, reduction of disulfide bonds occurs when the sperm established a pronase-resistant binding to the egg membrane, that is, prior to penetration into the vitellus. This observation will require further confirmation, however, since other investigators have suggested that changes in staining intensity of sperm nuclei, which is believed to be correlated to the extent to disulfide bond formation, occurs only after entry into the egg cytoplasm (Krzanowska, 1982).

Finally, it should be noted that the *in vitro* systems described above and listed in Table II are addressing only one or, at best, two aspects of male pronucleus formation—that of decondensation and removal of the protamine-like proteins. The studies address neither the critical steps of nuclear membrane disassembly and formation nor the mechanism of deposition of somatic histones on the sperm genome.

3. Acquisition by the Oocyte of the Ability to Form Mal⁻ Pronuclei

It has been recognized for some time that immature oocytes are not capable of normal pronuclear formation (Thibault and Gerard, 1970; Thibault *et al.*, 1975, 1976). The levels at which this block to pronuclear formation is manifested are not clear, even with respect to morphological changes. Complicating efforts to examine this apparent stage specificity of oocytes is the fact that "maturity" achieved *in vitro* does not reflect completely the normal *in vivo* maturation process with respect to developmental potential.

a. Germinal Vesicle Breakdown. The single most widely documented requirement for efficient pronuclear formation would appear to be breakdown of the germinal vesicle. This is seen regardless of whether sperm nuclei were introduced by typical fertilization or experimentally (Iwamatsu and Chang, 1972; Thadani, 1979; Berrios and Bedford, 1979; Usui and Yanagimachi, 1976; Thibault *et al.*, 1975, 1976;

Thibault and Gerard, 1970; Uehara and Yanagimachi, 1976; Niwa and Chang, 1973, 1975). Although mouse and rat ovarian oocytes with intact germinal vesicles can be penetrated by spermatozoa, particularly when the surrounding follicular cells are removed (Niwa and Chang, 1975), transformation of the fertilizing sperm into a male pronucleus has been shown to be retarded or to fail completely (Niwa and Chang, 1975; Iwamatsu and Chang, 1972). Hamster oocytes with intact germinal vesicles appear to be more readily penetrated by sperm, but, again, pronuclear formation is defective (Usui and Yanagimachi, 1976). The one mammal that appears to be an exception is the dog: canine ovarian oocytes fertilized *in vitro* were shown to be capable of decondensing sperm (Mahi and Yanagimachi, 1976); however, it is not known whether pronuclei were formed.

Similarly, placement of sperm into oocytes by microinjection showed that sperm nuclei remained intact unless germinal vesicle breakdown occurred (Thadani, 1979). In this study, an important distinction was made between a visible decondensation of the sperm nucleus and actual male pronucleus formation. Some decondensation of sperm chromatin has been reported in studies on germinal vesicle-intact rabbit oocytes fertilized *in vivo,* but critical events such as breakdown of the sperm nuclear membrane failed to occur (Berrios and Bedford, 1979). The ability to dissociate the nuclear membrane and totally decondense the penetrating sperm appears to be acquired gradually between germinal vesicle breakdown and formation of the metaphase II oocyte: most efficient decondensation is obtained when the meiotic processes are complete (Iwamatsu and Chang, 1972; Thibault *et al.,* 1976; Thadani, 1979). Decondensation would thus appear to be governed by factors that increase in amount (or activity) during the period of meiotic progression to metaphase II.

b. **Cytoplasmic Maturation.** Apparently even more sensitive to the maturational state of the oocyte is the phenomenon of functional pronucleus formation. Varying levels of decondensation and pronuclear formation can be achieved in oocytes that have been removed from follicles with the germinal vesicle intact and that have undergone meiotic maturation *in vitro.* However, the ability to support development appears to require factors present in metaphase II oocytes matured within the follicle (Chang, 1955; Thibault, 1977). Although there have been a few scattered reports of production of liveborns from oocytes matured *in vitro* (Cross and Brinster, 1970; Mukherjee, 1972), the majority of studies on fertilization of *in vitro*-matured oocytes reveal that meiotic maturation in culture media yields oocytes defective in factors necessary for ensuing pronuclear and embryonic development. Since few or no differences are seen in the progression of cytogenetic phenomena, these observations suggest that maturation is actually comprised of two parts—the meiotic progression (nuclear maturation) and the appearance of cytoplasmic factors necessary for development (cytoplasmic maturation).

The concept of the necessity of cytoplasmic maturation has been particularly emphasized by Thibault and co-workers (see Thibault, 1977, and references therein). Their efforts have been directed toward elucidation of the role of both the hormonal environment and the surrounding follicle cells on the ability of the oocyte to form the male pronucleus. In the rabbit, administration of testosterone or prolactin to *in vitro*-cultured follicles yielded oocytes capable of being fertilized and undergoing cleavage (Thibault *et al.*, 1975, 1976). They ascribed to this ability a "male pronucleus growth factor" (MPGF). In human oocytes, Soupart (1974) reported that culture of human oocytes first in estradiol and then in 17β-hydroxyprogesterone—a hormonal sequence that mimics the *in vivo* situation—yielded oocytes apparently capable of forming a male pronucleus. Whether the pronuclei thus formed were capable of supporting normal embryonic development could obviously not be ascertained. However, in a recent study by Nishimoto *et al.* (1982), pronuclei were formed in human oocytes matured *in vitro* in a chemically defined medium to which no exogenous hormones had been added. The authors did note some apparent variation in efficiency of penetration, depending upon the stage of the menstrual cycle of the individuals from whom the ovaries were recovered. In light of the scanty data available, even at the ultrastructural level, on the normal progression of the events in human fertilization, caution should be used in interpreting these observations.

4. Biological Universality of Egg Factors Involved in Pronuclear Formation.

An interesting corollary regarding the role of oocyte factors in male pronucleus formation has emerged recently. While some level of stage specificity with respect to appearance of such factors appears to be a widely observed phenomenon, a surprising amount of lack of species specificity of these factors has been noted. There are a few commonly known examples of the ability of the sperm of one species to fertilize and activate embryonic development of the oocyte of another species. This can result in viable offspring as in, for example, the production of a mule or hinny. The relatively recent use of two experimental approaches, namely (1) introduction of sperm by microsurgical techniques and (2) fertilization of zona-free eggs, has greatly expanded our understanding of the extent to which oocyte factors from one species can apparently form pronuclei from the sperm of evolutionarily quite separate species.

Results of studies in which these methods have been used in heterospecific combinations of selected mammals are summarized in Table III. Because of the technical difficulties involved with microinjection, the zona-free system has been used more frequently. In one of the earlier studies employing zona-free ova, ovulated ova of mice, rats, and golden hamsters were treated with hyaluronidase and trypsin or pronase to produce cumulus- and zona-free ova (Hanada and Chang, 1972). As noted in Table III, the zona-free eggs were then exposed to capacitated sperm from each of the three species. Although the extent of pronuclear formation varied, depending upon the nature of the combination, clearly interspecific decondensation and apparently normal pronuclear formation was possible (Hanada and Chang, 1972). Of the interspecies combinations thus far reported, ovulated hamster oocytes represent the most extensively used experimental system. Meiotically mature hamster oocytes have been shown to be capable of supporting the development of a male pronucleus from human sperm introduced by microinjection (Uehara and Yanagimachi, 1976) or by removal of the zona pellucida prior to exposure to capacitated spermatozoa (Yanagimachi *et al.*, 1976; Rogers *et al.*, 1979; Barros *et al.*, 1978; Binor *et al.*, 1980). For reasons that remain totally obscure, the human sperm–hamster oocyte combination appears to support development of pronuclei (Yanagimachi *et al.*, 1976), whereas a rat sperm–hamster oocyte combination does not (Hanada and Chang, 1972).

Caution should be used in assessing the biological implications of three aspects of this otherwise potentially very useful system (e.g., Rudak *et al.*, 1978; Rogers *et al.*, 1979; Binor *et al.*, 1980). First, as noted above, the extent to which an oocyte from any one species can accomplish pronuclear formation varies depending upon the species of the "fertilizing" sperm. Second, the progression of pronuclear formation is not dependent on the sperm per se since the same sperm in different oocyte cytoplasms behaves differently. Third, and probably most important, the extent to which such interspecies combinations accomplish all the events of pronuclear formation has not been established rigorously. Although decondensation of the sperm head (Rogers *et al.*, 1979) and visualization of the haploid chromosome complement (Rudak *et al.*, 1978) have been described, direct demonstration of a functional pronucleus capable of DNA synthesis and further development has not been established as far as this author is aware. The

TABLE III

Extent of Pronuclear Formation in Interspecific Sperm–Egg Combinations

Sperm	Egg	Method	Observations	Reference
Rat epid.[a] or uterine	Mouse	Zona-free	5% penetrated; decondensation of those penetrated; no pronuclei	Hanada and Chang, 1972
Hamster epid.	Mouse	Zona-free	2% penetrated; decondensation of those penetrated; no pronuclei	Hanada and Chang, 1972
Human ejac.[a]	Mouse	Zona-free	None penetrated	Quinn, 1979
Rat epid.	Mouse	Zona-free	20% penetrated; pronuclear formation not discussed	Quinn, 1979
Deer mouse epid.	Mouse	Intact	20% penetrated; no pronuclei	Fukuda et al., 1979
Hamster epid.	Rat	Zona-free	9% penetrated; decondensation of those penetrated; no pronuclei	Hanada and Chang, 1972
Mouse epid.	Rat	Zona-free	95% penetrated; male and female pronuclei	Hanada and Chang, 1972
Mouse epid.	Rat	Zona-free	50% penetrated; 25% to two-cell embryos	Quinn, 1979
Human ejac.	Rat	Zona-free	None penetrated	Quinn, 1979

(continued)

TABLE III—*Continued*

Sperm	Egg	Method	Observations	Reference
Mouse epid.	Rat	Zona-free	50% penetrated and with pronuclei (sperm at 1×10^6/ml); 10% embryos; 80% penetrated and with pronuclei (sperm at 1×10^4/ml); 80% two-cell embryos	Thadani, 1980
Mouse epid.	Rat	Microinjected	67–73% of those surviving microinjection had pronuclei; occasional two-cell embryos	Thadani, 1980
Deer mouse epid.	Rat	Microinjected	88% with pronuclei	Thadani, 1980
Rat epid., preincubated	Rabbit	Zona-free	92% penetrated; pronuclei not discussed	Hanada and Chang, 1976
Mouse epid., preincubated	Rabbit	Zona-free	67% penetrated between 1–11 hours postinsemination	Hanada and Chang, 1976
Rat epid. or uterine	Hamster	Zona-free	8–26% penetrated; decondensation of those penetrated; no pronuclei	Hanada and Chang, 1972
Guinea pig epid., not preincubated	Hamster	Zona-free	None penetrated	Yanagimachi, 1972
Guinea pig epid., preincubated	Hamster	Zona-free	100% penetrated; 1–6 pronuclei per egg	Yanagimachi, 1972
Rat epid., preincubated	Hamster	Zona-free	36–97% penetrated; 33–86% resume meiosis	Hanada and Chang, 1976

Mouse epid.	Zona-free	40% (1 hour) to 91% (2.5 hours) penetrated postinsemination; 67–85% resume meiosis	Hanada and Chang, 1976
Guinea pig, preincubated	Zona-free	All decondensed	Barros and Herrera, 1977
Human ejac. preincubated[b]	Zona-free	70–95% penetrated; "many" decondensed sperm heads and pronuclei	Yanagimachi et al., 1976
Human ejac. preincubated[b]	Zona-free	Complete decondensation; pronuclei	Barros et al., 1978
Human ejac. preincubated[b]	Zona-free	75% penetrated; 50% decondensation and haploid chromosomes visualized	Rudak et al., 1978
Human ejac. preincubated[b]	Zona-free	14–100% decondensation	Rogers et al., 1979
Human ejac. preincubated[b]	Zona-free	80%–100% decondensation or pronuclei (sperm conc. optimum, 3×10^6 motile sperm/ml)	Binor et al., 1980
Human ejac. preincubated[b]	Zona-free	23–89% penetrated; 60% decondensation or pronuclei	Tyler et al., 1981
Human ejac. washed	Microinjected	50–72% decondensation or pronuclei	Uehara and Yanagimachi, 1976

[a] epid., epididymal; ejac., ejaculated.
[b] Only fertile males.

importance of this distinction lies in the fact that, as noted in earlier discussion, it is these later stages of pronuclear formation that are most sensitive to control by oocyte factors. One might speculate, therefore, that such factors would probably be important for activation of normal embryonic development.

IV. MACROMOLECULAR SYNTHETIC ACTIVITIES FOLLOWING FERTILIZATION

Profound alterations in the pattern of gene expression accompany early embryonic development in mammals. Whereas amphibian embryos, for example, can proceed through several cell divisions in the absence of transcriptional activity by the embryo, mouse zygotes are arrested at two to four cells in the presence of inhibitors of RNA synthesis (reviewed in Johnson, 1981). Furthermore, since transcriptional activity clearly occurs by the two-cell stage and probably earlier, at least in mouse zygotes (Clegg and Pikó, 1982), distinction should be made between the ability of the zygote to undergo one or two cell divisions and the ability to trigger and continue the program for normal embryonic development. Protein synthesis is known to occur immediately following fertilization in all of the mammalian species in which it has been studied (Sherman, 1979; Magnuson and Epstein, 1981). Identification and characterization of discrete changes in the patterns of proteins synthesized have been enhanced tremendously by the recent use of high-resolution, two-dimensional gel electrophoresis and exquisitely sensitive methods for separating and detecting polypeptides. Mouse and rabbit ova and embryos have been analyzed in some detail with respect to changes in the patterns of polypeptides being synthesized at the time of and immediately following fertilization. Notably absent are comparably detailed observations on the RNA synthetic activities at concomitant stages of development of these species. Finally, neither protein nor RNA synthesis has been characterized in the ova and embryos of higher primates, including man.

A. Changes in Polypeptide Patterns following Fertilization.

The observations presented here will describe only very briefly changes in the patterns of polypeptides and rates of protein synthesis that occur at fertilization. This topic has been reviewed in detail by Sherman (1979), Johnson (1981), and Magnuson and Epstein (1981), among others. Initial attempts to detect qualitative and quantitative differences in the patterns of proteins synthesized by the ovulated ovum, zygote, and two-cell embryo in the mouse were only partially successful. With the exception of one study by Schultz et al. (1979), the majority of analyses of overall rates of total protein synthesis detect only slight changes at the time of fertilization. A net increase in protein synthesis was demonstrated to occur as the two-cell embryo develops to eight cells (e.g., Monesi and Salfi, 1967; Tasca and Hillman, 1970; Brinster, 1971; Abreu and Brinster, 1978). Recently, more sensitive detection procedures and higher resolution techniques have shown both the appearance of new proteins in one-cell mouse zygotes (Howe and Solter, 1979; Cullen et al., 1980) as well as the production of distinct quantitative changes in the amounts of proteins present (Chen et al., 1980). Some proteins appear and disappear within the first day after fertilization of mouse ova (Cullen et al., 1980). In a quantitative study where the synthesis of 95 individual polypeptides was monitored before and after fertilization, six polypeptide spots showed significant increases in the ratio of their synthesis while 11 appeared to decrease in synthesis (Chen et al., 1980). Thus clear quantitative and qualitative differences can be detected when individual species of polypeptides are examined, although the most notable changes are seen during development from the two-cell to four- to eight-cell stages (e.g., Van Blerkom and Brockway, 1975; Levinson et al., 1978; Handyside and Johnson, 1978; Howe and Solter, 1979).

A slightly different situation appears to exist following fertilization in the rabbit, although it is difficult to draw firm conclusions since the data are far less extensive. In contrast to the changes seen in two-cell mouse embryos, the patterns of polypeptides synthesized by fertilized rabbit ova through to the eight- to 16-cell stages closely resemble those of the unfertilized ovum (Van Blerkom and McGaughey, 1978; Van Blerkom, 1979). Interestingly, a few of the distinct changes that occur at the 16-cell stage appear to be fertilization-autonomous (Van Blerkom, 1979); that is, the new proteins appear at time intervals corresponding to the 16-cell stage regardless of whether fertilization has taken place. An analogous observation was made by Petzholdt et al. (1980) at the two-cell stage in mouse. They compared the proteins synthesized in enucleated-fertilized eggs versus intact two-cell embryos and found that the patterns were remarkably similar whether or not the nucleus was present. The significance of these observations in terms of the role of maternal mRNA in early embryogenesis is discussed in the ensuing section.

B. RNA Synthesis following Fertilization

The most fundamental question of the time of onset of expression of the embryonic mammalian genome remains unanswered. This question may actually be divided into several parts. First, there is the problem of determining when transcription is first detectable. Second, it remains to be established when new mRNAs first appear. Third, it must be shown that new RNAs have some structural or regulatory function, as inferred from the appearance of macromolecules coded for by the embryonic genome or by sensitivity of ensuing development to inhibitors of RNA synthesis.

1. Earliest Detection of Transcriptional Activity

Incorporation of RNA precursors into RNase-sensitive material by two-cell mouse embryos has been clearly established (Mintz, 1964; Bernstein and Mukherjee, 1972; Knowland and Graham, 1972; Moore, 1975). Nascent RNA transcripts were seen by direct visualization of chromatin spreads from mouse (Hughes *et al.,* 1979; Petrov *et al.,* 1980) and rabbit two-cell embryos (Cotton *et al.,* 1980). However, the question of when transcription first occurs following fertilization is still a matter of controversy. Mintz (1964) reported incorporation of [³H]uridine (and [³H]cytidine and [³H]adenosine) into the pronuclei of mouse zygotes. Several subsequent studies failed to detect synthesis. No RNA polymerase activity was detected in the *in vitro* assays described by Moore (1975) in which [³H]UMP is used as a substrate. In the chromatin visualization studies of Hughes *et al.* (1979), no mention was made of the presence of nascent RNA transcripts in the pronuclei. Although a low level of [³H-uridine incorporation occurred in one-cell mouse zygotes within 3 hours postfertilization, no label could be detected over pronuclei following autoradiography (Young *et al.,* 1978). In this study, the site of RNA synthetic activity was postulated to be a polar body, although direct experimental proof of this contention was not presented. No incorporation of [³²P]phosphate into RNA by one-cell embryos was detected in experiments by Young and Sweeney (1978), although the possibility that transcription occurred but was not measureable could not be excluded since the [³²P]phosphate was not incorporated into the triphosphates in the α-position. That transcription of pronuclei existed but that the level of synthesis was too low to be detected remained, therefore, a formal possibility (Young *et al.,* 1978; Knowland and Graham, 1972).

Very recently, a study appeared which may partially resolve these discrepancies. Clegg and Pikò (1982), using [³H]adenosine as the radioactive RNA precursor, were able to demonstrate transcriptional activity at the pronuclear stage. The sensitivity of detection of transcription was tremendously enhanced by the fact that [³H]adenosine is taken up ~ 1000 times more efficiently than is [³H]uridine. Thus, at least in the mouse zygote, it does appear that transcription of pronuclei occurs, although how soon after fertilization must still be determined.

2. Characterization of Transcripts Early in Embryogenesis

Only mouse and rabbit embryos have been characterized to any extent with respect to transcription. Several lines of evidence are accumulating that suggest that initiation of synthesis of high-molecular-weight heterodisperse nuclear RNA (hnRNA) and tRNA procedes that of ribosomal RNA precursors. Synthesis of polyadenylated RNA transcribed from the embryonic genome was detected as early as the two-cell stage in mouse by affinity chromatography to oligo(dT)cellulose (Levey *et al.*, 1978). In studies visualizing transcription complexes in mouse embryos, Hughes *et al.* (1979) reported nascent hnRNA-type transcripts in two-cell embryos but failed to detect rRNA-type transcription complexes until the four- to eight-cell stage. Biochemical analyses, however, suggest that rRNA precursor molecules can be resolved at the two-cell stage (Knowland and Graham, 1972; Clegg and Pikó, 1982). Cytogenetic analysis in which silver-staining methods were used to detect transcriptionally active nucleolus organizer regions revealed positive chromosome staining at the two-cell stage (Engel *et al.*, 1977).

In the rabbit, early studies indicated the existence of a period (up to the 16-cell stage) during which no RNA synthesis could be detected (Manes, 1969). More recently, visulatization of chromatin has revealed that nascent non-rRNA transcripts can be found from the two- to four-cell stage on (Cotton *et al.*, 1980). The failure to detect the presence of newly synthesized molecules in the earlier studies was most likely due to a lower level of sensitivity of detection—a common problem in all of the investigations, as noted previously.

3. Evidence for Functional Transcription

All the biochemical analyses cited above examined total RNA rather than separated nuclear and cytoplasmic components. There exists the possibility that the early transcripts never enter, or are at least delayed in entering, the cytoplasm of the embryo. This would eliminate their serving as functional mRNAs but would still leave open a possible nuclear regulatory role.

One approach which has been used to address the question of the

time of appearance and role of embryonic RNAs involves exposure of
the fertilized ovum to inhibitors of RNA synthesis such as α-amanitin,
actinomycin D, and cordycepin. Two aspects are then examined: (1) the
effects of the inhibition of RNA synthesis on embryonic progression;
and (2) differences in the proteins produced in the presence or absence
of concomitant RNA synthesis. The results of experiments that used
this approach are discussed in much greater detail in reviews by
Schultz and Church (1975), Sherman (1979), and Johnson (1981).

With any experiment in which drugs are used to inhibit a cellular
function, one is faced with the problem of separating pharmacological
and biological effects. In a recent study by Petzholdt *et al.* (1980), the
effects of enucleation of embryos, so that there can be no genomic
contribution, were observed on patterns of protein synthesis. There
were remarkable similarities in the pattern of polypeptides produced
by two-cell embryos with and without nuclei. The investigators suggested that the common proteins, which were fertilization-dependent
with respect to time of appearance, could have resulted from stored or
"masked" mRNAs. Two other investigations lend support to this conclusion. Braude *et al.* (1979) examined the mRNAs of fertilized and
unfertilized mouse eggs by cell-free translation *in vitro*. They found
that unfertilized ova contain mRNAs for proteins that are usually only
expressed after fertilization. These were believed to be of oocyte, not
embryonic, origin, since α-amanitin did not change the polypeptide
pattern. The oocyte origin of these proteins is also supported by the
observations of Petzholdt and Hoppe (1980) who showed that equivalent changes in polypeptide patterns were produced by both fertilized
and parthenogenetically activated embryos. Thus, there is the very
straightforward observation that newly synthesized RNA appears very
early in mouse embryogenesis, most likely at the pronuclear stage and
clearly by the two-cell stage, but there is an ambiguity in determination of the genetic (transcriptional) origin of concomitantly synthesized proteins.

The most direct test of the contribution of the embryonic genomes in
the production of functional mRNAs coding for proteins is the demonstration of the synthesis of the specific polypeptides from these messages. In order to distinguish translation of newly synthesized mRNAs
from translation of stored maternal mRNAs, the most widely used
approach has been to identify manifestations of the gene products
coded for by alleles contributed by the paternal complement. This body
of information, identifying a male genetic contribution by the four- to
eight-cell stage, has been reviewed by Magnuson and Epstein (1981)
and Johnson (1981). However, very recently, evidence has been pre-

sented that demonstrates, for the first time, a contribution of the paternal genome at the two-cell stage (Sawicki *et al.*, 1981). Synthesis of β_2-microglobulin of paternal genetic origin was detected with direct immunoprecipitation and two-dimensional gel electrophoresis. It remains to be determined when, following fertilization, the β_2-microglobulin mRNA is transcribed.

V. CONCLUDING REMARKS

It has been my intent to focus attention on the alterations in genetic activity of the gametes at the time of and immediately following fertilization in mammals. While advances in high resolution of minute quantities of macromolecules, polypeptides in particular, have greatly enhanced our understanding of the biochemistry of very early embryogenesis in the laboratory mouse, there are glaring gaps in our understanding of the activation of development in a general sense. The pronuclear stage, in particular, remains a virtual black box with respect to our understanding of the molecular biology of the changes in chromatin structure and onset of transcription and replication. The role of the oocyte in accomplishing these events is open to speculation. Finally, the available biochemical information regarding early embryogenesis is limited almost exclusively to the mouse, with a small amount of data being available on the rabbit. Given the differences in macromolecular synthetic activities that have been shown between these two species and the recent advent of the use of *in vitro* fertilization and embryo transfer in animal husbandry and in medical practice, the time would seem ripe to extend studies to include other mammals, including primates.

ACKNOWLEDGMENTS

This work was supported by grants from The Irma T. Hirschl Trust and The Andrew W. Mellon Foundation. Special thanks are extended to Brian Gavin and James Eberwine for their help and patience during the preparation of this manuscript.

REFERENCES

Abramczuk, J., and Sawicki, W. (1975). Pronuclear synthesis of DNA in fertilized and parthenogenetically activated mouse eggs. *Exp. Cell Res.* **92**, 361–372.
Abreu, S. L., and Brinster, R. L. (1978). Synthesis of tubulin and actin during the preimplantation development of the mouse. *Exp. Cell Res.* **114**, 135–141.

Alfert, M. (1958). Cytochemische Untersuchungen an basichen Kernproteinen wahrend der Gametenbildung, Befruchtung, und Entwicklung. *Ges. Physiol. Chem. Colloq.* **9,** 73–84.

Barros, C., and Herrera, E. (1977). Ultrastructural observations of the incorporation of guinea pig spermatozoa into zona-free hamster oocytes. *J. Reprod. Fertil.* **49,** 47–50.

Barros, C., Gonzalez, J., Herrera, E., and Bustos-Obregon, E. (1978). Fertilizing capacity of human spermatozoa evaluated by actual penetration of foreign eggs. *Contraception* **17,** 87–92.

Bedford, J. M., Bent, M. J., and Calvin, H. I. (1973). Variations in structural character and stability of the nuclear chromatin in morphologically normal human spermatozoa. *J. Reprod. Fertil.* **33,** 19–29.

Bellvé, A. R. (1979). The molecular biology of mammalian spermatogenesis. *Oxford Rev. Reprod. Biol.* **1,** 159–261.

Bernstein, R. M., and Mukherjee, B. B. (1972). Control of RNA synthesis in 2-cell and 4-cell mouse embryos. *Nature (London)* **238,** 457–459.

Berrios, M., and Bedford, J. M. (1979) Oocyte maturation: Aberrant post-fusion responses of the rabbit primary oocyte to penetrating spermatozoa. *J. Cell Sci.* **39,** 1–12.

Binor, Z., Sokoloski, J. E., and Wolf, D. P. (1980). Penetration of the zona-free hamster egg by human sperm. *Fertil. Steril.* **33,** 321–327.

Bloch, D. P., (1969). A catalog of sperm histones. *Genetics* **61**(1), Suppl., 93–111.

Brackett, B. G., Oh, Y. K., Evans, J. F., and Donawick, W. J. (1980). Fertilization and early development of cow ova. *Biol. Reprod.* **23,** 189–205.

Braude, P. R., Pelham, H. R. B., Flach, G., and Lobatto, R. (1979). Post-transcriptional control in the early mouse embryo. *Nature (London)* **282,** 102–105.

Brinster, R. L. (1971). Uptake and incorporation of amino acids by the pre-implantation mouse embryo. *J. Reprod. Fertil.* **27,** 329–338.

Calvin, H. I. (1976). Comparative analysis of the nuclear basic proteins in rat, human, guinea pig, mouse, and rabbit spermatozoa. *Biochim. Biophys. Acta* **434,** 377–389.

Calvin, H. I., and Bedford, J. M. (1971). Formation of disulfide bonds in the nucleus and accessory structures of mammalian spermatozoa during maturation in the epididymis. *J. Reprod. Fertil.* Suppl. 13, 65–75.

Chang, M. C. (1955). Fertilization and normal development of follicular oocytes in the rabbit. *Science* **121,** 867–869.

Chang, T. S. K., and Zirkin, B. (1978). Proteolytic degradation of protamine during thiol-induced nuclear decondensation in rabbit spermatozoa. *J. Exp. Zool.* **204,** 283–289.

Chen, H. Y., Brinster, R. L., and Merz, E. A. (1980). Changes in protein synthesis following fertilization of the mouse ovum. *J. Exp. Zool.* **212,** 355–360.

Chevaillier, P., and Philippe, M. (1976). In situ detection of a DNA-polymerase activity in the nuclei of mouse spermatozoa. *Chromosoma* **54,** 33–37.

Clegg, K. B., and Pikó, L. (1982). RNA synthesis and cytoplasmic polyadenylation in the one-cell mouse embryo. *Nature (London)* **295,** 342–345.

Coelingh, J. P., and Rozihn, T. H. (1975). Comparative studies on the basic nuclear proteins of mammalian and other spermatozoa. *Biol. J. Linn. Soc.* **7,** 245–256.

Cotton, R. W., Manes, C., and Hamkalo, B. A. (1980). Electron microscopic analysis of RNA transcription in preimplantation rabbit embryos. *Chromosoma* **79,** 169–178.

Cross, P. C., and Brinster, R. L. (1970). *In vitro* development of mouse oocytes. *Biol. Reprod.* **3,** 298–307.

Cullen, B., Emigholz, K., and Monahan, J. (1980). The transient appearance of specific proteins in one-cell mouse embryos. *Dev. Biol.* **76,** 215–221.

Donahue, R. P. (1972). Fertilization of the mouse oocyte: Sequence and timing of the two-cell stage. *J. Exp. Zool.* **180,** 305–318.

Ecklund, P. S., and Levine, L. (1975). Mouse sperm basic nuclear protein. *J. Cell Biol.* **66,** 251–262.

Engel, W., Zenzes, M. T., and Schmid, M. (1977). Activation of mouse ribosomal RNA genes at the two-cell stage. *Hum. Genet.* **38,** 57–63.

Evenson, D. P., Witkin, S. S., DeHarven, E., and Bendich, A. (1978). Ultrastructure of partially decondensed human spermatozoal chromatin. *J. Ultrastructure Res.* **63,** 178–187.

Evenson, D. P., Darzynkiewicz, Z., and Melamed, M. R. (1980). Comparison of human and mouse sperm chromatin structure by flow cytometry. *Chromosoma* **78,** 225–238.

Fukuda, Y., Maddock, M. B., and Chang, M. C. (1979). *In vitro* fertilization of two species of deer mouse eggs by homologous or heterologous sperm and penetration of laboratory mouse eggs by deer mouse sperm. *J. Exp. Zool.* **207,** 481–490.

Gall, W. E., and Ohsumi, Y. (1976). Decondensation of sperm nuclei *in vitro*. *Exp. Cell Res.* **102,** 349–358.

Gusse, M., and Chevaillier, P. (1980). Electron microscope evidence for the presence of globular structures in different sperm chromatins. *J. Cell Biol.* **87,** 280–284.

Hanada, A., and Chang, M. C. (1972). Penetration of zona-free eggs by spermatozoa of different species. *Biol. Reprod.* **6,** 300–309.

Hanada, A., and Chang, M. C. (1976). Penetration of hamster and rabbit zona-free eggs by rat and mouse spermatozoa with special reference to sperm capacitation. *J. Reprod. Fertil.* **46,** 239–241.

Handyside, A. H., and Johnson, M. H. (1978). Temporal and spatial patterns of the synthesis of tissue specific polypeptides in the preimplantation mouse embryo. *J. Embryol. Exp. Morphol.* **44,** 191–199.

Hecht, N. B. (1974). A DNA polymerase isolated from bovine spermatozoa. *J. Reprod. Fertil.* **41,** 345–354.

Howe, C. C., and Solter, D. (1979). Cytoplasmic and nuclear protein synthesis in preimplantation mouse embryos. *J. Embryol. Exp. Morphol.* **52,** 209–225.

Hughes, M. E., Burki, K., and Fakan, S. (1979). Visualization of transcription in early mouse embryos. *Chromosoma* **73,** 179–190.

Hunter, R. H. F. (1972). Fertilization in the pig: Sequence of nuclear and cytoplasmic events. *J. Reprod. Fertil.* **29,** 395–406.

Iwamatsu, T., and Chang, M. C. (1972). Sperm penetration *in vitro* of mouse oocytes at various times during maturation. *J. Reprod. Fertil.* **31,** 237–247.

Jackson, V., and Chalkley, R. (1981). A new method for the isolation of replicative chromatin: Selective deposition of histone on both new and old DNA. *Cell* **23,** 121–134.

Johnson, M. H. (1981). The molecular and cellular basis of preimplantation mouse development. *Biol. Rev. Cambridge Philos. Soc.* **56,** 463–498.

Kaye, P. L., and Wales, R. G. (1981). Histone synthesis in preimplantation mouse embryos. *J. Exp. Zool.* **216,** 453–459.

Kierszenbaum, A. L., and Tres, L. L. (1975). Structural and transcriptional features of the mouse spermatid genome. *J. Cell Biol.* **65,** 258–270.

Kierszenbaum, A. L., and Tres, L. L. (1978). RNA transcription and chromatin structure during meiotic and postmeiotic stages of spermatogenesis. *Fed. Proc. Fed. Am. Soc. Exp. Biol.* **37,** 2512–1516.

Knowland, J., and Graham, C. (1972). RNA synthesis at the two-cell stage of mouse development. *J. Embryol. Exp. Morphol.* **27,** 167–176.

Kolk, A. H. J., and Samuel, T. (1975). Isolation, chemical, and immunological characterization of two strongly basic nuclear proteins from human spermatozoa. *Biochim. Biophys. Acta* **393,** 307–319.

Kopecny, V., and Pavlok, A. (1975a). Autoradiographic study of mouse spermatozoan arginine-rich nuclear protein in fertilization. *J. Exp. Zool.* **191,** 85–96.

Kopecny, V., and Pavlok, A. (1975b). Incorporation of arginine-³H into chromatin of mouse eggs shortly after sperm penetration. *Histochemistry* **45,** 341–345.

Krishna, M., and Generoso, W. M. (1977). Timing of sperm penetration, pronuclear formation, pronuclear DNA synthesis, and first cleavage in naturally ovulated mouse eggs. *J. Exp. Zool.* **202,** 245–252.

Krzanowska, H. (1982). Toluidine blue staining reveals changes in chromatin stabilization of mouse spermatozoa during epididymal maturation and penetration of ova. *J. Reprod. Fertil.* **64,** 97–101.

Laird, C. D., Wilkinson, L. E., Foe, V. E., and Chooi, W. Y. (1976). Analysis of chromatin-associated fiber arrays. *Chromosoma* **58,** 169–192.

Levey, I. L., Stull, G. B., and Brinster, R. L. (1978). Poly (A) and synthesis of polyadenylated RNA in the preimplantation mouse embryo. *Dev. Biol.* **64,** 140–148.

Levinson, J., Goodfellow, P., Vadeboncoeur, M., and McDevitt, H. (1978). Identification of stage-specific polypeptides synthesized during preimplantation development. *Proc. Natl. Acad. Sci. U.S.A.* **75,** 3332–3336.

Longo, F. J. (1973). Fertilization: A comparative ultrastructural review. *Biol. Reprod.* **9,** 149–215.

Longo, F. J., and Anderson, E. A. (1969). Cytological events leading to the formation of the two-cell stage in the rabbit: Association of the maternally and paternally derived genomes. *J. Ultrastructure Res.* **29,** 86–118.

Longo, F. J., and Kunkle, M. (1978). Transformations of sperm nuclei upon insemination. *Curr. Top. Dev. Biol.* **12,** 149–184.

Lopata, A., Sathananthan, A. H., McBain, J. C., Johnston, W. I. H., and Spiers, A. L. (1980). The ultrastructure of the preovulatory human egg fertilized *in vitro. Fertil. Steril.* **33,** 12–20.

Lung, B. (1972). Ultrastructure and chromatin disaggregation of human sperm head with thioglycolate treatment. *J. Cell Biol.* **52,** 179–186.

Luthardt, F. W., and Donahue, R. P. (1973). Pronuclear DNA synthesis in mouse eggs. *Exp. Cell Res.* **82,** 143–151.

McGaughey, R. W., and Chang, M. C. (1969). Meiosis of mouse eggs before and after sperm penetration. *J. Exp. Zool.* **170,** 397–410.

McKnight, S. L., and Miller, O. L., Jr. (1977). Electron microscopic analysis of chromatin replication in the cellular blastoderm *Drosophila melanogaster* embryo. *Cell* **12,** 795–804.

McKnight, S. L., and Miller, O. L., Jr. (1979). Post-replicative nonribosomal transcription units in *D. melanogaster* embryos. *Cell* **17,** 551–563.

McLaren, A. (1979). The impact of pre-fertilization events on post-fertilization development in mammals. *In* "Maternal Effects in Development" (D. R. Newth and M. Balls, eds.), pp. 287–320. Cambridge Univ. Press, London and New York.

Magnuson, T., and Epstein, C. J. (1981). Genetic control of very early mammalian development. *Biol. Rev. Cambridge Philos. Soc.* **56,** 369–408.

Mahi, C. A., and Yanagimachi, R. (1975). Induction of nuclear decondensation of mammalian spermatozoa *in vitro. J. Reprod. Fertil.* **44,** 293–296.

Mahi, C. A., and Yanagimachi, R. (1976). Maturation and sperm penetration of canine ovarian oocytes *in vitro. J. Exp. Zool.* **196,** 189–196.

Manes, C. (1969). Nucleic acid synthesis in preimplantation rabbit embryos. I. Quantitative aspects, relationship to early morphogenesis and protein synthesis. *J. Exp. Zool.* **172**, 311–322.

Marushige, Y., and Marushige, K. (1975). Enzymatic unpacking of bull sperm chromatin. *Biochim. Biophys. Acta* **403**, 180–191.

Marushige, Y., and Marushige, K. (1978). Dispersion of mammalian sperm chromatin during fertilization: An *in vitro* study. *Biochim. Biophys. Acta* **519**, 1–22.

Masui, Y., and Clarke, H. J. (1979). Oocyte maturation. *Int. Rev. Cytol.* **57**, 185–282.

Matheson, R. C., and Schultz, G. A. (1980). Histone synthesis in preimplantation rabbit embryos. *J. Exp. Zool.* **213**, 337–349.

Miller, M. A., and Masui, Y. (1982). Changes in the stainability and sulfhydryl level in the sperm nucleus during sperm-oocyte interaction in mice. *Gamete Res.* **5**, 167–179.

Mintz, B. (1964). Synthetic processes and early development in the mammalian egg. *J. Exp. Zool.* **157**, 85–100.

Monesi, V., and Salfi, V. (1967). Macromolecular synthesis during early development in the mouse embryo. *Exp. Cell Res.* **46**, 632–635.

Moore, G. P. M. (1975). The RNA polymerase activity of the preimplantation mouse embryo. *J. Embryol. Exp. Morphol.* **34**, 291–298.

Motlik, J., Kopecny, V., and Pivko, J. (1978). The fate and role of macromolecules synthesized during mammalian oocyte meiotic maturation. Autoradiographic topography of newly synthesized RNA and protein in the germinal vesicle of the pig and rabbit. *Ann. Biol. Anim., Biochim., Biophys.* **18**, 735–746.

Motlik, J., Kopecny, V., Pivko, J., and Fulka, J. (1980). Distribution of proteins labelled during meiotic maturation in rabbit and pig eggs at fertilization. *J. Reprod. Fertil.* **58**, 415–419.

Mukherjee, A. B. (1972). Normal progeny from fertilization *in vitro* of mouse oocytes matured in culture and sperm capacitated *in vitro*. *Nature (London)* **237**, 397–398.

Nishimoto, T., Yamada, I., Niwa, K., Nishimura, T., and Iritani, A. (1982). Sperm penetration in vitro of human oocytes matured in a chemically defined medium. *J. Reprod. Fertil.* **64**, 115–119.

Niwa, K., and Chang, M. C. (1973). Fertilization in vitro of rat eggs as affected by the maturity of the females and sperm concentration. *J. Reprod. Fertil.* **35**, 577–580.

Niwa, K., and Chang, M. C. (1975). Fertilization of rat eggs *in vitro* at various times before and after ovulation with special reference to fertilization of ovarian oocytes matured in culture. *J. Reprod. Fertil.* **43**, 435–451.

O'Brien, D. A., and Bellvé, A. R. (1980). Protein constituents of the mouse spermatozoon. I. An electrophoretic characterization. *Dev.Biol.* **75**, 386–404.

Petrov, P., Raitchera, E., and Tsanev, R. (1980). Nucleosomes and non-ribosomal RNA transcription in early mouse embryo. An electron microscope study. *Eur. J. Cell Biol.* **22**, 708–713.

Petzholdt, U., and Hoppe, P. C. (1980). Spontaneous parthenogenesis in *Mus musculus:* Comparison of protein synthesis in parthenogenetic and normal preimplantation embryos. *Mol. Gen. Genet.* **180**, 547–552.

Petzholdt, U., Hoppe, P. C., and Illmensee, K. (1980). Protein synthesis in enucleated fertilized and unfertilized mouse eggs. *Wilhelm Roux's Arch. Dev. Biol.* **189**, 215–219.

Puwaravutipanich, T., and Panyim, S. (1975). The nuclear basic proteins of human testis and ejaculated spermatozoa. *Exp. Cell Res.* **90**, 153–163.

Quinn, P. (1979). Failure of human spermatozoa to penetrate zona free mouse and rat ova *in vitro. J. Exp. Zool.* **210**, 497–506.

Richards, J. M., and Witkin, S. S. (1978). A nuclear DNA polymerase in bull spermatozoa. *J. Reprod. Fertil.* **54**, 43–47.

Rodman, T. C., and Bachvarova, R. (1976). RNA synthesis in preovulatory mouse oocytes. *J. Cell Biol.* **70**, 251–257.

Rodman, T. C., and Barth, A. H. (1979). Chromosomes of mouse oocytes in maturation: Differential trypsin sensitivity and amino acid incorporation. *Dev. Biol.* **68**, 82–95.

Rodman, T. C., Pruslin, F. H., Hoffmann, H. P., and Allfrey, V. G. (1981). Turnover of basic chromosomal proteins in fertilized eggs: A cytoimmunochemical study of events *in vivo. J. Cell Biol.* **90**, 351–361.

Rogers, B. J., Van Campen, H., Ueno, M., Lambert, H., Bronson, R., and Hale, R. (1979). Analysis of human spermatozoal fertilizing ability using zona-free ova. *Fertil. Steril.* **32**, 664–670.

Rudak, E., Jacobs, P. A., and Yanagimachi, R. (1978). Direct analysis of the chromosome constitution of human spermatozoa. *Nature (London)* **274**, 911–913.

Samuel, T., Kolk, A. H. J., Rumke, P., Aarden, L. A., and Bustin, M. (1976). Histone and DNA detection in swollen spermatozoa and somatic cells, by immunofluorescence. *Clin. Exp. Immunol.* **24**, 63–71.

Sato, K., and Blandau, R. J. (1979). Second meiotic division and polar body formation in mouse eggs fertilized *in vitro. Gamete Res.* **2**, 283–293.

Sawicki, J. A., Magnuson, T., and Epstein, C. J. (1981). Evidence for expression of the paternal genome in the two-cell mouse embryo. *Nature (London)* **294**, 450–451.

Schultz, G. A., and Church, R. B. (1975). Transcriptional patterns in early mammalian development. *In* "The Biochemistry of Animal Development" (R. Weber, ed.), Vol. 3, pp. 47–90. Academic Press, New York.

Schultz, R. M., LeTourneau, G. E., and Wassarman, P. M. (1979). Program of early development in the mammal: Changes in patterns and absolute rates of tubulin and total protein synthesis during oogenesis and early embryogenesis in the mouse. *Dev. Biol.* **68**, 341–359.

Shalgi, R. and Kraicer, P. F. (1978). Timing of sperm transport, sperm penetration, and cleavage in the rat. *J. Exp. Zool.* **204**, 353–360.

Sherman, M. I. (1979). Developmental biochemistry of preimplantation mammalian embryos. *Annu. Rev. Biochem.* **48**, 443–470.

Sipski, M. L., and Wagner, T. E. (1977). The total structure and organization of chromosomal fibers in eutherian sperm nuclei. *Biol. Reprod.* **16**, 428–440.

Siracusa, G., Coletta, M., and Monesi, V. (1975). Duplication of DNA during the first cell cycle in the mouse embryo. *J. Reprod. Fertil.* **42**, 395–398.

Sobhon, P., Thungkasemvathana, P., and Tanphaichitr, N. (1981). Electron microscope studies of rat sperm heads treated with urea, dithiothreitol, and micrococcal nuclease. *Anat. Rec.* **201**, 225–235.

Soupart, P. (1974). The need for capacitation of human sperm; functional and ultrastructural observations. *In* "Biology of Spermatozoa" (E. Hafez and C. Thibault, eds.), pp. 182–191. Karger, Basel.

Szollosi, D. (1965). Time and duration of DNA synthesis in rabbit eggs after sperm penetration. *Anat. Rec.* **154**, 209–212.

Szollosi, D., and Hunter, R. H. F. (1973). Ultrastructural aspects of fertilization in the domestic pig: Sperm penetration and pronuclear formation. *J. Anat.* **116**, 181–206.

Tanphaichitr, N., Sobhon, P., Taluppeth, N., and Chalermisarachai, P. (1978). Basic nuclear proteins in testicular cells and ejaculated spermatozoa in man. *Exp. Cell Res.* **117**, 347–356.

Tanphaichitr, N., Sobhon, P., Chalermisarachai, P., and Patilantakarnkool, M. (1981). Acid-extracted nuclear proteins and ultrastructure of human sperm chromatin as revealed by differential extraction with urea, mercaptoethanol, and salt. *Gamete Res.* **4**, 297–315.

Tasca, R. J., and Hillman, N. (1970). Effects of actinomycin D and cycloheximide on RNA and protein synthesis in cleavage stage mouse embryos. *Nature (London)* **225**, 1022–1025.

Thadani, V. (1979). Injection of sperm heads into immature rat oocytes. *J. Exp. Zool.* **210**, 161–168.

Thadani, V. (1980). A study of hetero-specific sperm-egg interactions in the rat, mouse, and deer mouse using *in vitro* fertilization and sperm injection. *J. Exp. Zool.* **212**, 435–453.

Thibault, C. (1977). Are follicular maturation and oocyte maturation independent processes? *J. Reprod. Fertil.* **51**, 1–15.

Thibault, C., and Gerard, M. (1970). Facteur cytoplasmique necessaire a la formation du pronucleus male dans l'ovocyte de lapin. *C. R. Hebd. Seances Acad. Sci., Ser. D.* **270**, 2025–2027.

Thibault, C., Gerard, M., and Menezo, Y. (1975). Preovulatory and ovulatory mechanisms in oocyte maturation. *J. Reprod. Fertil.* **45**, 605–610.

Thibault, C., Gerard, M., and Menezo, Y. (1976). Nuclear and cytoplasmic aspects of mammalian oocyte maturation *in vitro* in relation to follicle size and fertilization. *Prog. Reprod. Biol.* **1**, 233–240.

Tyler, J. P. P., Pryor, J. P., and Collins, W. P. (1981). Heterologous ovum penetration by human spermatozoa. *J. Reprod. Fertil.* **63**, 499–508.

Uehara, T., and Yanagimachi, R. (1976). Microsurgical injection of spermatozoa into hamster eggs with subsequent transformation of sperm nuclei into male pronuclei. *Biol. Reprod.* **15**, 467–470.

Usui, N., and Yanagimachi, R. (1976). Behavior of hamster sperm nuclei incorporated into eggs at various stages of maturation, fertilization, and early development. *J. Ultrastruct. Res.* **57**, 276–288.

Van Blerkom, J. (1979). Molecular differentiation of the rabbit ovum. III. Fertilization-autonomous polypeptide synthesis. *Dev. Biol.* **72**, 188–194.

Van Blerkom, J., and Brockway, G. O. (1975). Qualitative patterns of protein synthesis in the preimplantation mouse embryo. I. Normal pregnancy. *Dev. Biol.* **44**, 148–157.

Van Blerkom, J., and McGaughey, R. W. (1978). Molecular differentiation of the rabbit ovum II. During the preimplantation development of *in vivo* and *in vitro* matured oocytes. *Dev. Biol.* **63**, 151–164.

van Meel, F. C. M., and Pearson, P. L. (1979). Replacement of protamine by F1 histone during reactivation of fused human sperm nuclei. *Histochemistry* **63**, 329–339.

Wagner, T. E., Sliwinski, J. E., and Shewmaker, D. B. (1978). Subunit structure of eutherian sperm chromatin. *Arch. Androl.* **1**, 31–41.

Wassarman, P. M., and LeTourneau, G. E. (1976a). Meiotic maturation of mouse oocytes *in vitro:* Association of newly synthesized proteins with condensing chromosomes. *J. Cell Sci.* **30**, 549–568.

Wassarman, P. M., and LeTourneau, G. E. (1976b). RNA synthesis in fully-grown mouse oocytes. *Nature (London)* **261**, 73–74.

Wassarman, P. M., and Mrozak, S. (1981). Program of early development in the mammal: Synthesis and intracellular migration of histone H4 during oogenesis in the mouse. *Dev. Biol.* **84**, 364–371.

Wassarman, P. M., Schultz, R. M., and LeTourneau, G. E. (1979). Protein synthesis during meiotic maturation of mouse oocytes *in vitro:* Synthesis and phosphorylation of a protein localized in the germinal vesicle. *Dev. Biol.* **69,** 94–107.

Wassarman, P. M., Bleil, J. D., Cascio, S. M., LaMarca, M. J., LeTourneau, G. E., Mrozak, S. C., and Schultz,R. M. (1981). Programming of gene expression during mammalian oogenesis. *In* "Bioregulators of Reproduction" (G. M. Jagiello and H. J. Vogel, eds.), pp. 119–150. Academic Press, New York.

Wiesel, S., and Schultz, G. A. (1981). Factors which may affect removal of protamine from sperm DNA during fertilization in the rabbit. *Gamete Res.* **4,** 25–34.

Witkin, S. S., and Bendich, A. (1977). DNA synthesizing activity in normal human sperm. *Exp. Cell Res.* **106,** 47–54.

Witkin, S. S., Korngold, G. C., and Bendich, A. (1975). Ribonuclease-sensitive DNA-synthesizing complex in human sperm heads and seminal fluid. *Proc. Natl. Acad. Sci. U.S.A.* **72,** 3295–3299.

Witkowska, A. (1981). Pronuclear development and the first cleavage division in polyspermic mouse eggs. *J. Reprod. Fertil.* **62,** 493–498.

Wolf, D. P., Hanada, M., and Inoue, M. (1977). Kinetics of sperm penetration into and the zona reaction of mouse ova inseminated *in vitro. J. Exp. Zool.* **201,** 29–36.

Wolgemuth-Jarashow, D. J., and Jagiello, G. M. (1979). RNA synthesis during *in vitro* meiotic maturation of mammalian oocytes. *In* "Ovarian Follicular Development and Function" (A. R. Midgley, Jr. and W. A. Sadler, eds.), pp. 379–384. Raven Press, New York.

Woodland, H. R., and Adamson, E. D. (1977). The synthesis and storage of histones during the oogenesis of *Xenopus laevis. Dev. Biol.* **57,** 118–135.

Yanagimachi, R. (1972). Penetration of guinea pig spermatozoa into hamster eggs *in vitro. J. Reprod. Fertil.* **28,** 477–480.

Yanagimachi, R. (1978). Sperm-egg association in mammals. *Curr. Top. Dev. Biol.* **12,** 83–105.

Yanagimachi, R., Yanagimachi, H., and Rogers, B. J. (1976). The use of zona-free animal ova as a test-system for the assessment of the fertilizing capacity of human spermatozoa. *Biol. Reprod.* **15,** 471–476.

Young, R. J. (1979). Rabbit sperm chromatin is decondensed by a thiol-induced proteolytic activity not endogenous to its nucleus. *Biol. Reprod.* **20,** 1001–1004.

Young, R. J., and Sweeney, K. (1978). Mammalian ova and one-cell embryos do not incorporate phosphate into nucleic acids. *Eur. J. Biochem.* **91,** 111–117.

Young, R. J., and Sweeney, K. (1979). The structural organization of sperm chromatin. *Gamete Res.* **2,** 265–282.

Young, R. J., Sweeney, K., and Bedford, J. M. (1978). Uridine and guanosine incorporation by the mouse one-cell embryo. *J. Embryol. Exp. Morphol.* **44,** 133–148.

Zirkin, B. R., Chang, T. S. K., and Heaps, J. (1980). Involvement of an acrosin-like proteinase in the sulfhydryl-induced degradation of rabbit sperm nuclear protamine. *J. Cell Biol.* **85,** 116–121.

10

The Interaction of Mammalian Gametes in the Female

HARRY D. M. MOORE and J. MICHAEL BEDFORD

I. INTRODUCTION

The essential elements of vertebrate and invertebrate fertilization consist of a series of interactions between the spermatozoon and ovum which lead ultimately to their union and the combination of their genomes. The main steps are sperm binding to and penetration of the egg vestments, incorporation of the spermatozoon into the ooplasm, and the activation of the egg followed by syngamy (see Austin and Bishop, 1957). At first, this basic sequence of events remained unaltered with the adoption of internal fertilization, but the relationship between the gametes and their environment then became increasingly complex, at least in eutherian mammals. In the present discussion, the term "mammals" alludes to eutherian mammals except where otherwise stated.

453

Mechanism and Control of Animal Fertilization
Copyright © 1983 by Academic Press, Inc.
All rights of reproduction in any form reserved.
ISBN 0-12-328520-8

The mode of fertilization in mammals differs in several important aspects from that observed in other animals. After leaving the testis, the mammalian spermatozoon must undergo a maturation phase in the epididymis and then subtle changes in the female tract which confer on it the ability to penetrate and fertilize the egg (see Gwatkin, 1976; Bedford and Cooper, 1978). The latter process, capacitation, initiates in the spermatozoon the acrosome reaction and a modification in the pattern of motility, both of which appear to be important for fertilization.

The gametes of eutherian mammals exhibit other new features. In the sperm head, the nucleus has a keratin-like rigid nature, and the whole inner membrane and posterior equatorial segment of the acrosome are unusually stable (Bedford and Calvin, 1974; Bedford et al., 1979). The ovum is encased at ovulation by cumulus cells embedded in a gel and, compared with that of other vertebrates, has a thick and resilient zona pellucida. Furthermore, in eutherian mammals the spermatozoon penetrates the egg vestments and is incorporated into the vitellus in a manner which is unique, and is not even shared by the other therian group—the marsupials (Rodger and Bedford, 1982).

This chapter considers the preparation that mammalian spermatozoa undergo in the female tract before interacting with the ovum and the specific processes involved in fertilization of the egg. In a wider context, the character of fertilization in Eutheria will be discussed in relation to gamete morphology and function in mammals in general.

II. CAPACITATION

As the spermatozoon is transported through the female tract, an essential change in its functional state occurs over several hours, which allows fertilization to proceed. The need for this process, capacitation, has been recognized for 30 years (Austin, 1951; Chang, 1951). It appears to be ubiquitous among the Eutheria, at least, although the specific alterations in the spermatozoon associated with this phenomenon have yet to be firmly established. Capacitation is now commonly recognized, however, as the process in the female (or *in vitro*) that prepares the spermatozoon to undergo the acrosome reaction and also quite probably to develop a whiplash or hyperactivated motility that may enhance ability to penetrate the zona pellucida (Yanagimachi, 1970). In general terms, the physiological environments in which capacitation can occur both *in vivo* and *in vitro* have been discussed (for reviews, see Bedford, 1972b; Barros, 1974; Chang and Hunter, 1975; Yanagimachi, 1977; Rogers, 1978). It is still not clear what the factors are in the female tract that promote the changes in spermatozoa. Nevertheless, we can ascertain the character of capacitation *in vivo* by determining how the process is influenced by the female environment.

Successive regions of the female tract differ in their potential to capacitate spermatozoa. For some species, the fallopian tube is more effective than the uterus (see Bedford, 1969; Chang and Hunter, 1975), but the time required for capacitation, as judged by the moment when spermatozoa first exhibit the ability to fertilize, is normally minimal when they are allowed to pass naturally along the whole of the female tract (Bedford, 1969; Hunter and Hall, 1974). This indicates that a synergism exists in that respect between the uterine and tubal environments. In the rodents where whole semen is deposited *in utero,* it is questionable whether spermatozoa can be effectively capacitated in the uterus alone (Hunter, 1969). Thus, their transport to the oviductal ampulla at about the time of ovulation (Braden and Austin, 1954; Yanagimachi and Chang, 1963; Moore and Bedford, 1978b) may possibly also signify an important functional correlation between the completion of capacitation and the presence of eggs in the oviduct. In this context, guinea pig spermatozoa and hamster spermatozoa observed *in situ* in the oviduct at the time of ovulation show the characteristic activated motility (Yanagimachi and Mahi, 1976; Katz and Yanagimachi, 1981) which is associated with the capacitated state (Yanagimachi, 1970).

The ability of the female tract to capacitate spermatozoa is altered by the endocrine status of the female. High plasma estrogen levels tend to promote capacitation in the uterus, while high progesterone levels will suppress it (see Bedford, 1974c). The capacitating potential of the oviduct is less easily regulated. That of an induced ovulator like the rabbit resists all manner of endocrine manipulation (Chang, 1958; Bedford, 1974c). On the other hand, in the hamster, a short cycling species, this ability is seriously suppressed by progesterone (Viriyapanich and Bedford, 1981). Overall, the results of endocrine studies suggest that capacitation is mediated through definite factors in the female tract. Although the identity of these factors is unknown, they are not species specific. Cross-fertilization can occur between similar species (i.e., sheep and goat, rabbit and hare, mink and ferret; see Chang and Hancock, 1967), proving that spermatozoa can be capacitated in a heterologous tract, albeit closely related. More recently, the wider limits of capacitation specificity have been reexamined by the transfer of gametes into host females of very different species (De

Mayo *et al.*, 1980; Saling and Bedford, 1981). Thus, complete capacitation of squirrel monkey, rabbit, mouse, and hamster spermatozoa and subsequent fertilization of homologous eggs have been achieved in a foreign tract, confirming the conclusions drawn from some earlier studies (Baker and Coggins, 1969; Chang *et al.*, 1971). Furthermore, capacitation may be attained even where the environment itself is obviously deleterious to the metabolic functions of the spermatozoa (Saling and Bedford, 1981).

The plasmalemma has been the focus of much investigation because it is directly exposed to the capacitating environment and is involved directly in the regulation of motility and the acrosome reaction. Now, considerable circumstantial evidence points to its involvement during capacitation *in vivo*. For example, when exposed to an unusual rabbit seminal plasma, which contained powerful agglutinins, capacitated (12-hour uterine) spermatozoa were immediately immobilized where ejaculated or epididymal spermatozoa survived normally (Bedford, 1970). In addition, changes in the distribution and mobility of membrane surface components are claimed to occur during incubation of rabbit spermatozoa *in utero* (Gordon *et al.*, 1974; O'Rand, 1977a) and of guinea pig spermatozoa *in vitro* (Kinsey and Koehler, 1978). Capacitation has been reported to bring a reduction in the net negative charge of spermatozoa (Vaidya *et al.*, 1971); however, in a more recent study conducted through whole cell isoelectric focusing, no change was detected in the mean surface charge of rabbit and hamster spermatozoa incubated in the uterus for 12 and 4 hours, respectively, or incubated in capacitating media (Moore, 1979). This result is perhaps not surprising as a population of spermatozoa is heterologous and the proportion completing capacitation at any one time may be quite small. Lack of species specificity appears to negate the possibility that spermatozoa acquire components from the female tract secretions and, instead, adds weight to the notion that components are removed or modified at the sperm surface. This should be simple to demonstrate with immunological techniques if the components involved are glycoproteins acquired from the secretions of the epididymis. Whatever the nature of the change, the modifications to the plasmalemma may result in a rearrangement of intrinsic proteins (O'Rand, 1979) which permit the acrosome reaction to take place (see next section) and possibly alter sperm motility. It is of interest that the minimum time for the capacitation of spermatozoa is a species characteristic and remains fairly constant *in vivo* or *in vitro*, regardless of the specific character of the environment (see Chang and Hunter, 1975; Saling and Bedford, 1981). This most likely reflects inherent species differences in the properties of the sperm membranes such as surface components (see Bedford and Cooper, 1978) and lipid composition (Scott, 1973) which affect the movement of intercalated proteins. The molecular mechanisms that might be involved are discussed in Chapter 4 in this volume.

The biological significance of capacitation has remained uncertain, possibly because of the lack of precise information on events *in vivo*. Our understanding of many of the changes in spermatozoa during capacitation comes from *in vitro* studies and, although these investigations have been of great value, they do not allow certain examination of the relationship between spermatozoa and the female tract. Indeed, it is not known whether the mechanisms involved in capacitation *in vitro* are the same as those occurring *in vivo*. For instance, the rate of capacitation varies in different regions of the female tract and can be modified by hormones (Bedford, 1972b), while *in vitro* the process appears to proceed spontaneously if a suitable but nonspecific environment is found. Much of the information on capacitation in the female tract is drawn from the studies in the rabbit. However, it is the capacitation environment in the oviduct of the spontaneous ovulator such as the hamster that appears to be the more malleable, its capacitation potential being severely depressed during progesterone dominance in the luteal phase (Viriyapanich and Bedford, 1981). Analysis of differences in the oviducal milieu during the estrous cycle in these animals or, more likely, in those with longer cycles may provide an indication of the nature of capacitation factors *in vivo*.

Since, in some species at least, capacitated and acrosome-reacted spermatozoa have only a limited fertile life (see Bedford, 1972b; Fleming and Yanagimachi, 1982), it would seem to be expedient and perhaps critical that the completion of capacitation is synchronized both temporally and physically with ovulation. Indeed, this correlation is probably reflected in the stepwise processes in the female tract of the rodent and the rabbit in which motile spermatozoa complete capacitation, as judged by the acrosome reaction and activated motility, only after they have entered the oviduct (Bedford, 1969; Hunter, 1969; Yanagimachi and Mahi, 1976; Overstreet and Cooper, 1979). It might seem logical to speculate, therefore, that capacitation in mammals has emerged as a means of regulating the occurrence and timing of the acrosome reaction (Bedford, 1983), a mechanism which in other groups is normally governed by the egg. The general mode of invertebrate fertilization, for instance, requires the initiation of the acrosome reaction at or close to the egg surface by specific products of the egg coat in conjunction with calcium (see Chapter 6, this volume). As discussed in the next section, it seems doubtful that the eutherian egg can undertake this function. On the other hand, the concentration of calcium ions in the fluids of the mammalian female tract (Hamner, 1975) is sufficient to evoke an acrosome reaction and possibly a change that confers an activated motility pattern on spermatozoa once they are fully capacitated. Hence, the need for capacitation may have evolved in response to an absence of a controlling mechanism from the eutherian oocyte, as well as in response to the development of formidable vestments that the spermatozoon must penetrate (Bedford, 1983). Why the eutherian egg has undergone such evolutionary change with the emergence of the eutherian mammals is not known.

III. ACROSOME REACTION

While the precise significance of the role of the acrosome reaction is not yet wholly clear, it is apparent that it must occur before the spermatozoon can fertilize. The reaction involves a series of point fusions between the plasmalemma and the outer acrosomal membrane beneath it, forming gaps through which the acrosome content can diffuse (for reviews, see Bedford and Cooper, 1978; Meizel, 1978; Green, 1978b). Compared with the reaction in invertebrate spermatozoa (Colwin and Colwin, 1967; Epel and Vacquier, 1978), these pores are more numerous in eutherian mammals, creating a fenestrated shroud around the reacted sperm head that may remain for some time. This arrangement allows the acrosomal contents to be released while retaining much of the plasma membrane overlying the acrosome and its putative receptors for binding to the zona pellucida. The acrosome reaction is limited to the membrane overlying the rostral region of the acrosome and progresses caudally only as far as the anterior margin of the equatorial segment, where fusion between the remaining outer acrosomal and plasma membranes ensures continuity of the sperm head surface (Barros et al., 1967; Bedford, 1968). The equatorial segment has a number of particular features that may prevent the participation of its membranes in the acrosome reaction. The inner and outer acrosomal membranes display an unusual pentalaminar structure (Roomans, 1975; Moore and Bedford, 1978a), while the material between them is ladderlike or septate (Bedford et al., 1979). Freeze-fracture studies have demonstrated that this appearance is due to a hexagonal array of intermembrane bridges (Phillips, 1977; Russell et al., 1980), which stabilize the equatorial segment to an extent that it resists detergents that disrupt the remainder of the acrosome (Wooding, 1973; Russell et al., 1980). This stability is reflected in its persistence for some time after fertilization, even when the sperm nucleus has decondensed (Bedford, 1972a; Usui and Yanagimachi, 1976). The plasmalemma overlying the equatorial segment also has properties that distinguish it from that in the more apical region. Investigations with antibiotic probes such as polymixin B and filipin have shown that, preceding the acrosome reaction, the rostral plasmalemma is rich in anionic lipid, a constituent which increases membrane fluidity and the likelihood of fusion (Bearer and Friend, 1981). By contrast, the plasma membrane in the stable equatorial segment has much lower concentrations of anionic lipid, but how the spermatozoon maintains these different membrane domains is not entirely clear. The surface of the plasmalemma in the equatorial segment has at least one different antigenic component compared with those in other regions, as indicated by the specific binding of lectins (see Bedford and Cooper, 1978; Nicolson and Yanagimachi, 1979) or antibodies (Hjort and Hansen, 1971; Tung, 1977). These surface moieties, if retained during capacitation, may help to conserve a particular lipid composition. But, since enzymatic removal of guinea pig sperm surface neuraminic acid fails to affect lipid domains (Bearer and Friend, 1981), submembrane constituents, such as those noted previously, or integral membrane components, may be more important in maintaining membrane lipid composition. Interestingly, intramembrane particles of the inner and outer acrosomal membranes of the equatorial segment in boar spermatozoa are arranged in a similar array to the intermembrane bridges (Russell *et al.,* 1980), possibly signifying a relationship between the two patterns.

As discussed in the last section, changes in the sperm membranes associated with capacitation predispose the spermatozoon to the acrosome reaction, but the origin and the nature of the factors that specifically initiate membrane fusion *in vivo* are still unknown. A number of substances present under normal conditions at ovulation may facilitate or even trigger the acrosome reaction, but most of these factors are not essential to the process. For example, follicular fluid (Yanagimachi, 1969) and the cumulus oophorus (Gwatkin *et al.,* 1972) both appear to stimulate spermatozoa to undergo the acrosome reaction. However, fertilization of washed ova will occur *in vivo* and *in vitro* in the absence of follicular products (Bedford and Chang, 1962; Pavlok and McLaren, 1972; Overstreet and Bedford, 1974; Moore and Bedford, 1978b). The factors responsible do not appear to emanate from the egg either. Pretreatment of rabbit eggs with neuraminidase, trypsin, chymotrypsin, or antiprogesterone antiserum failed to block sperm penetration *in vivo* (Overstreet and Bedford, 1975). Furthermore, Overstreet and

Cooper (1979) have recovered motile acrosome-reacted rabbit spermatozoa from the ampulla of the rabbit oviduct in the absence of ovulation. This observation shows that, in the rabbit at least, the environment of the oviduct alone is sufficient to induce the acrosome reaction. Certainly, substances essential or important for the acrosome reaction *in vitro*, i.e., Ca^{2+}, albumin, pyruvate, and lactate are present in adequate concentrations in oviducal fluid (Hamner, 1975).

A characteristic of the acrosome reaction in mammalian spermatozoa is the heterogeneity of the response both *in vitro* and in the female tract. Under appropriate conditions, a solution of egg jelly may initiate an immediate reaction in the great majority of the spermatozoa of a particular invertebrate within 1 minute (Decker *et al.*, 1976; Kinsey *et al.*, 1979). By contrast, after the minimum time for complete capacitation *in vitro*, only 5–10% of a population of mammalian spermatozoa may undergo an acrosome reaction, with the proportion rising to possibly 50% of motile cells over 2 to 4 hours according to the species (Yanagimachi and Usui, 1974; Talbot and Franklin, 1976; Rogers, 1981). Such asynchrony is also observed in the rabbit female tract where not more than 20% of the motile population of spermatozoa in the oviducal ampulla have undergone the acrosome reaction, whether sampled 6, 10, 12, or 18 hours after insemination (Overstreet and Cooper, 1979). Clearly, the staggered induction of the acrosome reaction in a sperm population throughout the period that unfertilized eggs arrive in the oviduct carries an obvious advantage, maximizing the chance of fertilization. This may be important, particularly in species that are spontaneous ovulators, where the time between coitus and ovulation may be variable. The heterogeneity of reaction time in spermatozoa *in vivo* probably reflects not only inherent differences in individual cells but also in the time they spend in each region of the female tract.

Although the molecular mechanisms pertaining specifically to the acrosome reaction are still poorly understood, some general concepts relating to membrane fusion events are beginning to emerge which also appear to apply to spermatozoa. The results of investigations in a number of mammalian cell types favor the idea that membrane fusion is preceded by the formation of protein-free zones of lipid bilayer due to the aggregation of intrinsic proteins (Ahkong *et al.*, 1975). These particle-free areas of membrane, if opposing one another and sufficiently close ($\simeq 10$ Å), will intermingle in focal fusion (Lucy, 1978). The evidence from freeze-fracture studies in guinea pig spermatozoa would seem to corroborate this view. Just prior to the acrosome reaction, spermatozoa display membrane clearances of protein particles in the anterior acrosomal region (Friend *et al.*, 1977) and particularly at the border with the equatorial segment where fusion of the plasma and acrosomal membrane is essential for the integrity of the cell. The appearance of these areas would indicate that the lateral mobility of proteins increases in the plasmalemma and outer acrosomal membrane overlying the anterior acrosome. This may be due to changes in the lipid composition of the membranes, such as a local reduction of cholesterol or other steroids (Friend, 1980), which might increase membrane fluidity. Alternatively, modifications to intramembrane proteins during capacitation may remove constraints to their movement (O'Rand, 1979).

Whatever the precise events that result in membrane fusion, extracellular Ca^{2+} has been shown to be essential for the acrosome reaction (Yanagimachi and Usui, 1974). In this respect, the mammalian reaction is similar to that of invertebrates, which requires Ca^{2+} even when exposed to an inducing factor contained in the egg jelly coat (Dan, 1967). After incubation in capacitating media depleted of Ca^{2+} or with the ionophore A23187 (which elicits a rise in intracellular calcium concentration), the addition of extracellular Ca^{2+} will initiate a normal acrosome reaction in a proportion of spermatozoa within a few minutes (Yanagimachi and Usui, 1974; Talbot *et al.*, 1976; Green, 1978a). This reaction is probably due to an influx of calcium permitted by change in head membrane permeability. But the exact role of Ca^{2+} during membrane fusion still remains unclear. Since the ionophore will induce an acrosome reaction in guinea pig spermatozoa in the presence of protease inhibitors (Green, 1978b; Perreault *et al.*, 1982), implying that acrosomal proteases are not involved, it seems likely that Ca^{2+} has a direct influence on fusion, possibly by destabilization of lipid bilayers (Papahadjopoulos, 1978), rather than through the action of acrosomal enzymes as suggested by Meizel (1978). Calmodulin, a specific calcium-binding protein involved in cell regulatory processes (see Means and Dedman, 1980), has been localized in rabbit and guinea pig spermatozoa (Jones *et al.*, 1980). This protein receptor may possibly be the functional mediator through which calcium acts. Certainly, it has been implicated in membrane exocytosis/fusion processes (Steinhardt and Alderton, 1982). Furthermore, if the Ca^{2+} signal is amplified through the activation of specific protein kinases, it is perhaps not surprising that substances such as catecholamines, adenylate cyclase, and cyclic AMP (see Meizel, 1978; Yanagimachi, 1981) also may propagate the acrosome reaction. Papahadjopoulous (1978) has speculated that Ca^{2+}, acting either directly or indirectly, might induce phase transitions in the membrane, creating crystalline and non-crystalline areas between which unstable regions would promote fusion. This process may be influenced in spermatozoa by the action of phospholipases (Hirao and Yanagimachi, 1978). Unfortunately, however, it must be admitted that the precise mechanisms by which sperm membranes are perturbed to a point compatible with fusion are far from being understood.

IV. GAMETE SURFACE INTERACTIONS

At the surface of the oocyte, spermatozoa of monotreme and marsupial mammals are faced only by the zona pellucida. In order for the spermatozoa of eutherian mammals to reach the newly ovulated ovum, however, they must first pass through the cumulus oophorus, a cellular investment of granulosa/follicular cells and mucopolysaccharide matrix which varies considerably between species in size and character. Ultrastructural and biochemical studies indicate that the relationship with granulosa cells is of major importance in regulating oocyte maturation (see Masui and Clarke, 1979), but it has yet to be demonstrated that these cells play a positive role during fertilization as such. Fertilization of cumulus-denuded ova has been carried out *in vitro* in chemically defined media (see Rogers, 1978, for literature), and ova devoid of granulosa cells can be fertilized readily *in vivo* (Harper, 1970; Moore and Bedford, 1978b). In addition, the cumulus does not have the essential role suggested for it in capacitation of spermatozoa in the oviduct (Gwatkin *et al.*, 1972; Gwatkin, 1976). Finally, ova may be fertilized *in vitro* or *in vivo* in the absence of any follicular products (Bavister, 1969; Moore and Bedford, 1978b). Thus, while it is possible that both the cumulus oophorus and follicular fluid may benefit spermatozoa in the fallopian tube (Bedford and Chang, 1962; Moore and Bedford, 1978b), there is no evidence to suggest that they are essential in this respect.

It appears that spermatozoa must be capacitated to penetrate the intact cumulus, and it has been generally thought that this passage is assisted by hyaluronidase and other acrosomal hydrolases that can act to disperse its matrix (for reviews, see Bedford, 1974a; McRorie and Williams, 1974). This hypothesis depends on these enzymes being released from the acrosome in a controlled manner at or near the outer vestments of the egg or remaining associated with the sperm surface if released in some other region of the oviduct. In support of such an argument, acrosome-reacted motile spermatozoa which have not entered the cumulus have been recovered from the oviducts of several species (Austin and Bishop, 1958; Yanagimachi and Mahi, 1976; Overstreet and Cooper, 1979). Morton (1975, 1977) has shown that acrosome-denuded spermatozoa retain some hyaluronidase activity, probably on the inner acrosomal membrane. Although intact spermatozoa have been seen at the zona surface (Bedford, 1972a), these preparations were recovered some hours after ovulation at a point when cumulus disintegration had begun. It is very clear, however, that fertilization may often occur in rabbit and hamster, for example, before any noticeable change in the state of the cumulus. While the claim cannot be discounted that (hamster) spermatozoa may release hyaluronidase without any detectable acrosome reaction (Talbot and Franklin, 1974), it is difficult to see how hyaluronidase can emanate from spermatozoa whose plasma and outer acrosomal membranes remain intact. Thus, there is no real consensus at present as to the precise means by which spermatozoa penetrate the egg vestments, and the role of the various acrosomal enzymes at different points in the sperm's progress toward the oocyte surface is proving extremely difficult to elucidate to everyone's satisfaction. It is interesting, however, that although the ovum of the opossum has no cumulus investment and a trivial zona pellucida (see Rodger and Bedford, 1982), its acrosome contains as great, and in some instances greater, amounts of enzymes (Rodger and Young, 1982) of the type believed to facilitate penetration of the eutherian egg vestments. Further investigations are required to clarify our understanding in this area. In this respect, the culture systems of Bavister (1979) using 1:1 sperm/egg ratios could be useful in establishing the sequence of events of a single spermatozoon as it penetrates the egg and in assessing the importance of other factors, such as motility.

The point at which the acrosome reaction occurs in the fertilizing spermatozoon also has a direct bearing on the next event of fertilization—sperm attachment to the zona pellucida. It is important here to distinguish the semantics of "intact," "reacted," and "acrosome loss" (Fig. 1). Must a fertilizing spermatozoon meet the zona surface with its plasma membrane intact (Fig. 1a; see also Saling and Storey, 1979), or can it undergo the acrosome reaction prior to attachment and still penetrate the egg? Rabbit spermatozoa without acrosomes are observed both remote from and in the vicinity of the ovum (Bedford, 1968, 1972a). Ultrastructural investigations have, nonetheless, consistently shown that spermatozoa generally adhere by the reacted acrosomal complex to the zona surface during fertilization *in vivo* (Fig. 1b) and that the discarded acrosome of the penetrating rabbit spermatozoon associates tenaciously with the zona (Bedford, 1972a; Gwatkin, 1976; Phillips and Shalgi, 1980) and may remain thereafter

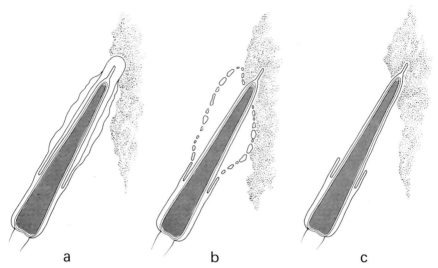

Fig. 1. Diagram of three possible situations that could exist between sperm and egg at the surface of the eutherian zona pellucida, as seen in thin sections in the transmission electron microscope. The arrangement depicted in (a) is likely to occur only rarely in a biological situation, since the fertilizing sperm probably must undergo the acrosomal reaction to penetrate the intact cumulus oophorus that invests newly ovulated oocytes. The situation depicted in (b) is considered to represent that existing at the moment a fertilizing reacted spermatozoon binds to the zona surface. Such binding of the reacted complex to the zona may well provide a stable base from which the sperm head can intrude itself into the zona pellucida. The impression that the reacted vesicles are separated from each other and from the leading border of the equatorial segment is an erroneous one created by the plane of the thin section. Though fenestrated throughout, the surface remains as a continuous sheet. (c) A spermatozoon is depicted that has lost the acrosomal complex and is adhering to the zona surface. This situation is believed not to occur in actuality, since it is highly unlikely that specific receptors for zona substance exist at the surface of the inner acrosomal membrane. As a corollary, a motile spermatozoa having lost the reacted acrosomal complex before zona contact seems unlikely to be able to fertilize. A possible exception is raised by light microscope observation of the interaction of apparently acrosomeless guinea pig spermatozoa with the zona pellucida (Yanagimachi, 1981; Huang et al., 1981).

at the zona surface. Not surprisingly, mouse spermatozoa may become attached to the zona pellucida *in vitro* prior to the acrosome reaction in the absence of the cumulus oophorus (Saling and Storey, 1979), that binding being mediated by a Ca^{2+}-dependent mechanism involving the plasma membrane (Heffner *et al.*, 1980). But, since the cumulus was not present in all these experiments, it represents a situation quite different from that which the fertilizing spermatozoon faces *in vivo*. Recently, Huang *et al*. (1981) have stated categorically that only the guinea pig spermatozoon that has lost the acrosomal complex can bind to the zona pellucida *in vitro* (Fig. 1c). The acrosome is easily identified in guinea pig spermatozoa, but whether the finding is applicable *in vivo* remains to be confirmed, and whether this is true for other species seems doubtful. Certainly, evidence in the rabbit (Fig. 8 in Bedford, 1972a) shows clearly that the acrosomal complex is left adhering to the zona surface by a sperm in the act of penetrating the zona pellucida.

Observations *in vitro* are complicated further by the fact that epididymal and ejaculated spermatozoa may attach to the zona even though they must undergo capacitation before zona penetration. Normally, only spermatozoa in which capacitation is complete or well underway, would be present at the site of fertilization *in vivo*. Hence, zona attachment by uncapacitated spermatozoa *in vitro* need not necessarily be functional and, as has been reported by Hartmann and co-workers (1972; Hartmann and Hutchison, 1974, 1977), could involve different components than those present during sperm penetration *in vivo*. In fact, recent evidence in the mouse suggests that the affinity of spermatozoa for the homologous zona pellucida increases after capacitation (Swenson and Dunbar, 1982).

The initial interaction between the spermatozoon and the zona pellucida is believed to involve specific recognition sites on the sperm and zona surface, but the nature of these receptors has not been fully elucidated. For practical reasons, most investigations have been undertaken using *in vitro* systems, and the molecular basis for these interactions are reviewed in Chapter 7 in this volume.

The components involved in sperm binding to the zona must be present at an early stage of oocyte maturation, in some species at least. Spermatozoa attach to and penetrate primary oocytes of the rabbit, dog, and hamster as freely as they do to ovulated eggs (Overstreet and Bedford, 1974; Mahi and Yanagimachi, 1976; Moore and Bedford, 1978a). Immature human oocytes also are readily penetrable by spermatozoa (Overstreet and Hembree, 1976; Overstreet *et al*., 1980). The reception system is maintained during aging of the ovum, in some cases at least. The zona remains penetrable at least 26 hours postovulation in ova incubated in oviducts of ovariectomized rabbits (which therefore do not secrete mucus) and for much longer in oviducts of normal hamsters (Viriyapanich and Bedford, 1981). Whether age-related changes in the zona of the mouse egg (Longo, 1981) actually prevent its penetration *in vivo* remains to be determined.

Less is known about the nature of the complementary binding components on the spermatozoon. A glycoprotein secreted by the proximal epididymis of the rabbit and localized on the plasmalemma overlying the anterior acrosome of cauda epididymal spermatozoa may possibly play a role in gamete interaction in this species (Moore, 1980). First, spermatozoa released from the proximal segment of the rabbit epididymis 10 days after low corpus ligation showed optimal sustained motility but did not penetrate or even adhere to the zona surface *in vivo* (Bedford, 1967). Second, when mature spermatozoa are incubated with specific univalent antibody to this glycoprotein component, they display a marked reduction in fertility in the oviduct (Moore, 1981) and, despite the maintenance of good motility, seldom attach to or penetrate eggs. Thus, the sperm moieties involved in zona attachment would appear to be antigenic in nature.

Notwithstanding the apparently indiscriminate adhesion of foreign spermatozoa to the zona surface, in many cases *in vitro* (Bedford, 1977; Peterson *et al.*, 1979; Gulyas and Schmell, 1980; Yanagimachi, 1981), they are normally excluded from penetrating the intact egg (for a discussion of this topic, see chapter 7, this volume). The basis for the specificity expressed at the stage of zona penetration is still unclear. However, its eventual elucidation may at the same time tell much about the normal mechanism of zona penetration (see below). Other factors currently considered to bear on zona penetration, namely sperm motility and hydrolytic enzymes (see next section), do not hold an obvious degree of specificity (Brown, 1982). The key to specificity may lie in the possibility that capacitated spermatozoa can bind in a stable fashion only to homologous eggs. The reason that a stable binding between sperm and egg is required for penetration to follow sperm/egg association is not at all clear as yet. It is quite possible, however, that a tenacious attachment of the reacted sperm plasma membrane to the zona surface may act as a stable base from which the narrow nuclear profile of the sperm head can intrude itself into the substance of the zona (Fig. 1b). Weak adhesive forces could then preclude penetration. The possibility has been raised from time to time that there may be a specific receptor-type interaction between zona and the inner acrosomal membrane, at least during the initial phase of penetration (as in Fig. 1c). It would seem impractical for the inner acrosome membrane to bind with zona receptors, however, when it must later move freely within the zona in creating a penetration slit. As explained below, how that slit is formed by the spermatozoon is very much open to question.

V. PENETRATION OF ZONA PELLUCIDA

The acrosome reaction is an essential prerequisite for sperm penetration of the zona pellucida (Austin and Bishop, 1958; Bedford, 1968), but it is still debatable what it is precisely about the reacted state that then permits the spermatozoon to pass through the zona substance (for reviews, see Bedford, 1974a; Yanagimachi, 1977). The most favored view has been that localized zona digestion by lysin(s) of acrosomal origin has an essential and major role in forming the characteristic penetration slit (see reviews by McRorie and Williams, 1974; Stambaugh, 1978). Ultrastructural studies showing that the matrix of the acrosome is always lost before penetration occurs (Bedford, 1968, 1972a; Yanagimachi and Noda, 1970a), necessitated the suggestion that the functional lytic moiety, presumably the trypsin-like enzyme acrosin (Stambaugh and Buckley, 1968; Zaneveld et al., 1968), is actually bound to the inner acrosomal membrane (Bedford, 1968; Pikó, 1969). In accordance with this viewpoint is the biochemical finding that a significant amount of acrosin remains with the spermatozoon after the acrosome has been removed (Brown and Hartree, 1974, 1978; Fritz et al., 1975; Brown et al., 1975) and the unlikely candidacy of the equatorial segment as a site in that respect. The consistent failure to localize proteases in the equatorial segment, despite their visualization in the rest of the acrosome (Yanagimachi and Teichman, 1972; Morton, 1975; Gould and Bernstein, 1975; Garner et al., 1977), and the intact state of the equatorial segment in some spermatozoa in the perivitelline space and in the fertilizing spermatozoon (Bedford, 1972a; Nicosia et al., 1977; Moore and Bedford, 1978a) would seem to rule out the possibility that this region contributes to zona penetration.

The means by which the spermatozoon penetrates the substance of the zona pellucida is a matter of contention now. The most common belief that the enzymic action of acrosomal proteases, particularly acrosin, is required is based mainly on the circumstantial evidence of reports that fertilization in vivo or in vitro can be suppressed when capacitated spermatozoa are exposed to naturally occurring or synthetic trypsin inhibitors (Stambaugh et al., 1969; Zaneveld et al., 1970, 1971). This belief has been sustained by investigations showing that acrosomal extracts or purified fractions of acrosin will eventually dissolve the zona pellucida in vitro (Srivastava et al., 1965; Stambaugh and Buckley, 1969; Zenveld et al., 1969; Polakoski and McRorie, 1973), and histochemical reaction product in the penetration slit has been interpreted as reflecting the presence there of acrosin (Stambaugh,

1976), a report not substantiated by a recent autoradiography study (Kopecny and Fléchon, 1981). In fact, although such reports may seem consistent with a lytic role for acrosin—and lysis is still viewed by a majority of investigators as the key to zona penetration—an accumulating literature raises serious doubts about that interpretation. First, the mode of action of trypsin inhibitors has not been satisfactorily resolved. In a number of experiments (Stambaugh et al., 1969; Zaneveld et al., 1971), ova were surrounded by cumulus oophorus, and so inhibition may have been exerted at the level of cumulus cells rather than the zona. Low-molecular-weight inhibitors, such as TLCK or p-aminobenzamidine, also effectively inhibit the acrosome reaction (Meizel and Lui, 1976) and halt the dispersal of the acrosomal matrix in mouse, guinea pig, and ram spermatozoa (Green, 1978b; Perreault et al., 1982; Fraser, 1982; W. V. Holt, personal communication). Contrary to a report by Wolf (1977), trypsin inhibitors applied in vitro will block fertilization of intact mouse and hamster eggs, while zona-free eggs are freely penetrated. This suggests that the enzymes are not required for sperm fusion and incorporation by the oocyte (Fraser, 1982; H. D. M. Moore, unpublished data). Soluble extracts may not be comparable with membrane-bound enzyme (Hartree, 1977), but the finding that an easily observed increase in the resistance of the zona pellucida to proteases after fertilization or lectin treatment has no effect on sperm penetration (Overstreet and Bedford, 1974; Bedford and Cross, 1978) does raise the possibility that acrosin may not be critical for penetration. Observations by Hartmann and Hutchison (1974) with hamster gametes and Saling (1981) with those of the mouse that protease inhibitors in the medium blocked zona binding, but not zona penetration, once spermatozoa had bound to the zona (Saling, 1981), raises the same question. It also seems curious that if acrosin really plays a key role in enabling the spermatozoon to penetrate the zona, acrosin purified from ram spermatozoa does not in any way affect the sheep zona pellucida (Brown, 1982). Lastly, because some inhibitors that have been used, e.g., TLCK, are somewhat nonspecific alkylating agents (Shaw and Springhorn, 1967), a number of other enzymes involved in penetration may also be rendered inactive by them. Indeed, crude acrosomal extracts appear more effective in dissolving the zona than might be anticipated from their acrosin content (Hartree, 1977), suggesting the presence of other lytic agents. Recently, Farooqui and Srivastava (1979, 1980) have demonstrated that combinations of acrosin with testicular aryl sulfatase or n-acetyl hexosaminidase are superior in dispersing the zona to acrosin acting alone. Furthermore, certain nontrypsin en-

zymes and disulfide reducing agents will also disrupt the zona substance (McRorie and Williams, 1974). The idea that a hyaluronidase-
proteinase complex may be involved (Stambaugh, 1972) is supported
by the observation that sodium aurothiomalate, an inhibitor of
hyaluronidase but not acrosin, will block fertilization of intact hamster
oocytes *in vitro* although the fertilization of zona-free ova is not affected (Perreault *et al.,* 1980).

Interpretation of the results of experiments in which inhibitors are
used *in vitro* is complicated, finally, by the apparent importance of the
development of activated motility for zona penetration (Fraser, 1981).
Where the presence of organic inhibitors in the medium is correlated
with a percentage reduction or absence of fertilization, it seems critical
that objective measurements should also show that the spermatozoa
were able to develop a quite normal form of activated motility. Only
then can effects seen be related exclusively to inhibition of acrosomal
lysin(s).

There seems little question, in fact, that sperm motility is important
for zona penetration, and a substantial propulsive force is probably
required for zona passage. It is of some interest, therefore, to consider
the way the sperm head and zona may interact from a mechanical
perspective. As noted earlier, some spermatozoa exhibit a most active
form of motility only after capacitation, just prior to interaction with
the egg (Yanagimachi, 1970). A comparable change in motility pattern
has been correlated with onset of the ability of mouse spermatozoa to
fertilize (Fraser, 1981). The pattern of activated motility of rodent
spermatozoa is characterized by rapid oscillations of the head (Katz *et
al.,* 1978), and as the spermatozoon attaches to the zona, such motion
becomes more symmetrical (Katz and Yanagimachi, 1981). Exactly
how this modifies the "push" the sperm exerts has not been analyzed
carefully as yet, but it may mechanically facilitate penetration by
maximizing the force of the sperm head against the zona material. In
considering the relative importance in penetration of the physical element of the sperm/zona interaction, one is intrigued in fact by how
much of the evolutionary change in the character of the eutherian
sperm head (e.g., flattened foreshortened form, increased nuclear
rigidity, keratinoid perforatorium, highly stable inner membrane of
the acrosome) can be interpreted as adaptation to forces incurred over
and above those that obtain in other groups of animals. It may even be
important in considering the consequences of the acrosome reaction
that in mammalian spermatozoa the profile of the anterior head region
is sharpened considerably by the acrosome reaction and the subse-

quent dissipation of acrosomal material (Green, 1978b), the human spermatozoon being the least extreme. In particular, the projection of a prominent perforatorium from the anterior region of the sperm head in the rabbit and rodent maximizes the force the sperm head can exert per unit of zona surface area. Yet this minimizes the area presenting to the zona substance at which a sperm lysin might act most directly (Fig. 2). It seems reasonable that a lytic activity would be of primary importance at the leading (A) rather than the lateral borders (B) of the sperm head.

In summation then, several features of the sperm head in Eutheria suggest that there has been some selection in this group for an ability to withstand physical forces in the process of entering the egg. These include the design of the head, its narrow profile, its oscillating movement, and the minimal area of the leading surface, in contrast to the whole acrosomal face that the marsupial (*Didelphis*) sperm presents to the zona material, as noted below. Together they hint at the possibility that the mode of egg coat penetration has changed in the Eutheria,

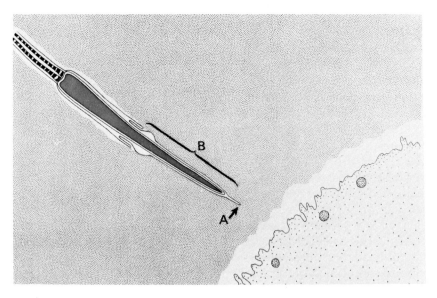

Fig. 2. Generalized diagram of a eutherian spermatozoon in the act of passing through the zona pellucida. Although the angle of approach to the oocyte may vary widely from sperm to sperm, the border (A) presents a relatively small area of inner acrosomal membrane to the zona substance opposing it. On the other hand, any lytic activity that persists on the lateral face of the sperm head (B) seems unlikely to be of major assistance in the penetration process. (See Bedford and Cross, 1978.)

perhaps because the coat itself has changed to an extent that a primarily lytic mechanism no longer is sufficient for rapid penetration.

Whereas the manner in which the spermatozoon penetrates the zona
pellucida in eutherian mammals remains uncertain, studies in the
opossum, a marsupial, strongly suggest an enzymatic mode of sperm
penetration (Rodger and Bedford, 1982). Not only does the whole area
of the acrosome appose the zona, the hole it makes in the flimsy zona

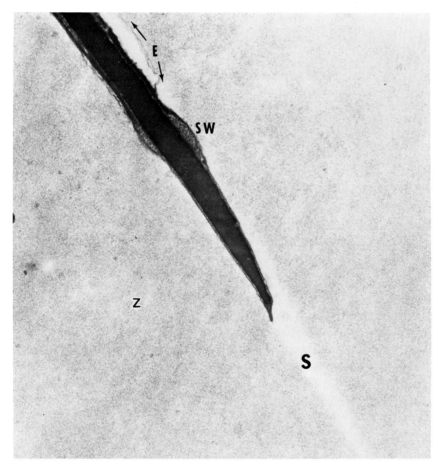

Fig. 3. Transmission electron micrograph of a rabbit sperm head in the process of
penetrating the zona pellucida (Z). This illustrates the situation seen sometimes where
the penetration slit(s) extends in front of the anterior limit of the sperm head. Note the
preequatorial swellings (SW) which we suggest may help in part to shield membranes
associated with the equatorial segment (E) posterior to it. × 32,000.

pellucida is large and has uneven edges, so differing markedly from the narrow discrete penetration slit the spermatozoa makes in the zona of eutherian eggs (Figs. 3 and 4). Moreover, the opossum zona pellucida is very susceptible to enzymatic digestion, being dissolved entirely in 2 to 3 seconds at 37°C with 0.1% bovine pancreatic trypsin, and in a few minutes by acrosomal extract (Rodger and Bedford, 1982). The significance of this difference between sperm penetration in eutherians and marsupials is discussed later in relation to the fine structure of the gametes.

VI. FUSION

Increasing evidence has emerged over the last few years that the rather complex process by which the oocytes of eutherian mammals incorporate the spermatozoon is unique to this single group among the Metozoa. What is now generally referred to as "mammalian" fertilization is a complicated interaction involving membrane fusion and then phagocytic engulfment (Fig. 5; see Bedford and Cooper, 1978). Since the way that eutherian eggs incorporate spermatozoa has been discussed recently (Bedford and Cooper, 1978; Bedford et al., 1979;

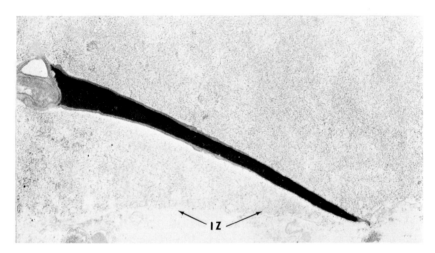

Fig. 4. Transmission electron micrograph of guinea pig sperm head emerging from the zona pellucida to pass into the perivitelline space. Note the narrow profile of the sperm nucleus and the angle of penetration. IZ, inner border of the zona pellucida. × 30,000.

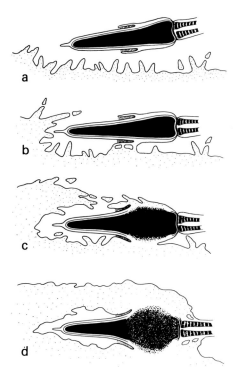

Fig. 5. Diagrammatic illustration of the successive stages of incorporation of a spermatozoon that has passed the zona pellucida. In (a), the fertilizing sperm approaches the
oolemma. The sperm then fuses with the oolemma by way of the membrane overlying
the equatorial segment of the sperm head (b). The zone of union then extends posteriorly
into the postacrosomal region (c), the sperm nuclear envelope disappears, and the begin-
nings of nuclear decondensation may have become evident already. Finally, movement
of the oocyte cortex anticipates the total engulfment of the acrosomal region of the head
shown complete in (d).

Yanagimachi, 1981), this treatment will be confined to the most pertinent points and to a comparison of events in marsupials and other
vertebrates.

    After passage of the fertilizing spermatozoon through the zona pel-
lucida, fusion with the oolemma normally follows within a short period. It is likely that the acrosome reaction (and thus, indirectly, capacitation) confers on the spermatozoon the ability to fuse with the egg
plasma membrane, perhaps by virtue of the change the reaction propagates in the sperm plasma membrane overlying the equatorial segment. For even zona-free ova incorporate only reacted spermatozoa

(Yanagimachi and Noda, 1970b; Noda and Yanagimachi, 1976). The molecular basis of this alteration is not known, although Friend and co-workers (1977; Friend, 1980) have observed the emergence of protein particle-free areas of membrane in the equatorial and postacrosomal region of guinea pig spermatozoa. Similar particle-free regions appear in fusing membranes undergoing exocytosis (Pinto da Silva and Nogueira, 1977).

It is very difficult to visualize precisely the initial moment of fusion between spermatozoon and vitellus in the electron microscope. However, the few observations of the earliest phases made so far in the rabbit, hamster, and guinea pig at least (Bedford, 1972a; Moore and Bedford, 1978a; Noda and Yanagimachi, 1976; Bedford et al., 1979), suggest that it is that segment of plasma membrane remaining over the restricted equatorial region of the spermatozoon that fuses first with the oolemma (Figs. 6 and 7) rather than sperm membrane of the postacrosomal region as initially reported (Bedford, 1970, 1972a; Yanagimachi and Noda, 1970a). A study by scanning electron microscopy (Fig. 8) also supports this view (Shalgi and Phillips, 1980). The earliest examples of this phase seen a decade ago gave the impression that fusion occurs by way of the postacrosomal region, and even now different authors writing about this (e.g., Yanagimachi, 1981; Talbot and Chacon, 1982) are unwilling to discard the idea that the postacrosomal (as well as equatorial) region takes part in the fusion event itself. However, the impression that the postacrosomal region takes part is, we feel, almost certainly a result of the fact that ooplasm immediately begins to flow posteriorly into the postacrosomal region (Figs. 6 and 7), dissecting the prominent —S—S— stabilized electron-dense material from the sperm plasma membrane that overlies it (see Bedford and Cooper, 1978). There is no question that the equatorial segment becomes disrupted in some spermatozoa "caught" at various points in the process of penetration, whether in the zona pellucida or in the perivitelline space. However, because it is seen intact in spermatozoa that fertilize (Bedford, 1972a; Moore and Bedford, 1978a; Berrios and Bedford, 1979; Anderson et al., 1975; Barros and Herrera, 1977), it seems very doubtful that the particular spermatozoa with disrupted equatorial segments remain functional. The characteristic pentalaminar structure of its membrane and septate appearance of the intermembrane content (Roomans, 1975) is particularly prominent in the equatorial segment of spermatozoa incorporated by immature oocytes (Fig. 9) (Moore and Bedford, 1978a; Berrios and Bedford, 1979). Together, therefore, present observations of the early stages of interaction suggest that gamete fusion probably occurs first over some point of

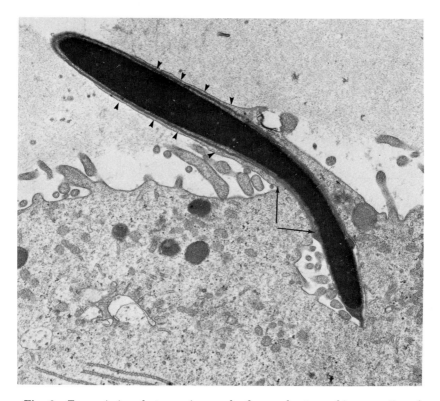

Fig. 6. Transmission electron micrograph of an early stage of incorporation of a hamster sperm head (see Fig. 5c, d), included to illustrate the obvious regional restriction of interaction (arrows) on one face within the limits of the anterior half of the equatorial region. Ooplasm, however, is beginning to penetrate posteriorly, dissecting away the dense perinuclear material from the surface membrane (arrow heads). Note that here (and in Fig. 7) fusion occurred before the head had really freed itself of the zona material. × 28,000.

the sperm plasmalemma within the limits of the equatorial region, to extend caudally as far as the postacrosomal region. The postacrosomal plasma membrane thus becomes continuous with the oolemma, as noted above, so giving the ooplasm access to the perinuclear material and the chromatin of the sperm nucleus (Bedford and Cooper, 1978; Bedford *et al.*, 1979). This sequence is shown diagrammatically in Fig. 5. Local activity of the egg cortex brings the spermatozoon further into the ooplasm, the flagellum being incorporated by a merging of the tail plasmalemma with oolemma (Bedford, 1972a). The remaining membranes of the acrosome are never themselves involved in the fusion reaction. They are brought within the oocyte through their envelop-

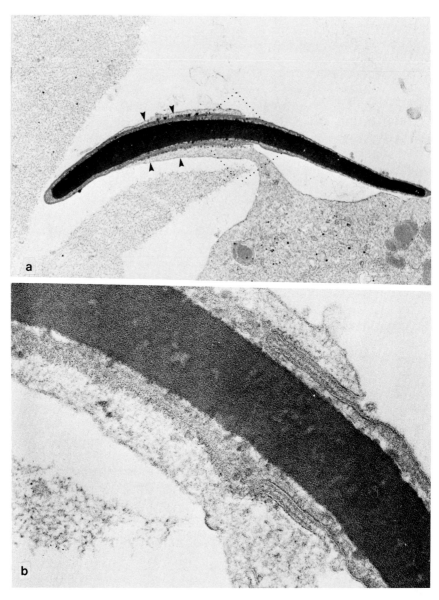

Fig. 7a,b. Transmission electron micrograph depicting the early interaction of a guinea pig spermatozoon with the oolemma of a follicular oocyte placed into the oviduct approximately 3 hours earlier. Note especially the emergent exit in the zona (lower left) and the narrow tongue extending from the oocyte surface that focuses on the equatorial region. As in Fig. 6, ooplasm extends posteriorly from it (arrow heads) separating dense postacrosomal material from surface membrane. The region within the hatched square is magnified in (b) to illustrate the typical configuration of intact equatorial segment of the acrosome. Note the appearance of an inner "sleeve" that finally creates the image of a distinct bilayer within the segment. a, × 26,000; b, × 130,000.

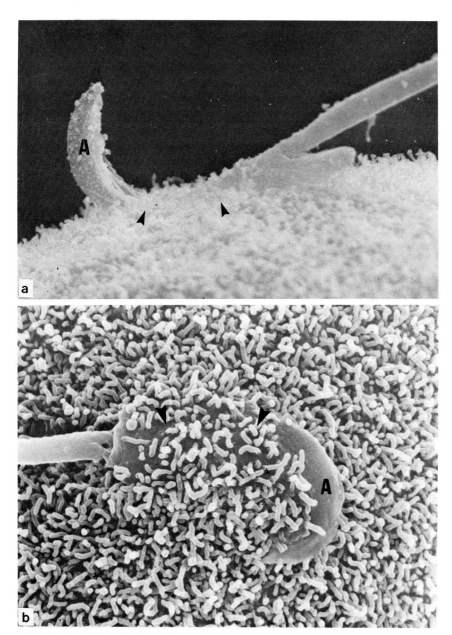

Fig. 8a,b. The early phase of gamete interaction immediately following fusion of the eutherian spermatozoon with the oolemma, as seen in the scanning electron microscope. (a) Shows a rat spermatozoon that has passed the zona pellucida and is now associating with the oolemma only by the midregion of the sperm head, here delineated by arrow heads. (b) Shows a hamster spermatozoon after passing the zona pellucida at approximately the same early stage of gamete interaction. Note that in both cases the surface of the sperm head covered by the inner acrosomal membrane (A) is not involved with oolemma. a, × 6,800; b, × 7,500.

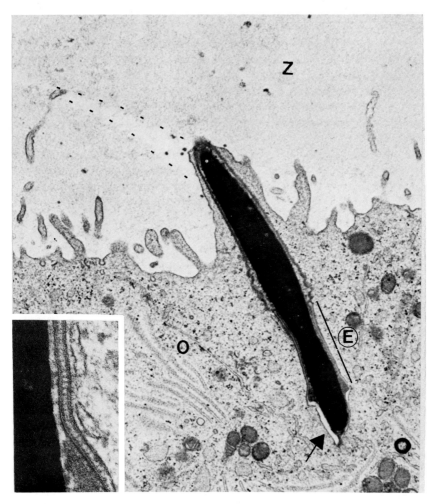

Fig. 9. Final stage of incorporation of a hamster spermatozoon that approximates that shown in Fig. 5d. Note the vesicle (arrow) around the rostral (acrosomal) region of the head, which is foreshortened in this section, and the intact equatorial region E. When magnified (inset), this exhibits characteristic bilayers and transmembrane bridges. Z, Zona pellucida; O, ooplasm. Dots delineate the penetration path in the zona pellucida. × 18,000; inset, × 50,000.

ment by folds of oolemma and actually form part of a vesicle around the front of the sperm head, composed of acrosomal and egg membrane (Figs. 6, 9). The stable nature of the inner acrosomal membrane is reflected in its resistance to detergent and MgCl$_2$ treatment (Wooding, 1973, 1975; Srivastava *et al.*, 1974) and its persistence within the egg.

This stability may possibly be due to its lower cholesterol content compared with the plasma membrane (Russell *et al.,* 1979).

Although the spermatozoon probably makes contact with the numerous microvilli on the surface of the vitellus, it is still unclear whether fusion is initiated at their tips (Austin, 1968) or at the intervillous regions (Bedford and Cooper, 1978), though more recent observations favor the former (Talbot and Chacon, 1982). Scanning electron micrographs also show microvilli over the equatorial region of the spermatozoon (Yanagimachi and Noda, 1972; Shalgi and Phillips, 1980). However, one cannot see beneath the sperm head where fusion is occurring, and the resolution achieved so far has been insufficient to determine the exact point of fusion. Endocytosis (a comparable membrane fusion event) normally takes place in the intervillous region where the membrane has apparently greater fluidity. By contrast, microvilli appear to be more stable structures and in mouse oocytes, for example, have a high membrane viscosity (Wassarman *et al.,* 1977). In this respect it is of interest that fusion between sea urchin eggs requires that the microvilli are first smoothed out by hypotonic medium (Bennett and Mazia, 1981). Similarly, fusion may be difficult in certain culture cell lines because their microvilli prevent the necessary apposition (Mercer and Schleger, 1979). Thus, it is very possible that it is indeed in intervillous regions that the oolemma possesses characteristics that favor fusion. The finding that spermatozoa will fuse readily with immature rabbit oocytes which have only a few microvilli (Berrios and Bedford, 1979) seems in agreement with this idea. However, we stress that the matter has to be resolved by observation rather than by conjecture.

Apart from its restriction to membrane over the equatorial region, it is likely that fusion in eutherians is similar at the molecular level to that proposed for other cell types (Ahkong *et al.,* 1975; Papahadjopoulous, 1978). As discussed earlier, this may require close apposition of membranes and the formation of protein-free zones of lipid bilayers. Calcium is an essential factor in this scheme, perhaps functioning to enhance the electrostatic attraction of adjacent membranes and to induce regions of destabilized membrane. In keeping with this proposal, sperm/egg fusion is Ca^{2+} dependent (Yanagimachi, 1978), and the oolemma of the unfertilized egg has a high viscosity (Johnson and Edidin, 1978). Indeed, in the presence of fusogenic agents such as glycerylmonooleate, mammalian spermatozoa fuse even with erythrocytes (Lucy, 1975; Holt and Dott, 1980). Using ram spermatozoa and chicken erythrocytes, Holt and Dott (1980) have demonstrated that this induced fusion closely parallels fertilization in that only the plasmalemma overlying the equatorial segment became involved, and a vesicle was formed from acrosomal and erythrocyte membrane around the apical sperm head. The pattern in this artificial system again suggests that the features characterizing sperm/egg fusion reflect regional qualities in the membranes of the spermatozoon, although clearly the receptivity of the oolemma to spermatozoa frequently expresses some species specificity (see review by Yanagimachi, 1981). Holt and Dott (1980) used fusogenic agents and, under normal conditions, mammalian gametes will not fuse with other cell types. Acrosome-reacted spermatozoa have been reported by Siroky *et al.* (1979) to fuse with fibroblasts, apparently in the absence of fusogenic agents, but the magnifications of their micrographs make it impossible to determine whether the interaction involved fusion or phagocytosis. Fusion between zona-denuded eggs and somatic cells has not been observed as far as we are aware, although oocytes may be fused together (Soupart *et al.*, 1979). This may mean that specific recognition mechanisms must exist between spermatozoon and egg as a prerequisite for fertilization. If this is the case, recognition must be rapid, as acrosome-reacted spermatozoa fuse with zona-denuded eggs very soon after contact (Usui and Yanagimachi, 1976). In the hamster, treatment of the oocyte with a variety of agents (trypsin, mercaptoethanol) fails to inhibit fusion (Hirao and Yanagimachi, 1978). The receptivity of the vitellus also is apparently not modified in any important way during the resumption of meiosis from the diplotene state, since primary oocytes readily incorporate spermatozoa *in vivo* (Moore and Bedford, 1978a; Berrios and Bedford, 1979) and *in vitro* (Usui and Yanagimachi, 1976). The relative lack of specificity and insensitivity to a variety of agents displayed by the oolemma of the hamster (see Yanagimachi, 1981), a major model for studies of fertilization in mammals, suggests the existence of real differences among species in the nature of the components involved (Yanagimachi and Nicolson, 1976). In the hamster, the first interactions may not be mediated to any important degree through protein or polysaccharide receptors on the vitellus, whereas the vitelline surfaces of the rabbit and mouse appear less receptive to heterologous spermatozoa (Hanada and Chang, 1978; Pavlok, 1979). In addition, anti-guinea pig sperm autoantigens will inhibit the fusion of acrosome-reacted spermatozoa with guinea pig vitellus (Yanagimachi *et al.*, 1981), implicating autoantigenic molecules in sperm-egg recognition here. Thus, although it reduces the specificity of gamete interactions at the oolemma, removal of the zona pellucida does not entirely remove the barrier to fusion, and compatibility expressed at the level of the zona pellucida does not necessarily mean that sperm reaching the perivitelline space will be incorporated into the vitellus (Thadani, 1980).

Although closely related in an evolutionary sense, fertilization in metatherian (marsupial) mammals differs in several of its aspects from that seen in eutherian mammals. While fine structural observations are limited yet to the American opossum, *Didelphis virginiana* (Rodger and Bedford, 1982), there is little doubt that the marsupial spermatozoon enters the egg by a simpler process, allied to that in non-mammalian vertebrates and invertebrates (Colwin and Colwin, 1967; Nicander and Sjöden, 1971; Okamura and Nishiyama, 1978). In the opossum, phase-contrast and electron microscope observations indicate that the inner acrosomal membrane of the reacted sperm head comes into apposition with the zona and, having penetrated it, fuses directly with the oolemma. Thus, the sperm nucleus is incorporated into the vitellus devoid of any membrane component (Rodger and Bedford, 1982), in marked contrast to the situation in Eutheria.

It has been suspected for some time that membrane components of the spermatozoon may be inserted into the egg membrane at fertilization. This view was really substantiated through the use of iso-anti-serum against whole rabbit spermatozoa (O'Rand, 1977b). Fertilized rabbit eggs were lysed when incubated with this preparation plus complement, whereas unfertilized eggs remained unaffected, indicating the exposure of sperm antigens on the fertilized egg surface. More recently, Menge and co-workers (1979) demonstrated that antiserum to sperm fractions is responsible for postfertilization infertility in rabbits. However, it is not clear whether this last effect was due to antigens originating from sperm plasmalemma or to *de novo* antigen transcribed from DNA-dependent RNA of the male genome. As well as its chromatin, a considerable proportion of the remainder of the eutherian spermatozoon is incorporated into the vitellus, including its perinuclear material and tail organelles. The contribution, if any, of these components to postfertilization events and to the development of the embryo is largely unknown.

VII. EVOLUTIONARY PERSPECTIVES ON THE MODE OF FERTILIZATION IN EUTHERIANS

Although the spermatozoa of eutherians may differ in the shape and relative proportions of their organelles according to species, all have morphological features unique to this group. Two structural characteristics set them apart from spermatozoa of subtherian vertebrates and marsupial or monotreme mammals. The differentiation of the posterior acrosome to form the equatorial segment is the more visible (Fig. 10). Delineated in the light microscope as a crescent extending across the center of the sperm head (Hancock, 1957), this has a distinctive ultrastructure which distinguishes it from the remainder of the acrosome (see Section III). Structural proteins between the membranes of the equatorial segment (Russell et al., 1979) appear to confer on it a particular stability, because of which it remains intact during the acrosome reaction, penetration of the zona pellucida, and fusion with the oolemma. A second structural feature, limited almost exclusively to eutherian spermatozoa among higher vertebrates, is the stabilization of chromatin and perinuclear material in the sperm head (Calvin and Bedford, 1971). This attribute gives it an extremely rigid character that may be significant in the face of barriers presented by the egg (Bedford and Calvin, 1974). Accompanying these two major changes in sperm structure is the radical alteration in the mode of fertilization in Eutheria. As we discussed earlier, eutherian spermatozoa cleave a narrow discrete slit through the zona pellucida and fuse with the

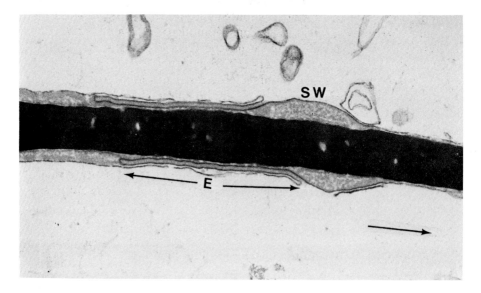

Fig. 10. Transmission electron micrograph of the midregion of a rabbit sperm head that has undergone the acrosome reaction and has shed the reacted complex. This is included to illustrate more clearly the way the preequatorial swellings (SW) might be disposed to protect the equatorial segment (E) from shear forces during forward progression (arrow) through the zona pellucida. × 54,000.

oolemma over the equatorial region followed by phagocytic engulfment of the persistent inner membrane of the acrosome into the vitellus. The spermatozoon of the marsupial *Didelphis virginiana,* by contrast, creates a relatively large, diffuse hole in the zona pellucida and appears to fuse then with the egg membrane by way of the inner acrosomal membrane (Rodger and Bedford, 1982: see Section V). Thus, the pattern in marsupial mammals essentially follows that typically seen in birds (Okamura and Nishiyama, 1978), amphibians (Picheral, 1977a,b), cyclostomes (Nicander and Sjöden, 1971), and even invertebrates (Colwin and Colwin, 1967).

In attempting to answer the natural question as to why this form of the sperm and the mode of fertilization has changed so radically in Eutheria alone, we should consider first an obvious correlate, the form of the female gamete. Apart from a reduction in size, the ovum remained largely unaltered during evolution of vertebrates to the point at which monotremes appeared (Hughes, 1977). In the Theria, however, the egg became substantially smaller and, of more importance, in Eutheria developed an unusually thick resilient zona pellucida surrounded by a cellular investment at ovulation (Austin and Bishop, 1958; Austin, 1961). In contrast, marsupial eggs at ovulation are encased only by a relatively thin, more diffusely organized zona pellucida, a tough vestment being acquired in this and many other vertebrate groups *after* fertilization. In some, e.g., teleosts, the tough coat or chorion possesses a micropyle obviating the need for spermatozoa to penetrate the substance of the coat. It is our belief that the special character of eutherian spermatozoa and the apparently unique mode by which they enter the egg in existing eutherians are evolutionary responses to alterations in the structural nature of the egg vestments. To penetrate the obdurate barriers of the outer investment, the head of the eutherian spermatozoon may have needed an intrinsically resistant quality (Bedford and Calvin, 1974; Bedford *et al.,* 1979).

The above viewpoint may allow us to speculate usefully about two special characteristics of eutherian spermatozoa. It is plausible that significant physical forces are generated during penetration of the eutherian zona, and the striking keratinoid nature of the sperm nucleus may also be a provision that enhances the intrinsic rigidity of the sperm head. The occasional electron microscopic observation of rabbit spermatozoa in which the nucleus has buckled while traversing the zona pellucida (Bedford and Calvin, 1974) and the crumpling of the DTT-treated sperm nuclei exposed to high-speed centrifugation through hyperosmolar solutions (Bedford and Rodgers, 1983) suggest that the keratinoid nature of the head allows it to withstand greater physical forces. The inner acrosomal membrane that must interact immediately with the resilient zona substance itself has acquired an unusual stability, one that may enable it to withstand the shear forces involved in penetrating the substance of the zona.

A consequence of the resilience or stability perhaps required of the inner acrosomal membrane may have been an inability to take part in fusion, and so the need arose to adopt another fusion strategy. Fusogenic membranes are generally organized so that intrinsic protein can move freely, while those that are not fusogenic have cytoskeletal anchors for intramembrane components (Bretscher and Raff, 1975). As described, the segment of plasma membrane overlying the equatorial segment, by way of which fusion occurs, has no visible submembranous material, unlike that of the rest of the reacted acrosome, and, therefore, probably can be more "labile." The appreciation that it is this region of plasmalemma that participates in the initial events of fusion also highlights the significance of the sperm's development of the equatorial segment of the acrosome, for its inherent inertness serves to halt the acrosome reaction at the rostral border to preserve plasmalemma for gamete fusion (Bedford *et al.*, 1979).

The present inference that sperm membranes need to be stable for zona penetration raises the question as to how the fusogenic plasmalemma of the equatorial segment survives during passage across the zona pellucida. In this connection, it is interesting that the sperm heads of a number of eutheria display a ridge or shoulder of perinuclear material at the rostral border of the equatorial segment, e.g., hamster (Moore and Bedford, 1978a), hare, rabbit (Fig. 10), guinea pig (Nicander and Bane, 1966), and bushbaby (Bedford, 1974b), or an abrupt narrowed waist in the region of the nucleus in which the equatorial segment sits, e.g., dog, bull, boar, ram (Nicander and Bane, 1966), musk shrew (Cooper and Bedford, 1976), and marmoset (Moore, *et al.*, 1983). Either arrangement must minimize the contact and sliding sheer forces between the equatorial surface and substance of the zona pellucida. Even the flared perforatorium on the anterolateral borders of the rat sperm head (Lalli and Clermont, 1981) would operate to relieve abrasive forces on the equatorial segment.

As well as specialized modifications, eutherian spermatozoa display more general structural changes which may be associated with their fertilization pattern. The discrete penetration slit in the zona pellucida probably reflects in part the oscillating motion which spermatozoa may utilize to cleave through the zona substance (Katz and Yanagimachi, 1981). For this mode of penetration, sperm heads with dorsoventrally flat profiles will be more effective than heads which are oval or round. Many acrosome-reacted eutherian spermatozoa do indeed show a marked asymmetry in this respect with ratios of cross-sectional dimensions exceeding 1:4 or 5 (Austin, 1976). In contrast, those of monotremes, nonmammalian vertebrates, or invertebrates have retained a vermiform or a rounded shape (see Afzelius, 1972), one seemingly unsuited to penetration that involves an oscillating cleaving movement. Marsupial spermatozoa display an intermediate form with some degree of dorsoventral flattening. This is quite marked in the Dasyuridae and Peramelidae but not in Phascolarctidae (Hughes, 1965). Perhaps of more importance is the position of the acrosome which usually lies on one aspect of the head surface. Such an arrangement is in keeping with a diffuse perforation of the zona pellucida resulting from the action of enzymes emanating from the one surface of the sperm head in contact with the zona substance, as is observed in *Didelphis* (Rodger and Bedford, 1982).

Within the Eutheria there has been a further divergence in sperm structure. An obvious feature is the acrosomal complex (acrosome and perforatorium) which has remained very similar in most mammalian groups, though the Rodentia display some extreme configurations, especially so the hystricomorphs (e.g., guinea pig, chinchilla) and Australian rodents (e.g., *Pseudomys*) (Phillips, 1975; Breed and Sarafis, 1979). The reason for this often bizarre acrosomal morphology in some rodents is not clear. In some instances, superficial correlations between acrosomal ultrastructure and the morphology of the ovum at fertilization are evident. For example, the massive acrosome of spermatozoa of the musk shrew, *Suncus murinus* (Green and Dryden, 1976; Cooper and Bedford, 1976), is stabilized by —S—S— bonds (Bedford *et al.*, 1983) and may in some way facilitate sperm passage through the peculiarly stable cumulus oophorus surrounding its ovum. But this is not a straightforward relationship of an increase in acrosome size furnishing a greater abundance of lytic enzymes to digest the egg investment, because the follicular cells in *Suncus* are insensitive to breakdown by hyaluronidase or proteases such as trypsin, due to the presence of structural junctions between them (Bedford *et al.*, 1983). The perforatorium is also prominent in spermatozoa of most rodents, reaching its largest dimensions in the rat where it forms a pyramidal structure (Fawcett, 1975). As already pointed out, in the acrosome-reacted cell this organelle is exposed first to the substance of the zona and has acquired an —S—S— dependent stability that may reflect a response to changing properties (resistance?) of the eutherian zona pellucida. It is of particular interest in that respect that all such structural attributes (shape, percentage of cysteine in nuclear protamine, lack of a perforatorium) are minimized together in the human sperm head. This suggests to us that penetration of the human zona may be a relatively less demanding activity in a physical sense.

While we feel it is reasonable to speculate that the prime mover for such changes in the structure and function of the eutherian spermatozoon may have been an increase in size and resistance of the zona pellucida, the underlying reason for that alteration is not clear. The value of a resilient vestment is understandable, since it will protect the oolemma, which by virtue of its fusogenic properties must have a "labile" nature. However, why the resilience of the vestment has been exaggerated or enhanced to such a degree in Eutheria alone is difficult to explain now. Perhaps the answer lies partly in the processes occurring immediately after fertilization. However, although a mucoid coat comes to surround the zygote of the rabbit and hare, the ova of most eutherian mammals do not acquire extraneous coats. In marsupials, where the zona pellucida is thinner and more delicate than in eutherian mammals, the large sperm penetration hole is sealed by mucoid deposited by the oviduct, followed in the uterus by a thin "shell." Such addition is obviously a common characteristic of other subtherian vertebrates.

VIII. CONCLUDING REMARKS

Despite the difficulties in the study of fertilization in mammals—for example, the need for capacitation, the cryptic nature of the fertilization site, the few eggs available—much has been learned about it in the last years. One critical factor has been the development of *in vitro* methods that allow dissection of the different steps. The possibilities these methods afford as well as acute manipulation performed within the environment of the fallopian tube already have led to more understanding of the determinants of the sperm's ability to unite with the egg. Some discoveries—for instance, that the acrosome reaction apparently propagates change in the adjacent intact sperm plasma membrane overlying the equatorial segment in a way appropriate to its fusion role—could not have been uncovered without pulling apart the process of fertilization *in vitro* and bypassing some of its steps. It should not be overlooked, on the other hand, that gamete interaction in mammals is in some respects very different from that in other groups and is subject to a variety of controls *in vivo*. It does not necessarily follow either that the demonstration of a phenomenon between eutherian gametes *in vitro* means it is of physiological interest. For example, the approach of potentially fertilizing spermatozoa through the female tract to the site of fertilization is a highly restrictive event, and so enumeration of the way large numbers interact with eggs *in vitro* seems unlikely to give much insight into the biology of conception. Recent studies indicate that spermatozoa reaching the oviduct of the homologous female select themselves in large part on the basis of their intrinsic motility, and that those that do so are no different in a genetic sense from the ejaculate as a whole. However, even the spermatozoa gaining the fertilization site naturally may not all be equivalent in a functional sense, since it is quite possible that individual spermatozoa reach a functionally capacitated state at different rates. A variety of treatments capacitate spermatozoa *in vitro* for most species in which this has been attempted, and capacitation is not species specific *in vivo*. Nonetheless, in a consideration of the nature of the capacitation factors that operate in the female tract, it should not be missed that the potential of its different regions may differ in this respect and that in some cases hormones may eliminate it. Thus, capacitation *in vivo* probably involves more than the provision of conditions generally appropriate to sperm survival and viability.

Currently, much interest centers on the underlying mechanisms that ordain the passage of spermatozoa through the vestments of the eutherian oocyte. We feel it needs to be emphasized now, therefore, that the egg vestment has changed remarkably in the transition to the eutherian state and that the spermatozoon may have developed new strategies in order to pass through it. Comparison of eutherian fertilization with that of a marsupial studied, illustrates why. The spermatozoa of marsupial (*Didelphis*) and eutherian mammals appear to have a similar complement of acrosomal hydrolases (Rodger and Young, 1982). However, the whole of the surface area of the marsupial acrosome binds directly to its zona, whereas the fertilizing eutherian spermatozoon has first to negotiate the matrix of the cumulus oophorus and probably must undergo a reaction (as distinct from a loss) of the acrosome to do so. Thus, while putative receptors for the zona are maintained at the surface of the reacted complex in Eutheria, much of the acrosomal content disperses before the zona has been reached. The eutherian zona is, even relative to its size, much more resistant to trypsin and acrosomal extract than the marsupial zona (Rodger and Bedford, 1982). Yet, at its leading surface, the eutherian spermatozoon presents a minimal area of inner acrosomal membrane to the zona substance. Such observations and the fact that the eutherian sperm head has in several respects become stabilized to an unusual degree suggest that a strong physical element has become the major factor responsible for passage of the eutherian spermatozoon through the zona pellucida. Although it is a difficult question to resolve by experiment, a similar case can be made for the view that an enhanced stability of eutherian sperm head organelles, and the inner acrosomal membrane in particular, has in turn necessitated the unusual strategy by which eutherian spermatozoa are incorporated into the oocyte.

ACKNOWLEDGMENT

Figures 4, 6, and 10 were given to us by Miguel Berrios, Fig. 6 by Luther Franklin, and Fig. 8 by David Phillips, to all of whom we are most grateful.

REFERENCES

Afzelius, B. A. (1972). Sperm morphology and fertilization biology. *In* "Edinburgh Symposium on the Genetics of the Spermatozoon" (R. A. Beatty and S. Gluecksohn-Waelsch, eds.), pp. 131–143. Edinburgh Univ. Press, Edinburgh.

Ahkong, Q. F., Fisher, D., Tampion, W., and Lucy, J. A. (1975). Mechanism of cell fusion. *Nature (London)* **253**, 194–195.

Anderson, E., Hoppe, P. C., Whitten, W. K., and Lees, G. S. (1975). *In vitro* fertilization and early embryogenesis: A cytological analysis. *J. Ultrastruct. Res.* **50**, 231–252.

Austin, C. R. (1951). Observations on the penetration of the sperm into the mammalian egg. *Aust. J. Sci. Res., Ser. B* **4**, 581–596.

Austin, C. R. (1961). "The Mammalian Egg." Thomas, Springfield, Illinois.

Austin, C. R. (1968). "Ultrastructure of Fertilization." Holt, New York.

Austin, C. R. (1976). Specialization of gametes. *In* "Reproduction in Mammals" (C. R. Austin and R. V. Short, eds.), Vol. 16, pp. 149–182. Cambridge Univ. Press, London and New York.

Austin, C. R., and Bishop, M. W. H. (1957). Fertilization in mammals. *Biol. Rev. Cambridge Philos. Soc.* **32**, 296–349.

Austin, C. R., and Bishop, M. W. H. (1958). Role of the rodent acrosome and perforatorium in fertilization. *Proc. R. Soc. London, Ser. B* **149**, 234–240.

Baker, R. D., and Coggins, E. G. (1969). Transport, survival and union of foreign gametes in the genital tract of the rabbit. *J. Reprod. Fertil.* **18**, 161–162.

Barros, C. (1974). Capacitation of mammalian spermatozoa. *In* "Physiology and Genetics of Reproduction" (E. M. Coutinho and F. Fuchs, eds.), Part B, pp. 3–24. Plenum, New York.

Barros, C., and Franklin, L. E. (1968). Behaviour of the gamete membranes during sperm entry into the mammalian egg. *J. Cell Biol.* **37**, C13–C18.

Barros, C., and Herrera, E. (1977). Ultrastructural observations of the incorporation of guinea pig spermatozoa into zona-free hamster oocytes. *J. Reprod. Fertil.* **49**, 47–50.

Barros, C., Bedford, J. M., Franklin, L. E., and Austin, C. R. (1967). Membrane vesiculation as a feature of the mammalian acrosome reaction. *J. Cell Biol.* **34**, C1–C5.

Bavister, B. D. (1969). Environmental factors important for *in vitro* fertilization in the hamster. *J. Reprod. Fertil.* **18**, 544–545.

Bavister, B. D. (1979). Fertilization of hamster eggs in vitro at sperm: egg ratios close to unity. *J. Exp. Zool.* **210,** 259–264.

Bearer, E. L., and Friend, D. S. (1981). Maintenance of lipid domains in guinea-pig sperm membranes. *J. Cell Biol.* **91,** 266a (abstr.).

Bedford, J. M. (1967). Effect of duct ligation on the fertilizing ability of spermatozoa from different regions of the rabbit epididymis. *J. Exp. Zool.* **166,** 271–282.

Bedford, J. M. (1968). Ultrastructural changes in the sperm head during fertilization in the rabbit. *Am. J. Anat.* **123,** 329–358.

Bedford, J. M. (1969). Limitations of the uterus in the development of the fertilizing ability (capacitation) of spermatozoa. *J. Reprod. Fertil., Suppl.* **8,** 19–26.

Bedford, J. M. (1970). Sperm capacitation and fertilization in mammals. *Biol. Reprod., Suppl.* **2,** 128–158.

Bedford, J. M. (1972a). An electron microscopic study of sperm penetration into the rabbit egg after natural mating. *Am. J. Anat.* **133,** 213–254.

Bedford, J. M. (1972b). Sperm transport, capacitation and fertilization. *In* "Reproductive Biology" (H. Balin and S. Glasser, eds.), pp. 338–392. Excerpta Medica, Amsterdam.

Bedford, J. M. (1974a). Mechanisms involved in penetration of spermatozoa through the vestments of the mammalian egg. *In* "Physiology and Genetics of Reproduction" (E. M. Coutinho and F. Fuchs, eds.), Part B, pp. 55–68. Plenum, New York.

Bedford, J. M. (1974b). Biology of primate spermatozoa. *In* "Reproductive Biology of Primates" (W. P. Luckett, ed.), Contrib. Primatol., Vol. 3, pp. 97–141. Karger, Basel.

Bedford, J. M. (1974c). Endocrine regulation of sperm capacitation. *Endocrinol., Proc. Int. Symp., 4th, 1973* pp. 939–943.

Bedford, J. M. (1977). Sperm/egg interaction: The specificity of human spermatozoa. *Anat. Rec.* **188,** 477–488.

Bedford, J. M. (1983). Functional significance of the need for sperm capacitation before fertilization in eutherian mammals. *Biol. Reprod.* (in press).

Bedford, J. M., and Calvin, H. I. (1974). The occurrence and possible functional significance of —s—s— cross links in sperm heads with particular reference to eutherian mammals. *J. Exp. Zool.* **188,** 137–156.

Bedford, J. M., and Chang, M. C. (1962). Fertilization of rabbit ova in vitro. *Nature (London)* **193,** 898–899.

Bedford, J. M., and Cooper, G. W. (1978). Membrane fusion events in the fertilization of vertebrate eggs. *Cell Surf. Rev.* **5,** 65–125.

Bedford, J. M., and Cross, N. L. (1978). Normal penetration of rabbit spermatozoa through a trypsin and acrosin resistant zona pellucida. *J. Reprod. Fertil.* **54,** 385–392.

Bedford, J. M., and Rodger, J. C. (1983). Determinants of gamete interaction in mammals. (In preparation.)

Bedford, J. M., Moore, H. D. M., and Franklin, L. E. (1979). Significance of the equatorial segment of the acrosome of the spermatozoon in eutherian mammals. *Exp. Cell Res.* **119,** 119–126.

Bedford, J. M., Cooper, G. W., and Dryden, G. L. (1983). Unusual aspects of the physiology of conception in an insectivore, the musk shrew (*Suncus murinus*). (In preparation).

Bennett, J., and Mazia, D. (1981). Interspecific fusion of sea urchin eggs. Surface events and cytoplasmic mixing. *Exp. Cell. Res.* **131,** 197–207.

Berrios, M., and Bedford, J. M. (1979). Oocyte maturation: Aberrant post-fusion responses of the rabbit oocyte to penetrating spermatozoa. *J. Cell Sci.* **39,** 1–12.

Braden, A. W. H., and Austin, C. R. (1954). The number of sperm about the eggs in mammals and its significance for normal fertilization. *Aust. J. Biol. Sci.* **7,** 541–551.

Breed, W. G., and Sarafis, V. (1979). On the phylogenetic significance of spermatozoal morphology and male reproductive tract anatomy in Australian rodents. *Trans. R. Soc. South Aust.* **103,** 127–135.

Bretscher, M. S., and Raff, M. C. (1975). Mammalian plasma membranes *Nature (London)* **258,** 43–49.

Brown, C. R. (1982). Effects of ram sperm acrosin on the investments of sheep, pig, mouse and gerbil eggs. *J. Reprod. Fertil.* **64,** 457–462.

Brown, C. R., and Hartree, E. F. (1974). Distribution of a trypsin-like proteinase in the ram spermatozoon. *J. Reprod. Fertil.* **36,** 195–198.

Brown, C. R., and Hartree, E. F. (1978). Studies on ram acrosin. Activation of proacrosin accompanying the isolation of acrosin from spermatozoa and purification of the enzyme by affinity chromatography. *Biochem. J.* **175,** 227–238.

Brown, C. R., Andani, Z., and Hartree, E. F. (1975). Studies on ram acrosin. Isolation from spermatozoa, activation by cations and organic solvents and influence of cations on its reaction with inhibitors. *Biochem. J.* **149,** 133–146.

Calvin, H. I., and Bedford, J. M. (1971). Formation of disulphide bonds in the nucleus and accessory structures of mammalian spermatozoa during maturation in the epididymis. *J. Reprod. Fertil., Suppl.* **13,** 65–75.

Chang, M. C. (1951). Fertilizing capacity of spermatozoa deposited into the fallopian tubes. *Nature (London)* **168,** 697.

Chang, M. C. (1958). Capacitation of rabbit spermatozoa in the uterus with special reference to the reproductive phases of the female. *Endocrinology* **63,** 619–623.

Chang, M. C., and Hancock, J. L. (1967). Experimental hybridization. *In* "Comparative Aspects of Reproductive Failure" (K. Benirschke, ed.), pp. 206–217. Springer-Verlag, Berlin and New York.

Chang, M. C., and Hunter, R. H. F. (1975). Capacitation of mammalian sperm: Biological and experimental aspects. *In* "Handbook of Physiology" (D. W. Hamilton and R. O. Greep, eds.), Sect. 7, Vol. V, pp. 339–351. Am. Physiol. Soc., Washington, D.C.

Chang, M. C., Hunt, D. M., and Marston, J. H. (1971). The capacitation time and fertilizing life of snowshoe hare spermatozoa in the female tract of the rabbit. *J. Reprod. Fertil.* **25,** 287–289.

Colwin, L. H., and Colwin, A. L. (1967). Membrane fusion in relation to sperm-egg association. *In* "Fertilization" (C. B. Metz and A. Monroy, eds.), Vol. I, pp. 295–367. Academic Press, New York.

Cooper, G. W., and Bedford, J. M. (1976). Asymmetry of spermiation and sperm surface charge patterns over the giant acrosome in the musk shrew *Suncus murinus. J. Cell Biol.* **69,** 415–428.

Dan, J. C. (1967). Acrosome reaction and lysin. *In* "Fertilization" (C. B. Metz and A. Monroy, eds.), Vol. I, pp. 237–295. Academic Press, New York.

Decker, G. L., Joseph, D. B., and Lennarz, W. J. (1976). A study of factors involved in induction of the acrosome reaction in sperm of the sea urchin *Arbacia punctulata. Dev. Biol.* **53,** 115–125.

De Mayo, F. J., Mizoguchi, H., and Dukelow, W. R. (1980). Fertilization of squirrel monkey and hamster ova in the rabbit oviduct (xenogenous fertilization). *Science* **208,** 1468–1469.

Epel, D., and Vacquier, V. D. (1978). Membrane fusion events during invertebrate fertilization. *Cell Surf. Rev.* **5,** 2–63.

Farooqui, A. A., and Srivastava, P. N. (1979). Isolation, characterization and the role of rabbit testicular arylsulfatase A in fertilization. *Biochem. J.* **181**, 332–337.

Farooqui, A. A., and Srivastava, P. N. (1980). Isolation of β-*N*-acetylhexosaminidase from the rabbit semen and its role in fertilization. *Biochem. J.* **191**, 827–834.

Fawcett, D. W. (1975). The mammalian spermatozoon. *Dev. Biol.* **44**, 394–436.

Fleming, A. D., and Yanagimachi, R. (1982). Motile life of guinea pig spermatozoa before and after the acrosome reaction. *J. Exp. Zool.* (in press).

Fraser, L. R. (1981). Dibutyryl cyclic AMP decreases capacitation time *in vitro* in mouse spermatozoa. *J. Reprod. Fertil.* **62**, 63–72.

Fraser, L. R. (1982). *p*-Aminobenzamidine, an acrosin inhibitor, inhibits mouse sperm penetration of the zona pellucida but not the acrosome reaction. *J. Reprod. Fertil.* **65**, 185–194.

Friend, D. S. (1980). Freeze fracture alterations in guinea pig membranes preceding gamete fusion. *In* "Membrane–Membrane Interactions"(N. B. Gilula, ed.), pp. 153–165. Raven Press, New York.

Friend, D. S., Orci, L., Perrelet, A., and Yanagimachi, R. (1977). Membrane particle changes attending the acrosome reaction in guinea pig spermatozoa. *J. Cell Biol.* **74**, 561–577.

Fritz, H., Schleuning, W.-D., Schiessler, H., Schill, W.-B., Wendt, V., and Winkler, G. (1975). Boar, bull and human sperm acrosin—isolation properties and biological aspects. *Cold Spring Harbor Conf. Cell Proliferation* **2**, pp. 715–736.

Garner, D. L., Reamer, S. A., Johnson, L. A., and Lesley, B. A. (1977). Failure of immunoperoxidase staining to detect acrosin in the equatorial segment of spermatozoa. *J. Exp. Zool.* **201**, 309–315.

Gordon, M., Dandekar, P. V., and Bartoszewicz, W. (1974). Ultrastructural localization of surface receptors for concanavalin A on rabbit spermatozoa. *J. Reprod. Fertil.* **36**, 211–214.

Gould, S. F., and Bernstein, M. H. (1975). The localization of bull sperm hyaluronidase. *Differentiation* **3**, 123–132.

Green, D. P. L. (1978a). The induction of the acrosome reaction in guinea pig spermatozoa by the divalent metal cation ionophone A 23187. *J. Cell Sci.* **32**, 137–151.

Green, D. P. L. (1978b). The mechanism of the acrosome reaction. *Dev. Mamm.* **3**, 65–82.

Green, J. A., and Dryden, G. L. (1976). Ultrastructure of epididymal spermatozoa of the asiatic musk shrew *Suncus murinus*. *Biol. Reprod.* **14**, 327–331.

Gulyas, B. J., and Schmell, E. D. (1980). Mammalian sperm-egg recognition and binding *in vitro*. I. Specificity of sperm interactions with live and fixed eggs in homologous and heterologous inseminations of hamster, mouse and guinea pig oocytes. *Biol. Reprod.* **23**, 1075–1085.

Gwatkin, R. B. L. (1976). Fertilization. *Cell Surf. Rev.* **1**, 1–54.

Gwatkin, R. B. L., Andersen, O. F., and Hutchison, C. F. (1972). Capacitation of hamster sperm *in vitro*, the role of cumulus components. *J. Reprod. Fertil.* **30**, 389–394.

Hamner, C. E. (1975). Oviducal fluid—composition and physiology. *In* "Handbook of Physiology" (R. O. Greep and E. B. Astwood, eds.), Sect. 7, Vol. II, pp. 141–151.

Hanada, A., and Chang, M. C. (1978). Penetration of the zona-free or intact eggs by foreign spermatozoa and the fertilization of deer mouse eggs *in vitro*. *J. Exp. Zool.* **203**, 277–286.

Hancock, J. L. (1957). Morphology of boar spermatozoa. *J. R. Microsc. Soc.* **76**, 84–97.

Harper, M. J. K. (1970). Factors influencing sperm penetration of rabbit eggs *in vivo*. *J. Exp. Zool.* **173**, 47–62.

Hartmann, J. F., and Hutchison, C. F. (1974). Contact between hamster spermatozoa and the zona pellucida releases a factor which influences early binding stages. *J. Reprod. Fertil.* **37**, 61–66.

Hartmann, J. F., and Hutchison, C. F. (1977). Involvement of two carbohydrate-containing components in the binding of uncapacitated spermatozoa to eggs of the golden hamster *in vitro. J. Exp. Zool.* **201**, 383–390.

Hartmann, J. F., Gwatkin, R. B. L., and Hutchison, C. F. (1972). Early contact interactions between mammalian gametes *in vitro:* Evidence that the vitellus influences adherence between sperm and zona pellucida. *Proc. Natl. Acad. Sci. U.S.A.* **69**, 2767–2799.

Hartree, E. F. (1977). Spermatozoa, eggs and proteinases. *Biochem. Soc. Trans.* **5**, 375–394.

Heffner, L. J., Saling, P. M., and Storey, B. T. (1980). Separation of calcium effects on motility and zona binding ability of mouse spermatozoa. *J. Exp. Zool.* **212**, 53–60.

Hirao, Y., and Yanagimachi, R. (1978). Effects of various enzymes on the ability of hamster egg plasma membranes to fuse with spermatozoa. *Gamete Res.* **1**, 3–12.

Hjort, T., and Hansen, K. B. (1971). Immunofluorescent studies on human spermatozoa. I. The detection of different spermatozoal antibodies and their occurrence in normal and infertile women. *Clin. Exp. Immunol.* **8**, 9–23.

Holt, W. V., and Dott, H. M. (1980). Chemically induced fusion between ram spermatozoa and avian erythrocytes: An ultrastructural study. *J. Ultrastruct. Res.* **71**, 311–320.

Huang, T. T. F., Fleming, A. D., and Yanagimachi, R. (1981). Only acrosome-reacted spermatozoa can bind to and penetrate zona pellucida. A study using the guinea pig. *J. Exp. Zool.* **217**, 287–278.

Hughes, R. L. (1965). Comparative morphology of spermatozoa from five marsupial families. *Aust. J. Zool.* **13**, 533–543.

Hughes, R. L. (1977). Egg membranes and ovarian function during pregnancy in monotremes and marsupials. *In* "Reproduction and Evolution" (J. H. Caloby and C. H. Tyndale Biscoe, eds.), pp. 281–291. Aust. Acad. Sci., Canberra.

Hunter, R. H. F. (1969). Capacitation in the golden hamster, with special reference to the influence of the uterine environment. *J. Reprod. Fertil.* **20**, 223–237.

Hunter, R. H. F., and Hall, J. P. (1974). Capacitation of boar spermatozoa synergism between uterine and tubal environments. *J. Exp. Zool.* **188**, 203–214.

Johnson, M. H., and Edidin, M. (1978). Lateral diffusion in plasma membrane of mouse egg is restricted after fertilization. *Nature (London)* **272**, 448–450.

Jones, H. P., Lenz, R. W., Palevitz, B. A., and Cormier, M. J. (1980). Calmodulin localization in mammalian spermatozoa. *Proc. Natl. Acad. Sci. U.S.A.* **77**, 2772–2776.

Katz, D. F., and Yanagimachi, R. (1981). Movement characteristics of hamster and guinea pig spermatozoa on attachment to the zona pellucida. *Biol. Reprod.* **25**, 785–791.

Katz, D. F., Yanagimachi, R., and Dresdner, R. D. (1978). Movement characteristics and power output of guinea-pig and hamster spermatozoa in relation to activation. *J. Reprod. Fertil.* **52**, 167–172.

Kinsey, W. H., and Koehler, J. K. (1978). Cell surface changes associated with *in vitro* capacitation of hamster sperm. *J. Ultrastruct. Res.* **64**, 1–13.

Kinsey, W. H., Segall, G. K., and Lennarz, W. J. (1979). The effect of the acrosome reaction on the respiratory activity and fertilizing capacity of echinoid sperm. *Dev. Biol.* **71**, 49–59.

Kopecny, V., and Fléchon, J. E. (1981). Fate of acrosomal glycoproteins during the acrosomal reaction and fertilization: A light and electron microscope autoradiographic study. *Biol. Reprod.* **24**, 201–216.

Lalli, M., and Clermont, Y. (1981). Structural changes of the head components of the rat spermatid during late spermiogenesis. *Am. J. Anat.* **160**, 419–434.

Longo, F. J. (1981). Changes in the zona pellucida and plasmalemma of aging mouse eggs. *Biol. Reprod.* **25**, 399–412.

Lucy, J. A. (1975). Aspects of the fusion of cells *in vitro* without viruses. *J.Reprod. Fertil.* **44**, 193–205.

Lucy, J. A. (1978). Mechanisms of chemically induced cell fusion. *Cell Surf. Rev.* **5**, 267–304.

McRorie, R. A., and Williams, W. L. (1974). Biochemistry of mammalian fertilization. *Annu. Rev. Biochem.* **43**, 777–801.

Mahi, G. A., and Yanagimachi, R. (1976). Maturation and sperm penetration of canine ovarian oocytes *in vitro*. *J. Exp. Zool.* **196**, 189–196.

Masui, Y., and Clarke, H. J. (1979). Oocyte maturation. *Int. Rev. Cytol.* **57**, 185–282.

Means, A. R., and Dedman, J. R. (1980). Calmodulin—an intracellular calcium receptor. *Nature (London)* **285**, 73–77.

Meizel, S. (1978). The mammalian sperm acrosome reaction, a biochemical approach. *Dev. Mamm.* **3**, 1–64.

Meizel, S., and Lui, C. W. (1976). Evidence for the role of trypsin-like enzyme in the hamster sperm acrosome reaction. *J. Exp. Zool.* **195**, 137–144.

Menge, A. C., Peegel, H., and Riolo, M. L. (1979). Sperm fractions responsible for immunologic induction of pre- and post- fertilization infertility in rabbits. *Biol. Reprod.* **20**, 931–937.

Mercer, W. E., and Schlegel, R. A. (1979). Phytohemagglutinin enhancement of cell fusion reduces polyethylene glycol cytoxicity. *Exp. Cell Res.* **120**, 417–420.

Moore, H. D. M. (1979). The net surface charge of mammalian spermatozoa as determined by isoelectric focusing. Changes following sperm maturation, ejaculation, incubation in the female tract and after enzyme treatment. *Int. J. Androl.* **2**, 449–462.

Moore, H. D. M. (1980). Localization of specific glycoproteins secreted by the rabbit and hamster epididymis. *Biol. Reprod.* **22**, 705–718.

Moore, H. D. M. (1981). Glycoprotein secretions of the epididymis in the rabbit and hamster: Localization on epididymal spermatozoa and the effect of specific antibodies on fertilization *in vivo*. *J. Exp. Zool.* **215**, 77–85.

Moore, H. D. M., Hartman, T. D., and Holt, W. Y. (1983). Sperm maturation in the common marmoset. *J. Anat.* (submitted).

Moore, H. D. M., and Bedford, J. M. (1978a). Ultrastructure of the equatorial segment of hamster spermatozoa during penetration of oocytes. *J. Ultrastruct. Res.* **62**, 110–117.

Moore, H. D. M., and Bedford, J. M. (1978b). An *in vivo* analysis of factors influencing the fertilization of hamster eggs. *Biol. Reprod.* **19**, 879–885.

Morton, D. B. (1975). Acrosomal enzymes: Immunochemical localization of acrosin and hyaluronidase in ram spermatozoa. *J. Reprod. Fertil.* **45**, 375–378.

Morton, D. B. (1977). Immunoenzymic studies on acrosin and hyaluronidase in ram spermatozoa. *In* "Immunobiology of Gametes" (M. Edidin and M. H. Johnson, eds.), pp. 115–155. Cambridge Univ. Press, London and New York.

Nicander, L., and Bane, A. (1966). Fine structure of the sperm head in some mammals with particular reference to the acrosome and the subacrosomal substance. *Z. Zellforsch. Mikrosk. Anat.* **72**, 496–515.

Nicander, L., and Sjöden, I. (1971). An electron microscopic study of the acrosomal complex and its role in fertilization in the river lamprey, *Lampetra fluviatilis*. *J. Submicrosc. Cytol.* **3**, 309–317.

Nicolson, G. L., and Yanagimachi, R. (1979). Cell surface changes associated with the epididymal maturation of mammalian spermatozoa. *In* "The Spermatozoon" (D. W. Fawcett and J. M. Bedford, eds.), pp. 187–194. Urban & Schwarzenberg, Munich and Baltimore.

Nicosia, S. V., Wolf, D. P., and Inoue, M. (1977). Cortical granule distribution and cell surface characteristics in mouse eggs. *Dev. Biol.* **57**, 56–74.

Noda, Y. D., and Yanagimachi, R. (1976). Electron microscopic observations of guinea pig spermatozoa penetrating eggs *in vitro*. *Dev. Growth Differ.* **18**, 15–23.

Okamura, F., and Nishiyama, H. (1978). Penetration of spermatozoon into the ovum and transformation of the sperm nucleus into the male pronucleus in the domestic fowl, *Gallus gallus*. *Cell Tissue Res.* **190**, 89–98.

O'Rand, M. G. (1977a). Restriction of a sperm surface antigen's mobility during capacitation. *Dev. Biol.* **55**, 260–290.

O'Rand, M. G. (1977b). The presence of sperm-specific surface isoantigens on the egg following fertilization. *J. Exp. Zool.* **202**, 267–273.

O'Rand, M. G. (1979). Changes in sperm surface properties correlated with capacitation. *In* "The Spermatozoon" (D. W. Fawcett and J. M. Bedford, eds.), pp. 195–204. Urban & Schwarzenberg, Munich and Baltimore.

Overstreet, J. W., and Bedford, J. M. (1974). Comparison of the penetrability of the egg vestments in follicular oocytes, unfertilized and fertilized ova of the rabbit. *Dev. Biol.* **41**, 185–192.

Overstreet, J. W., and Bedford, J. M. (1975). The penetrability of rabbit ova treated with enzymes and anti-progesterone antibody: A probe into the nature of a mammalian fertilizin. *J. Reprod. Fertil.* **44**, 273–284.

Overstreet, J. W., and Cooper, G. W. (1979). The time and location of the acrosome reaction during sperm transport in the female rabbit. *J. Exp. Zool.* **209**, 97–104.

Overstreet, J. W., and Hembree, W. C. (1976). Penetration of the zona pellucida of non-living human oocytes by human spermatozoa *in vitro*. *Fertil. Steril.* **27**, 815–831.

Overstreet, J. W., Yanagimachi, R., Katz, D. F., Hayashi, K., and Hanson, F. W. (1980). Penetration of human spermatozoa into the human zona pellucida and the zona-free hamster egg: A study of fertile donors and infertile patients. *Fertil. Steril.* **33**, 534–542.

Papahadjopoulos, D. (1978). Calcium induced phase changes and fusion in natural and model membranes. *Cell Surf. Rev.* **5**, 765–790.

Pavlok, A. (1979). Interspecies interaction of zona-free ova with spermatozoa in mouse rat and hamster. *Anim. Reprod. Sci.* **2**, 395–402.

Pavlok, A., and McLaren, A. (1972). The role of cumulus cells and the zona pellucida in fertilization of mouse eggs *in vitro*. *J. Reprod. Fertil.* **29**, 91–97.

Perreault, S. D., Zaneveld, L. J. D., and Rogers, B. J. (1980). Inhibition of fertilization in the hamster by sodium aurothiomalate, a hyaluronidase inhibitor. *J. Reprod. Fertil.* **60**, 461–467.

Perreault, S. D., Zirkin, B. R., and Rogers, B. J. (1982). Effect of trypsin inhibitors on acrosome reaction of guinea pig spermatozoa. *Biol. Reprod.* **26**, 343–352.

Peterson, R. N., Russell, L., Bundman, D., and Freund, M. (1979). Sperm-egg interaction: Evidence for boar sperm plasma membrane receptors for porcine zona pellucida. *Science* **207**, 73–74.

Phillips, D. M. (1975). Mammalian sperm structure. *In* "Handbook of Physiology" (R. O. Greep and D. W. Hamilton, eds.), Sect. 7, Vol. V, Chapter 19. Am. Physiol. Soc., Washington, D.C.

Phillips, D. M. (1977). Surface of the equatorial segment of the mammalian acrosome. *Biol. Reprod.* **16**, 128–137.

Phillips, D. M., and Shalgi, R. M. (1980). Surface properties of the zona pellucida. *J. Exp. Zool.* **213**, 1–8.

Picheral, B. (1977a). La Fécondation chez le triton pleurodele. II. La pénétration des spermatozoides et la réaction locade de l'oeuf. *J. Ultrastruct. Res.* **60**, 106–120.

Picheral, B. (1977b). La fécondation chez le triton pleurodele. I. La traversée des enveloppes de l'oeuf par les spermatozoides. *J. Ultrastruct. Res.* **60**, 181–202.

Pikó, L. (1969). Gamete structure and sperm entry in mammals. In "Fertilization" (C. Metz and A. Monroy, eds.), Vol. 2, pp. 325–403. Academic Press, New York.

Pinto da Silva, P., and Nogueira, M. L. (1977). Membrane fusion during secretion. *J. Cell Biol.* **73**, 161–181.

Polakoski, K., and McRorie, R. A. (1973). Boar acrosin. II. Classification inhibition and specificity studies of a proteinase from sperm acrosomes. *J. Biol. Chem.* **248**, 8183–8188.

Rodger, J. C., and Bedford, J. M. (1982). Separation of sperm pairs and sperm-egg interaction in the opossum *Didelphis virginiana*. *J. Reprod. Fertil.* **64**, 171–179.

Rodger, J. C., and Young, R. G. (1982). Glycosidase and cumulus dispersal activities of acrosomal extracts from opossum (marsupial) and rabbit (eutherian) spermatozoa. *Gamete Res.* **4** (in press).

Rogers, B. J. (1978). Mammalian sperm capacitation and fertilization in vitro. A critique of methodology. *Gamete Res.* **1**, 165–223.

Rogers, B. J. (1981). Factors affecting mammalian in vitro fertilization In "Bioregulators of Reproduction" (G. Jagiello and H. J. Vogel, eds.), pp. 459–486. Academic Press, New York.

Roomans, G. M. (1975). Calcium binding to the acrosomal membrane of human spermatozoa. *Exp. Cell Res.* **96**, 23–30.

Russell, L., Peterson, R., and Freund, M. (1979). Direct evidence for formation of hybrid vesicles by fusion of plasma and outer acrosomal membranes during the acrosome reaction in boar spermatozoa. *J. Exp. Zool.* **208**, 41–56.

Russell, L., Peterson, R. N., and Freund, M. (1980). On the presence of bridges linking the inner and outer acrosomal membranes of boar spermatozoa. *Anat. Rec.* **198**, 449–459.

Saling, P. M. (1981). Involvement of trypsin-like activity in binding of mouse spermatozoa to zonae pellucidae. *Proc. Natl. Acad. Sci. U.S.A.* **78**, 6231–6235.

Saling, P. M., and Bedford, J. M. (1981). Absence of species specificity for mammalian sperm capacitation in vivo. *J. Reprod. Fertil.* **63**, 119–123.

Saling, P. M., and Storey, B. T. (1979). Mouse gamete interactions during fertilization in vitro. *J. Cell Biol.* **83**, 544–555.

Scott, T. W. (1973). Lipid metabolism of spermatozoa. *J. Reprod. Fertil.* **18**, Suppl., 65–76.

Shalgi, R., and Phillips, D. (1980). Mechanics of sperm entry into cycling hamsters. *J. Ultrastruct. Res.* **71**, 154–161.

Shaw, E., and Springhorn, S. (1967). Identification of the histidine residue at the active centres of trypsin labelled by TLCK. *Biochem. Biophys. Res. Commun.* **27**, 391–397.

Siroky, J., Spurna, V., Kopecny, V., and Tradlecek, L. (1979). Acrosomal removal induces features analogous to fertilization during mouse sperm fusion with somatic cells. *J. Exp. Zool.* **208**, 245–255.

Soupart, P., Torbit, C. A., and Repp, J. E. (1979). Blastocysts obtained by fusion of mouse oocytes. *Soc. Study Reprod. Annu. Meet.* Abstract, p. 50A.

Srivastava, P. N., Adams, C. E., and Hartree, G. F. (1965). Enzymic action of acrosomal preparations on the rabbit ovum in vitro. *J. Reprod. Fertil.* **10**, 61–67.

Srivastava, P. N., Munnell, J. F., Yang, C. H., and Foley, C. W. (1974). Sequential release of acrosomal membranes and acrosomal enzymes of ram spermatozoa. *J. Reprod. Fertil.* **36**, 363–372.

Stambaugh, R. (1972). Acrosomal enzymes and fertilization. *In* "Biology of Mammalian Fertilization and Implantation" (K. S. Moghissi and E. S. E. Hafez, eds.), pp. 166–212. Thomas, Springfield, Illinois.

Stambaugh, R. (1976). Sperm proteinase release during fertilisation of rabbit ova. *J. Exp. Zool.* **197**, 121–125.

Stambaugh, R. (1978). Enzymatic and morphological events in mammalian fertilization. *Gamete Res.* **1**, 65–85.

Stambaugh, R., and Buckley, J. (1968). Zona pellucida dissolution enzymes of the rabbit sperm head. *Science* **161**, 585–586.

Stambaugh, R., and Buckley, J. (1969). Identification and subcellular location of the enzymes effecting penetration of the zona pellucida by rabbit spermatozoa. *J. Reprod. Fertil.* **19**, 423–432.

Stambaugh, R., Brackett, B. G., and Mastroianni, L. (1969). Inhibition of *in vitro* fertilization of rabbit ova by trypsin inhibitors. *Biol. Reprod.* **1**, 223–227.

Steinhardt, R. A., and Alderton, J. M. (1982). Calmodulin confers calcium sensitivity on secretory exocytosis. *Nature (London)* **295**, 154–155.

Swenson, C. E., and Dunbar, B. S. (1982). Specificity of sperm-zona interaction. *J. Exp. Zool.* **219**, 97–104.

Talbot, P., and Chacon, R. S. (1982). Ultrastructural observations on binding and membrane fusion between human sperm and zona pellucida-free hamster oocytes. *Fertil. Steril.* **37**, 240–248.

Talbot, P., and Franklin, L. E. (1974). Hamster sperm hyaluronidade. II. Its release from sperm *in vitro* in relation to the degenerative and normal acrosome reaction. *J. Exp. Zool.* **189**, 321–332.

Talbot, P., and Franklin, L. E. (1976). Morphology and kinetics of the hamster sperm acrosome reaction. *J. Exp. Zool.* **198**, 163–176.

Talbot, P., Summers, R. G., Hylander, B. L., Keough, E. M., and Franklin, L. E. (1976). The role of calcium in the acrosome reaction. An analysis using ionophore A23187. *J. Exp. Zool.* **198**, 383–392.

Thadani, V. M. (1980). A study of hetero-specific sperm-egg interactions in the rat, mouse and deer mouse using *in vitro* fertilization and sperm injection. *J. Exp. Zool.* **212**, 435–453.

Tung, K. S. K. (1977). The nature of antigens and pathogenetic mechanisms in autoimmunity to sperm. *In* "Immunobiology of Gametes" (M. Edidin and M. H. Johnson, eds.), pp. 157–185. Cambridge Univ. Press, London and New York.

Usui, N., and Yanagimachi, R. (1976). Behaviour of hamster sperm nuclei incorporated into eggs at various stages of maturation, fertilization and early development. *J. Ultrastruct. Res.* **57**, 276–288.

Vaidya, R. A., Glass, R. H., Dandekar, P., and Johnson, K. (1971). Decrease in the electrophoretic mobility of rabbit spermatozoa following intrauterine incubation. *J. Reprod. Fertil.* **24**, 299–301.

Viriyapanich, P., and Bedford, J. M. (1981). Sperm capacitation in the fallopian tube of the hamster and its suppression by endocrine factors. *J. Exp. Zool.* **217**, 403–407.

Wassarman, P. M., Ikena, T. E., Josefowicz, W. J., and Karnovsky, M. J. (1977). Assymetrical distribution of microvilli in cytochalasin B-induced pseudocleavage of mouse oocytes. *Nature (London)* **265**, 742–745.

Wolf, D. P. (1977). Involvement of a trypsin-like activity in sperm penetration of zona-free mouse ova. *J. Exp. Zool.* **199**, 149–156.

Wooding, F. B. P. (1973). The effect of Triton X-100 on the ultrastructure of ejaculated boar spermatozoa. *J. Ultrastruct. Res.* **42**, 502–516.

Wooding, F. B. P. (1975). Studies on the mechanism of the hyamire-induced acrosome reaction in ejaculated bovine spermatozoa. *J. Reprod. Fertil.* **44**, 185–192.

Yanagimachi, R. (1969). *In vitro* capacitation of hamster spermatozoa by follicular fluid. *J. Reprod. Fertil.* **18**, 275–286.

Yanagimachi, R. (1970). The movement of golden hamster spermatozoa before and after capacitation. *J. Reprod. Fertil.* **23**, 193–196.

Yanagimachi, R. (1977). Specificity of sperm-egg interaction. *In* "Immunobiology of Gametes" (M. Edidin and M. H. Johnson, eds.), pp. 255–295. Cambridge Univ. Press, London and New York.

Yanagimachi, R. (1978). Calcium requirement for sperm-egg fusion in mammals. *Biol. Reprod.* **19**, 949–958.

Yanagimachi, R. (1981). Mechanisms of fertilization in mammals. *In* "Fertilization and Embryonic Development *in vitro*" (L. Mastroianni, Jr. and J. D. Biggers, eds.), pp. 81–182. Plenum, New York.

Yanagimachi, R., and Chang, M. C. (1963). Sperm ascent through the oviduct of the hamster and rabbit in relation to the time of ovulation. *J. Reprod. Fertil.* **6**, 413–420.

Yanagimachi, R., and Mahi, C. A. (1976). The acrosome reaction and fertilization in the guinea pig. A study *in vivo*. *J. Reprod. Fertil.* **46**, 49–54.

Yanagimachi, R., and Nicolson, G. L. (1976). Lectin binding properties of hamster egg zona pellucida and plasma membrane during maturation and pre-implantation development. *Exp. Cell Res.,* **100**, 249–257.

Yanagimachi, R., and Noda, Y. D. (1970a). Physiological changes in the hamster sperm head during fertilization. *J. Ultrastruct. Res.* **31**, 465–485.

Yanagimachi, R., and Noda, Y. D. (1970b). Physiological changes in the post nuclear cap region of mammalian spermatozoa: A necessary preliminary to the membrane fusion between sperm and egg cells. *J. Ultrastruct. Res.* **31**, 486–493.

Yanagimachi, R., and Noda, Y. D. (1972). Scanning electron microscopy of golden hamster spermatozoa before and during fertilization. *Experientia* **28**, 69–72.

Yanagimachi, R., and Teichman, R. J. (1972). Cytochemical demonstration of acrosomal proteinase in mammalian and avian spermatozoa by a silver proteinate method. *Biol. Reprod.* **6**, 87–97.

Yanagimachi, R., and Usui, N. (1974). Calcium dependence of the acrosome reaction and activation of the guinea pig spermatozoon. *Exp. Cell Res.* **89**, 161–174.

Yanagimachi, R., Okada, A., and Tung, K. S. K. (1981). Sperm autoantigens and fertilization. II. Effects of anti-guinea pig serum autoantibodies on sperm-ovum interactions. *Biol. Reprod.* **24**, 512–518.

Zaneveld, L. J. D., McRorie, R. A., and Williams, W. L. (1968). A sperm enzyme that removes the corona radiata from ova and its inhibition by decapacitation factor. *Fed. Proc., Fed. Am. Soc. Exp. Biol.* **27**, 567.

Zaneveld, L. J. D., Srivastava, P. M., and Williams, W. L. (1969). Relationship of a trypsin-like enzyme in rabbit spermatozoa to capacitation. *J. Reprod. Fertil.* **20**, 337–339.

Zaneveld, L. J. D., Robertson, R. I., and Williams, W. L. (1970). Synthetic enzyme inhibitors as anti-fertility agents. *FEBS Lett.* **11**, 345–347.

Zaneveld, L. J. D., Robertson, R. I., Kessler, M., and Williams, W. L. (1971). Inhibition of fertilization *in vivo* by pancreatic and seminal plasma trypsin inhibitors. *J. Reprod. Fertil.* **25**, 387–392.

11

Transport of Gametes in the Reproductive Tract of the Female Mammal

JAMES W. OVERSTREET

I. INTRODUCTION

The generation of a new individual begins with the joining of male and female gametes during fertilization. In those vertebrates in which there is internal fertilization, initiation of this union is controlled by mechanisms that transport the sperm and ova through the female tract. In view of the critical importance of these processes, it may seem

Mechanism and Control of Animal Fertilization
Copyright © 1983 by Academic Press, Inc.
All rights of reproduction in any form reserved.
ISBN 0-12-328520-8

surprising that our knowledge of these events is quite limited, and our understanding of their physiology remains superficial. These limitations are particularly apparent in studies of sperm transport, which have not advanced far beyond the level of description and phenomenology addressed initially by Heape (1905). Application of modern technology and sophisticated methodology in this area has been frustrated by incomplete descriptions of the gamete transport phenomena and by a lack of agreement in the literature even when observations have been made. Considerable physiological differences among species and absence of any comprehensive description of the process in single species have resulted in the lack of a "model" system for intensive study. Nevertheless, recent research reports have begun to indicate a great complexity in the physiology of gamete transport. As we begin to appreciate this complexity, it may stimulate the interest of scientists with more diversified skills and perspectives.

The great diversity of gamete transport phenomena in different species of mammals has been documented in a relatively large body of literature. Since our state of knowledge today remains largely at the descriptive level, virtually all of this material remains of current interest. This literature has been reviewed a number of times in the past 15 years. Readers interested in sperm transport should consult the reviews of Ahlgren (Ahlgren *et al.,* 1975), Bedford (1972), Blandau (1969, 1973a,b), Davajan *et al.* (1970), Hafez (1976, 1980), Hunter (1975a, 1980), Mattner (1973), Moghissi (1973, 1977), Mortimer (1978), Overstreet and Katz (1977, 1981), and Thibault (1972). Those who are interested in ovum transport should see reviews by Blandau (1969, 1973b), Croxatto (1974), Croxatto and Ortiz (1975), Humphrey (1969), and Pauerstein and Eddy (1979).

In this chapter the greatest emphasis will be placed on gamete transport in humans and in rabbits. Sperm behavior in the cervix has been studied more extensively in humans than in any other mammal. Sperm and ovum transport in the oviduct have been studied most intensively in the rabbit, and for this species there is now a large body of data on the transport of both gametes which is available for integration. Important differences among species will be pointed out where they are known and appropriate references to the literature will be given in such cases. In describing the biology of ovum transport, this chapter will be limited to those events which may control fertilization. The transport of the embryo and the fate of the unfertilized ovum will not be discussed here.

II. THE EARLY EVENTS OF SPERM TRANSPORT

A. Insemination

In many mammalian species including primates, ruminants, rabbits, and some rodents, semen is ejaculated into the vagina of the female. In women the vaginal acidity is usually pH 5 or less (Kroeks and Kremer, 1977), which is deleterious for sperm survival (Miller and Kurzrok, 1932). However, the buffering capacity of human seminal plasma can raise the vaginal pH to more than 7 within the first 8 seconds after ejaculation (Fox *et al.*, 1973). In at least some cases, an elevated vaginal pH and good sperm motility may persist for as long as 2 hours (Masters and Johnson, 1966). Human semen is usually ejaculated in a specific sequence, the majority of spermatozoa and the prostatic secretions forming the initial fraction, with the bulk of the remaining fluid being supplied by the seminal vesicles (Eliasson and Lindholmer, 1974). The human ejaculate coagulates almost immediately after its constituents have been mixed within the vagina, and it spontaneously liquefies within the next 20 minutes (Sobrero and MacLeod, 1962). The biochemistry of human semen coagulation has been studied, but it remains poorly understood (Koren and Lukac, 1979; Lukac and Koren, 1979; Tauber *et al.*, 1980), and the physiological significance of coagulation is uncertain. Motile sperm have been observed swimming freely in the cervical mucus within 90 seconds after ejaculation, long before the liquefaction of the coagulum (Sobrero and MacLeod, 1962). Clearly, these sperm entered the mucus before coagulation of the semen was completed. This initial sperm entry into the cervix is associated with rapid sperm transport and is facilitated by the pressure gradient across the cervix resulting both from penile thrusting and female visceral contractions (Section II,B,2). The human semen coagulum may be analogous in some respects to a copulation plug, which in some mammals may act as a physical and/or chemical stimulus for contractions of the female viscera.

The biology of insemination in humans and rabbits is similar in many respects; the two species were placed in the same category by Walton (1960) on the bases of the common vaginal site of insemination and the presence of incipient seminal plug or slight coagulation. However, the duration of sperm survival in the vagina differs significantly for the two species. Human sperm live for no more than a few hours in the vaginal environment (Masters and Johnson, 1966), while rabbit sperm survive there for the entire 12 hours of sperm transport (Overstreet *et al.*, 1978). A second important difference between these species is the virtual absence of mucus in the rabbit cervix (Parker, 1931; Blandau, 1973a, 1977). This absence contrasts with the abundant cervical mucus of humans, which is thought to play a primary role in sperm passage through the lower reproductive tract in women.

Walton's (1960) classification of mammalian species on the basis of copulation and insemination patterns placed the ruminants within a second group, with intravaginal deposition of a semen containing little accessory fluid and high sperm concentration. Many other mammals were thought to ejaculate semen directly into the uterus, but the lack of critical evidence for this assumption has been emphasized (Freund, 1973). There is no good reason to contradict the long-standing descriptions of direct intrauterine insemination in the horse, dog, and pig (Hunter, 1975a), although the latter species has been the most carefully studied in this regard (Hunter, 1975b).

In classical descriptions, the uterus was also described as the site of insemination for rats (Walton, 1960). The early events of sperm transport in this species have recently received careful study, the results of which illustrate how our long-held assumptions can be altered when old problems receive new attention. In his classical study of sperm transport in rats, Blandau (1945) postulated that the "sperm mass . . . is ejaculated with considerable force and is catapulted into the uterine cornua." Blandau also recognized that the female played an active role in the early transport process and that the copulation plug probably mediated this interaction, since males unable to produce a copulation plug ejaculated into the vagina, and spermatozoa did not reach the uterus (Blandau, 1945). Nevertheless, until recently, the prevailing view held that male rats ejaculate directly into the uterus with the female tract playing a facilitating role (e.g., Hunter, 1975a; Blandau, 1977).

In contrast, recent studies have suggested that the normal site of sperm deposition in rats is the vagina rather than the uterus, and that sperm passage to the uterus may take place over an interval of 6 to 10 minutes (Matthews and Adler, 1977, 1978). The critical role of the female tract in this transport process was emphasized by the altered transport observed in female rats which were manipulated during the first few minutes after mating; sperm transport across the cervix in such cases was often significantly impeded (Adler and Zoloth, 1970). The stimuli initiating sperm transport in rats include both the intromissions of the male and the position of the copulation plug after ejaculation (Chester and Zucker, 1970; Matthews and Adler, 1978). The latter may be a source of chemical and/or physical stimulation to the female tract (Matthews and Adler, 1978).

Notwithstanding its importance in the rat, the copulation plug seems to play a less essential role in the transport of guinea pig and mouse sperm. Removal of the plug shortly after mating in guinea pigs does not adversely affect fertility (Martan and Shepherd, 1976), nor does removal of the coagulating glands from male mice (Pang *et al.*, 1979). The fact that intravaginal artificial insemination is successful in guinea pigs (Martan and Shepherd, 1976) suggests that sperm deposition may also be intravaginal in that species. There appears to be no comparable experimental evidence on the site of insemination in mice.

B. Rapid Sperm Transport

1. Prevalence in Mammalian Species

In his discussions of sperm passage through the female reproductive tract, Hunter (1975a) has drawn attention to the distinction between sperm transport, which implies a passive movement of cells through the female tract, and sperm migration, which depends upon the intrinsic motility of the sperm cells. With closer study of sperm passage phenomena, it has become increasingly apparent that a combination of sperm transport and migration probably occurs at almost every level of sperm ascent. However, during the interval immediately following insemination, passive sperm transport by the female is most evident, and during this phase of rapid sperm transport, a role for sperm motility has not been clearly established.

During rapid sperm transport, there is almost instantaneous passage of the sperm cells along the entire length of the reproductive tract and into the peritoneal cavity. This rate of transport cannot be explained by the swimming speeds of the sperm cells; therefore, it has been assumed to reflect a passive transfer resulting from female visceral contractions. Over the past 50 years, rapid sperm transport phenomena have been observed in every species of mammal examined (Table I). Yet the existence of the process and its biological significance remain subjects of contemporary debate. Studies of the distribution of small particles (spermatozoa) within a relatively large, contractile, tubular system (the female tract) must be undertaken with great care. Much of the current disagreement has been centered on the choice of experimental methodology and whether observations of the occurrence

TABLE I

Elapsed Time between Insemination and Sperm Recovery from the
Mammalian Oviduct

Species	Recovery time (minutes)	Reference
Cow	2	VanDemark and Moeller, 1951
Dog	2	Whitney, 1937
Guinea pig	15	Martan and Shepherd, 1976
Hamster	2	Yamanaka and Soderwall, 1960
Human	5	Settlage et al., 1973
Mouse	15	Lewis and Wright, 1935
Pig	15	First et al., 1968
Rabbit	1	Overstreet and Cooper, 1978
Rat	15	Blandau and Money, 1944
Sheep	5	Mattner and Braden, 1963

or absence of rapid sperm transport in a given species might be the
result of experimental artifacts. In the majority of studies, the experimental animal has been sacrificed or laparotomized at specified intervals after insemination, specific regions of the reproductive tract have
been isolated, and each has been flushed in order to recover its complement of sperm cells. The major sources of artifact in such experiments
are those resulting from manipulation of the tract before its division
(stimulation of the viscera and redistribution of their contents), the
relative insensitivity of the flushing and counting techniques (a population of cells might be missed if small in number), and the possibility
that contamination of instruments and/or media could lead to false
positive results.

Those researchers who have been skeptical of the conclusions drawn
from flushing studies have generally used alternative methods. For
example, Thibault (1972; Thibault et al., 1975) has questioned the
existence of rapid sperm transport in sheep and cattle on the basis of
his search for sperm heads in serial sections of genital tracts fixed at
intervals after coitus. Hunter (Hunter et al., 1980) has also expressed
reservations concerning rapid sperm transport in the ewe, in light of
his finding that surgical transection of the oviducts, as late as 6 hours
after mating, prevented subsequent fertilization. However, not even
these types of experimental study are free from artifact or from the
confounding effects of unsuspected biological factors. The way in which
such factors may interact is illustrated by experiments with rabbits
carried out in my laboratory.

Although evidence of rapid sperm transport had been reported for a number of species, it was thought for many years that this was not a feature of reproduction in rabbits (e.g., Bedford, 1972; Freund, 1973). This conclusion dated from the classical studies of Braden (1953) in which spermatozoa were not recovered from the oviduct until a number of hours after mating. This notion was reinforced by subsequent flushing studies (El-Banna and Hafez, 1970; Krehbiel *et al.*, 1972; Morton and Glover, 1974), and gained additional support from the experiments of Adams (1956) and Greenwald (1956), which demonstrated that ligation of the rabbit oviduct within 3 hours of mating prevented conception.

In contrast, our studies of rapid sperm transport in rabbits (Overstreet and Cooper, 1978) revealed the presence of spermatozoa in the upper oviduct of every animal examined at 1 minute postcoitus (pc). This unexpected finding was primarily attributable to improvements in methodology. More sensitive flushing and counting methods were employed, greater care was taken to avoid redistribution of the luminal contents during division of the tract, and the surfaces of the oviductal fimbriae and ovaries also were flushed for spermatozoa. The latter addition proved to be of critical importance, since more than 95% of the sperm recovered from the upper tract at 1 minute pc were associated with the fimbriae and ovaries (Overstreet and Cooper, 1978). The apparent conflict between our findings and the previous ligation studies was explained in part by our observation that the vast majority of rabbit spermatozoa recovered at these early times were immotile, disrupted, and obviously nonviable (Overstreet and Cooper, 1978). We also discovered that the viable spermatozoa which subsequently entered the oviduct (first detected at 90 minutes pc) were confined for hours in the oviductal isthmus within a few millimeters of the uterotubal junction, a location which may have lead to their exclusion from the oviduct after ligation.

Although sperm have been flushed from the oviducts of cows and ewes within minutes of coitus (Table I), studies of histological sections have failed to confirm this in either species (sheep: Thibault and Winterberger-Torres, 1967; cattle: Thibault *et al.*, 1975). If the biology of rapid sperm transport in rabbits and ruminants were similar, an explanation for these discrepant observations could be offered. After rapid transport, rabbit spermatozoa are located almost exclusively in the most cranial regions of the oviduct (Overstreet and Cooper, 1978). During the next several hours, these cells gradually disappear (presumably they are cleared from the oviduct to the peritoneal cavity), and spermatozoa cannot be detected again in the upper oviduct until the periovulation period (Overstreet *et al.*, 1978). If similar phenomena occur in sheep and cattle, it would not be surprising that rapidly transported sperm were not detected in histological studies of the lower oviduct shortly after mating and/or of the upper oviducts several hours later.

The question of whether or not rapid sperm transport occurs in women is also a subject of contemporary debate. Spermatozoa have been recovered from the human fallopian tubes within 5 minutes after artificial insemination (Settlage *et al.*, 1973). There is also experimental evidence demonstrating the ability of the human female tract mechanically to transport inert particles along its length (e.g., Egli and Newton, 1961; De Boer, 1972). However, other experiments have failed to demonstrate the passage of radiopaque material across the human cervix (e.g., Masters and Johnson, 1966). These apparent conflicts can probably be explained by the unique rheologic properties of the cervical mucus, which permit the forced permeation of small microparticles such as spermatozoa, but prevent bulk passage of fluids such as radiopaque media or seminal plasma (Katz and Overstreet, 1982). The idea of a rapid phase of sperm transport in women has also met resistance from those who cite the lack of association between pregnancy and orgasm in women (Moghissi, 1977). However, rapid sperm transport has been demonstrated after artificial insemination both in humans (Settlage *et al.*, 1973) and rabbits (Overstreet and Cooper, 1978; Overstreet and Tom, 1982), and it appears likely that the mechanism of rapid sperm transport is initiated independently of the occurrence of orgasm (see Section II,B,2).

In summary, rapid sperm transport has not been unequivocally demonstrated in every mammalian species. However, there is substantial evidence that the phenomenon is found widely among species which show significant variation among other features of sperm transport. This suggests that rapid sperm transport could have universal and fundamental biological importance in the regulation of mammalian fertility.

2. The Mechanism of Rapid Sperm Transport

Rapid sperm transport after artificial insemination of dead spermatozoa has been demonstrated in cows (VanDemark and Moeller, 1951), pigs (First *et al.*, 1968), and rabbits (Overstreet and Tom, 1982). These findings show clearly, in these species at least, that rapid sperm passage to the oviducts can be accomplished entirely through a mechanism of passive transport by the female tract. Experiments with rabbits suggested that rapid transport might be initiated by the seminal plasma, since artificial insemination of nonmotile spermatozoa in seminal plasma was always followed by rapid transport, whereas rapid transport never occurred when nonmotile sperm were inseminated in saline (Overstreet and Tom, 1982). Seminal plasma is known to contain a number of poorly characterized "spasmogens" (Freund, 1973) including prostaglandins, which are present in the semen of some species (Kelly, 1981). These compounds could stimulate contraction of smooth muscle in the female reproductive tract (Freund, 1973). Such a localized action on the vaginal and/or cervical musculature could result in passive transport of sperm cells into the cervical canal and perhaps as far as the uterine lumen (Blandau, 1977). Thus, a parallel appears to exist between the initial events of sperm transport in rabbits and those occurring in rodents such as the rat (Section II,A). In both species, components of the seminal plasma appear to act as chemical stimulants of the reproductive tract. A principal difference between these mammals appears to involve the contractile activity of the cervix. The cervical muscles of the rat are presumed to relax during sperm transport, allowing bulk passage of millions of spermatozoa from the vagina (Hunter, 1975a; Blandau, 1977). In contrast, the valvelike cervix of the rabbit (Blandau, 1977) efficiently blocks the passage of all but a few thousand sperm cells (Overstreet and Cooper, 1978).

The rapid transport of spermatozoa into the oviducts appears to be mediated by uterine contractions. There is no evidence that significant amounts of seminal plasma reach the rabbit uterus (Asch *et al.*, 1977a), and it is likely that other stimuli initiate and control the uterine activity. We observed rapid transport of rabbit sperm when there was no seminal plasma in the inseminate (Overstreet and Tom, 1982). However, whereas sperm motility was not required for rapid transport when seminal plasma was present, only motile sperm were transported to the upper oviduct when seminal plasma was absent. This suggests that when passive transport across the cervix was not induced by seminal plasma, the spermatozoa had to traverse the cervical canal by swimming. Since the time between insemination and sperm recovery (15 minutes) was insufficient for sperm to swim to the oviduct, their transit beyond the uterine lumen was presumably accomplished by independent contractions of the uterus and oviducts (Overstreet and Tom, 1982).

The observations of Fuchs (1972) suggest that the sympathetic nervous system is of principal importance in regulating the intrauterine pressure changes associated with mating in rabbits, and thus the early events of sperm transport. This notion is supported by recent experiments in which rapid sperm transport was blocked by the α-adrenergic blocking agent phenoxybenzamine (Overstreet and Tom, 1982). Under conditions of natural mating, uterine contractions (Fuchs, 1972) and oviductal contractions (Westman, 1926) may be initiated by pressure or stretch receptors in the vagina (Fuchs *et al.,* 1965), perhaps through a spinal reflex (Cross, 1958). Ascending contractions of the uterus could result in electrical activation of the lower isthmus (Ruckebusch, 1975), with propagation of contractile waves into and through the oviduct (DeMattos and Coutinho, 1971).

Oxytocin is released from the pituitary gland at the time of mating in cattle (Hays and VanDemark, 1953), sheep (Roberts and Share, 1968), goats (McNeilly and Ducker, 1972), and humans (Fox and Knaggs, 1969). However, there appears to be no significant release of oxytocin during the mating of rabbits (Sharma and Chaudhury, 1970). There is also experimental evidence to suggest that oxytocin is not involved in the uterine pressure changes associated with the mating in rabbits (Fuchs, 1972). Experiments in goats (McNeilly and Ducker, 1972) and sheep (Lightfoot, 1970) have cast doubt on the role of oxytocin in sperm transport for these species as well.

Uterine contractions continue for 2 to 5 minutes after mating in rabbits (Fuchs, 1972), and passive sperm transport to the oviduct may continue during this interval (Overstreet and Cooper, 1978). Thereafter, the uterine activity is relatively quiescent for 1 to 3 hours (Fuchs, 1972). However, the female remains sensitive to genital stimuli, and a second insemination will result in a second episode of rapid sperm transport to the oviducts (Overstreet and Tom, 1982). If additional matings do not occur, the rapidly transported spermatozoa disappear from the upper oviduct during the next 4 to 6 hours (Overstreet and Cooper, 1978). At the same time, a second population of sperm begins migrating from the lower reproductive tract and gradually accumulates in the isthmus of the oviduct (see Section III,C). It is from this second sperm population that the fertilizing spermatozoa will ultimately derive.

3. The Biological Significance of Rapid Sperm Transport

Nearly all spermatozoa recovered from the rabbit oviduct after rapid transport were immotile. Ninety-eight percent had visible disruptions of the acrosome and 15% had separated into heads and tails (Overstreet and Cooper, 1978). Comparable studies in other species are lacking, but there is circumstantial evidence that the damaging effects of rapid sperm tansport may not be limited to rabbits. A conflict between the results of sperm recovery studies and postcoital ligation experiments recurs frequently in descriptions of mammalian sperm transport. Ligation or transection of the lower oviduct shortly after mating reduces or prevents fertility in rats (Leonard, 1950; Sharma *et al.,* 1969), hamsters (Yanagimachi and Chang, 1963), rabbits (Adams, 1956; Greenwald, 1956), and sheep (Hunter *et al.,* 1980). Yet, an early appearance of sperm in the oviduct has been reported in all of these species (Table I). Such conflicts could be explained if a high rate of sperm mortality were universally associated with rapid sperm transport.

The destruction of rapidly transported spermatozoa would seem to preclude their direct participation in fertilization. Moreover, rapid sperm transport appears to be a feature of reproduction in species which become receptive to the male many hours before ovulation (Hunter, 1975b, 1981), as well as in the rabbit, a reflex ovulator with a 10-hour delay between rapid sperm transport and ovulation (Harper, 1961b). The fact that several hours of capacitation in the female tract are required for sperm fertility in most species (Bedford, 1970) would also seem to preclude any immediate involvement of these spermatozoa in fertilization, even on those occasions when insemination followed ovulation. What then is the biological significance of rapid transport? The possibility must be considered that rapid sperm transport is merely an epiphenomenon, a consequence of the pericoital contractions of the female tract with no inherent biological significance. In my opinion, this possibility is not likely, if for no other reason than the widespread occurrence and apparent similarity of rapid transport among mammals. The notion must also be entertained that the biological significance of the phenomenon relates to events occurring in the lower tract and not to sperm passage through the oviduct. Thus, the early appearance of spermatozoa in the oviducts could be an "overshoot" phenomenon resulting from rapid filling of the cervix and/or uterus. In humans, immediate sperm escape to the cervix from the hostile vagina is of obvious biological advantage (Overstreet and Katz, 1981). Bulk passage of semen to the uterus in species such as pigs may be an evolutionary adaptation for temporary retention of very large ejaculate volumes (Hunter, 1975b). However, one is still left to ponder the commonality of oviductal rapid transport in these species as well as in the rabbit, where no biological motivation for the process is apparent.

Since the events of gamete transport and fertilization are of primary importance for reproduction, it seems certain that during the evolution of internal fertilization a number of complex mechanisms arose to control and facilitate union of the gametes. Reproductive biologists have often viewed the sperm transport process as the simple movement of inert particles through a conduit system. Since we are now beginning to appreciate the complexity of the sperm–female interaction, it is appropriate to consider what is known of other, better studied, luminal transport systems. The gastrointestinal system is an interesting model for comparison, particularly since smooth muscle in the reproductive tract and in the gastrointestinal tract may share unique substances thought to be local hormones (Helm *et al.*, 1981). Even the most superficial examination of gastrointestinal physiology reveals amazing complexity in control of the transport process (Jerzy Glass, 1980). Among the myriad signals and receptors which are known to coordinate passage of the products of digestion, there are many examples of the transported material (e.g., amino acids) serving as local messengers to receptors along the tract. Recently there have been tentative suggestions that the rapidly transported sperm cells could serve a similar function as local messenger to the female reproductive tract (Overstreet and Katz, 1977; Hunter, 1980).

The reproductive tract is active in the transport of gametes during only a fraction of the animal's life. At other times its principal function is to defend this portal of entry against other invading microorganisms. It is a reasonable hypothesis that this shift in function, which begins with insemination, could be signaled by the rapid transport event. The messenger could be a part of the sperm cells. There are many such components with functions which are still unknown. Some, such as the hCG-like substance (Asch *et al.*, 1977b), the fibronectin-like material (Koehler *et al.*, 1980), and calmodulin (Jones *et al.*, 1980) are associated with the sperm membranes, while others could be released as a consequence of acrosomal disruption during rapid sperm transport (cf. Hartree, 1977). Another rich source of messengers is the seminal plasma (Freund, 1973) which, recent studies have suggested, could reach the oviduct in small amounts (Einarsson *et al.*, 1980). The search for these messengers and their receptors in the female should be an exciting area for future research.

III. THE REGULATION OF SPERM MIGRATION

A. The Cervix

1. The Cervix as a Site of Sperm Storage

The active migration of spermatozoa through the female depends not only on the flagellar activity of the cells but also on their interaction with the structures and secretions which line the tract. Muscular contractions continue to play an important role, but the epithelial surfaces, cilia, and luminal fluids assume greater importance during sperm migration than during the initial passive phase of rapid transport. In many descriptions of this active phase of sperm migration, the female tract has been viewed as a site for temporary sperm retention as well as a conduit for sperm passage (e.g., Hafez, 1976; Overstreet and Katz, 1981). In species with intravaginal insemination, the cervix has long been thought to function as a sperm reservoir. Quinlan *et al.* (1932) were the first to suggest that the cervix of the ewe could store spermatozoa, and this notion has been subsequently expanded and extended (Quinlivan and Robinson, 1969; Robinson, 1973). Mattner (1963, 1966, 1968) has also commented extensively on the possibility of sperm storage in the ruminant cervix. The cervix has been suggested to be a site of sperm storage in humans (Tredway *et al.*, 1975; Insler *et al.*, 1980) and in other primates (Jaszczak and Hafez, 1973), as well as in rabbits (El-Banna and Hafez, 1970; Bedford, 1971; Morton and Glover, 1974).

In the attempt to understand the biology of mammalian sperm interaction with the cervix, we must make a distinction between species such as ruminants and primates whose cervical lumen is filled with mucus and the rabbit which has virtually no mucus (Parker, 1931; Blandau, 1973a) and only a potential cervical canal (Blandau, 1977). Although there appear to be many similarities of sperm–cervical interaction across these species lines, the cervical secretion, when present, is thought to be the primary modulator of sperm behavior in this region and may be the principal site of sperm storage (Overstreet and Katz, 1981).

2. Sperm Entry into the Cervical Mucus

Sperm–cervical mucus interaction has been studied most extensively in humans, where such observations are clinically significant in an evaluation of infertility (Davajan *et al.*, 1970). It seems likely that many normal phenomena described in humans have biological relevance to other mammals with abundant mucus in the cervix. The mechanical contractions of the female viscera and the associated pressure changes (Section II,B,2) appear to be important mediators of initial sperm entry into the mucus. The human cervical mucus is subjected to intermittent shearing forces during coitus as a consequence of pressure differences across the cervix (Fox *et al.*, 1970). The first fraction of the ejaculate, which contains the majority of the sperm cells, may be passively transported into the mucus before coagulation of the semen is complete, but the unique physical properties of the mucus preclude appreciable mixing of semen and mucus (Katz and Overstreet, 1982). After the visceral contractions have subsided and the semen coagulum has liquefied, proteases in the seminal plasma may assist the remaining sperm in swimming across the semen–mucus interface. Preincubation of mucus with seminal proteases has been shown to alter its physical properties and increase the efficiency of sperm entry (Moghissi and Syner, 1970). Simple dilution of the seminal plasma with Tyrode solution reduces sperm penetration into the mucus, in spite of the fact that the vigor of sperm motility is increased by such dilution (Overstreet et al., 1980b). There is no good evidence to suggest that the acrosomal enzymes of the sperm cell contribute to sperm penetration of the mucus (Beyler and Zaneveld, 1979). Microscopic observations of sperm passage from semen into mucus suggest that physical contact between spermatozoa and the semen–mucus interface may facilitate later entry of sperm cells arriving at the same location (D. F. Katz and T. R. Bloom, unpublished observations).

The duration of the interval during which human spermatozoa continue to migrate from the vagina into the cervical mucus is uncertain. Observations following intravaginal artificial insemination suggest that sperm numbers in the cervix may reach a maximum by 15–20 minutes after liquefaction of the semen (Tredway et al., 1975, 1978). Thus, active colonization of the human cervix by spermatozoa must occur very quickly. In the rabbit, cervical filling is equally rapid (Overstreet et al., 1978) and a complement of sperm cells which is adequate for fertility is present within 5 minutes of mating in the rabbit (Bedford, 1971).

3. Sperm Migration in Cervical Mucus

The cervical mucus is a heterogeneous secretion with a liquid (plasma) phase and a solid (mucin) phase. The biophysical characteristics of the mucus result primarily from the interaction and orientation of glycoprotein-dominated macromolecules of the mucin (Gibbons and Sellwood, 1973). During the preovulatory and luteal phases of the cycle, the water content of the mucus is relatively low, the orientation of the macromolecules may be random, and there is little space between them (Odeblad, 1968). Such a mucus structure is virtually impermeable to spermatozoa. At the time of ovulation, the water content of the mucus increases and, consequently, the spaces between the macromolecules enlarge (Odeblad, 1968; Tam et al., 1982). When ovulatory mucus is stretched on a microscope slide or in a capillary tube, the mucin backbone is aligned, forming channels along which the sperm may swim in a linear orientation (Tampion and Gibbons, 1962; Mattner, 1966).

The *in vitro* swimming speeds of human sperm in stretched cervical mucus typically range from 25 to 50 μm per second (Katz and Overstreet, 1980). If sperm migration along the cervical canal conformed to this simple model of straight-line swimming, the first sperm cells to reach the uterine cavity would do so approximately 20 minutes after their passage from the vagina. However, many factors are known to complicate sperm–cervical mucus interaction. The interstices of the mucus microstructure measure only a few micrometers (Katz and Berger, 1980; Tam *et al.*, 1982). Thus, spermatozoa must swim in very close proximity to the mucus macromolecules, where significant physical and hydrodynamic interactions must occur (Katz and Berger, 1980). This relationship results both in modification of the flagellar undulations (Katz *et al.*, 1978) and perhaps in an electrochemical interaction between the sperm surface and the mucus microstructure. Recent high-speed cinemicrographic studies of sperm interaction with cervical mucus from cows (Katz *et al.*, 1981) and women (Katz *et al.*, 1982) demonstrated that "vanguard" sperm, which first penetrated the mucus, swam faster than "following" sperm which arrived at the same location later in time. Since the flagellar beats of the vanguard and following sperm were not different, the alteration in swimming speed was attributed to a change in mucus properties effected by passage of the vanguard sperm cells (Katz *et al.*, 1981, 1982). Little is understood about the adherent and repulsive forces which affect the interaction of the sperm head with the mucus microstructure, but these factors may be involved in the increased cervical mucus resistance which occurred after initial passage of the vanguard sperm (Katz and Overstreet, 1982).

Although we now appreciate the probable complexity of sperm–mucus interaction *in vivo,* our working hypotheses must continue to derive primarily from experiments with the simple *in vitro* models. A number of years ago, investigators studying sperm interaction with bovine and ovine mucus hypothesized that cervical mucus, if aligned during outflow down the cervical canal, could form a system of linear channels similar to those observed in capillary tubes (Mattner, 1966; Gibbons and Mattner, 1971). They supposed that spermatozoa, if guided along these passages, would reach the mucosal folds of the cervix and remain there temporarily before continuing their upward migration. A more recent hypothesis has envisioned organized "strings" of low-viscosity mucus, along which spermatozoa migrate to particular cervical "crypts" (Hoglund and Odeblad, 1977). Recent evidence suggests that the spermatozoa do not experience the cervical mucus as a homogeneous substance, but rather they encounter a mosaic of heterogeneous regions (Overstreet and Katz, 1981; Katz and Overstreet, 1982). Mucus heterogeneity may result in part from secretion of different types of mucus by different glands within the cervix (Odeblad, 1968; Odeblad and Rudolfsson, 1973). This mosaic structure may have a profound effect on the speed and direction of sperm migration within the mucus. Some regions of the cervical mucus are readily penetrated by sperm, while adjacent regions are not (Katz and Overstreet, 1982). The mucus is secreted in the form of granules less than 1 μm in diameter. Intermolecular bonding is established between these granules near the epithelial surface, as the network of the mucus is established (Wergin, 1979; Meyer and Silberberg, 1980). Once the mucus begins its outward flow toward the vagina, physical forces dominate the organization of its structure. A linear alignment of the microstructure probably occurs in some regions, as proposed with *in vitro* models (Gibbons and Mattner, 1971). However, mechanical forces related to visceral contractions or even to intraabdominal pressure changes would compress and shear the mucus to a much greater extent than the forces resulting from bulk mucus flow (Overstreet and Katz, 1981). Thus, the overall organization of the mucus *in vivo* depends upon the rate of mucus secretion, the effects of external forces, and the tendency of the mucus to "heal" itself. These effects are varied, nonuniform, and probably result in a heterogeneous and largely disordered column of mucus within the cervix.

It has been presumed that the aggregation of spermatozoa in the crypts between the mucosal villi reflects a storage mechanism, and that spermatozoa may subsequently terminate this association and continue their upward migration (Mattner, 1966, 1968). There is no understanding of the mechanism by which spermatozoa could be retained and released from a cervical reservoir. The properties of the cervical mucus may be different on or near the epithelial surface and this might possibly play a role in cervical sperm retention (Katz and Overstreet, 1982). In the rabbit, a species with little cervical mucus and only potential space in the cervical canal (Blandau, 1977), sperm may be stored in the cervix by a combination of inhibited flagellar activity and reversible adhesion to the mucosal surface (Cooper *et al.*, 1979). A similar pattern of inhibited sperm motility has been reported to occur within crypts of the human cervix, although no experimental data have been provided (Hoglund and Odeblad, 1977).

4. The Cervix as a Site of Sperm Restriction

The active migration of spermatozoa toward the site of fertilization is characterized by a decrease in the number of cells reaching each level of the tract. As a consequence of this restriction, only a few hundred sperm cells out of the millions ejaculated actually have the opportunity to fertilize ova (Blandau, 1969). For many years, the biological importance of this phenomenon has been attributed to the decreased risk of polyspermic fertilization afforded by the mechanism (Braden and Austin, 1954a). More recently, it has been suggested that the spermatozoa reaching the site of fertilization may not be a random sample of the ejaculate but rather a population of sperm cells selected by the female tract on the basis of unique and presumably favorable characteristics (Cohen, 1969; Cohen and Tyler, 1980). There is good reason to believe that the human cervical mucus may act as a biological filter, restricting the passage of morphologically abnormal sperm from the semen (Perry *et al.*, 1977; Fredricsson and Bjork, 1977; Hanson and Overstreet, 1981). Otherwise, experiments with mammals have been inconclusive and neither support nor refute the notion that sperm selection may occur during transport through the female tract (Overstreet and Katz, 1977; Mortimer, 1978; Fischer and Adams, 1981).

The progressive reduction in sperm numbers during transport occurs primarily at the anatomical sites, which are also presumed to serve as sperm reservoirs. Thus, for species with intravaginal insemination, a significant restriction of sperm migration occurs at the cervix. One cause for this restriction is mechanical. In the rabbit, the cervix may function as a valve with only a potential space between its apposing mucosal surfaces (Blandau, 1977). In species with an anatomical canal, the limited space within the cervical lumen is filled by a "plug" of mucus which may serve to hinder sperm passage. The association of the sperm cells with the cervical mucosa may provide another mechanism for restricting sperm ascent. The majority of the cervical sperm population does not appear to be free within the lumen but, rather, is associated with the cervical epithelium. Most of these mucosal sperm cannot be recovered from either the rabbit cervix (Overstreet *et al.*, 1978) or from the ruminant cervix (Mattner, 1966, 1968; Edey *et al.*, 1975) unless detergent is used, presumably because the cells are sequestered from the cervical lumen in the cervical crypts and/or they are adhering to the cervical epithelium (Kanawaga and Hafez, 1973; Overstreet *et al.*, 1978).

Those rabbit spermatozoa which can be flushed from the cervical lumen tend to have a lower flagellar beat frequency and generally poorer motility than do sperm cells recovered from the vagina or uterus (Cooper *et al.*, 1979). Sperm motility in the cervical mucus of ruminants appears to be excellent (Quinlan *et al.*, 1932) and motile sperm cells may persist in human cervical mucus for a number of days after insemination (Austin, 1975; Hanson *et al.*, 1982). The difference between the activity of spermatozoa recovered from the rabbit cervix compared with that of other species may be related to the scant volume of mucus in the rabbit cervix and the apparent absence of a true cervical lumen (Blandau, 1977). Thus, a higher proportion of the cervical sperm population may be associated with the mucosal surface in rabbits than in species with abundant mucus. There is good evidence that depression of rabbit sperm motility occurs at a second site of sperm restriction and/or storage in the oviductal isthmus, and that modulation of sperm motility may be important for control of sperm migration in the oviduct (Section III,C,1). A similar depression of sperm motility may occur at the mucosal surface of rabbit cervix (Cooper et al., 1979) and human cervix (Hoglund and Odeblad, 1977), but conclusive experimental evidence is lacking.

The kinetics of sperm migration through the cervix has not been carefully studied in any species. Our most detailed information has been obtained in rabbits (Braden, 1953; Overstreet et al., 1978), where the cervical sperm population appears to be established within minutes of mating, presumably as a result of passive transport by the same muscular contractions of the female tract which simultaneously carry spermatozoa to the upper oviduct (Section II,B,2). Thereafter, the cervical population remains relatively stable while the number of spermatozoa in the uterus and oviducts increases (Overstreet et al., 1978). Sperm numbers in the different anatomical compartments of the rabbit reproductive tract (i.e., cervix, uterus, oviduct) appear to reach a "steady state" by approximately 6 hours after mating and remain virtually unchanged for the last 6 hours of sperm transport (Overstreet et al., 1978). We have carried out experiments in which rabbit semen labeled with fluorescent dye (cf. Overstreet and Bedford, 1974) was introduced into the vagina during this steady state interval. In some cases, labeled spermatozoa were subsequently recovered from the oviduct (L. L. Johnson and J. W. Overstreet, unpublished observations). This suggests that the sperm populations within the rabbit female tract may remain in equilibrium for 6 hours preceding fertilization and that exchange of spermatozoa between compartments could occur during this interval. These observations further suggest that the rabbit vagina as well as the cervix may serve as a reservoir for sperm storage (cf. Blandau, 1977).

Much of our thinking with regard to the cervical reservoir has been influenced by the widely held belief that the vaginal environment is deleterious to the sperm survival. This has been long considered the case in ruminants (Quinlan et al., 1932) and in humans (MacLeod et al., 1959). Some investigators have erroneously assumed that a similar situation could exist in rabbits (El-Banna and Hafez, 1970; Morton and

by contractile waves of the myometrium, which effectively mix the
semen and uterine fluids and propel the sperm cells almost instantane-
ously into contact with the uterotubal junction (Hunter, 1975a). Infil-
tration of leukocytes appears to begin shortly after insemination and
active phagocytosis of the sperm cells ensues. Within a few hours, the
cervix relaxes and the uterine contents are evacuated. This appears to
be the case in rodents (Blandau and Odor, 1949; Austin, 1957), pigs
(Hunter, 1975b), and horses (Mann et al., 1956). The situation in dogs
could be different, since a high concentration of spermatozoa may remain in the uterus for several days after mating (Doak et al., 1967);
important sites of sperm storage may, therefore, exist within the
lumen or in the uterine glands (Griffiths and Amoroso, 1939). In species where whole semen enters the uterus, the uterotubal junction
(UTJ) must serve as an important regulator of sperm entry into the
oviduct. This function of the UTJ has been studied most carefully in
pigs, where its edematous polyploid processes probably function as a
mechanical valve, resisting the bulk passage of semen into the oviduct
(Fléchon and Hunter, 1981). The folds of the UTJ may also serve as the
site of a sperm reservoir in pigs (du Mesnil du Buisson and Dauzier,
1955a; Rigby, 1966). However, it seems likely that this storage site
may only be of temporary importance after mating, since within 1 to 2
hours of insemination, sufficient numbers of sperm have entered the
pig oviduct to ensure 100% fertilization (Hunter, 1981).

   In mammals with an efficient cervical barrier to sperm transport, it
is unlikely that more than a few percent of the spermatozoa ejaculated
ever migrate upward from the vagina (i.e., sheep: Mattner, 1963; cattle: Dobrowolski and Hafez, 1970; rabbits: Morton and Glover, 1974).
In the rabbit, as many as 80% of the sperm in the ejaculate may be
expelled from the vagina within minutes of mating (Morton and
Glover, 1974), and most of the human ejaculate appears to be similarly
lost following coitus (Perloff and Steinberger, 1964). Those rabbit spermatozoa which reach the uterus may be frequently associated with
ciliated epithelial cells (Motta and Van Blerkom, 1975a). When recovered in suspension, sperm cells from the rabbit uterus are vigorously active (Cooper et al., 1979), and it seems likely that their transit through the uterus is accomplished both by their flagellar activity
and by the uterine contractions (Fuchs, 1972). Within a few hours of
insemination, many polymorphonuclear leukocytes invade the rabbit
uterine lumen (Soupart, 1970), and most uterine sperm are thereafter
associated with leucocytes. However, few of the uterine sperm which
encounter leukocytes are actively phagocytized (Bedford, 1965). Many
appear to be capable of dissociation from the sperm–leucocyte complex

and thus remain potentially available for continued upward migration (Overstreet *et al.,* 1978).

In rabbits, the accumulation of spermatozoa in the uterus and lower isthmus of the oviduct are coincidental (Overstreet *et al.,* 1978), beginning slowly during the period of uterine quiescence which follows mating and then accelerating when uterine activity increases 2 to 4 hours postcoitus (Fuchs, 1972). The efficacy of sperm restriction by the UTJ is probably enhanced after mating as the uterine-directed contractions of the tubal isthmus increase (Salomy and Harper, 1971; Maistrello, 1971; Bourdage and Halbert, 1980) and the isthmic lumen is narrowed (Blair and Beck, 1976). The anatomical barriers presented by the UTJ and the tubal isthmus appear to have complimentary but clearly different roles in controlling sperm migration in the rabbit. The UTJ reduces the number of spermatozoa entering the oviduct by two to three orders of magnitude (Overstreet *et al.,* 1978), while the tubal isthmus completely restricts sperm passage beyond the lower oviduct until the time of ovulation (Overstreet and Cooper, 1979).

During the passive phase of rapid sperm transport, the UTJ appears to offer little resistance to sperm passage. However, in the subsequent phases of active sperm migration, the flagellar activity of the sperm cells seems to be required for negotiating this barrier. There is disagreement in the literature as to whether or not the UTJ acts at this time as an absolute barrier to inert particles and dead sperm cells, but the balance of evidence indicates that motile spermatozoa have a definite advantage over immotile cells in passing the barrier (see Gaddum-Rosse, 1981). Sperm selection at the UTJ on the basis of variation in head morphology has been described in mice (Krzanowska, 1974; De Boer *et al.,* 1976). The genotype of the sperm cell may also play a role in sperm passage across this barrier (Olds, 1970; Tessler and Olds-Clarke, 1981). The mechanism of this genetic influence is not understood, but it could be mediated by effects on sperm motility (Tessler *et al.,* 1981) or on the sperm surface (Hash and Wolfe, 1979). Direct observations have been made of rat spermatozoa passing out of the excised uterine cornua via the cut end of the oviductal isthmus (Gaddum-Rosse, 1981). Vigorously motile sperm emerged head first from the cut oviduct and into the bath of culture medium. When trypan blue was also present in the uterus, the dye did not cross the UTJ (Gaddum-Rosse, 1981), suggesting that passive transport by uterine contractions was minimal. When immature epididymal rat sperm were inseminated into the uterine lumen, these were not successful in passing the UTJ (Gaddum-Rosse, 1981). The characteristic circular pattern of motility exhibited by such sperm (Blandau and Rumery, 1964) was assumed to be responsible for their failure to negotiate the UTJ (Gaddum-Rosse, 1981).

In summary, the balance of evidence would seem to indicate that the uterus is more of a conduit than an active regulator of sperm migration, although it must be remembered that the role of this region in the sperm transport process of species with an efficient cervical barrier has not received extensive attention. The uterus may serve as a temporary source of sperm supply for the lower oviduct in most species, and the UTJ may be a region which is specialized to accomplish this function. There seems to be little evidence in support of the once widely held notion that the UTJ itself is a major sperm reservoir in mammals (e.g., Braden, 1953; Thibault, 1973). Rather, this function seems to be exercised by the lower isthmus of the oviduct in a variety of species (see below). The role of the UTJ in restricting sperm passage to the oviduct has been well established in many mammals, and there is good reason to suppose that this restriction is selective in the sense that "normal" sperm with vigorous motility have a distinct advantage in passing the barrier. Sperm restriction at the UTJ is particularly important in species where large quantities of semen enter the uterus, but the UTJ seems also to play a similar role in species where the cervix exercises the major restriction to sperm ascent.

C. Sperm Migration through the Oviduct

1. The Isthmic Reservoir

The isthmus of the oviduct appears to function as a site of sperm retention in most mammals. There is evidence for isthmic sperm storage and/or restriction in rabbits (Harper, 1973; Overstreet *et al.*, 1978), guinea pigs (Yanagimachi and Mahi, 1976), rats (Shalgi and Kraicer, 1978), mice (Olds, 1970; Nicol and McLaren, 1974), pigs (Hunter, 1981), sheep (Hunter *et al.*, 1980), and perhaps in cattle (Thibault *et al.*, 1975). The biology of sperm accumulation and storage in the isthmic reservoir is at least as complicated as that occurring in the cervix. Yet, because of its relative inaccessibility, the isthmic sperm reservoir has received far less attention.

The details of sperm–isthmic interaction have been studied most extensively in rabbits, in which an absolute restriction to sperm ascent appears to be exercised by this region during most of the interval of sperm migration (Overstreet *et al.*, 1978). The entry of spermatozoa into the rabbit isthmus is evident within 90 minutes of mating, and sperm accumulation in the isthmic reservoir continues for the first 6 hours after mating. During the final 6 hours of sperm transport (i.e., from 6 to 12 hours pc), the reservoir is apparently filled, since sperm numbers in this compartment are invariable throughout this interval (Overstreet *et al.*, 1978). The site of the reservoir in rabbits appears to lie within a few millimeters of the uterotubal junction, and virtually no spermatozoa are found above this region until the periovulatory period (Harper, 1973; Overstreet *et al.*, 1978).

Sperm retention in the isthmic reservoir probably results from a combination of mechanical and physiological factors. The lumen of the lower isthmus in rabbits is extremely narrow; for much of its length the mucosal surfaces are closely apposed (Jansen and Bajpai, 1982; G. W. Cooper and J. W. Overstreet, unpublished). A similar isthmic morphology is evident in other mammalian species (mouse: Nilsson and Reinius, 1969; pig: Fléchon and Hunter, 1981; rat: Gaddum-Rosse, 1981). The water content of the rabbit oviductal tissues increases rapidly after mating (Overström *et al.*, 1980), and this edema may contribute to the anatomical restriction of sperm passage through the lower oviduct. Rabbit spermatozoa have a special affinity for ciliated epithelial cells (Motta and Van Blerkom, 1975a), and spermatozoa in the isthmic reservoir may frequently adhere to such cells (Cooper *et al.*, 1979). However, this is unlikely to be a universal feature of sperm–isthmic interaction, since the degree of ciliation in the oviductal isthmus is highly variable among mammals (Gaddum-Rosse and Blandau, 1976). In the pig, sperm association with isthmic cilia appears to be the exception rather than the rule (Fléchon and Hunter, 1981). An additional barrier to sperm migration in rabbits may arise from uterine-directed oviductal contractions (Westman, 1926), which appear to be strongest in the lower isthmus (Talo, 1975) and have been shown to increase in frequency following the mating stimulus (Bourdage and Halbert, 1980). The oviductal cilia beat toward the uterus in most mammals (Gaddum-Rosse and Blandau, 1976). Interestingly, there is also a proovarian ciliary current in rabbits, but this appears to be confined to the lower 2 to 3 cm of the isthmus, and the ciliary beat cranial to the isthmic reservoir is uniformly prouterine (Gaddum-Rosse and Blandau, 1973). A tenacious, mucuslike secretion has been described in the oviductal isthmus of the rabbit (Jansen, 1978; Jansen and Bajpai, 1982) and human (Jansen, 1980). The secretion has been likened to cervical mucus and its appearance may be transitory during the period of sperm transport (Jansen and Bajpai, 1982). However, its role, if any, in impeding or facilitating sperm migration has not been established.

A number of studies in my laboratory have indicated that rabbit spermatozoa become temporarily immobilized within the isthmic reservoir. This was first suggested by experiments in which the isthmic contents were flushed with culture medium. The flagellar activity of the recovered sperm was found to be greatly subdued in comparison with sperm populations obtained from adjacent regions of the female tract (Overstreet and Cooper, 1975; Cooper et al., 1979). When the isthmus was flushed with mineral oil, in order to recover the sperm cells in their native fluid, sperm were found to be virtually motionless (Johnson et al., 1981). After dilution with appropriate culture media or with oviductal fluid, the flagellar beat frequency of isthmic sperm increased to levels seen elsewhere in the tract (Overstreet et al., 1980a). These experiments suggest that the depression of flagellar activity in the isthmic reservoir is reversible and that modulation of sperm motility may be important for control of sperm migration through the rabbit oviduct. There is no information on the occurrence of similar phenomena in other mammalian species.

The physiological mechanisms by which the female tract modulates sperm movement are undoubtedly complex, but recent experiments have begun to examine the biological factors which might be involved. Vigorous flagellar activity was induced in sperm populations recovered from the rabbit isthmus by flushing with 300 mOsm sucrose in distilled water (Johnson and Overstreet, 1982). Since this flushing medium contained neither ions nor substrate, it would appear that the induction of active sperm motility resulted from dilution of an inhibitory factor rather than from a stimulatory effect of the medium. There is some evidence to suggest that potassium ions might play a role in the inhibition of flagellar activity in the rabbit isthmic reservoir. In humans and in mice potassium concentrations have been shown to be higher in the oviductal fluid than in blood plasma (Borland et al., 1977, 1980), and we have evidence to suggest that potassium concentrations may be fourfold higher in the rabbit oviduct (30 mM) than in the uterine fluid (Johnson and Overstreet, 1982). Experiments in which we were able to induce a reversible depression of isthmic sperm motility by altering potassium levels (Johnson and Overstreet, 1982) lend further support to the notion that this ion may play an important role in oviductal sperm physiology.

2. Sperm Ascent to the Site of Fertilization

Studies in many mammals have demonstrated a close association between ovulation and the final ascent of spermatozoa from the isthmic reservoir to the site of fertilization (rabbit: Harper, 1973; Overstreet and Cooper, 1979; guinea pigs: Yanagimachi and Mahi, 1976;

rats: Shalgi and Kraicer, 1978; mice: Zamboni, 1972; pigs: Hunter, 1981; sheep: Hunter et al., 1980). This view is in agreement with classical observations that sperm transport into and through the oviducts is accelerated when mating occurs near the time of ovulation (rabbits: Braden and Austin, 1954b; Turnbull, 1966; hamster: Yanagimachi and Chang, 1963; sheep: Dauzier and Winterberger, 1952; pigs: du Mesnil du Buisson and Dauzier, 1955b; Ito et al., 1959).

The migration of rabbit spermatozoa from the isthmic reservoir may depend upon a number of independent biological factors. These include ovulation-associated alterations in the physiology of the female tract, changes in the flagellar activity of the sperm cells which are related to the capacitation phenomena, and, possibly, chemotactic attraction between spermatozoa and the products of ovulation. The association between ovulation and sperm escape from the isthmic reservoir was demonstrated in rabbits by experiments in which sperm distribution in the oviduct was studied in animals that were artificially inseminated but not induced to ovulate (Overstreet and Cooper, 1979). Sperm numbers and motility in the isthmic reservoir of these animals were similar to those of animals that were induced to ovulate. However, in the absence of ovulation, few spermatozoa reached the site of fertilization (Overstreet and Cooper, 1979). The synchronization of sperm ascent with ovulation is probably related to changes in the contractility of the oviductal musculature. The amplitude and frequency of rabbit oviductal contractions undergo significant changes around the time of ovulation (Salomy and Harper, 1971; Talo, 1974). Experiments with pigs (Blandau and Gaddum-Rosse, 1974), rats (Blandau, 1978), and hamsters (Battalia and Yanagimachi, 1979, 1980) have demonstrated a coordinated proovarian propulsive movement of the oviductal isthmus in the periovulatory period which resulted in the passive transport of inert particles to the upper oviduct. It is unlikely that sperm ascent under biological conditions involves such a simple mass movement of the isthmic contents, since only a relatively small number of sperm cells reach the site of fertilization, and most of the oviductal sperm population appears to remain sequestered in the isthmic reservoir at the time of fertilization (e.g., Overstreet et al., 1978). Complex interactions involving these muscular contractions and tissue edema (Overström et al., 1980; Spilman, 1980) may be involved in limiting the number of sperm cells released from the reservoir. There is evidence that suggests that the ascending sperm population in rabbits may be transported en masse to the site of fertilization and beyond, since many reach the ovarian surface and peritoneal cavity (Motta and Van Blerkom, 1975b; Overstreet et al., 1978). It also appears that this interval of sperm ascent is limited and ends shortly after ovulation, since by 4 to 6 hours after ovulation there is no longer any evidence of sperm on the ovarian surface (Overstreet *et al.,* 1978).

The synchronization of these oviductal functions with ovulation is likely to be mediated by changes in ovarian steroid secretion which occur before, during, and after ovulation (Hilliard *et al.,* 1964, 1974; Waterson and Mills, 1976). These hormones could reach the isthmus via the systemic circulation, although it is possible that specialized local vascular pathways may exist within the oviducts of some species (Hunter, 1980). Hormonal control of tubal contractility is probably mediated by the autonomic nervous system. The mammalian oviduct contains many adrenergic receptors (Black, 1974), which are known to be influenced by estrogen and progesterone (Paton *et al.,* 1978). The complexity of the hormonal–neural interactions which may be involved is well illustrated by the experiments of Battalia and Yanagimachi (1980), who found that the proovarian transport of inert particles from the isthmus of the hamster oviduct was most effectively induced by a combination of progesterone administration and estrogen withdrawal.

In addition to convincing evidence for the importance of oviductal physiology in the synchronization of sperm and ovum transport, there is also reason to believe that specific movements of the sperm cell may be involved in its ascent to the site of fertilization. In a number of rodents and in the rabbit, a unique pattern of sperm movement termed activated motility or hyperactivated motility is associated with the completion of capacitation and the acrosome reaction (Yanagimachi, 1981). Activated rabbit sperm do not appear in the oviductal flushings until 6 hours or more after mating (Cooper *et al.,* 1979) and, by the time of fertilization, more than 90% of rabbit ampullar sperm are activated (Suarez and Katz, 1982). For rabbit sperm, the shift from preactivated to activated motility involves a 20-fold increase in power output, an energy expenditure which may be necessary for escape from the isthmic reservoir (Johnson *et al.,* 1981). In the rabbit, activated motility is characterized *in vitro* by episodes of nonprogressive swimming with large amplitude, whiplashlike flagellar undulations, alternating with other episodes of lower amplitude, progressive swimming (Cooper *et al.,* 1979; Johnson *et al.,* 1981). Observations made through the relatively transparent wall of the hamster oviduct have suggested how the swimming behavior of such spermatozoa, which appears to be nonprogressive *in vitro,* may be translated into directed movement *in vivo* (Katz and Yanagimachi, 1980). The flagellar beat frequencies and shapes which resulted in nonprogressive swimming by hamster sper-

matozoa *in vitro* produced rapid swimming along the epithelial surfaces of the oviduct, which both guided the sperm trajectory and increased its velocity (Katz and Yanagimachi, 1980).

Experimental evidence which implicates activated motility in sperm
ascent to the site of fertilization was obtained in studies of delayed
mating in rabbits (Overstreet and Cooper, 1979). Coitus with a vasec-
tomized male was used as an ovulation-inducing stimulus, but mating
with the fertile male was not allowed for an additional 8 hours. Thus,
when ovulation and its associated endocrine changes were occurring,
the spermatozoa had been present in the tract for only 2 to 4 hours, an
insufficient time for completion of capacitation (Bedford, 1970). In
spite of the fact that many spermatozoa were present in the isthmic
reservoir, none reached the site of fertilization (Overstreet and Cooper,
1979). Since spermatozoa with activated motility were not observed in
the upper isthmus, it was suggested that, lacking this special type of
movement, spermatozoa were incapable of ascending to the site of fertilization (Overstreet and Cooper, 1979).

However, the control of sperm release from the isthmic reservoir
may be even more complex. Batalia and Yanagimachi (1979) observed
a puzzling difference in the proovarian transport of inert particles out
of the hamster isthmus in mated versus nonmated animals, the process
being significantly more efficient in mated animals. The initial events
of sperm transport may involve delivery of messages to the oviduct
(Section II,B,3). It is possible, therefore, that the failure of sperm ascent which we observed after delayed mating could still be related in
part to the contractile activity of the female tract, i.e., asynchrony of
the rapid transport message and the ovulation-inducing stimulus led
to inefficient sperm transport from the reservoir at the time of ovulation. We have shown in subsequent experiments that spermatozoa recovered from the rabbit isthmus at 4 hours after mating can be activated *in vitro* when removed from the isthmic environment (Overstreet
et al., 1980a). The mechanism of sperm motility activation *in vivo* is
unknown, and it remains a mystery why activation did not take place
in the few sperm that were released from the lower isthmus in delayed
mated rabbits (Overstreet and Cooper, 1979).

Chemically mediated interaction between spermatozoa and ova has
been demonstrated in plants and in a number of invertebrate animals
(Miller, 1977). Notwithstanding a previous claim for chemotaxis of
rabbit spermatozoa (Dickmann, 1963), the phenomenon has never
been convincingly demonstrated in any mammal (Yanagimachi, 1981).
However, there has never been a serious attempt to demonstrate
chemotaxis in mammals with appropriate material (spermatozoa and

ova from the oviducts), sensitive recording devices, and adequate mathematical analysis. Therefore, the possibility cannot be ruled out that the products of ovulation could directly stimulate sperm ascent (Harper, 1973). It is unlikely, however, that these are the only stimuli, since sperm ascent has been observed in some rabbits as early as 2 hours before the expected time of ovulation (Overstreet et al., 1978).

IV. OVUM TRANSPORT

A. Ovum Passage from the Ovarian Surface to the Oviduct

Like sperm transport, ovum transport has been frequently described as occurring in steps or stages (e.g., Blandau, 1969; Croxatto, 1974). The first step of the process involves the passage of the oocyte from the ruptured ovarian follicle into the distal end of the oviduct. Subsequent stages involve its transport through the oviductal ampulla and a period of ovum retention at the ampullar–isthmic junction. In most, if not all, mammals, fertilization is believed to occur during these early stages of the transport process (Austin and Bishop, 1957). Subsequently, the embryo passes through the oviductal isthmus, pausing in some species at the uterotubal junction before entering the uterine cavity (Blandau, 1969).

The biology of ovum passage from the ovarian surface to the ostium of the oviduct is highly variable among species. The factors involved in mediating these events include the contractile activity of the muscular structures supporting the ovaries and oviducts, the ciliary activity of the oviductal fimbriae, and the physical properties of the oocyte investments. In species such as mice, hamsters and rats the ovaries are enclosed in a periovarial sac, and there may be no direct contact between the fimbrial and ovarian surfaces (Alden, 1942; Wimsatt and Waldo, 1945). In these rodents, the oocytes float freely in the periovarial fluid and quickly contact cilia of the tubal infundibulum (Blandau, 1969).

In other species, including rabbits and primates, the ovary is not enclosed within an anatomical bursa and the extent of fimbrial–ovarian communication varies with the stage of the ovarian cycle. In some species, the fimbria may expand to cover virtually all of the ovarian surface by the time of ovulation (Blandau, 1969). For those mammals without an anatomical bursa, the oocyte does not float freely away from the ovary but rather remains attached to its surface by the sticky cumulus oophorus (rabbits: Blandau, 1969; primates: Dukelow, 1975).

Contractions of smooth muscle fibers in the supporting structures of the ovary and fimbria enable contact between the cumulus mass and the ciliated fimbria, and facilitate the entry of the oocyte into the tubal ostium (Blandau, 1969). Some investigators have suggested that negative pressure could be generated within the tubal ampulla and that this could result in the "insuck" of the oocyte (Westman, 1952; Austin, 1963a; Maia and Coutinho, 1970). However, both direct observations (Blandau, 1969) and experimental ligation of the ampulla (Clewe and Mastroianni, 1958) have indicated that the movement of particles into the tubal ostium can be accounted for by ciliary activity alone.

In spite of compelling evidence that the foregoing descriptions accurately portray the normal biology of oocyte capture, there are equally convincing observations to indicate that other mechanisms may also be effective. Notwithstanding the normal function of the fimbria in capture of the oocyte, pregnancies have been obtained with rabbits after bilateral fimbriectomy (Metz and Mastroianni, 1979; Beyth and Winston, 1981; Halbert and Patton, 1981). Although the oocyte is thought to remain on the ovarian surface until pickup by the fimbria, it may also be captured from the peritoneal cavity. On rare occasions pregnancies have been reported in women with one ovary and a contralateral oviduct (First, 1954), and ova have been recovered from human oviducts contralateral to the corpus luteum-bearing ovary (Doyle et al., 1966). In spite of the preeminent role of oviductal cilia in ovum capture, some women with immotile cilia do become pregnant (Afzelius et al., 1978; Jean et al., 1979).

B. Ovum Transport through the Oviductal Ampulla

The passage of the cumulus mass from the infundibulum to the ampullar isthmic junction has generally been viewed as an extremely rapid event (e.g., Blandau, 1969). This is undoubtedly true for the rabbit, in which direct observations of ovum passage through the ampulla have indicated a total transit time of only a few minutes (Harper, 1961a, 1962; Blandau, 1969). However, the rabbit model may not be typical, since considerably longer ampullar transit times may occur in other species, including humans (Croxatto et al., 1978), cattle (Crisman et al., 1980), and sheep (Holst and Braden, 1972).

The physiological regulation of this phase of transport is complex and poorly understood, although it is generally agreed to rely primarily on the muscular contractions and ciliary activity of the ampulla. Observations of ovum transport in the rabbit oviduct indicated that the muscular contractions were discontinuous and segmental;

peristaltic rushes were interspersed with antiperistaltic contractions, which at times moved the oocytes back toward the ovary (Harper, 1961a, 1962; Blandau, 1969). The cilia of the rabbit ampulla beat uniformly toward the uterus (Gaddum-Rosse and Blandau, 1973), and these are capable of transporting ova rapidly through the ampulla when muscular contractions are blocked (Halbert *et al.*, 1976a, b). On the other hand, women with immotile cilia in their oviducts can become pregnant (Afzelius *et al.*, 1978; Jean *et al.*, 1979), so that ciliary beating is not in itself essential.

It has long been appreciated that the cumulus mass is important for efficient transport by the oviductal cilia (Blandau, 1969). Experimental studies have since shown that the tips of rabbit cilia contain anionic sites which, when blocked with poly-L-lysine, become ineffective in transporting ova (Norwood *et al.*, 1978; Norwood and Anderson, 1980). These studies have suggested that such sites on the cilia may be essential for adhesion of the cumulus to the epithelium and, thus, are necessary for efficient transport. This fact would appear to resolve the apparent discrepancy between reports of the association of oviductal deciliation with infertility on the one hand and immotile cilia and fertility on the other (Pauerstein and Eddy, 1979). Providing that immotile cilia have a normal number of adhesive sites, they could function adequately to facilitate muscular transport of the oocyte (Norwood and Anderson, 1980).

There is a good reason to believe that contractions of the oviductal musculature are related to changes in the levels of circulating steroids (e.g., Bourdage and Halbert, 1980; Battalia and Yanagimachi, 1980). There have also been recent suggestions that hormones could directly affect ciliary activity (Verdugo *et al.*, 1980). The hormonal-neural control of tubal contractility has been studied in relationship to ovum transport. However, there are widely differing patterns of steroid secretion in the periovulatory period in different mammals, and the species also vary in their oviductal response to exogenous hormone injections (Croxatto and Ortiz, 1975). It is unlikely, therefore, that a common endocrine-mediated regulatory mechanism for ovum transport exists, and none has yet been proposed. There is significant variation among species in the retention of the granulosa cell investment during ovum transport, but, in virtually all eutherian mammals, the oocyte appears to be invested with a cumulus oophorus during transport to the site of fertilization (Austin, 1963b). The importance of these vestments seems well established and is related primarily to the physical interaction between the cumulus mass and the ciliated tubal epithelium. There is an intriguing possibility that chemical and/or physical messages between the oocyte and oviduct might also modulate ovum transport. Blandau (1969) suggested that the cumulus itself might initiate oviductal contractions within its immediate proximity. There is suggestive evidence, for some species, that the developing embryo may "communicate" with the oviduct, since fertilized and unfertilized ova are transported differently (see Croxatto, 1974). There are no data to suggest that such interactions occur during the transport of oocytes prior to fertilization, and, if such occur, the effects are likely to be subtle, since inert particles and oocytes are transported in virtually the same manner, providing their physical properties are similar (Harper et al., 1960; Croxatto et al., 1973).

There is as yet no integrated description of the mechanism of ovum passage through the ampulla. In fact, it has been suggested that completely random movements of the oviductal musculature could result in directed transport of oocytes (Portnow et al., 1977). In such a situation, prouterine ciliary activity would be required to prevent return of oocytes to the peritoneal cavity; the relative inactivity of musculature at the ampullar-isthmic junction could then arrest the progress of the oocytes as they enter this region (Portnow et al., 1977).

C. Retention of Ova at the Ampullar–Isthmic Junction

The site of fertilization has been classically located in the lower ampulla (Austin and Bishop, 1957), although the interaction between spermatozoa and ova probably begins higher in the oviduct and may even be initiated on the ovarian surface prior to ovum pickup (cf. Fig. 17a of Motta and Van Blerkom, 1975b). Oocytes are retained in the lower ampulla at the ampullar–isthmic junction for 24 to 48 hours in many species (Humphrey, 1969), although no structural basis for this "physiological sphincter" has been demonstrated (Greenwald, 1961). Explanations which have been advanced include pressure differentials (Braudin, 1964), subserosal edema (Edgar and Asdell, 1960; Overström et al., 1980), ciliary and secretory activity (Koester, 1970; Spilman, 1980), and differential peristaltic forces (Winterberger-Torres, 1961). Recent studies of myoelectrical activity in rabbits (Talo and Hodgson, 1978) and mice (Talo, 1980) lend support to the theory that muscular activity of the oviduct is the primary factor involved in ovum retention at the ampullar–isthmic function. It has been observed that muscular contractions do not appear to spread from the ampulla to the isthmus (Blandau, 1969; Talo, 1980). There is also an indication that electrical excitability is lower at the ampullar-isthmic junction than at either of the adjacent regions (Talo, 1980). In the mouse, at least, there may also be an adjacent region of the isthmus from which contractions propagate toward the ovary, thus preventing premature transport of the ova toward the uterus (Talo, 1980). Release of fertilized ova from the ampullar–isthmic junction is presumed to occur in response to alterations in oviductal contractions mediated by hormonal neural signals, since in some species administration of exogenous hormones will result in the "locking" of ova in this location (Croxatto and Ortis, 1975). After fertilization, embryos and unfertilized eggs are transported differently in some species (see Croxatto, 1974). Furthermore, there is a growing suspicion that the early embryo may transmit physiological signals to the female tract (Smart et al., 1981). A direct role for the fertilized ovum in the control of its subsequent transport must, therefore, be entertained.

IV. CONCLUDING REMARKS

The complexity of gamete transport is apparent even from the brief survey presented in this review. The fragmentary observations and experimental results which are currently available do not suggest·a complete or unified description of mammalian gamete transport biology. Considerable variation among species has been shown to exist. The degree of biological variation in these transport systems may well be greater than that in many of the other physiological processes involved in fertilization. Clearly, the details of sperm and ovum transport in one mammal cannot be applied to other species without experimental verification. Much greater scientific effort will be necessary, therefore, in this area of reproductive biology.

In attempting to synthesize the body of information already accumulated, we should keep in mind several general principles. The biological significance of results obtained by experimental manipulation must always be assessed with great care. In view of the primary importance of gamete transport in the reproductive process, a number of different mechanisms may exist to faciliate union of sperm and ova, with several parallel or redundant systems being available for many steps in the process. This complexity may underlie much of the lack of agreement and apparent confusion pertaining to questions such as the relative importance of sperm motility and female visceral contractions in sperm transport and the roles of muscular and ciliary activity in ovum transport.

In our studies of the biology of mammalian sperm transport, we should also bear in mind the dual role assumed by the female tract during the evolution of internal fertilization. It is reasonable to assume that the capacity for high sperm production would offer competitive advantage to many male mammals. The same logic would suggest that those females most efficient in conserving spermatozoa (i.e., prolonging transport to ensure the collision of mature sperm and ova at the appropriate site) would also be favored. However, mechanisms must also have evolved in parallel to protect the ova from the large numbers of spermatozoa which would often enter the tract (i.e., protection against polyspermic fertilization). It has been shown that pregnancy may result when rabbits are inseminated intravaginally with sperm numbers which are four orders of magnitude lower than in normal semen (cf. Overstreet and Katz, 1977). We must consider, therefore, the possibility that completely different sets of signals and responses are generated, depending upon whether the female is confronted by a large or small number of sperm, and upon the time of insemination in relation to ovulation. Gamete transport phenomena have never been carefully studied with these variables manipulated. Such studies may give us deeper insights into the mechanisms controlling the transport and union of the gametes.

ACKNOWLEDGMENTS

I wish to express my thanks to Dr. David Katz, Dr. Susan Suarez, and Dr. Lani Johnson for reading and criticizing the manuscript and to Ms. Patricia Blondheim for preparation of the manuscript. I wish to acknowledge a Research Career Development Award from the National Institute of Child Health and Human Development (HD 00224). The unpublished studies reported in this chapter were also carried out with support from NICHD (HD 11186 and HD 15149 to J. W. Overstreet and HD 12971 to D. F. Katz).

REFERENCES

Adams, C. E. (1956). A study of fertilization in the rabbit: The effect of post-coital ligation of the fallopian tube or uterine horn. *J. Endocrinol.* **13**, 296–308.

Adler, N. T., and Zoloth, S. R. (1970). Copulatory behavior can inhibit pregnancy in female rats. *Science* **168**, 1480–1482.

Afzelius, B. A., Camner, P., and Mossberg, B. (1978). On the function of cilia in the female reproductive tract. *Fertil. Steril.* **29**, 72–74.

Ahlgren, M., Boxtrom, K., and Malmqvist, R. (1975). Sperm transport and survival in women with special reference to the fallopian tube. *In* "The Biology of Spermatozoa" (E. S. E. Hafez and C. G. Thibault, eds.), pp. 63–73. Karger, Basel.

Alden, R. H. (1942). The periovarial sac in the albino rat. *Anat. Rec.* **83**, 421–435.

Asch, R. H., Balmaceda, J., and Pauerstein, C. J. (1977a). Failure of seminal plasma to enter the uterus and oviducts of the rabbit following artificial insemination. *Fertil. Steril.* **28**, 671–673.

Asch, R. H., Fernandez, E. O., and Pauerstein, C. J. (1977b). Immunodetection of a human chorionic gonadotropin-like substance in human sperm. *Fertil. Steril.* **28**, 1258–1262.

Austin, C. R. (1957). Fate of spermatozoa in the uterus of the mouse and rat. *J. Endocrinol.* **14**, 335–342.

Austin, C. R. (1963a). Fertilization and transport of the ovum. *In* "Mechanisms Concerned with Conception" (C. G. Hartman, ed.), pp. 285–320. Macmillan, New York.

Austin, C. R. (1963b). "The Mammalian Egg." Blackwell, Oxford.

Austin, C. R. (1975). Membrane fusion events in fertilization. *J. Reprod. Fertil.* **44**, 155–166.

Austin, C. R., and Bishop, M. W. H. (1957). Fertilization in mammals. *Biol. Rev. Cambridge Philos. Soc.* **32**, 296–349.

Battalia, D. E., and Yanagimachi, R. E. (1979). Enhanced and co-ordinated movement of the hamster oviduct during the periovulatory period. *J. Reprod. Fertil.* **56**, 515–520.

Battalia, D. E., and Yanagimachi, R. (1980). The change in oestrogen and progesterone levels triggers adovarian propulsive movement of the hamster oviduct. *J. Reprod. Fertil.* **59**, 243–247.

Bedford, J. M. (1965). Effect of environment on phagocytosis of rabbit spermatozoa. *J. Reprod. Fertil.* **9**, 249–256.

Bedford, J. M. (1970). Sperm capacitation and fertilization in mammals. *Biol. Reprod.* **2**, Suppl. 2, 128–158.

Bedford, J. M. (1971). The rate of sperm passage into the cervix after coitus in the rabbit. *J. Reprod. Fertil.* **25**, 211–218.

Bedford, J. M. (1972). Sperm transport, capacitation and fertilization. *In* "Reproductive Biology" (H. Balin and S. Glasser, eds.), pp. 338–392. Excerpta Medica, Amsterdam.

Beyler, S. A., and Zaneveld, L. J. D. (1979). The role of acrosin in sperm penetration through human cervical mucus. *Fertil. Steril.* **32**, 671–675.

Beyth, Y., and Winston, R. M. L. (1981). Ovum capture and fertility following microsurgical fimbriectomy in the rabbit. *Fertil. Steril.* **35**, 464–466.

Black, D. L. (1974). Neural control of oviduct musculature. *In* "The Oviduct and Its Functions" (A. D. Johnson and C. W. Foley, eds.), pp. 65–118. Academic Press, New York.

Blair, W. D., and Beck, L. R. (1976). Demonstration of postovulatory sphincter action by isthmus of rabbit oviduct. *Fertil. Steril.* **27**, 431–441.

Blandau, R. J. (1945). On the factors involved in sperm transport through the cervix uteri of the albino rat. *Anat. Rec.* **77**, 253–272.

Blandau, R. J. (1969). Gamete transport—Comparative aspects. *In* "The Mammalian Oviduct" (E. S. E. Hafez and R. J. Blandau, eds.), pp. 129–162. Univ. of Chicago Press, Chicago, Illinois.

Blandau, R. J. (1973a). Sperm transport through the mammalian cervix: Comparative aspects. *In* "Biology of the Cervix" (R. J. Blandau and K. S. Moghissi, eds.), pp. 285–304. Univ. of Chicago Press, Chicago, Illinois.

Blandau, R. J. (1973b). Gamete transport in the female mammal. *In* "Handbook of Physiology" (R. O. Greep, E. B. Astwood, and S. R. Geiger, eds.), Sect. 7, Vol. II, Part 2, Chapter 38, pp. 153–163. Am. Physiol. Soc., Washington, D.C.

Blandau, R. J. (1977). Comparative morphology and physiology of the cervix in several different animals and their relationship to sperm transport. *In* "The Uterine Cervix in Reproduction" (V. Insler and G. Bettendorf, eds.), pp. 36–43. Thieme, Stuttgart.

Blandau, R. J. (1978). Gamete transport in oviducts of rats. *Anat. Rec.* **190**, 593 (abstr.).

Blandau, R. J., and Gaddum-Rosse, P. (1974). Mechanism of sperm transport in pig oviducts. *Fertil. Steril.* **25**, 61–67.

Blandau, R. J., and Money, W. L. (1944). Observations on the rate of transport of spermatozoa in the female genital tract of the rat. *Anat. Rec.* **90**, 255–260.

Blandau, R. J., and Odor, D. L. (1949). The total number of spermatozoa reaching various segments of the reproductive tract in the female albino rat at intervals after insemination. *Anat. Rec.* **103**, 93–110.

Blandau, R. J., and Rumery, R. E. (1964). The relationship of swimming movements of epididymal spermatozoa to their fertilizing capacity. *Fertil. Steril.* **15**, 571–579.

Borland, R. M., Hazra, S., Biggers, J. D., and Lechene, C. P. (1977). The elemental composition of the environments of the gametes and preimplantation embryo during the initiation of pregnancy. *Biol. Reprod.* **16**, 147–157.

Borland, R. M., Biggers, J. D., Lechene, C. P., and Taymor, M. L. (1980). Elemental composition of fluid in the human fallopian tube. *J. Reprod. Fertil.* **58**, 479–482.

Bourdage, R. J., and Halbert, S. A. (1980). In vivo recording of oviductal contractions in rabbits during the periovulatory period. *Am. J. Physiol.* **239**, 332–336.

Braden, A. W. H. (1953). Distribution of sperms in the genital tract of the female rabbit after coitus. *Aust. J. Biol. Sci.* **6**, 693–705.

Braden, A. W. H., and Austin, C. R. (1954a). The number of sperms about the eggs in mammals and its significance for normal fertilization. *Aust. J. Biol. Sci.* **7**, 543–551.

Braden, A. W. H., and Austin, C. R. (1954b). Fertilization of the mouse egg and the effect of delayed coitus and hot shock treatment. *Aust. J. Biol. Sci.* **7**, 552–565.

Brudin, J. (1964). A functional block in the isthmus of the rabbit fallopian tube. *Acta Physiol. Scand.* **60**, 295–296.

Chester, R. V., and Zucker, I. (1970). Influence of male copulatory behavior on sperm transport, pregnancy and pseudopregnancy in female rats. *Physiol. Behav.* **5**, 35–43.

Clewe, T. H., and Mastroianni, L., Jr. (1958). Mechanisms of ovum pickup. I. Functional capacity of rabbit oviducts ligated near the fimbria. *Fertil. Steril.* **9**, 13–17.

Cohen, J. (1969). Why so many sperms? An essay on the arithmetic of reproduction. *Sci. Prog. (Oxford)* **57**, 23–41.

Cohen, J., and Tyler, K. R. (1980). Sperm populations in the female genital tract of the rabbit. *J. Reprod. Fertil.* **60**, 213–218.

Cooper, G. W., Overstreet, J. W., and Katz, D. F. (1979). The motility of rabbit spermatozoa recovered from the female reproductive tract. *Gamete Res.* **2**, 35–42.

Crisman, R. O., McDonald, L. E., and Wallace, C. E. (1980). Oviduct (uterine tube) transport of ova in the cow. *Am. J. Vet. Res.* **41**, 645–647.

Cross, B. A. (1958). The motility and reactivity of the oestrogenized rabbit uterus in vivo; with comparative observations on milk ejection. *J. Endocrinol.* **16**, 237–260.

Croxatto, H. B. (1974). The duration of egg transport and its regulation in mammals. *In* "Physiology and Genetics of Reproduction" (E. G. Coutinho and F. Fuchs, eds.), Part B, pp. 159–166. Plenum, New York.

Croxatto, H. B., and Ortiz, M.-E. S. (1975). Egg transport in the fallopian tube. *Gynecol. Invest.* **6**, 215–225.

Croxatto, H. B., Vogel, C., and Vasquez, J. (1973). Transport of microspheres in the genital tract of the female rabbit. *J. Reprod. Fertil.* **33**, 337–341.

Croxatto, H. B., Ortiz, M. E., Diaz, S., Hess, R., Balmaceda, J., Croxatto, H.-D. (1978). Studies on the duration of egg transport by the human oviduct. II. Ovum location at various intervals following luteinizing hormone peak. *Am. J. Obstet. Gynecol.* **132**, 629–634.

Dauzier, L., and Winterberger, S. (1952). Recherches sur la fécondation chez les mammiferes: Durée du pouvoir fécondant des spermatozides de bélier dans le tractus génital de la brébis et durée de la période de fécondité de l'oeuf après l'ovulation. *C. R. Seances Soc. Biol. Ses Fil.* **146**, 660–663.

Davajan, V., Nakamura, R. M., and Kharma, K. (1970). Spermatozoan transport in cervical mucus. *Obstet. Gynecol. Surv.* **25**, 1–43.

De Boer, C. H. (1972). Transport of particulate matter through the human female genital tract. *J. Reprod. Fertil.* **28**, 295–297.

De Boer, P., Van Der Hoeven, F. A., and Chardon, J. A. P. (1976). The production, morphology, karyotypes and transport of spermatozoa from tertiary trisomic mice and the consequences for egg fertilization. *J. Reprod. Fertil.* **48**, 249–256.

DeMattos, C. E. R., and Coutinho, E. M. (1971). Effects of the ovarian hormones on tubal motility of the rabbit. *Endocrinology* **89**, 912–917.

Dickmann, Z. (1963). Chemotaxis of rabbit spermatozoa. *J. Exp. Biol.* **40**, 1–5.

Doak, R. L., Hall, A., and Dale, H. E. (1967). Longevity of spermatozoa in the reproductive tract of the bitch. *J. Reprod. Fertil.* **13**, 51–58.

Dobrowolski, W., and Hafez, E. S. E. (1970). Transport and distribution of spermatozoa in the reproductive tract of the cow. *J. Anim. Sci.* **31**, 940–943.

Doyle, L. L., Lippes, J., Winters, H. S., and Margolis, A. J. (1966). Human ova in the fallopian tube. *Am. J. Obstet. Gynecol.* **95**, 115–117.

Dukelow, W. F. (1975). The morphology of follicular development and ovulation in nonhuman primates. *J. Reprod. Fertil., Suppl.* **22**, 23–51.

du Mesnil du Buisson, F., and Dauzier, L. (1955a). Distribution et resorption du sperme dans le tractus genital de la truie: Survie des spermatozoides. *Ann. Endocrinol.* **16**, 413–422.

du Mesnil du Buisson, F., and Dauzier, L. (1955b). La remontée des spermatozoides du verrat dans le tractus genital de la truie en oestrus. *C.R. Seances Soc. Biol. Ses Fil.* **149**, 76–79.

Edey, T. N., Thwaites, C. J., Pigott, F. A., and O'Shea, T. (1975). Fertility and sperm transport in Merino ewes at the first oestrous following embryonic death. *J. Reprod. Fertil.* **43**, 485–494.

Edgar, D. G., and Asdell, S. A. (1960). Spermatozoa in the female genital tract. *J. Endocrinol.* **21**, 321–326.

Egli, G. E., and Newton, M. (1961). The transport of carbon particles in the human female reproductive tract. *Fertil. Steril.* **12**, 151–155.

Einarsson, S., Jones, B., Larsson, K., and Viring, S. (1980). Distribution of small- and medium-sized molecules within the genital tract of artificially inseminated gilts. *J. Reprod. Fertil.* **59**, 453–457.

El-Banna, A. A., and Hafez, E. S. E. (1970). Sperm transport and distribution in rabbit and cattle female tract. *Fertil. Steril.* **21**, 534–540.

Eliasson, R., and Lindholmer, C. (1974). Effects of human seminal plasma on sperm survival and transport. *Colloq.—Inst. Natl. Sante Rech. Med.* **26**, 219–230.

First, A. (1954). Transperitoneal migration of ovum or spermatozoon. *Obstet. Gynecol.* **4**, 431–434.

First, N. L., Short, R. E., Peters, J. B., and Stratman, F. W. (1968). Transport of boar spermatozoa in estrual and luteal sows. *J. Anim. Sci.* **27**, 1032–1036.

Fischer, B., and Adams, C. E. (1981). Fertilization following mixed insemination with 'cervix-selected' and 'unselected' spermatozoa in the rabbit. *J. Reprod. Fertil.* **62**, 337–343.

Fléchon, J.-E., and Hunter, R. H. F. (1981). Distribution of spermatozoa in the uterotubal junction and isthmus of pigs, and their relationship with the luminal epithelium after mating: A scanning electron microscope study. *Tissue Cell* **13**, 127–139.

Fox, C. A., and Knaggs, G. S. (1969). Milk ejection activity (oxytocin) in peripheral venous blood in man during lactation and in association with coitus. *J. Endocrinol.* **45**, 145–146.

Fox, C. A., Wolff, H. S., and Baker, J. A. (1970). Measurement of intravaginal and intrauterine pressure during human coitus by radiotelemetry. *J. Reprod. Fertil.* **22**, 243–251.

Fox, C. A., Meldrum, S. J., and Watson, B. W. (1973). Continuous measurement by radiotelemetry of vaginal pH during human coitus. *J. Reprod. Fertil.* **33**, 69–75.

Fredricsson, B., and Bjork, G. (1977). Morphology of postcoital spermatozoa in the cervical secretion and its clinical significance. *Fertil. Steril.* **28**, 841–845.

Freund, M. (1973). Mechanisms and problems of sperm transport. *In* "The Regulation of Mammalian Reproduction" (S. J. Segal, R. Crozier, P. A. Corfman, and P. G. Confliffe, eds.), pp. 352–361. Thomas, Springfield, Illinois.

Fuchs, A. R. (1972). Uterine activity during and after mating in the rabbit. *Fertil. Steril.* **23**, 915–923.

Fuchs, A. R., Olsen, P., and Petersen, K. (1965). Effect of distension of uterus and vagina on uterine motility and oxytocin release in puerperal rabbits. *Acta Endocrinol. (Copenhagen)* **50**, 239–248.

Gaddum-Rosse, P. (1981). Some observations on sperm transport through the uterotubal junction of the rat. *Am. J. Anat.* **160**, 333–341.

Gaddum-Rosse, P., and Blandau, R. J. (1973). In vitro studies on ciliary activity within the oviducts of the rabbit and pig. *Am. J. Anat.* **136**, 91–104.

Gaddum-Rosse, P., and Blandau, R. J. (1976). Comparative observations on ciliary currents in mammalian oviducts. *Biol. Reprod.* **14**, 605–609.

Gibbons, R. A., and Mattner, P. F. (1971). The chemical and physical characteristics of the cervical secretion and its role in reproductive physiology. *In* "Pathways to Conception" (A. I. Sherman, ed.), pp. 143–155. Thomas, Springfield, Illinois.

Gibbons, R. A., and Sellwood, R. A. (1973). The macromolecular biochemistry of cervical secretions. *In* "Biology of the Cervix" (R. J. Blandau and K. S. Moghissi, eds.), pp. 251–266. Univ. of Chicago Press, Chicago, Illinois.

Greenwald, G. S. (1956). Sperm transport in the reproductive tract of the female rabbit. *Science* **124**, 586.

Greenwald, G. S. (1961). A study of the transport of ova through the rabbit oviduct. *Fertil. Steril.* **12**, 80–95.

Griffiths, W. F. B., and Amoroso, E. C. (1939). Pro-oestrus, oestrus, ovulation and mating in the greyhound bitch. *Vet. Rec.* **61**, 771–776.

Hafez, E. S. E. (1976). Transport and survival of spermatozoa in the female reproductive tract. *In* "Human Semen and Fertility Regulation in Men" (E. S. E. Hafez, ed.), pp. 107–129. Mosby, St. Louis, Missouri.

Hafez, E. S. E. (1980). The cervix and sperm transport. *In* "Human Reproduction. Conception and Contraception" (E. S. E. Hafez, ed.), 2nd ed., pp. 221–252. Harper & Row, Hagerstown, Maryland.

Halbert, S. A., and Patton, D. L. (1981). Ovum pick-up following fimbriectomy and infundibular salpingostomy in rabbits. *J. Reprod. Med.* **26**, 299–304.

Halbert, S. A., Tam, P. Y., and Blandau, R. J. (1976a). Egg transport in the rabbit oviduct: The roles of cilia and muscle. *Science* **191**, 1052–1053.

Halbert, S. A., Tam, P. Y., Adams, R. J., and Blandau, R. J. (1976b). An analysis of the mechanisms of egg transport in the ampulla of the rabbit oviduct. *Gynecol. Invest.* **7**, 306–320.

Hanson, F. W., and Overstreet, J. W. (1981). The interaction of human spermatozoa with cervical mucus in vivo. *Am. J. Obstet. Gynecol.* **140**, 173–178.

Hanson, F. W., Overstreet, J. W., and Katz, D. F. (1982). A study of the relationship of motile sperm numbers in cervical mucus 48 hours after artificial insemination with subsequent fertility. *Am. J. Obstet. Gynecol.* **143**, 85–90.

Harper, M. J. K. (1961a). The mechanisms involved in the movement of newly ovulated eggs through the ampulla of the rabbit fallopian tube. *J. Reprod. Fertil.* **2**, 522–524.

Harper, M. J. K. (1961b). The time of ovulation in the rabbit following the injection of luteinizing hormone. *J. Endocrinol.* **22**, 147–152.

Harper, M. J. K. (1962). Egg movement through the ampullar region of the fallopian tube of the rabbit. *Proc. Int. Congr. Anim. Reprod., 4th, 1961* pp. 375–380.

Harper, M. J. K. (1973). Stimulation of sperm movement from the isthmus to the site of fertilization in the rabbit oviduct. *Biol. Reprod.* **8**, 369–377.

Harper, M. J. K., Bennett, J. P., Boursnel, J. P., and Rowson, L. E. A. (1960). An autoradiographic method for the study of egg transport in the rabbit fallopian tubes. *J. Reprod. Fertil.* **1**, 249–267.

Hartree, E. F. (1977). Spermatozoa, eggs, and proteinases. *Biochem. Soc. Trans.* **5**, 375–394.

Hash, D. C., and Wolfe, H. F. (1979). Pink-eyed dilution alleles affect negative surface charges of mouse spermatozoa. *Dev. Genet.* **1**, 61–68.

Hays, R. L., and VanDemark, N. L. (1953). Effects of stimulation on the reproductive organs of the cow on the release of an oxytocinlike substance. *Endocrinology* **52**, 634–637.

Heape, W. (1905). Ovulation and degeneration of ova in the rabbit. *Proc. R. Soc. London, Ser. B* **76**, 260–268.

Helm, G., Ottesen, B., Fahrenkrug, J., Larsen, J.-J., Owman, C., Sjöberg, N.-O., Stolberg, B., Sundler, F., and Walles, B. (1981). Vasoactive intestinal polypeptide (VIP) in the human female reproductive tract: Distribution and motor effects. *Biol. Reprod.* **25**, 227–234.

Hilliard, J., Hayward, J. N., and Sawyer, C. H. (1964). Post coital patterns of secretion of pituitary gonadotropin and ovarian progestin in the rabbit. *Endocrinology* **75**, 957–963.

Hilliard, J., Scaramuzzi, R. J., Pang, C.-N., Penardi, R., and Sawyer, C. H. (1974). Testosterone secretion by rabbit ovary in vivo. *Endocrinology* **94**, 267–271.

Hoglund, A., and Odeblad, E. (1977). Sperm penetration in cervical mucus, a biophysical and group-theoretical approach. *In* "The Uterine Cervix in Reproduction" (V. Insler and G. Bettendorf, eds.), pp. 129–134. Thieme, Stuttgart.

Holst, P. J., and Braden, A. W. H. (1972). Ovum transport in the ewe. *Aust. J. Biol. Sci.* **25**, 167–173.

Humphrey, K. W. (1969). Mechanisms concerned with ovum transport. *Adv. Biosci.* **4,** 133–148.

Hunter, R. H. F. (1975a). Transport, migration and survival of spermatozoa in the female genital tract: Species with intra-uterine deposition of semen. *In* "The Biology of Spermatozoa" (E. S. E. Hafez and C. G. Thibault, eds.), pp. 145–155. Karger, Basel.

Hunter, R. H. F. (1975b). Physiological aspects of sperm transport in the domestic pig *Sus scrofa.* I. Semen deposition and cell transport. *Br. Vet. J.* **131,** 565–572.

Hunter, R. H. F. (1980). Transport and storage of spermatozoa in the female tract. *Proc. Int. Congr. Anim. Reprod. and Artif. Insem. 9th, 1980,*Vol. 2, pp. 227–233.

Hunter, R. H. F. (1981). Sperm transport and reservoirs in the pig oviduct in relation to the time of ovulation. *J. Reprod. Fertil.* **63,** 109–117.

Hunter, R. H. F., Nichol, R., and Crabtree, S. M. (1980). Transport of spermatozoa in the ewe: Timing of the establishment of a functional population in the oviduct. *Reprod., Nutr., Dev.* **20,** 1869–1875.

Insler, V., Glezerman, M., Zeidel, L., Bernstein, D., and Misgav, N. (1980). Sperm storage in the human cervix: A quantitative study. *Fertil. Steril.* **33,** 288–293.

Ito, S., Kudo, A., and Niwa, T. (1959). Studies on the normal oestrus in swine with special reference to proper time for service. *Ann. Inst. Natl. Rech. Agron., Ser. D,* ■, Suppl. 105–107.

Jansen, R. P. S. (1978). Fallopian tube isthmic mucus and ovum transport. *Science* **201,** 349–351.

Jansen, R. P. S. (1980). Cyclic changes in the human fallopian tube isthmus and their functional importance. *Am. J. Obstet. Gynecol.* **136,** 292–308.

Jansen, R. P. S., and Bajpai, V. K. (1982). Oviduct acid mucus glycoproteins in the estrous rabbit: Ultrastructure and histochemistry. *Biol. Reprod.* **26,** 155–168.

Jaszczak, S., and Hafez, E. S. E. (1973). Sperm migration through the uterine cervix in the macaque during the menstrual cycle. *Am. J. Obstet. Gynecol.* **115,** 1070–1082.

Jean, Y., Langlais, J., Roberts, K. D., Chapdelaine, A., and Bleau, G. (1979). Fertility of a woman with nonfunctional ciliated cells in the fallopian tubes. *Fertil. Steril.* **31,** 349–350.

Jerzy Glass, G. B. (1980). "Gastrointestinal Hormones." Raven Press, New York.

Johnson, L. L., and Overstreet, J. W. (1982). Potassium and pyruvate may be regulators of rabbit oviductal sperm motility. *Biol. Reprod.* **26,** Suppl. 1, 145A (abstr.).

Johnson, L. L., Katz, D. F., and Overstreet, J. W. (1981). The movement characteristics of rabbit spermatozoa before and after activation. *Gamete Res.* **4,** 275–282.

Jones, H. P., Lenz, R. W., Palevitz, B. A., and Cormier, M. J. (1980). Calmodulin localization in mammalian spermatozoa. *Proc. Natl. Acad. Sci. U.S.A.* **77,** 2772–2776.

Kanawaga, H., and Hafez, E. S. E. (1973). Kinocilia and sperm dynamics in the cervix uteri of the rabbit. *J. Reprod. Med.* **10,** 90–94.

Katz, D. F., and Berger, S. A. (1980). Flagellar propulsion of human sperm in cervical mucus. *Biorheology* **17,** 169–175.

Katz, D. F., and Overstreet, J. W. (1980). Mammalian sperm movement in the secretions of the male and female genital tracts. *In* "Testicular Development, Structure, and Function" (E. Steinberger and A. Steinberger, eds.), pp. 481–490. Raven Press, New York.

Katz, D. F., and Overstreet, J. W. (1982). The mechanisms and analysis of sperm migration through cervical mucus. *In* "Mucus in Health and Disease II" (E. Chantler and M. Elstein, eds.), pp. 319–330. Plenum, New York.

Glover, 1974), but direct observations have not supported this assumption (Cooper *et al.*, 1979). When there is a hostile vaginal environment, rapid sperm escape to the relative protection of the cervix would seem highly advantageous. On the other hand, progressive sperm motility may be maintained in the vagina of the ewe for as long as 6 hours (Quinlan *et al.*, 1932), by which time thousands of spermatozoa have reached the uterus (Mattner, 1963). Observations in fertile couples suggest that human spermatozoa may also maintain progressive motility in the vagina for as long as 4 hours (Masters and Johnson, 1966), and excellent sperm motility may persist in human cervical mucus for 48 hours or more after artificial insemination (Hanson and Overstreet, 1981; Hanson *et al.*, 1982). It is possible therefore, that in species with intravaginal insemination, there are sufficient viable spermatozoa in the cervical lumen and/or vagina to account for sperm numbers which subsequently reach the uterus and oviducts. There have never been direct observations of sperm dissociation from the cervical mucosa, and there are no experimental data with which to estimate the proportion of uterine or tubal sperm which was ever stored at this site in the cervix. Therefore, it cannot be concluded whether or not the sperm population associated with the cervical mucosa is stored within a reservoir, or whether these cells are irreversibly trapped and, thereby, restricted from subsequent upward migration.

B. The Uterus and Uterotubal Junction

The function of the uterus in sperm transport is related to the effectiveness of the cervix in initially blocking the passage of semen. For most species with intravaginal insemination, the cervix functions as an effective anatomical block to passage of the seminal plasma and most of the spermatozoa. In other species, including the horse, pig, and dog, the semen may be ejaculated directly into the uterus, thus completely bypassing the cervix. In some rodents, such as the rat, insemination may be intravaginal, but normally a bulk passage of semen from the vagina to the uterus rapidly follows insemination (Section II,A). For those species in which whole semen enters the uterus, the functions of sperm restriction and storage which are served by the cervix in ruminants, primates, and rabbits appear to be carried out by the uterine glands and the uterotubal junction. The physiology of sperm transport after uterine insemination has been recently reviewed by Hunter (1975a), and only general statements concerning sperm–uterine interaction in these species will be repeated here.

In general, bulk entry of the ejaculate into the uterus is accompanied

Katz, D. F., and Yanagimachi, R. (1980). Movement characteristics of hamster sper-matozoa within the oviduct. *Biol. Reprod.* **22,** 759–764.

Katz, D. F., Mills, R. N., and Pritchett, T. R. (1978). The movement of human sper-matozoa in cervical mucus. *J. Reprod. Fertil.* **53,** 259–265.

Katz, D. F., Bloom, T. D., and BonDurant, R. H. (1981). Movement of bull spermatozoa in cervical mucus. *Biol. Reprod.* **25,** 931–937.

Katz, D. F., Brofeldt, B. T., Overstreet, J. W., and Hanson, F. W. (1982). Alteration of cervical mucus by vanguard human spermatozoa. *J. Reprod. Fertil.* **65,** 171–175.

Kelly, R. W. (1981). Prostaglandin synthesis in the male and female reproductive tract. *J. Reprod. Fertil.* **62,** 293–304.

Koehler, J. K., Nudelman, E. D., and Hakomori, S. (1980). A collagen-binding protein on the surface of ejaculated rabbit spermatozoa. *J. Cell Biol.* **86,** 529–536.

Koester, H. (1970). Ovum transport. *In* "Mammalian Reproduction" (H. Gibian and E. J. Plotz, eds.), pp. 189–228. Springer-Verlag, Berlin and New York.

Koren, E., and Lukac, J. (1979). Mechanism of liquefaction of the human ejaculate. I. Changes of the ejaculate proteins. *J. Reprod. Fertil.* **56,** 493–499.

Krehbiel, E. B., Lodge, J. R., and Sharma, O. P. (1972). The effects of breeding stimuli on the rate of sperm transport in rabbits. *J. Reprod. Fertil.* **29,** 291–293.

Kroeks, M. V. A. M., and Kremer, J. (1977). The pH in the lower third of the genital tract. *In* "The Uterine Cervix in Reproduction" (V. Insler and G. Bettendorf, eds.), pp. 109–118. Thieme, Stuttgart.

Krzanowska, H. (1974). The passage of abnormal spermatozoa through the uterotubal junction of the mouse. *J. Reprod. Fertil.* **38,** 81–90.

Leonard, S. L. (1950). The reduction of uterine sperm and uterine fluid on fertilization of rat ova. *Anat. Rec.* **196,** 607–615.

Lewis, W. H., and Wright, E. S. (1935). On the early development of the mouse egg. *Contrib. Embryol. Carnegie Inst.* **25,** 115–143.

Lightfoot, R. J. (1970). The contractile activity of the genital tract of the ewe in response to oxytocin and mating. *J. Reprod. Fertil.* **21,** 376 (abstr.).

Lukac, J., and Koren, E. (1979). Mechanism of liquefaction of the human ejaculate. II. Role of collagenase-like peptidase and seminal proteinase. *J. Reprod. Fertil.* **56,** 501–506.

MacLeod, J., Martens, F., Silberman, C., and Sobrero, A. J. (1959). The post coital and post insemination cervical mucus and semen quality. *Stud. Fertil.* **10,** 41–57.

McNeilly, A. S., and Ducker, H. A. (1972). Blood levels of oxytocin in the female goat during coitus and in response to stimuli associated with mating. *J. Endocrinol.* **54,** 399–406.

Maia, H. S., and Coutinho, E. M. (1970). Peristalsis and antiperistalsis of the human fallopian tube during the menstrual cycle. *Biol. Reprod.* **2,** 305–314.

Maistrello, I. (1971). Extraluminal recording of oviductal contractions in the un-anesthetized rabbit. *J. Appl. Physiol.* **31,** 768–771.

Mann, T., Leone, E., and Polge, C. (1956). The composition of the stallion's semen. *J. Endocrinol.* **13,** 279–290.

Martan, J., and Shepherd, B. A. (1976). Role of copulatory plug in reproduction of guinea pig. *J. Exp. Zool.* **196,** 79–84.

Masters, W. H., and Johnson, V. E. (1966). "Human Sexual Response." Little, Brown, Boston, Massachusetts.

Matthews, M. K., Jr., and Adler, N. T. (1977). Facilitative and inhibitory influences of reproductive behavior on sperm transport in rats. *J. Comp. Physiol. Psychol.* **91,** 727–741.

Matthews, M. K., Jr., and Adler, N. T. (1978). Systematic interrelationship of mating, vaginal plug position, and sperm transport in the rat. *Physiol. Behav.* **20,** 303–309.

Mattner, P. E. (1963). Spermatozoa in the genital tract of the ewe. II. Distribution after coitus. *Aust. J. Biol. Sci.* **16,** 688–694.

Mattner, P. E. (1966). Formation and retention of the spermatozoan reservoir in the cervix of the ruminant. *Nature (London)* **212,** 1479–1480.

Mattner, P. E. (1968). The distribution of spermatozoa and leucocytes in the female genital tract in goats and cattle. *J. Reprod. Fertil.* **17,** 253–261.

Mattner, P. E. (1973). The cervix and its secretions in relation to fertility in ruminants. *In* "Biology of the Cervix" (R. J. Blandau and K. S. Moghissi, eds.), Chapter 18, pp. 339–350. Univ. of Chicago Press, Chicago, Illinois.

Mattner, P. E., and Braden, A. W. H. (1963). Spermatozoa in the genital tract of the ewe. I. Rapidity of transport. *Aust. J. Biol. Sci.* **16,** 473–481.

Metz, K. G. P., and Mastroianni, L., Jr. (1979). Dispensability of fimbriae: Ovum pickup by tubal fistulas in the rabbit. *Fertil. Steril.* **32,** 329–334.

Meyer, F. A., and Silberberg, A. (1980). The rheology and molecular organization of epithelial mucus. *Biorheology* **17,** 163–168.

Miller, E. G., and Kurzrok, R. (1932). Biochemical studies of human semen. III. Factors affecting migration of sperm through the cervix. *Am. J. Obstet. Gynecol.* **24,** 19–26.

Miller, R. L. (1977). Chemotactic behavior of the sperm of chitons (Mollusca: Polyplacophora). *J. Exp. Zool.* **202,** 203–212.

Moghissi, K. S. (1973). Sperm migration through the human cervix. *In* "Biology of the Cervix" (R. J. Blandau and K. S. Moghissi, eds.), Chapter 16, pp. 305–327. Univ. of Chicago Press, Chicago, Illinois.

Moghissi, K. S. (1977). Sperm migration through the human cervix. *In* "The Uterine Cervix in Reproduction" (V. Insler and G. Bettendorf, eds.), pp. 146–165. Thieme, Stuttgart.

Moghissi, K. S., and Syner, F. N. (1970). The effect of seminal protease on sperm migration through cervical mucus. *Int. J. Fertil.* **15,** 43–49.

Mortimer, D. (1978). Selectivity of sperm transport in the female genital tract. *In* "Spermatozoa, Antibodies and Infertility" (J. Cohen and W. F. Hendry, eds.), Chapter 5, pp. 37–53. Blackwell, Oxford.

Morton, D. B., and Glover, T. D. (1974). Sperm transport in the female rabbit: The role of the cervix. *J. Reprod. Fertil.* **38,** 131–138.

Motta, P., and Van Blerkom, J. V. (1975a). A scanning electron microscopic study of rabbit spermatozoa in the female reproductive tract following coitus. *Cell Tissue Res.* **163,** 29–44.

Motta, P., and Van Blerkom, J. (1975b). A scanning electron microscopic study of the luteo-follicular complex. II. Events leading to ovulation. *Am. J. Anat.* **143,** 241–264.

Nicol, A., and McLaren, A. (1974). An effect of the female genotype on sperm transport in mice. *J. Reprod. Fertil.* **39,** 421–424.

Nilsson, O., and Reinius, S. (1969). Light and electron microscopic structure of the oviduct. *In* "The Mammalian Oviduct" (E. S. E. Hafez and R. J. Blandau, eds.), pp. 57–84. Univ. of Chicago Press, Chicago, Illinois.

Norwood, J. T., and Anderson, R. G. W. (1980). Evidence that adhesive sites on the tips of oviduct cilia membranes are required for ovum pickup in situ. *Biol. Reprod.* **23,** 788–791.

Norwood, J. T., Hein, C. E., Halbert, S. A., and Anderson, R. G. W. (1978). Polycationic macromolecules inhibit cilia-mediated ovum transport in the rabbit oviduct. *Proc. Natl. Acad. Sci. U.S.A.* **75**, 4413–4416.

Odeblad, E. (1968). The functional structure of human cervical mucus. *Acta Obstet. Gynecol. Scand.* **47**, Suppl. 1, 59–79.

Odeblad, E., and Rudolfsson, C. (1973). Types of cervical secretions: Biophysical characteristics. *In* "Biology of the Cervix" (R. J. Blandau and K. Moghissi, eds.), pp. 267–284. Univ. of Chicago Press, Chicago, Illinois.

Olds, P. J. (1970). Effect of the T locus on sperm distribution in the house mouse. *Biol. Reprod.* **2**, 91–97.

Overstreet, J. W., and Bedford, J. M. (1974). Transport, capacitation and fertilizing ability of epididymal spermatozoa. *J. Exp. Zool.* **189**, 203–214.

Overstreet, J. W., and Cooper, G. W. (1975). Reduced sperm motility in the isthmus of the rabbit oviduct. *Nature (London)* **258**, 718–719.

Overstreet, J. W., and Cooper, G. W. (1978). Sperm transport in the reproductive tract of the female rabbit. I. The rapid transit phase of transport. *Biol. Reprod.* **19**, 101–114.

Overstreet, J. W., and Cooper, G. W. (1979). The time and location of the acrosome reaction during sperm transport in the female rabbit. *J. Exp. Zool.* **209**, 97–104.

Overstreet, J. W., and Katz, D. F. (1977). Sperm transport and selection in the female genital tract. *Dev. Mamm.* **2**, 31–65.

Overstreet, J. W., and Katz, D. F. (1981). Sperm transport and capacitation. *In* "Gynecology and Obstetrics" (L. Speroff and J. L. Simpson, eds.), Vol. V, Chapter 45, pp. 1–10. Harper, New York.

Overstreet, J. W., and Tom, R. A. (1982). Experimental studies of rapid sperm transport in rabbits. *J. Reprod. Fertil.* **66**, 601–606.

Overstreet, J. W., Cooper, G. W., and Katz, D. F. (1978). Sperm transport in the reproductive tract of the female rabbit. II. The sustained phase of transport. *Biol. Reprod.* **19**, 115–132.

Overstreet, J. W., Katz, D. F., and Johnson, L. L. (1980a). Motility of rabbit spermatozoa in the secretions of the oviduct. *Biol. Reprod.* **22**, 1083–1088.

Overstreet, J. W., Coats, C., Katz, D. F., and Hanson, F. W. (1980b). The importance of seminal plasma for sperm penetration of human cervical mucus. *Fertil. Steril.* **34**, 569–572.

Overström, E. W., Bigsby, R. M., and Black, D. L. (1980). Effects of physiological levels of estradiol-17β and progesterone on oviduct edema and ovum transport in the rabbit. *Biol. Reprod.* **23**, 100–110.

Pang, S. F., Chow, P. H., and Wong, T. M. (1979). The role of the seminal vesicles, coagulating glands and prostate glands on the fertility and fecundity of mice. *J. Reprod. Fertil.* **56**, 129–132.

Parker, G. H. (1931). The passage of sperm and egg through the oviducts in terrestrial vertebrates. *Philos. Trans. R. Soc. London* **219**, 381–419.

Paton, D. M., Widdicombe, J. H., Rheaume, D. E., and Johns, A. (1978). The role of the adrenergic innervation of the oviduct in the regulation of mammalian ovum transport. *Pharmacol. Rev.* **29**, 67–102.

Pauerstein, C. J., and Eddy, C. A. (1979). The role of the oviduct in reproduction; our knowledge and our ignorance. *J. Reprod. Fertil.* **55**, 223–229.

Perloff, W. H., and Steinberger, E. (1964). In vivo survival of spermatozoa in cervical mucus. *Am. J. Obstet. Gynecol.* **88**, 439–442.

Perry, G., Glezerman, M., and Insler, V. (1977). Selective filtration of abnormal spermatozoa by the cervical mucus in vitro. *In* "The Uterine Cervix in Reproduction" (V. Insler and G. Bettendorf, eds.), pp. 118–128. Thieme, Stuttgart.

Portnow, J., Talo, A., and Hodgson, B. J. (1977). A random walk model of ovum transport. *Bull. Math. Biol.* **39**, 349–357.

Quinlan, J., Mare, G. S., and Roux, L. L. (1932). The vitality of the spermatozoa in the genital tract of the Merino ewe, with special reference to its practical application in breeding. *Rep. Vet. Serv. Anim. Ind. S. Afr.* **18**, 831–870.

Quinlivan, T. D., and Robinson, T. J. (1969). Numbers of spermatozoa in the genital tract after artificial insemination of progesterone-treated ewes. *J. Reprod. Fertil.* **19**, 73–86.

Rigby, J. P. (1966). The persistence of spermatozoa at the uterotubal junction of the sow. *J. Reprod. Fertil.* **11**, 153–155.

Roberts, J. S., and Share, L. (1968). Oxytocin in plasma of pregnant, lactating and cycling ewes during vaginal stimulation. *Endocrinology* **83**, 272–278.

Robinson, J. (1973). Factors involved in the failure of sperm transport and survival in the female reproductive tract. *J. Reprod. Fertil., Suppl.* **18**, 103–109.

Ruckebusch, Y. (1975). Relationship between the electrical activity of the oviduct and the uterus of the rabbit in vivo. *J. Reprod. Fertil.* **45**, 73–82.

Salomy, M., and Harper, M. J. K. (1971). Cyclical changes of oviduct motility in rabbits. *Biol. Reprod.* **4**, 185–194.

Settlage, D. S. F., Motoshima, M., and Tredway, D. R. (1973). Sperm transport from the external cervical os to the fallopian tubes in women: A time and quantitation study. *Fertil. Steril.* **24**, 655–661.

Shalgi, R., and Kraicer, P. F. (1978). Timing of sperm transport, penetration and cleavage in the rat. *J. Exp. Zool.* **204**, 353–360.

Sharma, O. P., Lodge, J. R., and Hays, R. L. (1969). Fertilization after ligating the oviduct within minutes following mating. *J. Reprod. Fertil.* **18**, 179–180 (abstr.).

Sharma, S. C., and Chadhury, R. R. (1970). Studies on mating. I. The absence of release of oxytocin at mating in female rabbits. *Indian J. Med. Res.* **58**, 495–500.

Smart, Y. C., Roberts, T. K., Clancy, R. L., and Cripps, A. W. (1981). Early pregnancy factor: Its role in mammalian reproduction—research review. *Fertil. Steril.* **35**, 397–402.

Sobrero, A. J., and MacLeod, J. (1962). The immediate post-coital test. *Fertil. Steril.* **13**, 184–189.

Soupart, P. (1970). Leukocytes and sperm capacitation in the rabbit uterus. *Fertil. Steril.* **21**, 724–756.

Spilman, C. H. (1980). Fluid retention by the rabbit oviduct. *Proc. Soc. Exp. Biol. Med.* **165**, 133–136.

Suarez, S. S., and Katz, D. F. (1982). Movement characteristics and acrosomal status of populations of rabbit spermatozoa recovered at the site and time of fertilization. *Biol. Reprod.* **26**, Suppl. 1, 146A (abstr.).

Talo, A. (1974). Electric and mechanical activity of the rabbit oviduct in vitro before and after ovulation. *Biol. Reprod.* **11**, 335–345.

Talo, A. (1975). Amplitude variation of the pressure cycles in and between segments of rabbit oviduct in vitro. *Biol. Reprod.* **13**, 249–254.

Talo, A. (1980). Myoelectrical activity and transport of unfertilized ova in the oviduct of the mouse in vitro. *J. Reprod. Fertil.* **60**, 53–58.

Talo, A., and Hodgson, B. J. (1978). Spike bursts in rabbit oviduct. I. Effect of ovulation. *Am. J. Physiol.* **234**, 430–438.

Tam, P. Y., Katz, D. F., Sensabaugh, G. F., and Berger, S. A. (1982). Flow permeation analysis of bovine cervical mucus. *Biophys. J.* **38,** 153–159.

Tampion, D., and Gibbons, R. A. (1962). Orientation of spermatozoa in mucus of the cervix uteri. *Nature (London)* **17,** 465–478.

Tauber, P. F., Propping, D., Schumacher, G. F. B., and Zaneveld, L. J. D. (1980). Biochemical aspects of the coagulation and liquefaction of human semen. *J. Androl.* **1,** 280–288.

Tessler, S., and Olds-Clarke, P. (1981). Male genotype influences sperm transport in female mice. *Biol. Reprod.* **24,** 806–813.

Tessler, S., Carey, J. E., and Olds-Clarke, P. (1981). Mouse sperm motility affected by factors in the T/t complex. *J. Exp. Zool.* **217,** 277–285.

Thibault, C. (1972). Physiology and physiopathology of the fallopian tube. *Int. J. Fertil.* **17,** 1–13.

Thibault, C. (1973). Sperm transport and storage in vertebrates. *J. Reprod. Fertil.,* Suppl. **18,** 39–53.

Thibault, C., and Winterberger-Torres, S. (1967). Oxytocin and sperm transport in the ewe. *Int. J. Fertil.* **12,** 410–415.

Thibault, C., Gerard, M., and Heyman, Y. (1975). Transport and survival of spermatozoa in cattle. *In* "The Biology of Spermatozoa" (E. S. E. Hafez and C. G. Thibault, eds.), pp. 156–165. Karger, Basel.

Tredway, D. R., Settlage, D. S. F., Nakamura, R. M., Motoshima, M., Umezaki, C. V., and Mishell, D. R. (1975). Significance of timing for the post-coital evaluation of cervical mucus. *Am. J. Obstet. Gynecol.* **121,** 287–393.

Tredway, D. R., Buchanan, G. C., and Drake, T. S. (1978). Comparison of the fractional post-coital test and semen analysis. *Am. J. Obstet. Gynecol.* **130,** 647–652.

Turnbull, K. E. (1966). The transport of spermatozoa in the rabbit doe before and after ovulation. *Aust. J. Biol. Sci.* **19,** 1095–1099.

VanDemark, N. L., and Moeller, A. N. (1951). Speed of spermatozoan transport in reproductive tract of estrous cow. *Am. J. Physiol.* **165,** 674–679.

Verdugo, P., Rumery, R. E., and Tam, P. Y. (1980). Hormonal control of oviductal ciliary activity: Effect of prostaglandins. *Fertil. Steril.* **33,** 193–196.

Walton, A. (1960). Copulation and natural insemination. *In* "Marshall's Physiology of Reproduction" (A. S. Parkes, ed.), 3rd ed., Vol. I, Part 2, pp. 130–160. Longmans, Green, New York.

Waterston, J. W., and Mills, T. M. (1976). Peripheral-blood steroid concentrations in preovulatory rabbit. *J. Steroid Biochem.* **7,** 15–17.

Wergin, W. P. (1979). Cyclic changes in the surface structure of the cervix from the ewe as revealed by scanning electron microscopy. *Tissue Cell* **2,** 359–370.

Westman, A. (1926). A contribution to the question of the transit of the ovum from ovary to uterus in rabbits. *Acta Obstet. Gynecol. Scand.* **5,** 1–104.

Westman, A. (1952). Investigations into the transport of the ovum. *In* "Proceedings of the Conference on Studies on Testes and Ovary, Eggs, and Sperm" (E. T. Engle, ed.), pp. 163–175. Thomas, Springfield, Illinois.

Whitney, L. F. (1937). "How to Breed Dogs." Orange Judd Publ. Co., New York.

Wimsatt, W. A., and Waldo, C. M. (1945). The normal occurrence of a peritoneal opening the bursa ovarii of the mouse. *Anat. Rec.* **93,** 47–51.

Winterberger-Torres, S. (1961). Mouvements des trompes et progression des oeufs chez le brébis. *Ann. Biol. Anim., Biochim., Biophys.* **1,** 121–133.

Yamanaka, H. S., and Soderwall, A. L. (1960). Transport of spermatozoa through the female tract of hamsters. *Fertil. Steril.* **11,** 470–474.

Yanagimachi, R. (1981). Mechanisms of fertilization in mammals. *In* "Fertilization and Embryonic Development In Vitro" (L. Mastroianni, Jr. and J. D. Biggers, eds.), Chapter 5, pp. 81–182. Plenum, New York.

Yanagimachi, R., and Chang, M. C. (1963). Sperm ascent through the oviduct of the hamster and rabbit in relation to the time of ovulation. *J. Reprod. Fertil.* **6,** 413–420.

Yanagimachi, R., and Mahi, C. A. (1976). The sperm acrosome reaction and fertilization in the guinea pig: A study in vivo. *J. Reprod. Fertil.* **46,** 49–54.

Zamboni, L. (1972). Fertilization in the mouse. *In* "Biology of Mammalian Fertilization and Implantation" (K. S. Moghissi and E. S. E. Hafez, eds.), pp. 213–262. Thomas, Springfield, Illinois.

Index

A

Abalone, sperm, 297–298
Accessory sex gland, 185
Acetylcholine, 111
N-Acetyl-β-galactosidase, 102
β-N-Acetylglucosaminidase, 70
Acid phosphatase, 70
Acmaea, 240
Acrosin
  activation, 184, 186, 201–202, 204
  bindin modification, 299
  in capacitation, 201–202
  pH, 70, 201, 202
  properties, 70–71
  in sperm binding, 295, 352, 354
  in zona pellucida penetration, 145, 150,
    467–469
Acrosome
  as bindin component, 273
  components, 70
  enzymes, 56, 69–72, 102, 145, 150
  formation, 278–279
  Golgi apparatus and, 88–90
  granule, 290–291, 299–300
  lysosomal function, 70
  membrane, 299, 458–459, 460–462,
    466–467
  pH, 71, 196
  process, 273, 295

reaction, 69, 297–298, 326
  calcium ion in, 184–185, 203–205,
    305–306
  capacitation and, 178, 457–458, 459,
    461
  catecholamines in, 200–201
  complement in, 202–203
  cyclic nucleotides in, 288–289
  egg jelly in, 309–310, 384
  induction, 184, 186–187, 203–206,
    279–284, 357, 457, 460, 461
  inhibition, 195, 196, 198
  in vivo, 203–206
  ionic regulation, 284–287
  lipase activity in, 299
  location, 294–295
  molecular mechanisms, 460–462
  morphological events, 277–279
  penetration and, 463–465, 467–470,
    473–474
  plasma membrane in, 79, 80, 81, 82,
    105, 280–284
  zona pellucida in, 333–335
  during spermatogenesis, 90
  in sperm condensation, 432
  structure, 69, 71–72, 104, 105
Actin
  in cortical granule, 373
  in egg, 33–34, 45, 67, 69, 373
  functions, 33

CELL BIOLOGY: A Series of Monographs

EDITORS

D. E. Buetow

*Department of Physiology
and Biophysics
University of Illinois
Urbana, Illinois*

I. L. Cameron

*Department of Anatomy
University of Texas
Health Science Center at San Antonio
San Antonio, Texas*

G. M. Padilla

*Department of Physiology
Duke University Medical Center
Durham, North Carolina*

A. M. Zimmerman

*Department of Zoology
University of Toronto
Toronto, Ontario, Canada*

G. M. Padilla, G. L. Whitson, and I. L. Cameron (editors). THE CELL CYCLE: Gene-Enzyme Interactions, 1969

A. M. Zimmerman (editor). HIGH PRESSURE EFFECTS ON CELLULAR PROCESSES, 1970

I. L. Cameron and J. D. Thrasher (editors). CELLULAR AND MOLECULAR RENEWAL IN THE MAMMALIAN BODY, 1971

I. L. Cameron, G. M. Padilla, and A. M. Zimmerman (editors). DEVELOPMENTAL ASPECTS OF THE CELL CYCLE, 1971

P. F. Smith. The BIOLOGY OF MYCOPLASMAS, 1971

Gary L. Whitson (editor). CONCEPTS IN RADIATION CELL BIOLOGY, 1972

Donald L. Hill. THE BIOCHEMISTRY AND PHYSIOLOGY OF *TETRA-HYMENA*, 1972

Kwang W. Jeon (editor). THE BIOLOGY OF AMOEBA, 1973

Dean F. Martin and George M. Padilla (editors). MARINE PHARMACOGNOSY: Action of Marine Biotoxins at the Cellular Level, 1973

Joseph A. Erwin (editor). LIPIDS AND BIOMEMBRANES OF EUKARYOTIC MICROORGANISMS, 1973

A. M. Zimmerman, G. M. Padilla, and I. L. Cameron (editors). DRUGS AND THE CELL CYCLE, 1973

Stuart Coward (editor). DEVELOPMENTAL REGULATION: Aspects of Cell Differentiation, 1973

I. L. Cameron and J. R. Jeter, Jr. (editors). ACIDIC PROTEINS OF THE NU-CLEUS, 1974

Govindjee (editor). BIOENERGETICS OF PHOTOSYNTHESIS, 1975

James R. Jeter, Jr., Ivan L. Cameron, George M. Padilla, and Arthur M. Zimmerman (editors). CELL CYCLE REGULATION, 1978

Gary L. Whitson (editor). NUCLEAR–CYTOPLASMIC INTERACTIONS IN THE CELL CYCLE, 1980

Danton H. O'Day and Paul A. Horgen (editors). SEXUAL INTERACTIONS IN EUKARYOTIC MICROBES, 1981

Ivan L. Cameron and Thomas B. Pool (editors). THE TRANSFORMED CELL, 1981

Arthur M. Zimmerman and Arthur Forer (editors). MITOSIS/CYTOKINESIS, 1981

Ian R. Brown (editor). MOLECULAR APPROACHES TO NEUROBIOLOGY, 1982

Henry C. Aldrich and John W. Daniel (editors). CELL BIOLOGY OF *PHYSARUM* AND *DIDYMIUM*, Volume I: Organisms, Nucleus, and Cell Cycle, 1982; Volume II: Differentiation, Metabolism, and Methodology, 1982

John A. Heddle (editor). MUTAGENICITY: New Horizons in Genetic Toxicology, 1982

Potu N. Rao, Robert T. Johnson, and Karl Sperling (editors). PREMATURE CHROMOSOME CONDENSATION: Application in Basic, Clinical, and Mutation Research, 1982

George M. Padilla and Kenneth S. McCarty, Sr. (editors). GENETIC EXPRESSION IN THE CELL CYCLE, 1982

David S. McDevitt (editor). CELL BIOLOGY OF THE EYE, 1982

P. Michael Conn (editor). CELLULAR REGULATION OF SECRETION AND RELEASE, 1982

Govindjee (editor). PHOTOSYNTHESIS, Volume I: Energy Conversion by Plants and Bacteria, 1982; Volume II: Development, Carbon Metabolism, and Plant Productivity, 1982

John Morrow. EUKARYOTIC CELL GENETICS, 1983

John F. Hartmann (editor). MECHANISM AND CONTROL OF ANIMAL FERTILIZATION, 1983